26450
70C
4vols.
○6
P.B.

The Antigens

VOLUME III

Contributors

G. L. Ada

Anthony C. Allison

William H. Burns

P. L. Ey

S. Ferrone

Joel W. Goodman

Klaus Jann

George E. Kenny

David G. Marsh

M. A. Pellegrino

R. A. Reisfeld

Otto Westphal

The Antigens

VOLUME III

EDITED BY
MICHAEL SELA
Department of Chemical Immunology
The Weizmann Institute of Science
Rehovot, Israel

ACADEMIC PRESS   New York   San Francisco   London   1975
A Subsidiary of Harcourt Brace Jovanovich, Publishers

COPYRIGHT © 1975, BY ACADEMIC PRESS, INC.
ALL RIGHTS RESERVED.
NO PART OF THIS PUBLICATION MAY BE REPRODUCED OR
TRANSMITTED IN ANY FORM OR BY ANY MEANS, ELECTRONIC
OR MECHANICAL, INCLUDING PHOTOCOPY, RECORDING, OR ANY
INFORMATION STORAGE AND RETRIEVAL SYSTEM, WITHOUT
PERMISSION IN WRITING FROM THE PUBLISHER.

ACADEMIC PRESS, INC.
111 Fifth Avenue, New York, New York 10003

United Kingdom Edition published by
ACADEMIC PRESS, INC. (LONDON) LTD.
24/28 Oval Road, London NW1

Library of Congress Cataloging in Publication Data

Sela, Michael.
    The antigens.

    Includes bibliographies.
    1. Antigens and antibodies. 2. Immunochemistry.
I. Title. [DNLM: 1. Antigens.
2. Immunity. QW570 S464a H2 V2 v. 1-2)
QR186.5.S44   574.2'92   73-799
ISBN 0–12–635503–7

PRINTED IN THE UNITED STATES OF AMERICA

Dedicated to the memory of my beloved wife Margalit

Contents

List of Contributors xi
Preface xiii
Contents of Other Volumes. xv

Chapter 1 Microbial Polysaccharides
Klaus Jann and Otto Westphal

I. Introduction 1
II. Chemistry of Microbial Polysaccharide Antigens 3
III. Immunochemistry of Microbial Polysaccharide Antigens . . 49
IV. Immunobiology of Microbial Polysaccharide Antigens . . 83
V. Summary and Conclusions 108
References 110

Chapter 2 Antigenic Determinants and Antibody Combining Sites
Joel W. Goodman

I. Introduction 127
II. The Structural Specificity of Hapten–Antibody Interactions . 129
III. Antigenic Determinants 133
IV. The Antibody Combining Site 153
V. Immunogenic Determinants 162
VI. Concluding Remarks 179
References 183

Chapter 3 Lymphocytic Receptors for Antigens
G. L. Ada and P. L. Ey

I. Introduction 190
II. Historical 191

III.	Two Classes of Lymphocytes	193
IV.	The Lymphocyte Plasma Membrane	197
V.	Relevant Properties of Immunoglobulins.	201
VI.	Immunoglobulins on the Lymphocyte Plasma Membrane	206
VII.	The Binding of Antigen to Lymphocytes.	217
VIII.	Specificity and Immunocompetence of ABC	232
IX.	Receptors on Lymphocytes for Antigens	242
X.	Antigens, The Antigen–Receptor Complex, and Mitogens	251
XI.	Inside the B Cell	257
	References	260

Chapter 4 Allergens and the Genetics of Allergy

David G. Marsh

I.	Introduction	271
II.	Historical Development (1872–about 1960)	274
III.	Nomenclature	280
IV.	Modern Allergen Research	282
V.	Nature of Allergenic Sensitization and Stimulation	320
VI.	Genetics of Allergy	329
VII.	Practical Considerations	345
VIII.	Concluding Remarks	347
	References	350

Chapter 5 A Biologic and Chemical Profile of Histocompatibility Antigens

S. Ferrone, M. A. Pellegrino, and R. A. Reisfeld

I.	Introduction	362
II.	History	362
III.	Genetics	368
IV.	Serologic Detection of H Antigens	371
V.	Cell Surface Expression of H Antigens	385
VI.	Cross-Reactivity of H Antigens.	398
VII.	Extraction, Purification, and Biologic Activity of Soluble H Antigens	402
VIII.	Chemical and Molecular Nature of HL-A Antigens	418
IX.	Perspectives	431
	References	435

Chapter 6 Antigens of the Mycoplasmatales and Chlamydiae

George E. Kenny

I.	Introduction	449
II.	Classification and Nomenclature	450

III. Biology	451
IV. Phylogenetic Relationships	456
V. Antigenic Analysis of Mycoplasmata	459
VI. Antigenic Analysis of Chlamydiae	464
VII. Growth Inhibition and Mycoplasmacidal Activity of Serum	464
VIII. Antigenic Structure	467
References	476

Chapter 7 Virus Infections and the Immune Responses They Elicit

William H. Burns and Anthony C. Allison

I. Introduction	480
II. Viral Antigens	483
III. Humoral Responses	500
IV. Secretory Antibody Responses	506
V. Thymus Dependence of Viral Antigens	507
VI. B Lymphocyte Memory and "Original Antigenic Sin"	510
VII. Neutralization	512
VIII. Capacity of Macrophages to Support Virus Replication	519
IX. Ontogeny of Macrophage Resistance to Viral Infections	522
X. Surface Changes of Virus-Infected Cells	524
XI. Evidence for Cell-Mediated Immunity to Viral Antigens	532
XII. Persistence of Immunity to Viruses	541
XIII. Tolerance to Viral Antigens	543
XIV. Cooperative Effects of Viral Antigens on Immunogenicity	546
XV. Influence of Virus Infections on Immune Responses	549
XVI. Concluding Remarks	557
References	559

| Author Index | 575 |
| Subject Index | 612 |

List of Contributors

Numbers in parentheses indicate the pages on which the authors' contributions begin.

G. L. ADA (189), Department of Microbiology, The John Curtin School of Medical Research, The Australian National University, Canberra, Australia

ANTHONY C. ALLISON (479), Division of Cell Pathology, Clinical Research Centre, Middlesex, England

WILLIAM H. BURNS (479), National Institute for Dental Research, National Institutes of Health, Bethesda, Maryland

P. L. EY* (189), Department of Microbiology, The John Curtin School of Medical Research, The Australian National University, Canberra, Australia

S. FERRONE (361), Department of Molecular Immunology, Scripps Clinic and Research Foundation, La Jolla, California

JOEL W. GOODMAN (127), Department of Microbiology, University of California, San Francisco, California

KLAUS JANN (1), Max-Planck-Institut für Immunbiologie, Freiburg-Zähringen, Germany

GEORGE E. KENNY (449), Department of Pathobiology, School of Public Health and Community Medicine, University of Washington, Seattle, Washington

DAVID G. MARSH (271), Division of Clinical Immunology, Department of Medicine, The Johns Hopkins University School of Medicine at the Good Samaritan Hospital, Baltimore, Maryland

* Present address: Max-Planck-Institut für Immunbiologie, Freiburg-Zähringen, Germany

M. A. PELLEGRINO (361), Department of Molecular Immunology, Scripps Clinic and Research Foundation, La Jolla, California

R. A. REISFELD (361), Department of Molecular Immunology, Scripps Clinic and Research Foundation, La Jolla, California

OTTO WESTPHAL (1), Max-Planck-Institut für Immunbiologie, Freiburg-Zähringen, Germany

Preface

This is the third volume of a comprehensive treatise that covers all aspects of antigens and related areas of immunology, focusing its attention on the chemistry and biology of antigens as well as on their immunologic role and expression. Each contribution describes a particular subject in depth, keeping a historical perspective rather than dealing exclusively with developments of the past few years. It gives the reader an adequate key to the literature and at the same time summarizes succinctly the present status of the subject. Its ultimate purpose is to give an integrated picture that may help better understand immunologic phenomena.

The general plan of "The Antigens" is described in the Preface to Volume I. The first two volumes of this work were devoted to defined macromolecules as antigens and to immunoglobulins. The next two volumes are devoted primarily to more complex antigens and to antibodies.

The first chapter of this volume complements the antigenic macromolecules discussed in the previous volumes, as it gives a comprehensive and critical review of microbial polysaccharides as antigens. The second chapter deals with antigenic determinants and their specific reaction with antibody combining sites. The third chapter is devoted to the reaction of antigens with their specific receptors on lymphocytes. The next four chapters are concerned with several categories of more complex antigens which, in most cases, have not as yet been characterized adequately at a molecular level—allergens, histocompatibility antigens, antigens of Mycoplasmatales and chlamydiae, and animal viruses. They are all of crucial biologic importance, and progress in the elucidation of their structure and their biologic function is one of the exciting challenges to the immunologist.

It is a pleasure to acknowledge also on this occasion the cooperation of the staff of Academic Press in the preparation of this treatise.

MICHAEL SELA

Contents of Other Volumes

Volume I

Nucleic Acid Antigens
  B. David Stollar

Immunochemistry of Enzymes
  Ruth Arnon

Structure of Immunoglobulins
  Joseph A. Gally

Immunoglobulin Allotypes
  Rose Mage, Rose Lieberman, Michael Potter, and William D. Terry

The Evolution of Proteins
  Norman Arnheim

Phylogeny of Immunoglobulins
  R. T. Kubo, B. Zimmerman, and H. M. Grey

Chemistry and Biology of Immunoglobulin E
  Kimishige Ishizaka

AUTHOR INDEX – SUBJECT INDEX

Volume II

Protein Antigens: The Molecular Bases of Antigenicity and Immunogenicity
  Michael J. Crumpton

Blood Group Antigens
  Sen-itiroh Hakomori and Akira Kobata

Low Molecular Weight Antigens
  A. L. de Weck

The Application of Antibody to the Measurement of Substances of Physiological and Pharmacological Interest
  Edgar Haber and Knud Poulsen

Idiotypy of Antibodies
  Jacques Oudin

Immunoglobulin A
  J. F. Heremans

AUTHOR INDEX – SUBJECT INDEX

CHAPTER *1*

Microbial Polysaccharides*

KLAUS JANN AND OTTO WESTPHAL

I. Introduction	1
II. Chemistry of Microbial Polysaccharide Antigens	3
A. Methods	3
B. Bacterial Lipopolysaccharides	5
C. Capsular Polysaccharides	25
D. Other Polysaccharide Antigens	42
III. Immunochemistry of Microbial Polysaccharide Antigens . . .	49
A. Serologic Methods	49
B. Carbohydrate Determinants	50
C. Immunochemistry of O Antigen Factors	56
D. Significance of Mutations, Form Variations, and Lysogenic Conversions for the Immunochemical Analysis of Polysaccharide Antigens	62
E. Artificial Antigens with Carbohydrate Determinants . . .	68
F. Noncarbohydrate Determinants	74
G. Cross-Reactions between Microbial Polysaccharides . . .	76
IV. Immunobiology of Microbial Polysaccharide Antigens . . .	83
A. Parameters of Immunogenicity	83
B. Polysaccharide Antibodies with Restricted Heterogeneity . .	95
C. Myeloma Proteins with Anti-polysaccharide Specificity . .	99
D. Polysaccharides in Infection	103
V. Summary and Conclusions	108
References	110

I. Introduction

Microbial polysaccharides are located on the cell surface and are, therefore, of importance in recognition and immune response of a

* This article is dedicated to Professor Michael Heidelberger, New York, the great pioneer of polysaccharide immunochemistry.

higher organism to microbial infection. These polysaccharides are either an integral part of the cell wall, as this is known to be the case with the somatic lipopolysaccharides of gram-negative Enterobacteriaceae, or they may form large extracellular capsules like those of *Pneumococcus, Klebsiella,* and many *Escherichia coli.*

Polysaccharides of microorganisms have been studied chemically for a long time and much is known about their structure. They can be pure polysaccharides or complex ones. The most prominent and best studied complex polysaccharides are the somatic lipopolysaccharides. The biosynthesis of a number of microbial polysaccharides and lipopolysaccharides has been studied, and a coherent picture of the mechanism of polysaccharide biosynthesis has emerged from these studies.

The first immunologic approach to bacterial polysaccharides was achieved by Avery (1915), Goebel (1935, 1938, 1939), and Heidelberger (Heidelberger and Avery, 1923, 1924; Heidelberger and Kendall, 1929; for a review, see Heidelberger, 1960) at the Rockefeller Institute between 1920 and 1940. This was when, after the predominance of bacterial toxins, the importance of bacterial polysaccharides as antigens was shown in the studies of the capsular polysaccharides of *Pneumococcus.* The protective effect of pneumococcal polysaccharide against pneumonia infection (Heidelberger and McPherson, 1943a,b; MacLeod *et al.*, 1946; Heidelberger *et al.*, 1946, 1947) was proof of the immunologic importance of bacterial polysaccharides. The detection of oligosaccharidic serologic determinants was followed by their use as artificial antigens when coupled to protein (Goebel *et al.*, 1934a,b). Antisera obtained with these artificial antigens reacted with the native polysaccharides and also with the whole bacteria.

The promising start of the immunochemistry of microbial polysaccharides coincided with the beginning era of antibiotics. There is no doubt that antibiotics solved the problem not only of infection due to *Pneumococcus* but also of many other infections, but by the same token they created the severe problem of bacterial resistance to antibiotics, thus limiting their application. The early and quite spectacular results of antibiotic treatment, which seemed so simple, slowed down further development of the immunology of bacterial polysaccharides.

The topic of microbial polysaccharides as antigens gained renewed interest when it was found that the serologic classification of *Salmonella,* as laid down in the Kauffmann–White Scheme (Kauffmann, 1954, 1961) was based on the fine structure of the bacterial surface polysaccharides (for a review, see Lüderitz et al., 1966a, 1968a, 1971). The pioneering work of the Rockefeller group was taken up again and extended; new techniques were introduced and new perspectives opened.

In recent years important contributions were made to the problem of immunogenicity of polysaccharides, mainly on dextrans (Kabat and Bezer, 1958) and pneumococcal capsular polysaccharides (Howard et al., 1971a,b,c). It was found that most microbial polysaccharides can not be digested by mammalian enzymes so that they remain in the circulation and tissue for a long time. This became an important aspect in the immune response to microbial polysaccharides. Furthermore, antigenic specificity and the antigen–antibody reaction were analyzed in detail, which led to a better understanding of immunodominant sugars (Lüderitz et al., 1966a) and antigenic determinants. In the course of these studies, which were carried out by many research groups, antibodies with restricted heterogeneity (Kunkel et al., 1962; Krause, 1970; Haber, 1970) and myeloma proteins (Cohn, 1967; Cohen and Milstein, 1967; Potter, 1970) were found which are directed against microbial polysaccharides. This, of course, was a great help in studies of the kinetics of the antigen–antibody response and will be of importance with respect to its genetics. Also, the role of microbial polysaccharides in infection became more and more a topic of research, and in this context their relatedness to the polysaccharides of mammalian cells and to histocompatibility antigens has to be considered.

We review here the present state of microbial polysaccharide immunology by quoting relevant examples which, taken together, may give an up-to-date picture of results and problems in this field.

II. Chemistry of Microbial Polysaccharide Antigens

A. Methods

Chemical and physical methods may contribute to answer two questions: (1) What makes a polysaccharide immunogenic? (2) What is the chemical basis of its antigenicity (serologic specificity)? In any case it is desirable to know the structure of a polysaccharide as precisely as possible. Structural analysis has to clarify size and shape of the polysaccharide, its sugar composition, the sequence of sugar components, and the nature of their linkage (position of substitution and anomeric configuration). In the following the most widely used methods are mentioned.

Size and Shape. In general use are the Svedberg method (Kabat and Mayer, 1961; Svedberg and Pedersen, 1940; Schachman, 1959; Jann *et al.*, 1965, 1968) in which sedimentation and diffusion constants are measured with the ultracentrifuge, and the molecular weight is calculated from the data obtained. Similarly, sedimentation equilibrium may be used (Kabat and Mayer, 1961; Jann *et al.*, 1965, 1968; Archibald, 1947; Yphantis, 1960). For estimation of molecular weight, comparative gel chromatography may be used, but this is not reliable, since, in contrast to proteins, polysaccharides are mostly extended and their shape may vary greatly. The shape of polysaccharides can be assessed using their intrinsic viscosity (Kabat and Mayer, 1961; Jann *et al.*, 1965, 1968) or light scattering. In contrast to these physical methods there exist chemical methods for the determination of the molecular weight (chain length) of polysaccharides such as reaction with [^{14}C]cyanide (Isbell, 1951; Moyer and Isbell, 1958) or periodate oxidation (Abdel-Akher *et al.*, 1951; Unrau and Smith, 1957).

Sugar Composition. For qualitative determinations paper or thin-layer chromatography on total hydrolysates are run. According to more recent recommendations, the liberated sugar components are reduced to polyols, peracetylated, and then determined by gas–liquid chromatography (Sawardeker *et al.*, 1967). With the use of admixed reference substances, such as peracetyl-xylitol, this method is frequently performed on a quantitative basis. For enzymatic analysis total hydrolysates can be used.

Sequence. In order to gain information as to the sequence of the sugar constituents, oligosaccharides have to be isolated by partial acid hydrolysis or special techniques like Smith degradation (Goldstein *et al.*, 1959, 1965), acetolysis (Hanessian and Haskell, 1964; Kocourek and Ballou, 1969), or continuous hydrolysis and dialysis of the products (Painter, 1960; Painter and Morgan, 1961; Galanos *et al.*, 1969a) followed by chromatographic separation. The oligosaccharides are then analyzed using a variety of chemical and enzymatic methods that depend on the nature of the material under study. Their structure can also be established by methylation and gas chromatography followed by mass spectrometry (Kärkkäinen, 1970). From the results of oligosaccharide analyses the sequence in the polysaccharide can be reconstructed. Frequently, the oligosaccharides are methylated, hydrolyzed, and after subsequent reduction and acetylation subjected to combined gas chromatography and mass spectrometry (Björndal et al., 1970a).

Nature of Linkage. In a polysaccharide each sugar unit may be linked in one of two anomeric configurations (α or β) to any of the free hydroxyl groups of the next sugar unit. Thus, the variety is so large that reliable methods for linkage analysis are necessary. One of them consists in the oxidation of the polysaccharide with metaperiodate, followed by measurement of consumption of the reagent and determination of the reaction products, such as formic acid, acetaldehyde, etc. This method, which has been reviewed extensively (Goldstein et al., 1959; Smith and Montgomery, 1956; Hay et al., 1965), is rather complex and leads to ambiguous results. Nevertheless, it is useful and, in combination with other methods, widely in use. Presently the best method for linkage analysis is a combination of methylation, gas chromatography, and mass spectrometry. The methylation technique for polysaccharides and oligosaccharides has been repeatedly modified and is now a simple and reliable method (Hakomori, 1964; Hellerqvist et al., 1968; Björndal et al., 1970a). The methylated polysaccharide is hydrolyzed and the products are transformed into volatile derivatives which are subjected to gas chromatography. The various peaks that are eluted from the column with an inert carrier gas can be directly analyzed in a mass spectrometer (Kärkäinen, 1970; Hellerqvist et al., 1968). For certain components, such as hexuronic acids or amino sugars (Sandford and Conrad, 1966; Tarcsay et al., 1971; Lindberg et al., 1973a), special techniques have been worked out. In general it can be stated that linkage analysis in polysaccharides today has nearly reached perfection.

It is fair to say that the elaboration of the complete structure of any given polysaccharide is possible, in principle, and simply a matter of the availability and application of suitable refined analytic techniques.

B. *Bacterial Lipopolysaccharides*

Lipopolysaccharides (LPS) are found in the outer membrane (plastic layer of the cell envelope) of gram-negative bacteria, where they form complexes with protein and phospholipid of the kephaline type (Romeo et al., 1970, Rothfield and Romeo, 1971). They are the somatic antigens, and are thus the chemical basis for serologic classification of gram-negative bacteria (Kauffmann, 1966). Furthermore, they are receptors for many bacteriophages (Lindberg, 1973) and, therefore, play an important role in bacteriophage typing. Both properties of LPS are due to the polysaccharide moiety. Additionally,

LPS exert endotoxic activities for which the lipid moiety is responsible (Westphal *et al.*, 1952b; Eichenberger *et al.*, 1955; Lüderitz *et al.*, 1973).

Due to their manifold chemical and biologic aspects, LPS have been the subject of extensive studies through the last two decades. Consequently, many reviewing articles have been written (Lüderitz *et al.*, 1966a, 1968a, 1971; Nikaido, 1968, 1974; Osborn, 1969; Mäkelä and Stocker, 1969). For detailed information the reader is referred to these reviews.

1. Structural Features of LPS

It was found that the LPS of gram-negative bacteria, and especially those of enterobacteria are composed of three structural regions, I, II and III (Lüderitz *et al.*, 1971), as indicated in Fig. 1.

Region I is represented by the O-specific polysaccharide. This consists of oligosaccharide repeating units—a structural feature that seems to be common for most bacterial polysaccharides. This structural region of the LPS is distinguished by a great variability: many different sugar residues may be present in many combinations and glycosidic linkages.

Region II is an oligosaccharide that originally was found to be common for all *Salmonella* LPS and, therefore, called the "common core." It was found later that a number of different core oligosaccharides exist which are structurally closely related. These are but few, and there is a lower degree of structural freedom in region II than there is in region I. Through the core oligosaccharide the serologic R specificity is expressed.

Region III is the lipid moiety of the LPS which was termed lipid A. It is thought to be a structural component of the outer membrane of gram-negative bacteria. Thus the LPS are anchored in the outer membrane via their lipid component. Lipid A is a unique glycophospholipid, containing glucosamine, fatty acids, and phosphate. The structure of lipid A is practically the same in all enterobacteria.

As one compares the structure of many bacterial LPS, it will be obvious that structural variability becomes increasingly greater going from inner to outer parts of the molecule.

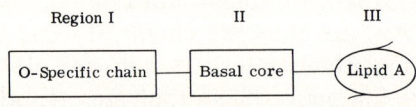

Fig. 1. Schematic diagram of the general structure of bacterial lipopolysaccharides. From Lüderitz *et al.* (1971).

There is evidence that several LPS units are linked together through pyrophosphodiester bridges in the lipid A moiety (region III). It was reported that three LPS units would form one large molecule on the bacterial surface (Romeo et al., 1970). By virtue of their amphiphilic character LPS, once isolated, tend to form large aggregates in aqueous solutions (Ribi et al., 1966). The physical state of LPS may influence their immunologic and biologic properties (Ribi et al., 1966; Whang et al., 1971).

2. Biochemistry and Genetic Determination of LPS

The biosynthesis of enterobacterial LPS is very complex, and only those steps are known which lead to the polysaccharide part of the molecule (regions I and II) (for a review, see Lüderitz et al., 1966a, 1968a, 1971). The main feature is the independent synthesis of the O-specific polysaccharide (region I) and the core oligosaccharide (region II). The latter is probably synthesized on the lipid A moiety (region III) as acceptor. It is itself the acceptor for the O-specific polysaccharide which is assembled from oligosaccharides on an intermediary acceptor and then transferred to the completed core oligosaccharide (Losick and Robbins, 1967; for a review, see Nikaido, 1968, 1974; Osborn 1969). The understanding of this mechanism is important for the appreciation of enterobacterial R mutants and SR mutants (Naide et al., 1965).

The enzymes responsible for the biosynthesis of LPS are determined by a number of genes or gene clusters on the bacterial chromosome. This was reviewed by Mäkelä and Stocker (1969). Briefly, the main gene loci and their functions are: *rfa* (closely linked to *xyl*, the locus determining xylose utilization) which codes for the synthesis of the core oligosaccharide; *rfb* (closely linked to *his*, the locus determining the synthesis of histidine) which codes for the synthesis of the oligosaccharide repeating units of the O-specific polysaccharide; and *rfc* (closely linked to *PMI*, the locus determining the enzyme phosphomannoseisomerase) which codes for a polymerase joining the O-specific oligosaccharide repeating units (Naide et al., 1965) to give the O-specific polysaccharide (region I). Until today nothing is known about the biosynthesis and genetic determination of lipid A (region III). The multiple genetic determination of one molecule by loci widely apart on the bacterial chromosome is a unique phenomenon and the reason for this is unknown.

3. Mutant LPS

Mutations affecting the *rfb* or *rfa* loci lead to bacterial forms which are termed R mutants. Correspondingly, their LPS are termed

R-LPS. Mutations in the *rfb* locus block the synthesis of the O-specific polysaccharide and such R (*rfb*) mutants have LPS which consist only of core oligosaccharide and lipid A (regions II and III). Mutations in the *rfa* locus interfere with the synthesis of the core oligosaccharide which remains more or less incomplete. Thus, the O-specific polysaccharide cannot be transferred and the resulting R (*rfa*) mutants have an LPS which, like those of *rfb* mutants, lack the O-specific polysaccharide and in addition have a defective core oligosaccharide.

Both types of mutations result in loss of O-specificity and in the appearance of a new specificity, the R specificity, which is cryptic in wild-type S forms. An intermediate, so-called SR form with only one O-specific oligosaccharide on the complete R core was originally predicted on theoretical grounds by Stocker and isolated soon afterwards (see Naide *et al.*, 1965).

Since in R mutants the (O-specific) polysaccharide is not present and the carbohydrate part of the LPS is only an oligosaccharide, it might be more appropriate to use the term lipooligosaccharide rather than LPS. Nevertheless, for simplicity, the general term of LPS is kept in use.

4. Isolation of LPS

The methods for isolation depend on the aim of research in connection with the antigenic, toxic, or pharmacologic properties of bacterial LPS. They have been dealt with in many review articles, and only a few shall be mentioned here.

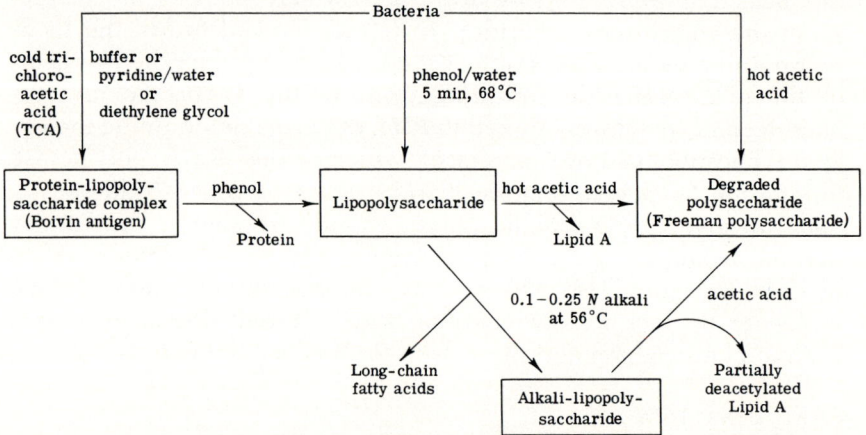

Fig. 2. Preparation of O-specific extracts from gram-negative bacteria.

1. Microbial Polysaccharides

The most widely used procedure to obtain the whole antigenic complex, containing LPS and protein, is the trichloroacetic acid extraction introduced by Boivin and Mesrobeanu (1935).

Pure protein-free LPS can be obtained by extraction with 45% aqueous phenol at 65°, which is applicable to all S forms and may also be used with R forms (Westphal et al., 1952a; Westphal and Jann, 1965). R forms can be specifically extracted with a mixture of phenol/chloroform/petroleum ether (Galanos et al., 1969b).

The O-specific polysaccharide moiety can be obtained by extraction of bacteria with 1% acetic acid at 100° (Freeman, 1942; Staub, 1965). Alternatively, the LPS may be treated (degraded) with 1% acetic acid at 100° with liberation of the water-insoluble lipid A. The water-soluble degraded polysaccharide (dPS) may then be obtained and purified by column gel chromatography (Müller-Seitz et al., 1968; Schmidt et al., 1969).

The isolation procedures and the products obtained are shown schematically in Figs. 2 and 3.

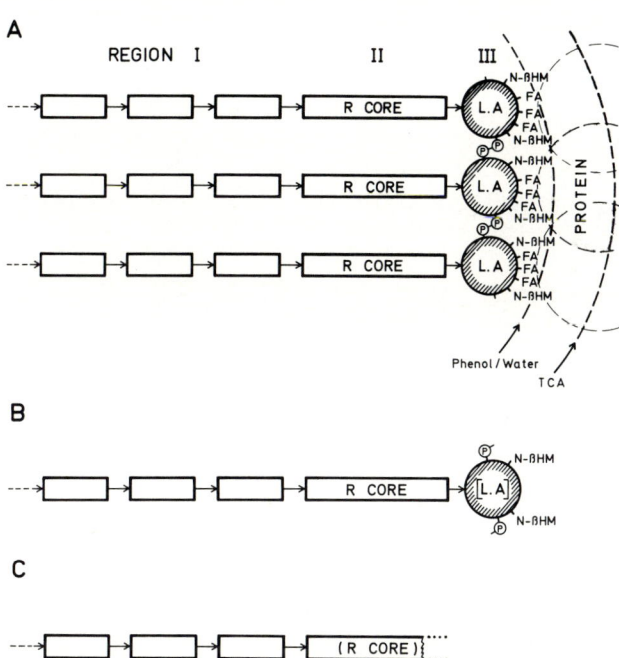

Fig. 3. O-specific preparations from Enterobacteriaceae. A, the complete O-antigenic complex; B, one chain of the alkali lipopolysaccharide; C, degraded (Freeman) polysaccharide; □→, O-specific oligosaccharide repeating unit; LA, lipid A; FA, long chain fatty acid; N-βHM, N-β-hydroxymyristoyl groups.

TABLE I

Sugar Constituents of Bacterial Lipopolysaccharides[a]

Type	Configuration	Trivial name	Occurrence
Pentoses	D-Ribose	—	*Salmonella*
	Ribose	—	*E. coli* O114
	Xylose	—	*Citrobacter*
Pentosamines	4-Amino-4-deoxy-L-arabinose	—	*Salmonella*
Hexoses	D-Glucose		Frequent
	D-Galactose		Frequent
	D-Mannose		Frequent
	D-Fructose		*V. cholerae*
4-Deoxyhexose[b]	D-Arabinose	—	*Citrobacter*
6-Deoxyhexoses	-L-Mannose	L-Rhamnose	Frequent
	-D-Mannose	D-Rhamnose	*Xanthomonas*
	-L-Galactose	L-Fucose	Frequent
	-L-Talose		*E. coli*
3,6-Dideoxyhexoses	D-*xylo*-(3,6-Dideoxy-D-galactose)	Abequose	*Salmonella, P. pseudotuberculosis, Citrobacter*
	L-*xylo*-(3,6-Dideoxy-L-galactose)	Colitose	*Salmonella, E. coli*
	D-*arabino*-(3,6-Dideoxy-D-mannose)	Tyvelose	*Arizona, Salmonella, P. pseudotuberculosis*
	L-*arabino*-(3,6-Dideoxy-L-mannose)	Ascarylose	*P. pseudotuberculosis*
	D-*ribo*-(3,6-Dideoxy-D-glucose)	Paratose	*Salmonella, P. pseudotuberculosis*
2-Amino-2-deoxyhexoses	-D-Glucose	Glucosamine	Frequent
	-D-Galactose	Galactosamine	Frequent
	-D-Mannose	Mannosamine	*Salmonella, E. coli, Arizona*
2-Amino-2,6-dideoxyhexoses	-D-Glucose	Quinovosamine	*Salmonella, Arizona, Proteus, Chromobacter, P. pseudotuberculosis*
	-D-Galactose	D-Fucosamine	

1. Microbial Polysaccharides

Category	Component	Occurrence
3-Amino-3,6-dideoxyhexoses	-L-Galactose	*E. coli* (frequent)
	-L-Mannose	*E. coli*
	-D-Glucose	*Citrobacter, Salmonella, E. coli*
	-D-Galactose	*Salmonella, Arizona, Brucella, Xanthomonas, E. coli*
4-Amino-4,6-dideoxyhexoses	-D-Glucose	*Chromobacter, E. coli*
	-D-Galactose	*E. coli*
	Viosamine	Frequent
	Thomosamine	*Chromobacter, Serratia, Proteus, Salmonella, E. coli*
Heptoses	L-Glycero-D-manno-	
	D-Glycero-D-manno-	*Chromobacter*
6-Deoxyheptose[c]	D-Glycero-D-galacto-	*Pasteurella pseudotuberculosis* group II
	D-Mannose	
Heptosamines	2-Amino-2-deoxyido (or deoxygulo-)-D-glyceroheptose	
Hexuronic acids	D-Glucuronic acid	*E. coli, Klebsiella*
	D-Galacturonic acid	*E. coli, Klebsiella*
Pentolusonic acid[d]	2-Keto-3-deoxypentonic acid	*Klebsiella*
Hexulusonic acid[e]	2-Keto-3-deoxygalactonic acid	*Azotobacter vinelandii*
Octulosonic acid	2-Keto-3-deoxyoctulosonic acid (3-Deoxy-D-mannooctulosonic acid)	"KDO" Frequent
Neuraminic acid	L-Fucosamine	*Salmonella, Citrobacter, Arizona, E. coli*
	L-Rhamnosamine	Rhodospirillaceae
O-Methyl sugars[f]	A number of O-methyl sugars (hexoses, hexosamine, pentoses and methylpentoses) were found in polysaccharides from	

[a] From Luderitz et al. (1971a) and Ashwell and Hickman (1971).
[b] From Keleti et al. (1970).
[c] From Hellerqvist et al. (1972).
[d] From Lindberg et al. (1973b).
[e] From Claus (1965).
[f] From Mayer et al. (1974).

5. Composition and Structure of the O-Specific Polysaccharide

The LPS of gram-negative bacteria can be composed of many different sugar constituents. Some Enterobacteriaceae can synthesize and incorporate into their cell wall polysaccharides up to eight or nine different sugars. The great variety of sugar constituents found in LPS is outlined in Table I.

The qualitative sugar composition of a given LPS was designated as *chemotype* by Kauffmann et al. (1960, 1962) and Westphal et al. (1960). No discrimination was made between the constituents of the 3 different regions shown in Figs. 1 and 3A. From the immunochemical point of view, it would appear today to be more appropriate if the sugar composition of the O-specific polysaccharide (region I) and of the R-specific core (region II) would be distinguished. In addition, glucosamine as a constituent of lipid A (region III) will always be found if the whole LPS is used for analysis.

The extensive work of many research groups on chemotyping of the LPS of gram-negative bacteria has already been reviewed by several authors (Lüderitz et al., 1966a, 1968a, 1971). In Table II chemotypes I-XLII are listed. This is based on the results of analyses of about 50 *Salmonella* and about 100 *E. coli* strains (Kauffmann et al., 1960; Ørskov et al., 1967) and extended to a greater number of genera (for a review, see Lüderitz et al., 1971). Of interest is the occurrence of 4 stereoisomeric 3,6-dideoxyhexoses in the LPS of *Salmonella* and of 6-deoxyhexosamines in *E. coli*. More recently, hexuronic acids were found as constituents of the LPS of many *E. coli* strains (Ørskov et al., 1971). Hexuronic acids were known to occur in the capsular (K) antigenic polysaccharides of *E. coli* (see below). Their presence also in the somatic LPS may render the definitions of the polysaccharide antigens of *E. coli* more ambiguous. The presence of charges in the surface polysaccharide antigens was the basis for a more recent immunochemical classification of *E. coli* strains using immunoelectrophoresis of saline extracts (Ørskov et al., 1971).

The specific polysaccharide moiety of the LPS is composed of oligosaccharidic repeating units—in fact, these polysaccharides were among the first on which this general structural feature was elaborated. The oligosaccharide units are linked such that either linear chains result or that nonreducing hexose units stick out of the polysaccharide main chain. In Table III the repeating units of a number of *Salmonella* LPS are given. These are biologic repeating units in the sense as discussed in Section II,B,2. With LPS the structure of

1. Microbial Polysaccharides

the biologic repeating unit cannot only be elaborated by biochemical studies (see Section II,B,2) but also by structural studies on R (*rfc*) mutants—also termed SR mutants—in which the specific polymerase is defective, and only one repeating unit is linked to the core (Naide *et al.*, 1965; Nikaido, 1968). Chemical repeating units as obtained by partial hydrolysis of the LPS listed in Table III would have L-Rha at the reducing end.

In all examples given here the polysaccharide main chain consists of a repeating sequence of Man → Rha → Gal. This group of closely related O-specific polysaccharides does not represent a general structural principle. There are many LPS having a quite different polysaccharide chain, a number of which are shown in Table IV.

The oligosaccharides in Table IV are chemical repeating units, obtained from the LPS by partial hydrolysis with acid or, in the case of *E. coli* O8, with a specific bacteriophage enzyme (Reske *et al.*, 1973). The O-specific polysaccharides of some LPS are homopolysaccharides. This was especially found in *Klebsiella* and *E. coli* of O groups 8 and 9 (Reske and Jann, 1972).

Recently, the structures of the O-specific polysaccharides of *Yersinia (Pasteurella) pseudotuberculosis*, serotypes I–VI were proposed by Samuelson *et al.* (1974). It is noteworthy that these polysaccharides contain not only all known 3,6-dideoxy sugars but some of them (serogroups I, II, IV) also 6-deoxy-D-mannoheptose.

6. COMPOSITION AND STRUCTURE OF THE R-SPECIFIC CORE OLIGOSACCHARIDE

R-LPS are the somatic antigens of bacterial R mutants. These do not occur frequently in nature, and are usually obtained by special techniques such as bacteriophage selection and mutagenesis (Schlosshardt, 1960, 1964; Lüderitz *et al.*, 1966b, 1971; Schmidt *et al.*, 1970b). *R-LPS with a complete core* can be isolated from *rfb* mutants. The first core oligosaccharide studied extensively was the one from *Salmonella* (for a review, see Lüderitz *et al.*, 1966a, 1968a, 1971). The structure which finally emerged from the results of many research groups is shown in Fig. 4. It can be divided into an inner core, consisting of heptose and KDO and an outer core consisting of hexoses and glucosamine. The inner core is substituted by phosphate and ethanolamine. This, taken together with the carboxyl groups of KDO, renders the inner core highly charged. In contrast, the outer core is neutral.

The core oligosaccharide structure (Fig. 4) was elaborated mainly

TABLE II

Qualitative Sugar Composition of Lipopolysaccharides of Various Enterobacteriaceae – Chemotypes[a]

Chemotype	4-Amino-4,6-dideoxyglucose	4-Amino-4,6-dideoxygalactose	3-Amino-3,6-dideoxyglucose	3-Amino-3,6-dideoxygalactose	2-Amino-2,6-dideoxymannose	2-Amino-2,6-dideoxyglucose	2-Amino-2,6-dideoxygalactose	Mannosamine	Galactosamine	Glucosamine	Ketodeoxyoctonic acid	L-Glycero-D-mannoheptose	Galactose	Glucose	Mannose	Fucose	Rhamnose	6-Deoxytalose	Ribose	Colitose	Abequose	Paratose	Tyvelose	Found in serotypes or serogroups
I										●	●	●	●	●										*Salmonella* V, X, Y; *E. coli* 14, 24, 28, 30, 42, 56, 64, 82, 83, 85, 118, 141; *Citrobacter* 5396/58; *Arizona* 8, 19, 26, 29; *Shigella sonnei* I, II, *S. boydii* 3, 7, 8, 15; *Salmonella* L, P, 51
II									○	●	●	●	●	●										*E. coli* 21, 22, 23, 27, 33, 37, 46, 61, 76, 81, 87; *Arizona* 16; *S. boydii* 16
III										●	●	●	●	●	○									*Salmonella* C, C, H; *E. coli* 8, 9, 40, 58, 73, 78, 93; *Arizona* 30
IV									○	●	●	●	●	●	○									*Salmonella* K, R; *E. coli* 6
V										●	●	●	●	●	○									*Salmonella* W; *E. coli* 41, 52
VI									○	●	●	●	●	●										*Salmonella* G, N, U; *E. coli* 80, 86, 90, 127, 128; *Arizona* 21, 25

VII						●	●	●	●	●			○							*Salmonella* 59; *E. coli* 1, 13, 18, 19, 31, 35, 39, 50, 53, 54, 60, 69, 99, 100, 102, 119, 129
																				Arizona 6; *S. flexneri* 1a–5a, 6
																				S. boydii 1, 2, 4, 9, 10, 11, 14
VIII					○	●	●	●	●	●			○							*Salmonella* 53, 57
																				E. coli 48, 49, 51, 117
IX					○	●	●	●	●	●					○					*Salmonella* 56
X						●	●	●	●	●						○				*Salmonella* O; *E. coli* O111
																				Arizona 9, 20
XI					○	●	●	●	●	●						○				*Salmonella* Z; *E. coli* 55
XII					○	●	●	●	●	●	○	○								*Salmonella* I; *E. coli* 11, 43, 125
XIII						●	●	●	●	●	○		○							*Salmonella* E, F, 54; *E. coli* 34, 68, 75, 79
																				Arizona 17; *S. boydii* 5, 12
XIV						●	●	●	●	●	○		○				○			*Salmonella* B, C_2, C_3; *Citrobacter* 139
XV						●	●	●	●	●	○		○					○		*Salmonella* A
XVI						●	●	●	●	●	○		○						○	*Salmonella* D_1, D_2
XVII						●	●	●		●	○									*E. coli* 44, 59, 77
XVIII						●	●	●	●	●	○	○								*E. coli* 126
XIX						●	●	●		●	○		○							*E. coli* 17
XX				○		●	●	●	●	●										*E. coli* 12, 15, 29, 57
XXI				○		●	●	●	●	●			○							*E. coli* 4, 16, 25, 26
XXII				○		●	●	●	●	●				○						*E. coli* 45
XXIII			○			●	●	●	●	●										*E. coli* 3
XXIV						●	●	●	●	●		○	○							*E. coli* 36
XXV						●	●	●	●	●					○					*Salmonella* 52; *Arizona* 15
XXVI						●	●	●	●	●	○			○						*E. coli* 66, 68
XXVII						●	●	●	●	●		○		○						*E. coli* 84
XXVIII		○				●	●	●	●	●										*E. coli* 74
XXIX		○				●	●	●	●	●			○							*E. coli* 2
XXX	○				○	●	●	●	●	●										*E. coli* 5, 65
XXXI	○				○	●	●	●	●	●		○								*E. coli* 70

TABLE II (Continued)[a]

Chemotype	4-Amino-4,6-dideoxyglucose	4-Amino-4,6-dideoxygalactose	3-Amino-3,6-dideoxyglucose	3-Amino-3,6-dideoxygalactose	2-Amino-2,6-dideoxymannose	2-Amino-2,6-dideoxyglucose	2-Amino-2,6-dideoxygalactose	Mannosamine	Galactosamine	Glucosamine	Ketodeoxyoctonic acid	L-Glycero-D-mannoheptose	Galactose	Glucose	Mannose	Fucose	Rhamnose	6-Deoxytalose	Ribose	Colitose	Abequose	Paratose	Tyvelose	Found in serotypes or serogroups
XXXII			O						O	●	●	●	●	●			O							*Salmonella* M (28, 28$_3$)
XXXIII			O							●	●	●	●	●					O					*E. coli* 71; *Citrobacter* 896
XXXIV										●	●	●	●	●										*E. coli* 114
XXXV						O		O		●	●	●	●	●										*Salmonella* J
XXXVI										●	●	●	●	●	O									*Salmonella* T
XXXVII									O	●	●	●	●	●	O	O								*Salmonella* 58; *Arizona* 1, 33
XXXVIII				O					O	●	●	●	●	●										*Salmonella* 5
XXXIX			O			O		O	O	●	●	●	●	●										*Salmonella* 55; *Arizona* 24
XL			O							●	●	●	●	●			O							*Salmonella* M (28$_1$, 28$_2$)
XLI		O								●	●	●	●	●			O							*E. coli* 10
XLII	O									●	●	●	●	●			O							*E. coli* 7

[a] Data extracted from Kauffmann et al. (1960), *Salmonella* chemotypes; Kauffmann et al. (1962) and Ørskov et al. (1967), *E. coli* chemotypes; Westphal et al. (1960) and Lüderitz et al. (1967, 1968a), *Arizona*, *Citrobacter*, and *Salmonella* chemotypes; Seltmann and Hofmann (1966) and Seltmann (1968), *S. boydii* chemotypes; Simmons (1957, 1962, 1966), *S. flexneri* chemotypes.

1. Microbial Polysaccharides

TABLE III

Biologic Repeating Units of Some Salmonella (Lipo)polysaccharides

Salmonella group (O factors)	Biologic repeating units	References
A S. paratyphi A (1, 2, 12)	$\xrightarrow{2}\text{Man}\xrightarrow[\alpha]{1,4}\text{Rha}\xrightarrow[\alpha]{1,3}\text{Gal}\xrightarrow[\alpha]{1}$ with Par $\xrightarrow[\alpha]{1,3}$ on Man(2), Glc $\xrightarrow[\alpha]{1,4}$ on Gal via 1,6, and OAc on Rha	Hellerqvist et al., 1971c
B S. bredeney (1, 4, 12)	$\xrightarrow{2}\text{Man}\xrightarrow[\alpha]{1,4}\text{Rha}\xrightarrow[\beta]{1,3}\text{Gal}\xrightarrow[\alpha]{1}$ with Abe $\xrightarrow[\alpha]{1,3}$ on Man(2), Glc $\xrightarrow[\alpha]{1,4}$ on Gal via 1,6	Bagdian et al., 1966; Hellerqvist et al., 1969c
S. typhimurium (4, 5, 12)	$\xrightarrow{2}\text{Man}\xrightarrow[\alpha]{1,4}\text{Rha}\xrightarrow[\beta]{1,3}\text{Gal}\xrightarrow[\alpha]{1}$ with 2-OAc-Abe $\xrightarrow[\alpha]{1,3}$ on Man(2), Glc $\xrightarrow[\alpha]{1,4}$ on Gal	Hellerqvist et al., 1968, 1969a
D_1 S. typhi (9, 12)	$\xrightarrow{2}\text{Man}\xrightarrow[\alpha]{1,4}\text{Rha}\xrightarrow[\alpha]{1,3}\text{Gal}\xrightarrow[\alpha]{1}$ with Tyv $\xrightarrow[\alpha]{1,3}$ on Man(2), (2-OAc-)Glc $\xrightarrow[\alpha]{1,4}$ on Gal	Tinelli and Staub, 1960a,b; Stirm et al., 1966a,b; Bagdian et al., 1969; Hellerqvist et al., 1969b
D_2 S. strassbourg ((9), 46)	$\xrightarrow{6}\text{Man}\xrightarrow[\alpha]{1,4}\text{Rha}\xrightarrow[\alpha]{1,3}\text{Gal}\xrightarrow[\alpha]{1}$ with Tyv $\xrightarrow[\alpha]{1,3}$ on Man(6), Glc $\xrightarrow[\alpha]{1,4}$ on Gal	
E_1 S. anatum (3, 10)	$\xrightarrow{6}\text{Man}\xrightarrow[\beta]{1,4}\text{Rha}\xrightarrow[\alpha]{1,3}\text{Gal}\xrightarrow[\alpha]{1}$ with {OAc} on Gal	Robbins and Uchida, 1962; Hellerqvist et al., 1971a
E_2 S. newington (3, 15)	$\xrightarrow{6}\text{Man}\xrightarrow[\beta]{1,4}\text{Rha}\xrightarrow[\alpha]{1,3}\text{Gal}\xrightarrow[\beta]{1}$	Robbins and Uchida, 1962; Hellerqvist et al., 1971b
E_3 S. illinois ((3), (15), 34)	$\xrightarrow{6}\text{Man}\xrightarrow[\beta]{1,4}\text{Rha}\xrightarrow[\alpha]{1,3}\text{Gal}\xrightarrow[\beta]{1}$ with Glc $\xrightarrow[\alpha]{1,4}$ on Gal	Robbins and Uchida, 1962
E_4 S. senftenberg (1, 3, 19)	$\xrightarrow{6}\text{Man}\xrightarrow[\beta]{1,4}\text{Rha}\xrightarrow[\alpha]{1,3}\text{Gal}\xrightarrow[\alpha]{1}$ with Glc $\xrightarrow[\alpha]{1,6}$ on Gal	Staub and Girard, 1965; Hellerqvist et al., 1971c

TABLE IV

Structures of the O-Specific Polysaccharides (Repeating Units) from Some O-Antigenic Lipopolysaccharides

Genus	O Group	Chemical repeating unit of O-specific polysaccharide	References
Klebsiella	1, 6	$\xrightarrow{3}$ Gal $\xrightarrow[\alpha]{1}$	Björndal et al. (1971)
	3	$\xrightarrow{3}$ Man $\xrightarrow[\alpha]{1,3}$ Man $\xrightarrow[\alpha]{1,2}$ Man $\xrightarrow[\alpha]{1,2}$ Man $\xrightarrow[\alpha]{1,2}$ Man $\xrightarrow{1}$	Curvall et al. (1973a)
	5^a	$\xrightarrow{3}$ Man $\xrightarrow[\alpha]{1,2}$ Man $\xrightarrow[\alpha]{1,3}$ Man $\xrightarrow[\alpha]{1,2}$ Man $\xrightarrow[\alpha]{1,2}$ Man $\xrightarrow{1}$	Lindberg et al. (1972b)
	4	$\xrightarrow{2}$ Ribf $\xrightarrow[\beta]{1,4}$ Galp $\xrightarrow[\alpha]{1}$	Björndal et al. (1972)
	7	$\xrightarrow{2}$ L-Rhap $\xrightarrow[\alpha]{1,2}$ Ribf $\xrightarrow[\beta]{1,3}$ L-Rhap $\xrightarrow[\alpha]{1,3}$ L-Rhap $\xrightarrow[\alpha]{1}$	Simmons et al. (1965c)
	8^b	2/6OAc 2 OAc 2/6OAc $\xrightarrow{3}$ Galp $\xrightarrow[\alpha]{1,3}$ Galf $\xrightarrow[\alpha]{1,3}$ Galp $\xrightarrow[\alpha]{1}$	Curvall et al. (1973b)
	9^b	2/4OAc 2/4OAc 2/4OAc $\xrightarrow{3}$ Galf $\xrightarrow{1,3}$ Galp $\xrightarrow{1,3}$ Galf $\xrightarrow{1,3}$ Galp $\xrightarrow{1}$ $\uparrow{1,3}$ Galp	Lindberg et al. (1972a)

1. Microbial Polysaccharides

		Structure	Reference
	10	$\rightarrow 3$ L-Rhap $\xrightarrow{1,3}_{\alpha}$ Ribf $\xrightarrow{1,4}_{\beta}$ L-Rha $\xrightarrow{1,3}_{\alpha}$ Ribf $\xrightarrow{1,4}_{\beta}$ L-Rha $\xrightarrow{1}_{\alpha}$	Björndal et al. (1970b)
E. coli	8[c]	$\rightarrow 3$ Man $\xrightarrow{1,2}_{\alpha}$ Man $\xrightarrow{1,2}_{\alpha}$ Man $\xrightarrow{1}_{\alpha}$	Reske and Jann (1972)
	86	$\rightarrow$ Gal $\xrightarrow{}$ GalNAc $\rightarrow$ GalNAc $\rightarrow$ ↑ ↑ L-Fuc Glc	Springer (1970)
	111	$\rightarrow$ GlcNAc $\xrightarrow{1,2}_{\beta}$ Glc $\xrightarrow{1,4}_{\alpha}$ Gal $\xrightarrow{1}_{\alpha}$ α ↑1,6 ↑ Col Col	Edstrom and Heath (1965)
Shigella flexneri	y	$\rightarrow 3$ GlcNAc $\xrightarrow{1,2}$ Rha $\xrightarrow{1,2/3}$ Rha $\xrightarrow{1,3/2}$ Rha $\xrightarrow{1}$	Lindberg et al. (1973a)
	G	$\rightarrow$ Gal $\xrightarrow{1,3}_{\beta}$ GalNAc $\xrightarrow{1,3}$ GalNAc $\rightarrow$ L-Fuc $\rightarrow$	Simmons et al. (1965a)
Salmonella	N	$\rightarrow$ Glc $\xrightarrow{1,3}_{\beta}$ GalNAc $\rightarrow$ L-Fuc $\rightarrow$ ↑ Glc	Simmons et al. (1965b)
	U	$\rightarrow$ Gal $\xrightarrow{1,3}$ GalNAc $\xrightarrow{1,3}$ GalNAc $\xrightarrow{1,4}$ L-Fuc $\rightarrow$ α ↑1,3 Gal	Simmons et al. (1965c)

[a] The O5 polysaccharide contains small amount of 3-O-methylmannose which is not present in the O3 polysaccharide.
[b] The dotted line indicates that the O-acetyl substituent is not present on all residues.
[c] The O8 polysaccharide contains small amounts of 3-O-methylmannose. The O9 polysaccharide contains likewise only mannose in -2 and -3 linkages, the fine structure differing from that of the O8 polysaccharide.

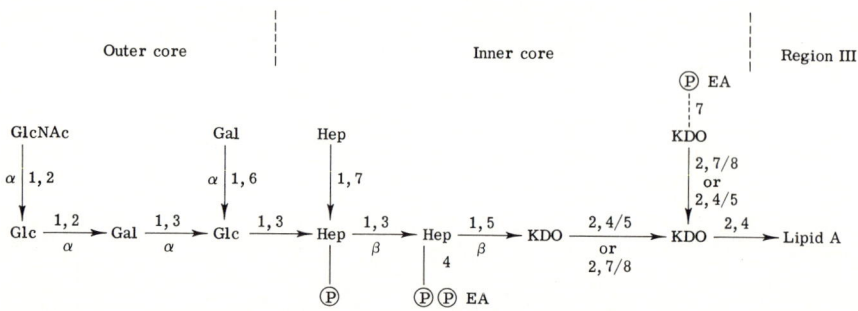

Fig. 4. Structure of the *Salmonella* core. ⓅEA and ⓅⓅEA, Phospho- and diphosphoethanolamine; KDO, 2-keto-3-deoxyoctonic acid; all linkages pyranosidic. After Lüderitz (1970) and Lüderitz et al. (1973).

on the R mutants of *S. minnesota* and *S. typhimurium*. In serologic studies, using cross-reactions as tool, it was found that all *Salmonella* LPS have the same R-core oligosaccharide (region II). Restricted to this genus, therefore, the term "common core" is correct. Later, other core oligosaccharides were found, especially in *E. coli*. In this genus there are now five distinct core types known (Schmidt et al., 1969, 1970a, 1974). There is partial cross-reaction with R cores of other genera, such as *Shigella*.

Differences between these types of complete core are not only found in sequence and linkage of sugar residues, but also in composition. Thus, the *Salmonella* core and *E. coli* core types 2 and 3 contain glucosamine, while *E. coli* core types 1 and 4 do not.

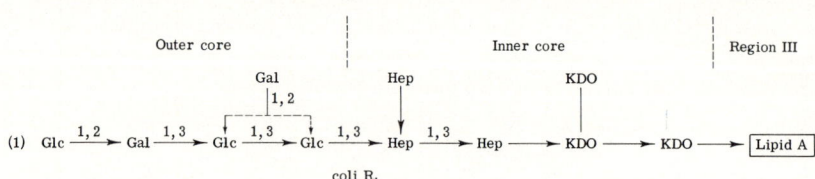

Fig. 5. Structures of the coli R1 and coli R2 core oligosaccharides. (1) From Jann et al. (1975); (2) from Hämmerling et al. (1970, 1971). Phosphate, phospho- and diphosphoethanolamine are present in unknown positions.

The structures of *E. coli* core types 1 (Jann *et al.*, 1975) and 2 (Hämmerling *et al.*, 1970, 1971) were elucidated recently. They are given in Fig. 5.

It should be mentioned that *E. coli* K12 and *E. coli* C have a complete core (Schmidt, 1973). *E. coli* K12 represents a type of its own and *E. coli* C seems to be identical with *E. coli* core type 1.

R-LPS with an incomplete core occur in *rfa* mutants. Through the action of mutagens on a given wild-type (S) strain, a number of R(*rfa*) mutants can be obtained which have more or less incomplete R-LPS. They can be characterized by bacteriophages and by their sensitivity to various dyes and antibiotics (Schlecht and Westphal, 1970). According to the completeness of the core structures (as expressed through sugar composition) the R(*rfa*) mutants were termed Ra, Rb, Rc, Rd, and Re, respectively (Lüderitz and Westphal, 1966). The lipopolysaccharides were used for biochemical studies which, together with structural investigations, provided a great help in establishing the structure of the complete core oligosaccharide (for a review, see Lüderitz *et al.*, 1966a, 1968a, 1971). The various structures of core oligosaccharides of *Salmonella rfa* mutants (Lüderitz, 1970) are shown in Table V. Johnston *et al.* (1968) have worked out the structure for the outer core pentasaccharide of a *Shigella flexneri* R mutant which is serologically closely related to coli R3.

More recently, *rfa* mutants of the *E. coli* R1 type were studied (Schmidt *et al.*, 1970b). The structures of the various incomplete core oligosaccharides, as elucidated by Jann *et al.* (1975), are shown in Table VI.

E. coli B is an R form with a *rfb* defect. The structure of its core oligosaccharide was established by Prehm *et al.* (1975), and is shown in Fig. 6.

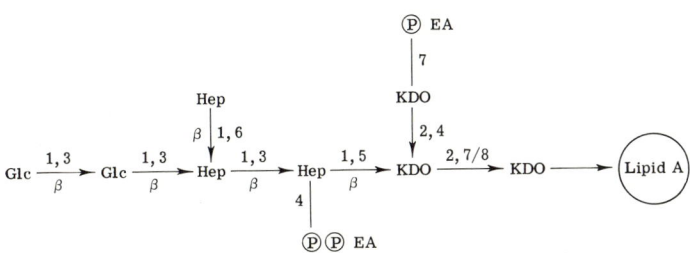

Fig. 6. Structure of the *E. coli* B lipopolysaccharide Ⓟ EA and ⓅⓅ EA, phospho- and diphosphoethanolamine; KDO, 2-keto-3-deoxyoctonic acid. From Prehm (1975).

TABLE V

Structure of Lipopolysaccharides of Core-Defective Salmonella R Mutants[a]

R chemotype	Oligosaccharide[b]
Ra	GlcNAc $\xrightarrow[\alpha]{1,2}$ Glc $\xrightarrow[\alpha]{1,2}$ Gal $\xrightarrow[\alpha]{1,3}$ Glc $\xrightarrow{1,3}$ Hep $\xrightarrow[\beta]{1,3}$ Hep $\longrightarrow$ (KDO)$_3$ $\longrightarrow$ Lipid A, with Gal $\xrightarrow{\alpha\,1,6}$ on Glc and Hep $\xrightarrow{1,7}$ on Hep
Rb	Glc $\longrightarrow$ Gal $\longrightarrow$ Glc $\longrightarrow$ Hep $\longrightarrow$ Hep $\longrightarrow$ (KDO)$_3$ $\longrightarrow$ Lipid A, with Gal on Glc and Hep on Hep
Rc	Glc $\longrightarrow$ Hep $\longrightarrow$ Hep $\longrightarrow$ (KDO)$_3$ $\longrightarrow$ Lipid A, with Hep on Hep
Rd$_1$	Hep $\longrightarrow$ Hep $\longrightarrow$ (KDO)$_3$ $\longrightarrow$ Lipid A
Rd$_2$	Hep $\longrightarrow$ (KDO)$_3$ $\longrightarrow$ Lipid A
Re	(KDO)$_3$ $\longrightarrow$ Lipid A

[a] From Lüderitz (1970).
[b] Substitution of the complete oligosaccharide by phosphoethanolamine is the same as shown in Fig. 4. Mutants have been isolated as P$^+$ (containing phosphoethanolamine) or P$^-$ forms.

7. Lipid A

Lipid A can be isolated by mild acid treatment of lipopolysaccharides (see Fig. 2), preferably of Re glycolipids (Galanos *et al.*, 1971a). Lipid A from *Salmonella* strains has the composition given in Table VII.

TABLE VI

Structure of the coli R1-Core Oligosaccharide and of Oligosaccharides from Core-Defective Mutants Derived from E. coli R1[a]

R chemotype	Oligosaccharide
Rb	Gal↓1,2 ; Hep↓ Glc →1,2 Gal →1,3 Glc →1,3 Glc →1,3 Hep →1,3 Hep ⟶ (KDO)$_3$ ⟶ Lipid A Gal↓1,2 ; Hep↓ Gal →1,3 Glc →1,3 Glc →1,3 Hep →1,3 Hep ⟶ (KDO)$_3$ ⟶ Lipid A
Rc	Hep↓ Glc →1,3 Hep →1,3 Hep ⟶ (KDO)$_3$ ⟶ Lipid A Glc →1,3 Hep →1,3 Hep ⟶ (KDO)$_3$ ⟶ Lipid A
Rd	Hep↓ Hep →1,3 Hep ⟶ (KDO)$_3$ ⟶ Lipid A Hep →1,3 Hep ⟶ (KDO)$_3$ ⟶ Lipid A

[a] From Jann and Jann (1975).

Lipid A was shown to consist of a highly substituted disaccharidic backbone: 4-phosphoglucosaminyl-β-1,6-glucosamine 1-phosphate (Gmeiner et al., 1969). The two amino groups of the glucosamine units are substituted with β-hydroxymyristic acid. One hydroxy position of the glucosamine disaccharide is substituted by 3-O-myristoyl-myristic ester (Rietschel et al., 1971). Studies of Lüderitz and his coworkers on the structure of lipid A (Lüderitz et al., 1973) led to the formula given in Fig. 7.

As a result of these many structural investigations on lipopolysaccharides of S forms, R forms, and on lipid A, the complete formula of several enterobacterial LPS could be elaborated. As an example, the structure of the LPS of *Salmonella typhimurium* is given in Fig. 8.

TABLE VII

The Constituents of Lipid A

Constituent	Molar ratio
Glucosamine	2
Phosphate	2
Amide-bound fatty acids	
D-β-Hydroxymyristic acid	2
Ester-bound fatty acids	
Lauric acid	1
Myristic acid	1
Palmitic acid	1
D-β-Hydroxymyristic acid	1

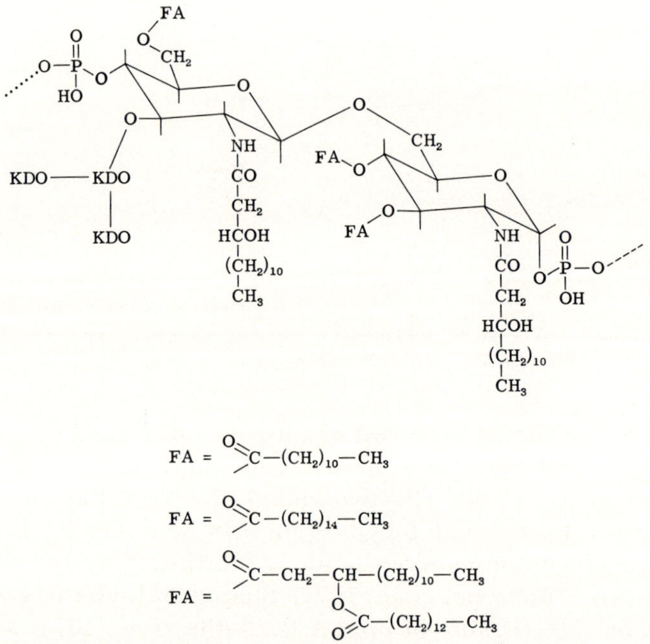

$$FA = \overset{O}{>}C-(CH_2)_{10}-CH_3$$

$$FA = \overset{O}{>}C-(CH_2)_{14}-CH_3$$

$$FA = \overset{O}{>}C-CH_2-\underset{\underset{\overset{|}{O}}{|}}{CH}-(CH_2)_{10}-CH_3$$
$$\overset{O}{\underset{O}{>}}C-(CH_2)_{12}-CH_3$$

Fig. 7. Structure of a *Salmonella* lipid A unit with an attached KDO trisaccharide. From Rietschel et al. (1971).

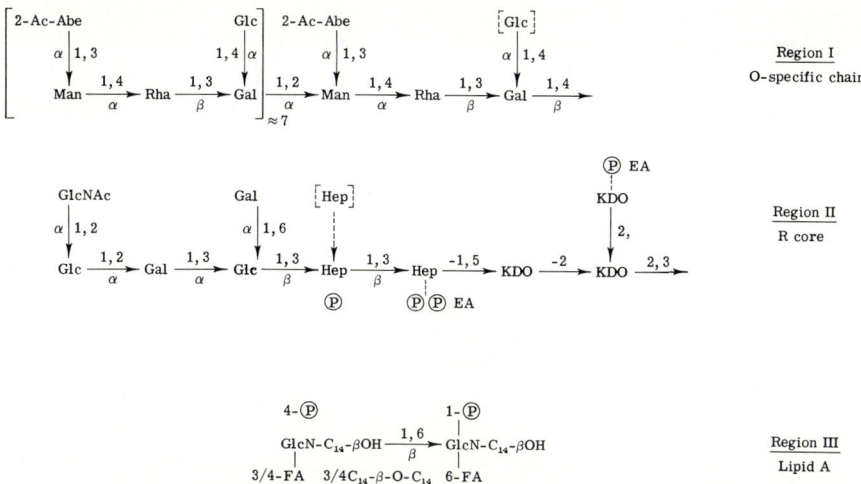

Fig. 8. Structure of the lipopolysaccharide of *S. typhimurium* according to present knowledge. After Lüderitz (1970) and Lüderitz *et al.* (1973).

C. Capsular Polysaccharides

Many bacteria can develop an envelope layer of considerable thickness which is termed capsule. The definition of a capsule is often arbitrary, since some are readily demonstrable in the light microscope with the India ink method (Bott *et al.*, 1936) or with the Neufeld swelling reaction using specific antibody (Neufeld, 1902), while others are not. Practically all bacterial capsules consist of polysaccharides charged with a high proportion of acidic constituents such as hexuronic acids, neuraminic acid, or pyruvate substitution (Lüderitz *et al.*, 1968a). This surface charge is used in the electron microscopic demonstration of capsules with ruthenium red as an electron-dense contrast medium (Springer and Roth, 1973).

Capsules are frequently found with bacteria obtained from pathogenic material, and the capacity of microorganisms to form a capsule may be lost on prolonged cultivation. In this context it should be mentioned that pathogenicity (virulence) of many bacteria in infection experiments can be increased by incorporation in hog gastric mucin, a charged and viscous mucopolysaccharide. This could mean that encapsulation—natural or artificial—by mucin, tends to increase the pathogenic properties of bacteria. The conclusion that encapsulation may in many cases (*E. coli*, *Klebsiella*, *Pneumococci*) be a parameter of pathogenicity is strengthened by the fact that capsules render bacteria resistant to phagocytosis and to the action of complement and antibody (Schwarzmann and Boring, 1971; Glynn, 1972).

For the isolation of capsular polysaccharides a number of methods may be used. They may be extracted with saline or buffer at temperatures between 20° and 50° or with 45% aqueous phenol (Westphal and Jann, 1965). Purification can be achieved by precipitation with cetavlon (Scott, 1960; Jann et al., 1965), ion-exchange chromatography (Yurewicz et al., 1971), or block electrophoresis in gels (Holmgren et al., 1969).

The purified capsular acidic polysaccharides have been used widely in immunologic studies. The pneumococcal polysaccharides (especially that from type III) are model substances for the study of stability and persistence in animals and man (Felton, 1949; Siskind et al., 1967; Howard et al., 1970a,b, 1972). They were recently found to be not only T cell independent antigens (Howard et al., 1971a,b; Howard, 1972), but also B cell mitogens (Coutinho and Möller, 1973). These properties, which they share with the somatic lipopolysaccharides, may be of importance in bacterial infections. Capsular acidic polysaccharides attach to erythrocytes and can then interfere with hemagglutination (Neter, 1962; Ceppelini and Landy, 1963). It is supposed that the effect is due to electrostatic repulsion of negatively charged cells (Ceppelini and Landy, 1963). Similarly, these capsular antigens may interfere in serologic typing of bacteria. This is well known in *E. coli*, where the presence of capsular polysaccharide antigens abolishes the agglutinability of bacterial cells in anti-O antisera (Kauffmann, 1954, 1966).

1. CAPSULAR POLYSACCHARIDE ANTIGENS OF
   Diplococcus pneumoniae (*Pneumococcus*)

More than 75 serologically distinct types of pneumococci can be differentiated by virtue of their capsular polysaccharide antigens. These types are designated as PnI, PnII, PnIII, etc., and the respective soluble polysaccharides as SI, SII, SIII, etc. The composition of some of these polysaccharides has been reported and is summarized in Table VIII. It is noteworthy that 17 out of the 19 polysaccharides listed are charged, either through hexuronic acid constituents or through phosphate or pyruvic acid substitution. Pyruvate was first reported to occur in an extracellular polysaccharide from *Xanthomonas campestris* (Sloneker and Orentas, 1962; Orentas et al., 1965) and in agar (Hirase, 1957), and has recently been found in many more polysaccharides. It is bound to the polysaccharide in a ketal linkage via its carbonyl group. The ketal linkage is very acid-

1. Microbial Polysaccharides

TABLE VIII
Composition of Some Capsular Polysaccharide Antigens of Diplococcus pneumoniae (Pneumococcus)

Polysaccharide	Amino sugar[a]	Neutral sugar	Hexuronic acid	Noncarbohydrate	Reference
SI	GlcN	—	GalUA	Acetate[b]	Heidelberger, 1960; Guy et al., 1967
SII	—	Glc Rha	GlcUA	—	Rebers and Heidelberger, 1961; Barker et al., 1966a; Barker et al., 1967
SIII	—	Glc	GlcUA	—	Adams et al., 1941; Reeves and Goebel, 1941
SIV	GalN ManN FucN	Gal	—	Pyruvate[c]	Higginbotham and Heidelberger, 1972
SV	FucN	Glc	GlcUA	—	Barker et al., 1966a,b
SVI	—	Gal Glc Rha	—	Ribitol phosphate	Rebers and Heidelberger, 1961; Tyler and Heidelberger, 1968
SVII	GalN GlcN	Gal Glc Rha	—	—	Heidelberger, 1960, 1967
SVIII	—	Gal Glc	GlcUA	—	Rao and Heidelberger, 1966
SIX	GalN GlcN ManN	Glc	GlcUA	—	Higginbotham and Heidelberger, 1972
SXI	—	Gal Glc	—	Glycerol phosphate	Heidelberger, 1960; Kennedy et al., 1969
SXIII	GlcN	Gal Glc	—	Ribitol phosphate	Shabarova et al., 1962
SXIV	GlcN	Gal Glc	—	—	Heidelberger, 1960
SVI	GalN GlcN	Gal Glc Rha	—	Glycerol phosphate	Shabarova et al., 1962
SXVIII	—	Gal Glc Rha	—	Glycerol phosphate	Estrada-Parra and Heidelberger, 1963
SXIX	ManN	Glc Rha	—	Phosphate	Miyuzaki and Yadomae, 1971
SXXVII	GlcN	Gal Glc Rha	—	Glycerol phosphate pyruvate[c]	Heidelberger et al., 1970
SXXXI	—	Gal Rha	GlcUA	—	Roy et al., 1970
SXXXIII	N.I.[d]	Gal Glc	GalUA	—	Mills and Smith, 1962
SXXXIV	—	Gal Glc	—	Ribitol phosphate, acetate	Dixon et al., 1966

[a] All amino sugars are N-acetylated. [b] Ester-bound. [c] Ketal-bound. [d] N.I., not identified.

TABLE IX

Structures of Some Type-Specific Capsular Polysaccharides of D. pneumoniae

Polysaccharides	Repeating unit	References
SIII	$\xrightarrow{3} GlcUA \xrightarrow[\beta]{1,4} Glc \xrightarrow{1}$	Heidelberger, 1960; Adams et al., 1941; Reeves and Goebel, 1941
SVI	$\xrightarrow{2} Gal \xrightarrow[\alpha]{1,3} Glc \xrightarrow[\beta]{1,3} L\text{-}Rha \xrightarrow{1,3} Ribitol \xrightarrow{1} P \longrightarrow$	Rebers and Heidelberger, 1959, 1961
SVIII	$\xrightarrow{4} GlcUA \xrightarrow[\beta]{1,4} Glc \xrightarrow[\alpha]{1,4} Glc \xrightarrow[\alpha]{1,4} Gal \xrightarrow[\alpha]{1}$	Heidelberger, 1960; Jones and Perry, 1957
SXI	$\xrightarrow{3} Gal \xrightarrow[\beta]{1,4} Glc \xrightarrow[\alpha]{1,6} Glc \xrightarrow[\alpha]{1,4} Gal \xrightarrow[\alpha]{1}$ $\|$ P-Glyc	Kennedy et al., 1969
SXIII	$\xrightarrow{4} Gal \xrightarrow[\beta]{1,4} Glc \xrightarrow[\beta]{1,3} Gal(f) \xrightarrow[\beta]{1,4} GlcNAc \xrightarrow{1,2} Ribitol \xrightarrow{1} P \longrightarrow$	Watson et al., 1972
SXVIII[a] or	$\xrightarrow{3} Gal \xrightarrow[\beta]{1,4} Glc \xrightarrow[\alpha]{1,6} Glc \xrightarrow[\alpha]{1,3} L\text{-}Rha \xrightarrow{1,4} Glc \xrightarrow{1}$ $\xrightarrow{3} Gal \xrightarrow[\beta]{1,4} Glc \xrightarrow[\alpha]{1,3} L\text{-}Rha \xrightarrow{1,4} Glc \xrightarrow[\alpha]{1,6} Glc \xrightarrow{1}$	Estrada-Parra and Heidelberger, 1963; Estrada-Parra et al., 1962
SXXXIV	$\xrightarrow{3} Gal \xrightarrow[\beta]{1,3} Glc \xrightarrow[\alpha]{1,2} Gal \xrightarrow[\beta]{1,3} Gal \xrightarrow{1,2} Ribitol \xrightarrow{1/5} P \longrightarrow$	Dixon et al., 1966; Chittenden et al., 1968

[a] To one of the proposed polysaccharide backbones glycerol phosphate is bound at an unknown place and one of the sugar residues (probably galactose) is O-acetylated.

labile, and for this reason pyruvic acid substitution has been overlooked for a long time.

There are only three different neutral sugar components in the pneumococcal polysaccharides, with a high incidence of L-rhamnose. The variability in amino sugar components is surprisingly great. In the genuine polysaccharides, amino sugars are N-acetylated.

In a number of cases the structures of pneumococcal polysaccharides have been completely elucidated, in some others partial structures were proposed. The structures of the type-specific polysaccharides SIII, SVI, SVIII, SXI, SXII, SXVIII, and SXXXIV are known. Their repeating units are shown in Table IX. For SXVIII two possible structures have been proposed for the main polysaccharide chain, to which glycerol phosphate is bound at an unknown site. The structure of SII was proposed by Lindberg (personal communication) as shown in Fig. 9. It should be pointed out, however, that results of a chemical (Larm et al., 1972) and serologic (Larm et al., 1972; Heidelberger et al., 1969) nature argue against this proposition. These studies established terminal disaccharide units of 6-O-(α-D-glucosyluronic)-D-glucose to be antigenic determinants—a fact that cannot be accommodated by the structure proposed and shown in Fig. 9. Recently, a structure has tentatively been assigned to SIX which is very complex insofar as a repeating unit with 14 monosaccharides has been suggested (Das et al., 1972). From a biochemical point of view this is rather surprising.

Partial structures of type-specific polysaccharides SI, SII, SV, SIX, SXIV, and SXIX have been suggested. From none of these can the respective genuine polysaccharide be reconstructed. Nevertheless, these oligosaccharide structures, which are shown in Table X, provide important information with respect to antigenic specificities and

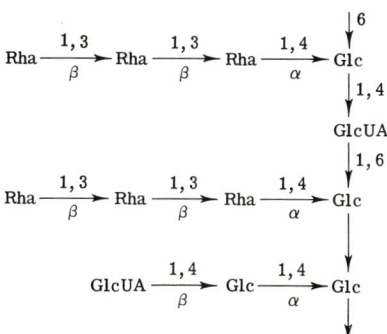

Fig. 9. Proposed structure of the capsular polysaccharide from *Pneumococcus* type II, as proposed by Lindberg (personal communication).

TABLE X

Oligosaccharides Obtained from Some Type-Specific Capsular Polysaccharides of D. pneumoniae

From polysaccharide	Oligosaccharide	References
SI	GalUA $\xrightarrow{1,3}$ GlcNAc $\xrightarrow{1,3}$ GalUA	Guy et al., 1967
SII	GlcUA $\xrightarrow[\alpha]{1,6}$ Glc; Rha $\xrightarrow{1,4}$ Glc	Larm et al., 1972
SV	GlcUA $\xrightarrow[\beta]{1,3}$ L-FucNAc	How et al., 1964
SIX	GlcUA $\longrightarrow$ GlcNAc; GlcUA $\xrightarrow{1,3}$ GalNAc; GlcUA $\xrightarrow{1,3}$ Glc	Higginbotham et al., 1972
SXIV	Gal $\xrightarrow[\beta]{1,4}$ Glc $\xrightarrow[\beta]{1,4}$ GlcNAc	Heidelberger, 1961
SXIX[a]	Rha $\xrightarrow[\alpha]{1,3}$ Glc $\xrightarrow[\alpha]{1,2}$ Rha	Miyuzaki and Jones, 1969

[a] The nonreducing terminal rhamnose is substituted in position 3 with phosphate.

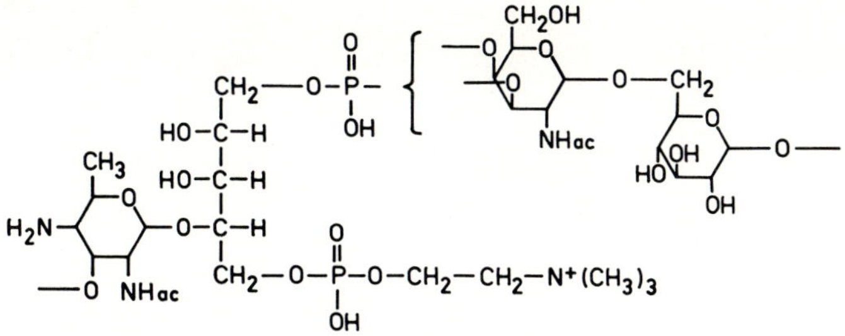

1. *Microbial Polysaccharides*   31

Fig. 10. Structure of the C polysaccharide from *Pneumococcus*. After Brundish and Baddiley (1968).

cross-reactivities of these polysaccharides.

Many strains of pneumococci produce a somatic polysaccharide that is not type-specific but rather species-specific. It was termed C polysaccharide and contains, like SVI and SXXXIV, ribitol phosphate. It is thus reminiscent of certain teichoic acids. In addition to ribitol phosphate, N-acetylgalactosamine, glucose, and a new amino sugar, 2-acetamido-4-amino-2,4,6-trideoxyhexose, were found in the C polysaccharide. The exact configuration is not yet known. Another component of the C polysaccharide is phosphoryl choline. This is also important with respect to bacteriophage receptor and cell division (Tomasz, 1967, 1968). The repeating unit of the C polysaccharide, as proposed by Brundish and Baddiley (1968), is shown in Fig. 10.

2. Capsular Polysaccharide Antigens of *Klebsiella*

In addition to the somatic lipopolysaccharides, all *Klebsiella* strains produce large capsules of acidic polysaccharides (K antigens) (Nimmich, 1968, 1971), which completely cover the O-antigenic lipopolysaccharides. The serologic individuality is, therefore, expressed by the capsular (K) antigens. There are only 12 O groups (12 different O antigens of which most are homopolysaccharides; see Table IV), but more than 80 different capsular polysaccharides. For this reason *Klebsiella* are serologically typed through their capsular polysaccharide antigens. In spite of this serologic variability, there are, nevertheless, only few sugar constituents found in the group of these polysaccharides, as shown in Table XI. Recently, pyruvate was found to be a substituent in some *Klebsiella* polysaccharides (Gormus and Wheat, 1971). Also, O-formyl and O-acetyl substitution occurs in some of these polysaccharides. There has, however, been no systematic search for such noncarbohydrate components. As will be shown later, these substituents may function as part of serologic

TABLE XI

Composition of Some Capsular Polysaccharide Antigens of Klebsiella

Type	Hexuronic acid	Gal	Glc	Man	Rha	Fuc	Noncarbohydrate[a]	Reference
1	GlcUA	−	+	−	−	+	Pyruvate	Barker et al., 1963
2	GlcUA	−	+	+	−	−	Pyruvate, formate, Acetate	Gormus et al., 1971 Gormus et al., 1971 Gahan et al., 1967
3	GalUA	+	−	+	−	−	Pyruvate	Gormus et al., 1971 Henriksen and Eriksen, 1962
4	N.I.	+	+	+	−	−	Pyruvate	Gormus et al., 1971 Eriksen, 1963
5	GlcUA	+	+	+	−	−	Pyruvate, acetate	Gormus et al., 1971 Henriksen et al., 1961
6	GalUA	−	+	+	−	+	Pyruvate	Gormus et al., 1971 Gormus and Wheat, 1971
8	GlcUA	+	+	−	−	−	Pyruvate, acetate	Gormus et al., 1971 Dudman and Wilkinson, 1956
9	GlcUA	+	−	−	+	−		Lindberg et al., 1972a,b,c
11	GlcUA	+	+	+	−	−		Thurow, 1973 Nimmich, 1969 Choy and Dutton, 1972

1. Microbial Polysaccharides

								Reference
20	GlcUA	+	−	+	−	−		Gormus et al., 1971
21	GlcUA	+	−	+	−	−	Pyruvate	Eriksen and Henriksen, 1963
23	GlcUA	−	+	−	−	−		Nimmich, 1969
26	N.I.	+	−	+	−	−		Dudman and Wilkinson, 1956
29	N.I.	+	−	+	−	−		Dudman and Wilkinson, 1956
32	−	+	−	−	+	−		Heidelberger et al., 1970
45	GlcUA	−	+	−	+	−		Nimmich, 1968
47	GlcUA	+	−	−	+	−		Heidelberger et al., 1970
52	GlcUA	+	−	−	+	−		Heidelberger et al., 1970
54	GlcUA	−	+	−	−	−	Acetate, formate	Dudman and Wilkinson, 1956
57	N.I.	+	−	+	−	−		Sutherland and Wilkinson, 1968
61	GlcUA	+	+	−	−	−		Dudman and Wilkinson, 1956
64	GlcUA	−	+	+	+	−		Nimmich, 1969
71	GlcUA	−	+	−	−	−		Barker et al., 1958
72	GlcUA	−	+	−	+	−		Nimmich, 1969

[a] Absence of noncarbohydrate in this list is not based on proof of absence, rather than absence of proof in the references given.

TABLE XII

Structures of Some Capsular Polysaccharide Antigens of Klebsiella

Type	Repeating unit	References
2	$\xrightarrow{3}$ Glc $\xrightarrow[\beta]{1,4}$ Man $\xrightarrow[\beta]{1,4}$ Glc $\xrightarrow[\alpha]{1}$ $\alpha \uparrow 1,3$ GlcUA	Gahan et al. (1967); Sutherland (1971a,b)
5[a]	$\xrightarrow{4}$ GlcUA $\xrightarrow[\beta]{1,4}$ Glc $\xrightarrow[\beta]{1,3}$ Man $\xrightarrow{1}$	Dutton and Yang (1972)
7[b]	$\xrightarrow{3}$ GlcUA $\xrightarrow[\rho]{1,2}$ Man $\xrightarrow[\alpha]{1,2}$ Man $\xrightarrow[\alpha]{1,3}$ Glc $\xrightarrow[\beta]{1}$ Gal 4,6 Py	Dutton (personal communication)
8	$\xrightarrow{3}$ Gal $\xrightarrow[\beta]{1,3}$ Gal $\xrightarrow[\alpha]{1,3}$ Glc $\xrightarrow[\beta]{1}$ $\alpha \uparrow 1,4$ GlcUA	Sutherland (1970)
9	$\xrightarrow{3}$ Gal $\xrightarrow[\alpha]{1,3}$ L-Rha $\xrightarrow[\alpha]{1,3}$ L-Rha $\xrightarrow[\alpha]{1,2}$ L-Rha $\xrightarrow[\alpha]{1}$ $\beta \uparrow 1,4$ GlcUA	Lindberg et al. (1972a,b,c)
11[c]	$\xrightarrow{3}$ Glc $\xrightarrow[\beta]{1,3}$ GlcUA $\xrightarrow[\beta]{1,3}$ Gal $\xrightarrow[\alpha]{1}$ $\alpha \uparrow 1,4$ Gal	Thurow (1973)
20	$\xrightarrow{2}$ Man $\xrightarrow[\alpha]{1,3}$ Gal $\xrightarrow{1}$ $\alpha \uparrow 1,3$ Gal $\beta \uparrow 1,3$ GlcUA	Choy and Dutton (1972)
21[c]	$\xrightarrow{3}$ GlcUA $\xrightarrow[\alpha]{1,3}$ Man $\xrightarrow[\alpha]{1,2}$ Man $\xrightarrow[\alpha]{1,3}$ Gal $\xrightarrow[\beta]{1}$ $\alpha \uparrow 1,4$ Gal	Choy and Dutton (1973)
38[d]	$\xrightarrow{\beta}$ Gal $\xrightarrow[\beta]{1,4}$ Gal $\xrightarrow[\alpha]{1,6}$ Glc $\xrightarrow[\beta]{1}$ $\beta \uparrow 1,2$ Glc	Lindberg et al. (1973b)

1. Microbial Polysaccharides

TABLE XII (Continued)

Type	Repeating unit	References
47	$\xrightarrow{3}$ Gal $\xrightarrow[\beta]{1,4}$ Rha $\xrightarrow{1}{\alpha}$ $\beta \uparrow 1,3$ GlcUA $\alpha \uparrow 1,4$ L-Rha	Björndal et al. (1973)
54	$\xrightarrow{6}$ Glc $\xrightarrow[\beta]{1,4}$ GlcUA $\xrightarrow[\alpha]{1,3}$ L-Fuc $\xrightarrow{1}$ $\beta \uparrow 1,4$ Glc	Conrad et al. (1966)

[a] Mannose is substituted (4, 6) with pyruvate.
[b] Part of the mannoses are substituted with galactose and part of the glucoses are substituted (4, 6) with pyruvate.
[c] Side chain galactose is substituted (4, 6) with pyruvate.
[d] Branching Gal is substituted with 3-deoxy-L-glyceropentulosonic acid

determinants and be responsible for cross-reactivity within *Klebsiella* polysaccharides and between polysaccharides from different genera.

The capsular polysaccharides (K antigens) of *Klebsiella* have been studied in some cases and the structures proposed are shown in Table XII.

3. Capsular Polysaccharide Antigens of *E. coli*

The K antigens of *E. coli* were divided into three groups (A,B,L) (for details, see Kauffmann, 1954), all of which comprise acidic polysaccharides. Distinctive features of A antigens are that they occur only together with the O antigens 8 and 9 (i.e., only with *E. coli* strains belonging to serogroups O8 and O9), that they form large capsules which can be lost upon mutation (Kauffmann, 1954), and that they are free of amino sugars. The sugar composition of some K antigens is shown in Table XIII. The structure of a few K-antigenic polysaccharides is shown in Table XIV. In principle, there is no difference in the structure between A, B, and L antigens. Like other microbial polysaccharides, they are all built up from repeating units.

As far as we know, the pattern of polysaccharide antigens in *E. coli* is more intricate than that in other genera. This is illustrated by the antigens of *E. coli* O100:K?(B):H12. The extracellular polysac-

TABLE XIII

Composition of Some Acidic Capsular Polysaccharides of E. coli[a]

Antigen type	Capsular type	Acidic sugar	Amino sugar	Composition							Noncarbohydrate
				Gal	Glc	Man	Fuc	Rha	Rib	
A	K26	GlcUA	—	+	—	—	—	+	—	Acetyl
	K27	GlcUA	—	+	+	—	+	—	—	Acetyl
	K29	GlcUA	—	—	+	+	—	—	—	Pyruvate
	K30	GlcUA	—	+	+	+	—	—	—	Acetyl
	K31	GlcUA	—	+	+	—	—	—	—	—
	K42	GalUA	—	+	—	—	+	—	—	—
B	K85	GlcUA	GlcN	—	—	—	—	—	—	—
	K87	GlcUA	GlcN, FucN	+	+	+	—	+	—	Acetyl
	K25	GlcUA	GalN	—	—	+	+	—	—	—
	K56	ManUA	—	—	+	—	—	—	—	—
	K57	GalUA	GlcN	+	+	—	—	—	—	—
L	K4	GalUA	GalN	—	+	—	—	—	—	—
	K8	GlcUA	GalN, GlcN	+	—	—	—	+	—	—
	K17	GlcUA	GlcN	+	—	—	—	—	—	—
	O45:K(L)[b]	NANA	—	—	+	—	—	—	—	—
	O56:K(L)[b]	NANA	GlcN	+	+	—	—	—	—	—
	O24:K(L)[b]	NANA	GalN	+	+	—	—	—	—	—
	K9	NANA	GalN	+	—	—	—	—	—	—
	K1	NANA	—	—	—	—	—	—	—	—

[a] From Lüderitz et al. (1968a) and Jann et al. (unpublished).
[b] K antigen is not numbered but known to be a L antigen.

1. Microbial Polysaccharides

TABLE XIV

Structures of Some Capsular Polysaccharides (K Antigens) of E. coli

Type	Repeating unit	References
K27	$\longrightarrow \text{Glc} \xrightarrow{1,3} \text{GlcUA} \xrightarrow{1,3} \text{L-Fuc} \xrightarrow{1}$ $\quad\quad\;\; {}^{1,3}\!\uparrow$ $\longrightarrow \text{Gal}$	Jann et al., 1968; Ørskov et al., 1963
K29(A)	$\xrightarrow{6} \text{Man} \xrightarrow{1,3} \text{Glc} \xrightarrow{1,6} \text{GlcUA} \xrightarrow{1,3} \text{Gal} \xrightarrow{1}$ $\quad\quad\quad\quad\quad\quad\quad\quad\;\;\uparrow$ $\quad\quad\quad\quad\quad\quad\text{Glc} \longleftarrow \text{Man-Pyruvate}$	Le-Ba Nhan et al., 1971, and unpublished; Fehmel, 1972
K30(A)[a]	$\xrightarrow{3} \text{Man} \xrightarrow{1,2} \text{GlcUA} \xrightarrow[\beta]{1,3} \text{Gal} \xrightarrow{1}$	Hungerer et al., 1967
K42(A)	$\xrightarrow{3} \text{Gal} \xrightarrow{1,3} \text{GalUA} \xrightarrow{1,2} \text{L-Fuc} \xrightarrow{1}$	Jann et al., 1965
K85(B)	$\longrightarrow \text{GlcUA} \xrightarrow[(1,4)]{(1,2)} \text{Man} \xrightarrow{1,3} \text{Man} \xrightarrow{1,3} \text{GlcNAc} \xrightarrow{1}$ $\quad\quad\quad\quad\quad\;\;\;\downarrow$ $\quad\quad\quad\quad\;\;\text{L-Rha}$	Jann et al., 1971
K87(B)[b]	$\xrightarrow{4} \text{GlcUA} \xrightarrow[\beta]{1,3} \text{L-FucNAc} \xrightarrow{1,3} \text{GlcNAc} \xrightarrow{1,6} \text{Gal} \xrightarrow{1}$ $\quad\quad\quad\quad\quad\quad\quad\quad\quad\quad\quad\;\; \beta\!\uparrow {}^{1,4}$ $\quad\quad\quad\quad\quad\quad\quad\quad\quad\quad\text{Glc} \cdots\cdots (2)\text{O-Ac}$	Tarcsay et al., 1971

[a] Contains approximately one O-acetyl group per 3 repeating units.
[b] The O-acetyl group is linked to the 2 position of either glucose or galactose.

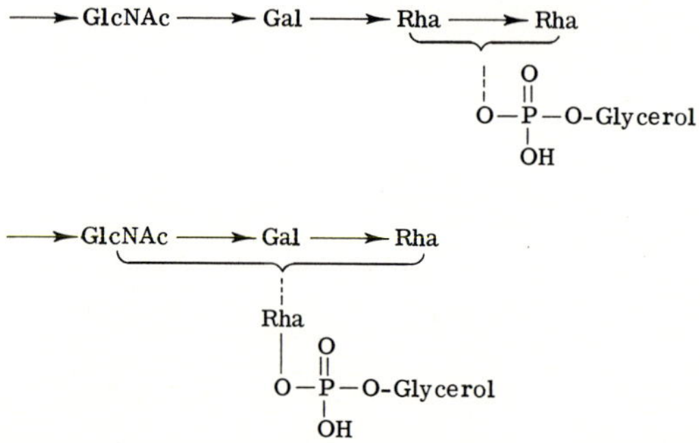

```
    ──▶ GlcNAc ──▶ Gal ──▶ Rha ──▶ Rha
                                 │   O
                                 │   ‖
                                 O—P—O—Glycerol
                                     │
                                     OH

    ──▶ GlcNAc ──▶ Gal ──▶ Rha
                           │
                           Rha
                           │   O
                           │   ‖
                           O—P—O—Glycerol
                               │
                               OH
```

Fig. 11. Alternative structures of the surface polysaccharide of *E. coli* O100. From Jann *et al.* (1970).

charide of this strain was assumed to be a K antigen, distinct from the somatic (O100-specific) lipopolysaccharide. It was found, however, that both polysaccharides have the same structure and also exert identical serologic specificity (Jann *et al.*, 1970). Two alternatives (Fig. 11) were proposed. It was found later that many O antigenic (lipo)polysaccharides (region I in Fig. 1) of *E. coli* are acidic, i.e., that they contain hexuronic acids as constituents (Ørskov *et al.*, 1971). Thus, from a chemical point of view there is no difference between an O-specific and a K-specific polysaccharide. This makes a differentiation of these polysaccharide antigens difficult. Antigenic complexity is further illustrated by the following finding. In *E. coli* O8:K87(B):H19 the acidic polysaccharide which is listed in Table XIV functions as K87 antigen. This is formed by the cells in addition to the O8 antigen. In *E. coli* (O32):K87(B):H45 the same polysaccharide is not only present as extracellular polysaccharide but also as the O-specific polysaccharide moiety of the somatic lipopolysaccharide (Jann *et al.*, 1972). Thus, with respect to antigenic diversity and regulation of polysaccharide biosynthesis, the genus *E. coli* provides a fascinating area of research.

The extracellular A antigens of *E. coli* may be compared to the K antigens of *Klebsiella* in some ways. In both genera these extracellular polysaccharides occur in few O groups and all of these are free of amino sugars. Additionally, the respective *E. coli* O antigens (O8 and O9) also bear resemblance to *Klebsiella* O antigens 5 and 3. All four lipopolysaccharides contain only mannose in addition to lipid A and core constituents (KDO, glucosamine, heptose, glucose, and galactose—see Lüderitz *et al.*, 1966a). As a corollary it was found that *E. coli* O8 cross-reacts with *Klebsiella* O5 and that *E. coli* O9 cross-reacts with *Klebsiella* O3.

TABLE XV

Composition of the Type-Specific Polysaccharides of H. influenzae

Type	Carbohydrate	Noncarbohydrate	References
a	Glc	Phosphate	Zamenhof and Leidy, 1954
b	Rib	Phosphate	Zamenhof and Leidy, 1954; Zamenhof et al., 1953; Rosenberg et al., 1961
c	Gal	Phosphate	Zamenhof and Leidy, 1954
d	GlcN, GlcNUA	–	Rosenberg et al., 1961
e	Hex, GlcN	–	Williamson and Zamenhof, 1963a; Schmidt, 1952
f	GalN	Phosphate	Williamson and Zamenhof, 1963b

4. CAPSULAR POLYSACCHARIDE ANTIGENS OF *Haemophilus*

In connection with studies on bacterial transformation by DNA preparations from autolyzed *H. influenzae* cultures, Zamenhof et al. isolated polyribose phosphate from *H. influenzae* type b (Zamenhof and Leidy, 1954; Zamenhof et al., 1953; Rosenberg et al., 1961). It was found that this was the type-specific capsular polysaccharide, and that another three of the six type-specific capsular antigens of *H. influenzae* (from types a, c, f) were polyhexose phosphate (Zamenhof and Leidy, 1954; Williamson and Zamenhof, 1963a,b). The polysaccharide antigen from type d is also an acidic polymer, its charge being due to *N*-acetylglucosaminuronic acid (Rosenberg et al., 1961). One type-specific polysaccharide proved to be neutral. The composition of the six type-specific polysaccharides from *H. influenzae* are shown in Table XV. Detailed structural studies of the type b capsular polysaccharide resulted in a structure (Zamenhof et al., 1953) which is shown in Fig. 12. The type b capsular antigen thus consists of double strands in which ribosyl-ribose disaccharides of the trehalose type are doubly joined through phosphate diester

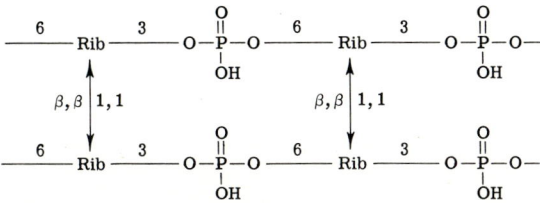

Fig. 12. Structure of the capsular polysaccharide of *H. influenzae* type b. After Zamenhof et al. (1953).

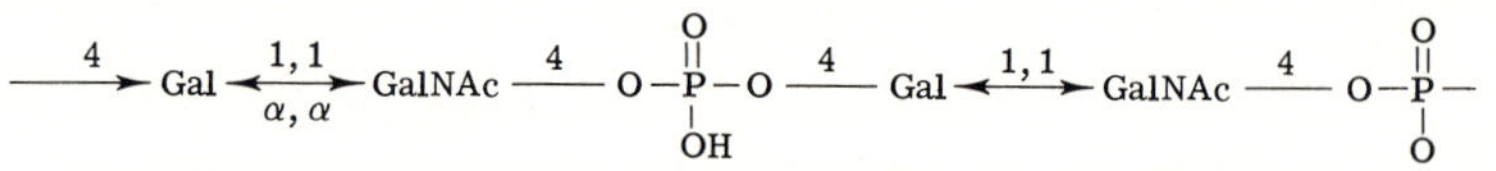

$$\xrightarrow{4} \text{Gal} \xleftarrow[\alpha,\alpha]{1,1} \text{GalNAc} \xrightarrow{4} \text{O} - \overset{\overset{\text{O}}{\|}}{\underset{\text{OH}}{\text{P}}} - \text{O} \xrightarrow{4} \text{Gal} \xleftarrow{1,1} \text{GalNAc} \xrightarrow{4} \text{O} - \overset{\overset{\text{O}}{\|}}{\underset{\text{O}}{\text{P}}} -$$

Fig. 13. Structure of the capsular polysaccharide of *H. parasuis*. From Williamson and Zamenhof (1964).

bridges. This intricate structure bears some resemblance to ribonucleic acid and is, in fact, hydrolyzed by ribonuclease (Zamenhof *et al.*, 1953). The other polysugar phosphates have not been studied hitherto.

In *H. parasuis* a capsular polysaccharide was shown to have a structure similar to the one of *H. influenzae* type b (Williamson and Zamenhof, 1964). Disaccharide units of the trehalose-type consisting of N-acetylglucosamine and a hexose (probably galactose) are joined by phosphodiester bridges to form single strands. This is shown in Fig. 13.

5. Capsular Staphylococcal Polysaccharide Antigen (SPA)

In the course of investigations on protective antibodies against *S. aureus*, it was found (Fisher, 1959) that from mucoid strains of *S. aureus* a vaccine could be produced which was mouse-protective. From such strains a highly potent immunizing capsular polysaccharide was obtained. This polysaccharide, which was termed staphylococcal polysaccharide antigen (SPA), actively protected mice against challenge infection when administered in low dose, but rendered the animals tolerant (and sensitive against challenge infection) when given in higher concentration (Fisher *et al.*, 1963). Subsequent structural studies showed that SPA is a polymer of glucosaminuronic acid. The monomeric units are alternatively N-substituted with acetyl and N-acetylalanyl groups. The structure of SPA is shown in Fig. 14.

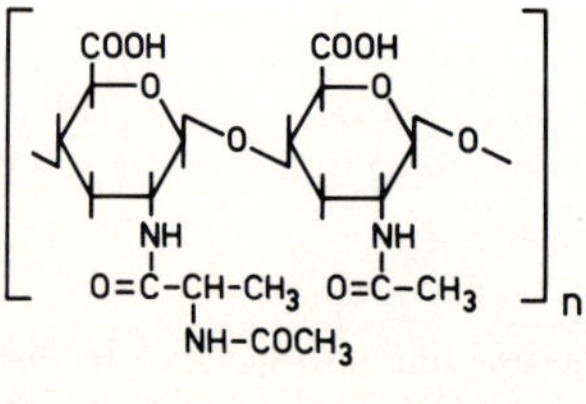

Fig. 14. Repeating unit of the staphylococcal polysaccharide antigen (SPA). From Hanessian and Haskell (1964).

6. M Antigen (Colanic Acid)

Many strains of gram-negative enteric bacteria, such as *Escherichia* or *Salmonella*, when grown under certain conditions (Anderson, 1961; Anderson and Rogers, 1963) form an extracellular polysaccharide antigen. This was termed M antigen ("mucus antigen") by Kauffmann (1954) and colanic acid by Goebel (1965). Strains that normally do not produce this antigen can be induced to do so by cultivation at room temperature instead of 37° or by addition of *p*-fluorophenylalanine to the growth medium (Kang and Markovitz, 1966). The genetic determination of this polysaccharide is complex and has been studied in detail (Markovitz, 1964; Markovitz and Rosenbaum, 1965). The polysaccharide consists of glucose, glucuronic acid, galactose, and L-fucose in molar ratios of 1:1:2:2. The structure that had remained obscure for a long time was elucidated recently (Garegg *et al.*, 1971a,b; Sutherland, 1969; Lawson *et al.*, 1969). It has a main chain of fucose and glucose to which trisaccharide side chains of galactosyl-glucuronosyl-galactose are attached. The terminal galactose carries a pyruvate substitution. During comparative studies on M antigen preparations from various sources, it was found that pyruvic acid is sometimes replaced by formaldehyde or acetaldehyde (Garegg *et al.*, 1971a). Therefore, what is commonly termed M antigen, actually represents a group of acidic polysaccharide antigens. They all have the same polysaccharide backbone, consisting of a branched hexasaccharide repeating unit. This may be substituted by formaldehyde (methylidene substitution), acetaldehyde (ethylidene substitution), or pyruvate (carboxyethylidene substitution). For all these substituents the terminal galactose of the side chain functions as acceptor. The structure of the different types of M antigens is generalized in Fig. 15. The substitution position in

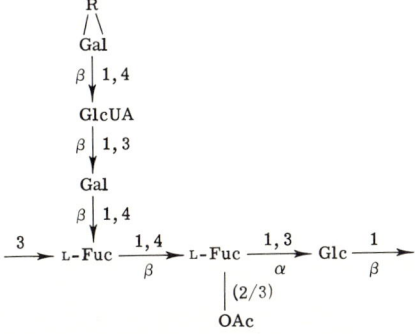

Fig. 15. Repeating unit of the M antigen. R is a carbonyl substituent of which nature and linkage are shown in Table XVI.

TABLE XVI

Substitutions of the Polysaccharide Backbone of M Antigens

$$\begin{array}{c} -O \\ -O \end{array} C \begin{array}{c} R_1 \\ R_2 \end{array}$$

Name	Substitution		Linkage position in galactose found	
	R_1	R_2	3,4	4,6
Methylidine	H	H	−	+
Ethylidene	CH_3	H	+	−
	H	CH_3	+	−
Carboxylethylidene	CH_3	COOH	+	+
	COOH	CH_3	+	+

the galactose moiety was found to be either 3,4 or 4,6. The different linkage types that specify the respective type of M antigen are shown in Table XVI. With one exception all these M antigens have an O-acetyl group in one of the fucose residues of the main chain.

7. Vi ANTIGEN

The Vi antigen, the only capsular polysaccharide of *Salmonella*, was first described in *S. typhi* by Felix and Pitt (1934a,b). It was first thought to cause virulence, a view that later proved to be incorrect (Kauffmann, 1966). The Vi antigen was also found in *Citrobacter* (*Paracolobactrum*) *ballerup* and *E. coli* (Kauffmann, 1941a,b; Webster et al., 1954). The isolated and purified material yielded, upon drastic acid hydrolysis, only D-galactosaminuronic acid (Clark et al., 1958). It was reported by Heyns and Kiessling (1967) that the Vi antigen is a homopolysaccharide which consists of D-N-acetylgalactosaminuronic acid linked α-1,4. The polysaccharide is partly O-acetylated.

D. Other Polysaccharide Antigens

1. POLYSACCHARIDE ANTIGENS OF *Streptococcus*

Streptococci are divided into groups (A, B, C, etc.—see Lancefield, 1933, 1940) that are characterized by specific polysaccharide an-

1. Microbial Polysaccharides

TABLE XVII

Sugar Composition of Some Group-Specific Polysaccharide Antigens of Streptococcus

Group	Rha	GlcN	GalN	Glc	Gal	References
A	+	+	−	−	−	McCarty, 1956; Schmidt, 1952
B	+	+	−	−	+	Curtis and Krause, 1964
C	+	−	+	−	+	Araujo and Krause, 1963; Bleiweis and Krause, 1965; Soprey and Slade, 1971
F	+	−	+	+	−	Willers et al., 1964
G	+	−	+	−	+	Curtis and Krause, 1964 Chionglo and Hayashi, 1969
L	+	+	−	−	+	Karakawa et al., 1971
R	+	+	−	+	+	Soprey and Slade, 1972

tigens. The groups can be further subdivided into immunologic types. Some type-specific antigens are polysaccharides, others are proteins (M proteins). We will consider here only hemolytic *Streptococci* which bear some significance in pathogenic conditions of humans. These groups together with the composition of their respective polysaccharides are listed in Table XVII.

The type-specific streptococcal polysaccharides have not been studied in detail. The sugar composition of the polysaccharides from types I, II, and III is listed in Table XVIII. These type antigens occur in different groups of *Streptococci*. This is indicated also in Table XVIII. It should be remembered that there are several different type

TABLE XVIII

Sugar Composition of Some Type-Specific Polysaccharide Antigens from Streptococcus

Type	(Group)	Rha	GlcN	GalN	Glc	Gal	Others	References
I	(D)	+	+	+	−	+	−	Bleiweis and Krause, 1965
II	(F)	+	−	+	+	+	−	Michel and Krause, 1967
III	(B)	−	+	−	+	+	GlcUA	Rusell and Norcross, 1972

antigens in many (but not all) groups, and that not all of them are polysaccharides. Some type-specific antigens, e.g., type I, were claimed to be associated with virulence of the respective organism. Antisera, specific for these antigens, will passively protect mice against infection with the homologous streptococcal type. It is obvious that rhamnose is an essential component of all these polysaccharides. With one exception (group E) all polysaccharides also contain hexosamines. The best studied group antigens are those of groups A and C. From these groups variant strains were isolated (McCarty and Lancefield, 1955; Krause and McCarty, 1962). These form polysaccharides that do not contain the hexosamines found in the respective related wild strain. Bacteria of group A are serologically distinct from those of group A-variant and, likewise, bacteria of group C are serologically distinct from those of group C-variant. The sugar compositions of these four strains are listed in Table XIX.

The detailed structure of streptococcal polysaccharides remains to be established. Only gross structural concepts for the polysaccharides from groups A, A-variant, C, and C-variant were suggested (Krause, 1963) which are based on enzymatic reactions and on immunologic interpretations, and have to be considered as preliminary. From other polysaccharides partial structures were worked out and studied serologically. Those from groups E and F are shown in Table XX. From the oligosaccharides of group E polysaccharide a trisaccharide repeating unit may be inferred.

2. TEICHOIC ACIDS

Teichoic acids represent a group of surface antigens that are firmly bound to the mucopeptide and which occur in some gram-positive bacteria such as staphylococci, streptococci, or lactobacilli. Ac-

TABLE XIX

Sugar Composition of the Polysaccharide Antigens from Streptococcal Groups A, C, and Their Variants[a]

Group antigen	Rha (%)	GlcNAc (%)	GalNAc (%)
A	60	30	—
A variant	83	3	—
C	43	4	35
C variant	86	4	2

[a] From Araujo and Krause (1963).

TABLE XX

Oligosaccharides Obtained from the Specific Polysaccharide Antigens of Streptococcus Groups E and F

Group	Oligosaccharide	References
E	Glc $\xrightarrow[\beta]{1,2}$ Rha	Soprey and Slade, 1971
	Glc $\xrightarrow{1,2}$ Rha $\xrightarrow{1,4}$ Rha	
	Rha $\xrightarrow{1,4}$ Rha $\xrightarrow{1,4}$ Glc	
	Rha $\xrightarrow{1,4}$ Rha $\xrightarrow{1,4}$ Glc $\xrightarrow{1,2}$ Rha	
F	Glc $\xrightarrow[\beta]{1,3}$ Gal	Willers et al., 1964
	Glc $\xrightarrow[\beta]{1,3}$ Gal $\longrightarrow$ Glc $\xrightarrow[\beta]{1,3}$ Gal	

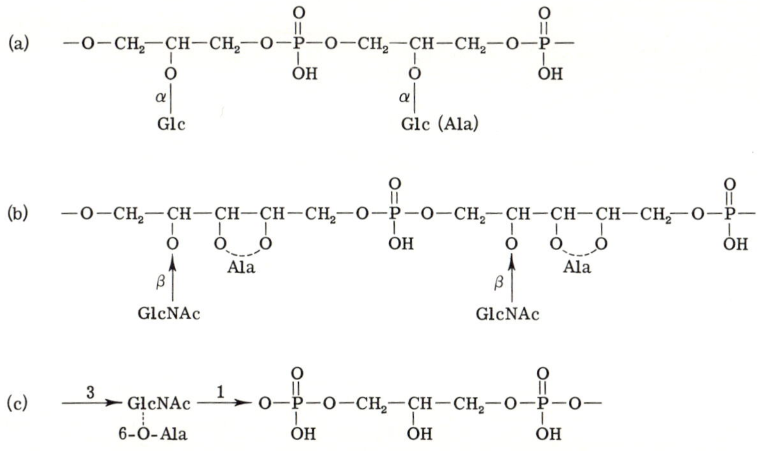

(a)
```
    —O—CH₂—CH—CH₂—O—P(=O)(OH)—O—CH₂—CH—CH₂—O—P(=O)(OH)—
               |                              |
               O                              O
               α|                             α|
              Glc                           Glc (Ala)
```

(b)
```
    —O—CH₂—CH—CH—CH—CH₂—O—P(=O)(OH)—O—CH₂—CH—CH—CH—CH₂—O—P(=O)(OH)—
            |   \ /                           |   \ /
            O    O                            O    O
            |    |                            |    |
            β    Ala                          β    Ala
            |                                 |
          GlcNAc                            GlcNAc
```

(c)
```
    —³→ GlcNAc —¹→ O—P(=O)(OH)—O—CH₂—CH—CH₂—O—P(=O)(OH)—O—
        6-O-Ala                        |
                                       OH
```

Fig. 16. Structure of the teichoic acid from (a) *Lactobacillus buchneri*, (b) *Staphylococcus aureus* H, and (c) *Streptococcus lactis* 13. From Shaw and Baddiley (1964), Baddiley *et al.* (1962), and Archibald *et al.* (1965).

cording to Baddiley (1962, 1968) there are three structural types: (1) linear polymers of glycerophosphate (1,3-linked) which are substituted with glycosyl and/or alanyl residues at position 2 of varying numbers of glycerol units; (2) linear polymers of ribitol phosphate (1,5-linked) in which all ribitol phosphate units carry glycosyl and alanyl substituents; and (3) linear copolymers of sugar units and glycerol or ribitol phosphate. These structural types are shown in Fig. 16. Thus, teichoic acids are a heterogeneous group of bacterial surface antigens. They range from polyglycerol phosphate, which is not a polysaccharide, to structures analogous to type 3 (Fig. 16), which are in close structural relation to certain capsular polysaccharides and the C polysaccharide of *Diplococcus pneumoniae* (see Fig. 10 and Table IX), and which *sensu stricto* cannot be called teichoic acids. The immunologically most important structural feature of teichoic acids is their glycosyl substitution.

3. DEXTRANS

These are formed as exopolysaccharides by some gram-positive bacteria such as *Leuconostoc mesenteroides*, *L. dextranicum*, or

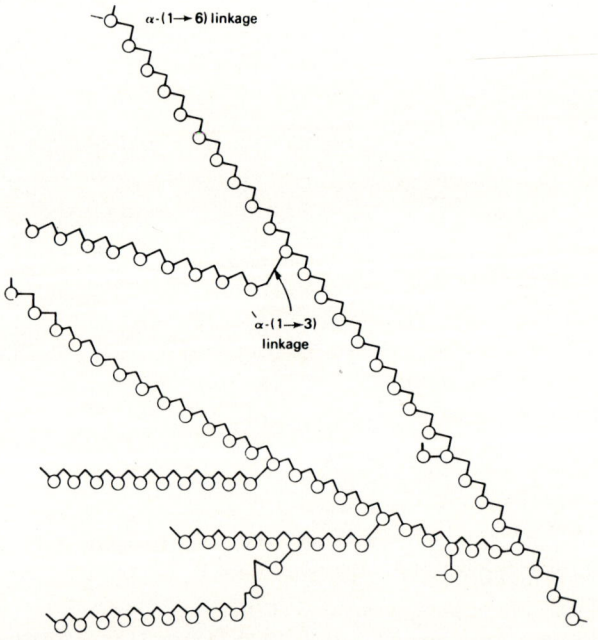

Fig. 17. Schematic representation of a small portion of a molecule of NRRL B 512 dextran. From Kabat (1968).

Streptococcus viridans. They are polymers of glucose with molecular weights of several million. The predominant linkage is α-1,6, which leads to very long chains. Some bacterial strains produce dextrans in which also other types of linkages occur (α-1,2, α-1,3, α-1,4), giving rise to more or less branched dextran molecules. One of the dextrans that was extensively studied by Kabat (Kabat and Berg, 1953) — dextran NRRL B 512 — is formed by *L. mesenteroides*. About 96% of its glucose units are α-1,6-linked, about 4% are α-1,3-linked. These linkages occur in statistical distribution. As a result the polysaccharide is built up of longer and shorter side chains of α-1,6-linked glucose units which are bound through α-1,3-linkages to a main chain of α-1,6-bound glucose units. This is shown schematically in Fig. 17.

4. Levans

Like dextrans, levans are bacterial exopolysaccharides. They are produced by plant pathogenic bacteria like *Pseudomonas* and *Xanthomonas* as well as by some genera of gram-positive bacteria such as *Bacillus* and *Streptococcus*. Levans are linear polymers of D-fructose in which predominantly β-2,6-ketosidic linkages occur. The molecular weight of levans is below 50,000. They are extremely sensitive to low pH and may, therefore, undergo partial degradation during handling.

5. Mannans

Bound to protein, mannans form the outermost layer of yeast cells, such as *Saccharomyces cerevisiae* (Northcote and Horne, 1952; Mill, 1966). *Micrococcus lysodeikticus* contains a mannan associated with the cell membrane (Scher *et al.*, 1967). The mannan from *S. cerevisiae* was the subject of intensive structural (Lee and Ballou, 1965; Steward *et al.*, 1969; Jones and Ballou, 1969a;b) and immunochemical (Suzuki *et al.*, 1968; Suzuki and Sunayama, 1968, 1969; Ballou, 1970) studies. With the aid of adapted enzymes and by acetolysis, series of oligomannans were isolated which contain α-1,2, α-1,3, and α-1,6 bonds. A composite structure of the polysaccharide shows a backbone of α-1,6-linked mannoses to which a number of short side chains are linked through α-1,2 linkages. These side-chain oligosaccharides, which differ in size and linkage type, can be enzymatically split off from the backbone. The structure of the *S. cerevisiae* mannan is indicated in Fig. 18. All yeast mannans seem to have an identical backbone of α-1,6-linked mannoses and differ in type and relative amounts from their oligosaccharidic side chains. There are also phosphorylated mannans in some yeast strains, such as *Kluyveromyces brevis* (Thieme and Ballou, 1971; Raschke and Ballou, 1971). The phosphate group is substituent of a mannan with a structure as shown in Fig. 18.

Another mannan was isolated from *Kloeckera lactis* (Ballou, 1970; Raschke and Ballou, 1972) which has side chains like S. cerevisiae and, in addition, tetrasaccharide side chains containing N-acetylglucosamine linked to the subterminal mannose unit. The structure of this mannan is also included in Fig. 18. More recently, other yeasts, belonging to *Saccharomyces* and *Hansenula* were also analyzed and additional variations in antigenic specificities were found (Ballou *et al.*, 1974; Lipke *et al.*, 1974).

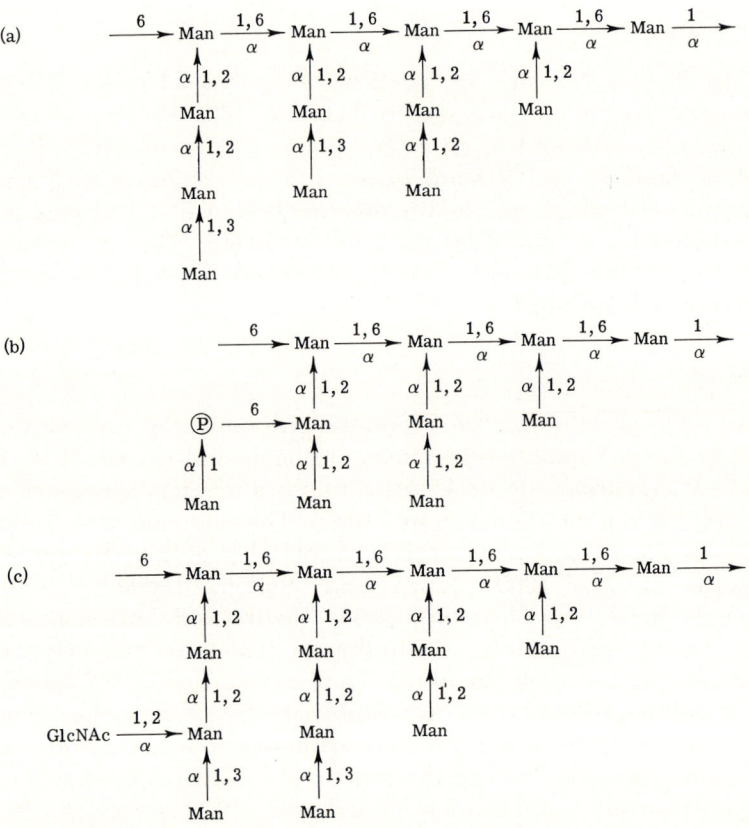

Fig. 18. Composite structures of the mannans from (a) *Saccharomyces cerevisiae* ×2180 (b) *Kloeckera brevis* 55-45, and (c) *Kluyveromyces lactis* NRRL 1140. From Raschke and Ballou (1972).

III. Immunochemistry of Microbial Polysaccharide Antigens

A. Serologic Methods

The antigenic specificities of polysaccharides may be assessed with the aid of many serologic reactions. These are not restricted to polysaccharides and have been reviewed in detail (Kabat and Mayer, 1961; Kabat, 1968). Therefore, they are only briefly mentioned here. With multivalent antigens direct methods such as precipitation (Heidelberger and Kendall, 1929), agglutination and passive hemagglutination (Neter, 1956; Neter et al., 1956), or complement fixation (Wasserman and Levine, 1961) can be used. Precipitation may be carried out in gels of agar and agarose (Ouchterlony, 1958; Hanson, 1959), and the lines formed give information concerning homogeneity of an antigen preparation. This method is very useful for the comparison of antigens and also for examination of antisera. In passive hemagglutination erythrocytes are coated with the polysaccharide antigen (Lüderitz et al., 1957). They will then agglutinate with antisera directed against the polysaccharide. Not all polysaccharides attach to red cells. Their affinity to erythrocytes can be greatly increased by partial acylation (Hämmerling and Westphal, 1967; Slade and Hämmerling, 1968; Pavlovskis and Slade, 1971). Charged polysaccharides such as capsular polysaccharides of *Pneumococcus* can also be attached to red cells using chromium chloride (Baker et al., 1969).

The reaction of polyvalent antigens with homologous antibody molecules can be inhibited with mono- or divalent haptens. Such substances of smaller molecular weight are obtained from the intact antigens by degradative procedures. Also antigen-binding studies using either equilibrium dialysis (Pinckard and Weir, 1973) or binding of a hapten to an antibody and precipitation of the antibody–hapten complex with ammonium sulfate (Minden and Farr, 1973) or anti-antibody (Schalch and Parker, 1964, Minden et al., 1969) can be applied. In the latter studies the hapten has to be labeled, e.g., with a radioactive substituent.

In combination with chemical analyses the serologic methods mentioned help to describe the immunologic message laid down in the structure of a polysaccharide.

B. Carbohydrate Determinants

The aim of the immunochemical analysis of polysaccharide antigens is to define an oligosaccharide structure within the polysaccharide as chemical expression of its serologic character. This can be studied either by inhibition of a suitable serologic reaction with oligosaccharides of different size and structure, as described in the previous chapter, or by use of oligosaccharide-specific antisera raised with artificial oligosaccharide antigens in the direct serologic reactions.

1. Inhibition with Oligosaccharides

Kabat (1957, 1960, 1966), Schlossman and Kabat (1962), Mage and Kabat (1963a,b), and Gelzer and Kabat (1964) compared the inhibitory capacities in dextran anti-dextran precipitating systems of oligosaccharides of the isomaltose series. With human immune sera it was found that the inhibitory power of isomaltooligosaccharides increased until the length of a hexa- or heptasaccharide was reached. Further extension of the oligosaccharides did not increase the inhibitory capacity substantially. The results are illustrated in Fig. 19. Since the inhibition data were obtained under equilibrium conditions, one can assume that at comparable points of the individual inhibition curves the relative inhibitory capacity of the various oligosaccharides is proportional to the free energy (F^0) in their antibody-binding reaction (Kabat, 1968; Gelzer and Kabat, 1964). On this basis Kabat estimated

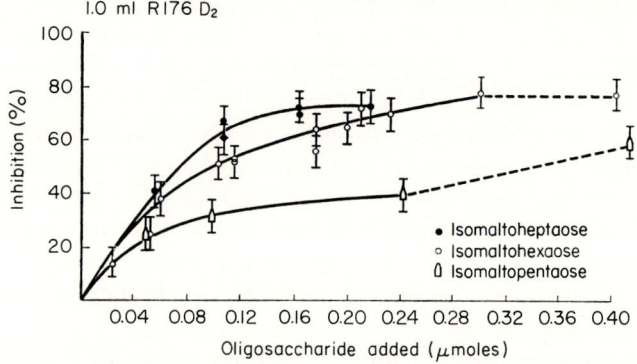

Fig. 19. Inhibition of the precipitation of human anti-dextran with dextran by isomaltopentaose, isomaltohexaose, and isomaltoheptaose. From Kabat (1960).

that the nonreducing terminal glucose unit contributed most to the antigen–antibody binding reaction with each succeeding glucose unit contributing a smaller increment (Kabat, 1968). The inhibition studies mentioned above were performed with α-1,6-dextrans and oligosaccharides of the corresponding isomaltose series. An oligosaccharide with one of the internal glucose units α-1,4-linked was a much poorer inhibitor than the corresponding "all-α-1,6"-linked oligosaccharide.

The results described can be interpreted that antigenic specificities of polysaccharides center around single hexose units (terminal, α-linked glucose in the above examples) and extend along the polysaccharide chain over regions of different lengths. According to a proposition of Staub and Heidelberger, the sugar unit that contributes most to serologic specificity was termed "immunodominant sugar" (Lüderitz *et al.*, 1966a). Complementary to antigenic determinants of different sizes around one immunodominant sugar of a polysaccharide antigen, the corresponding antiserum consists of many antibody molecules with different size of combining sites directed toward the same determinant region. Thus, the size of an antigenic determinant (mono- or oligosaccharide) and that of an antibody combining site are but two aspects of the same phenomenon: antigenic expression of a polysaccharide. This was also shown by specific absorption-elution experiments in which Sephadex was used as immunoadsorbent for anti-dextran antibodies (Gelzer and Kabat, 1964). After adsorption onto Sephadex the antibodies were successively eluted with oligosaccharides of the isomaltose series with increasing size. This resulted in separation of the antisera into fractions of antibody with different size of combining sites specific for partial substructures of α-1,6-specific dextran. With some overlap, mainly two fractions were obtained from human anti-dextran antisera: one population with a mostly small combining site (complementary to about the size of isomalto*triose*) and one with a mostly large combining site (complementary to about the size of isomalto*hexaose* (Gelzer and Kabat, 1964). Isomaltohexaose inhibited the reaction of dextran with the latter fraction much better than did isomaltotriose. On the other hand, with the anti-dextran possessing the smaller sized combining site, there was no difference in inhibitory capacity between isomaltotriose and isomaltohexaose. These results were recently confirmed with fluorescence quenching techniques (Harrisdangkul and Kabat, 1972) in which use was made of emission spectra of flavazole derivatives (description of the reaction in Section

III,E,1) of isomaltose oligosaccharides in combination with antibody which was quenched with the free oligosaccharides. In contrast to most other fluorescence probes, the flavazole portion of the molecule is remote from the immunodominant reducing sugar unit.

2. REACTIONS WITH OLIGOSACCHARIDE-SPECIFIC ANTISERA

As the studies by Goebel *et al.* (1934b) have shown, mono- and disaccharides may trigger a specific immune response when conjugated to a protein carrier. Antibodies obtained against them show specificity for the introduced saccharide with respect to the nature of the monosaccharide(s) and glycosidic links between them. Such reactions were frequently used to evaluate immunodominance of a given sugar (Lüderitz *et al.*, 1966a, 1968a, 1971). Also, precipitating systems could be established with polyvalent antigens such as triglycosylated phloroglucinols (Gleich and Allan, 1965), which precipitated homologous antibody and could be used in comparative inhibition studies (Gleich and Allan, 1965). Alternatively, isomaltose and isomaltotriose were oxidized to the respective aldonic acids and then coupled to protein (see Section III,E). With the respective artificial antigens thus obtained, antibodies were raised which were then studied with α-1,6-specific dextran. It should be mentioned that in the preparation of these derivatives the reducing monosaccharide units were lost with respect to specificity, due to change as a result of the coupling reaction. The α-maltosyl-specific rabbit antiserum (antibody to b of Fig. 27) reacted with the dextrans, whereas the α-glucosyl-specific rabbit antiserum (antibody to a of Fig. 27) did not (Arakatsu *et al.*, 1966). This illustrates that the smallest determinant of dextran recognized by antibody exceeds that of a single glucose unit. There are special cases known in which an antibody is directed against a single immunodominant sugar and its glycosidic bond. From the studies of Springer and Williamson (1962) on blood group substances, one can infer that the specifically recognized region on a saccharide might even be smaller than the dimension of a hexose ring.

3. DETERMINANT SITE ON THE POLYSACCHARIDE

Many polysaccharides are branched. This raises the question whether the branch or oligosaccharidic sequences within the main chain represent antigenic determinants in a branched polysac-

1. Microbial Polysaccharides

charide. It was found that in branched polysaccharides the side chains are usually immunodeterminant. The mannan antigens of yeast, which have been thoroughly studied, (Ballou, 1970; Raschke and Ballou, 1972; Suzuki et al., 1968; Suzuki and Sunayama, 1968) are a recent example. As can be seen from Fig. 18, these are highly branched structures. It was found that the predominant contribution to the serologic specificities of many strains of yeasts comes from the terminal nonreducing mannoses. In the mannan of S. cerevisiae the terminal α-1,3-mannose unit is immunodominant, the internal α-1,6-linked mannose units being of no serologic importance (Raschke and Ballou, 1972). A similar situation was found with the mannans of Candida strains: serologic specificity resides in the side chains of these branched polysaccharides (Summers et al., 1964; Hasenclever and Mitchell, 1964; Mitchell and Hasenclever, 1970).

It should be stressed, however, that serologic specificity of branched polysaccharides is by no means restricted to the side chains and substituent monosaccharide units alone. This became evident from the studies on the (lipo)polysaccharides of Salmonella (see Section III,C) and the capsular polysaccharides of pneumococci (for review, see Heidelberger, 1967; How et al., 1964).

4. INFLUENCE OF CHARGE

Negatively charged constituents of polysaccharides such as hexuronic acid, phosphate or KDO isomers (Lüderitz et al., 1966a, 1968a, 1971) and KDO analogues (Lindberg et al., 1973b; Dhir et al., 1972) are in most cases immunodominant. With the K-specific capsular polysaccharides of E. coli it was found (Jann et al., 1968; Le-Ba Nhan et al., 1971) that carboxyl reduction of hexuronic acid within the polysaccharide chain to the corresponding hexose (Hungerer et al., 1967) in some cases was detrimental to the serologic specificity of the polysaccharide and in other cases was not (see Figs. 20 and 21). Conversely, neutral immunodominant sugar constituents may be oxidized at their C-6 position to carboxylic acids, and this introduction of charge then monitored serologically. This has recently been done with the capsular polysaccharide of Pneumococcus type XIV (Estrada-Parra and Gomez, 1972). Enzymatic oxidation of the immunodominant galactose at C-6 to an aldehyde function did not interfere with serologic specificity at all, as judged by immune precipitation, and further chemical oxidation to a carboxylic acid only slightly reduced the SXIV specificity (see Fig. 22).

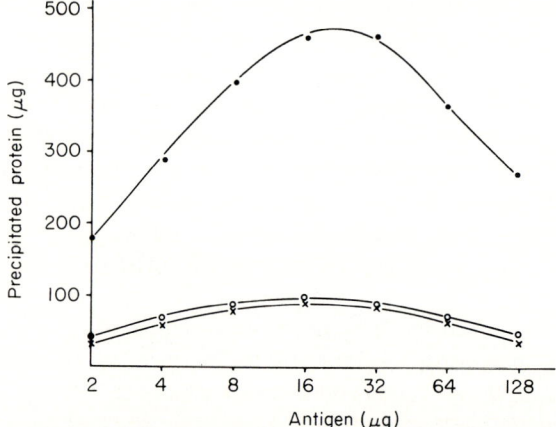

Fig. 20. Precipitation of preparations of the capsular polysaccharide from *E. coli* O9:K29 with anti-K29 antiserum. ●, capsular polysaccharide; ○, capsular polysaccharide after periodate oxidation; ×, capsular polysaccharide after carboxyl reduction. From Le-Ba Nhan *et al.* (1971).

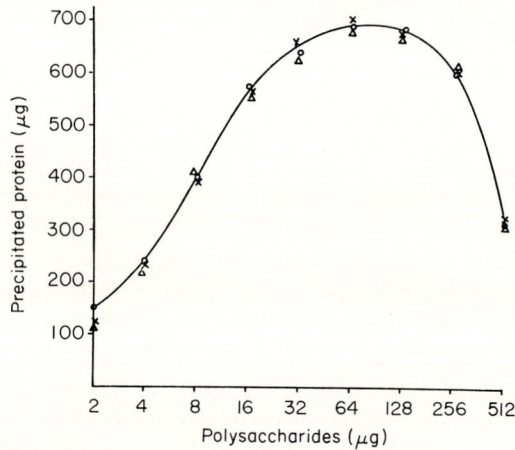

Fig. 21. Precipitation of preparations of the capsular polysaccharide from *E. coli* O8:K27 in anti-K27 antiserum. ○, capsular polysaccharide; ×, capsular polysaccharide after alkali treatment; △, capsular polysaccharide after carboxyl reduction. From Jann *et al.* (1968).

5. Possible Influence of Superstructure

In addition to these structural determinants which are expressed by sequence and linkage of a few sugar residues, there may exist a second type of determinant, which could be termed "conformational determinant" (Sela *et al.*, 1967). It depends on a structure of secon-

1. Microbial Polysaccharides

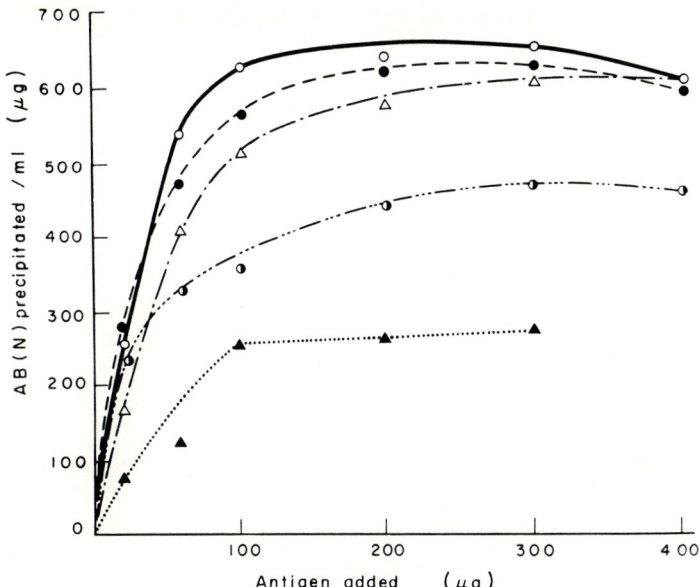

Fig. 22. Precipitation of preparations of the capsular polysaccharide from *Pneumococcus* type XIV in anti-XIV antiserum. ○, capsular polysaccharide; △ and ●, capsular polysaccharide treated with different concentrations of galactose oxidase; ◐, capsular polysaccharide treated with galactose oxidase and ClO_2; ▲, capsular polysaccharide after periodate oxidation. From Estrada-Parra and Gomez (1972).

dary order, like interchain links or helix formation. With proteins such superstructures and their role in serologic expression are known. Interchain links have been reported for certain acidic polysaccharide antigens of *E. coli* (Jann *et al.*, 1965, 1968; Le-Ba Nhan *et al.*, 1971; Hungerer *et al.*, 1967). Recently, conformational changes concomitantly occuring with bacteriophage-induced glucosylation of the *S. johannesburg* lipopolysaccharide (40a, 40b, 40c → 1_H, 40b, 1_{40}) have been used in the explanation of changes in carbohydrate specificity. In this context the term "conformational determinant" was used (Girard and Staub, 1974). Helical superstructures have been studied systematically with gelating polysaccharides of plant origin, like alginates and pectins (Rees, 1969, 1972) with respect to physical properties like optical measurements in induced metachromasia or optical rotatory dispersions via amide transitions in amino sugar containing polysaccharides (for a review, see Rees, 1972). However, information concerning the influence of conformation on the antigenicity of polysaccharides has not been studied. It may well be that conformational determinants as opposed to structural determinants also play a role in polysaccharides (see Kabat, 1966).

C. Immunochemistry of Antigen Factors

It is known that the oligosaccharide structures of the polysaccharide moiety (region I in Fig. 1) of the O-antigenic lipopolysaccharides are responsible for serologic specificity. The basis for immunochemical studies is a comparative serologic analysis of the O antigens of related microorganisms. For the O antigens of some genera of Enterobacteriaceae serologic classifications have been worked out. The pioneering example is the Kauffmann—White scheme of *Salmonella* in which the specificities of determinants on the O-specific chains (region I, Fig. 1) are expressed as *O factors* with numbers 1,2,3, etc. Serologically closely related *serotypes* (species) represent members of a *serogroup* A,B,C, etc., which is defined by the presence of a common strong O-determinant factor, such as O factor 2 for *Salmonella* group A, O factor 4 for *Salmonella* group B, O factor 9 for *Salmonella* group D, etc.

With serologic techniques (absorptions, cross-agglutination, etc.) Kauffmann has found that often several O factors can be present in the somatic antigen of a given serotype, such as 2,12 or 1,2,12 in Group A, 4,12, 1,4,12, or 4,5,12 in Group B, and 9,12 or 1,9,12 in Group D (see Kauffmann, 1954).

Systematic and extended analyses were first performed by the group of Staub in Paris in the fifties, partly in cooperation with the group of Lüderitz and Westphal in Freiburg, followed by many other research groups all over the world. These studies have already been extensively reviewed (Lüderitz *et al.*, 1966a, 1968a, 1973). In this chapter we, therefore, refer only to selected data from which certain general principles may be derived.

In the course of these studies the special contribution of monosaccharide substituents on the O-specific main chain became apparent. As examples, we refer to the immunodominant function of 3,6-dideoxyhexoses as unusual sugars and of glucose as one of the most common sugar constituents in O antigens. Besides spatially exposed sugars, as nonreducing substituents of the polysaccharide chains, it was later found that structures present in the main O-specific chain can also exert immunodominant function. One and the same immunodominant sugar—be it located as nonreducing substituent of a polysaccharide chain or in the main chain—can display more than one immunodominant function, according to the side from which the antibody approaches the determinant carbohydrate region. It is well understandable that different specificities would thus be expressed. Examples have been described and discussed by Staub (in Lüderitz

1. Microbial Polysaccharides

et al., 1971). Finally, noncarbohydrate substituents like O-acetyl groups, can strongly affect the serologic specificity of such immunodominant sugar constituents.

1. O FACTORS WITH 3,6-DIDEOXYHEXOSES

After the discovery of the class of 3,6-dideoxyhexoses in the O-specific (lipo)polysaccharides of gram-negative bacteria (for review, see Westphal and Lüderitz, 1960), Staub and her co-workers demonstrated their immunodominant role in many O factors. For inhibition studies the periodate-oxidized polysaccharides were used frequently, because glycosidically linked 3,6-dideoxyhexoses are resistant to periodate due to lack of two neighboring hydroxy groups, while other O factors are periodate-sensitive. Such systems allowed the elaboration of the role of 3,6-dideoxyhexoses in O specificity (O factors). Results of such inhibition studies are summarized in Table XXI.

Because 3,6-dideoxyhexose-containing oligosaccharides were not available, the anomeric configuration (α or β, pyranosidic or furanosidic) could only be estimated on the basis of quantitative inhibition studies with synthetic α- and β-3,6-dideoxyhexosides. In Table XXII an example is given of the inhibitory power of α- and β-abequosides in a *Salmonella* 4/anti-4 system clearly demonstrating that anti-4 antibodies are specifically adapted to the α-pyranosidic configuration of abequose.

As can be seen from Table XXI abequose and colitose each occur in two serologically non-cross-reacting groups of O antigens. This indicates that a single (terminal) immunodominant sugar, inhibitory in both precipitating polysaccharide/anti-polysaccharide systems, does not represent the *whole* determinant group, and that adjacent sugar constituents also play an important role. In fact, more refined structural analyses revealed (see for review, Lüderitz *et al.*, 1971: Tables IV and VI) that abequose is bound α-1,3 to D-mannose in *Salmonella* group B and α-1,3 to L-rhamnose in group C_2. In Table XXI the adjacent sugar constituent of the main chain, to which the 3,6-dideoxyhexose is linked as nonreducing substituent, is indicated.

The structural difference of factors 9 and 46 in *Salmonella* groups D_1 and D_2 (see Table XXI) shows that not only the adjacent sugar (mannose) contributes to specificity, but also its linkage within the main chain: α-mannose in factor 9, β-mannose in factor 46. Analogous findings apply for many other O factors. These facts clearly indicate that for a whole O determinant (O factor), besides the im-

TABLE XXI

Immunodominant Role of 3,6-Dideoxyhexoses in O-Specific Factors of Enterobacteriaceae[a]

Genus, serogroup	O Factor	Immunodominant sugar	Attached to	References
Salmonella A	2	Paratose (3,6-Dideoxy-D-glucose)	$\xrightarrow{}$ Man	Staub et al. (1959)
Salmonella B	4	Abequose (3,6-Dideoxy-D-galactose)	$\xrightarrow[\alpha]{3}$ D-Man	Staub and Tinelli (1957)
Citrobacter 4, 5	4			Staub et al. (1959)
P. pseudotub. 4, 27	4			Stirm et al., (1966a)
Salmonella C$_2$	8		$\xrightarrow[\alpha]{3}$ L-Rha	Staub et al. (1959)
Salmonella D$_1$	9	Tyvelose (3,6-Dideoxy-D-mannose)	$\xrightarrow[\alpha]{3}$ Man[b]	Staub and Tinelli (1957) Staub et al. (1959) Stirm et al. (1966a)
Salmonella D$_2$	46		$\xrightarrow[\alpha]{3}$ Man[c]	Nghiem et al. (1967)
Salmonella O Arizona	35 20	Colitose (3,6-Dideoxy-L-galactose)	$\xrightarrow[\alpha]{4}$ Glc	Lüderitz et al. (1958, 1960) Staub et al. (1959) Westphal et al. (1960) Stirm et al. (1966a)
E. coli	111		$\xrightarrow{\alpha}$	Edstrom and Heath (1965)
Salmonella Z	50			Schwarzmüller (1972)
Arizona	9			
E. coli	55			

[a] For the more complete structures of the 3,6-dideoxyhexose-containing O antigens see Lüderitz et al. (1971, Tables IV and VI).
[b] In the main chain the mannose residue is linked α-glycosidically.
[c] In the main chain the mannose residue is linked β-glycosidically.

1. Microbial Polysaccharides

TABLE XXII

Inhibition of the Precipitation of S. paratyphi B Polysaccharide (Factors 1, 4, 12) and S. paratyphi B Antiserum by Abequose and Abequosides[a]

Inhibitor	Amount of inhibitor (μmoles)	Inhibition (%)
Abequose	2	5
	10	18
	50	32
p-Nitrophenyl-α-abequoside (pyranoside)	0.4	30
	2	40
	10	60
p-Nitrophenyl-β-abequoside (pyranoside)	0.4	2
	2	5
	10	15

[a] After Lüderitz et al. (1966a, p. 208) (Table 9) and Westphal and Lüderitz (1961).

munodominant sugar, neighboring sugars and their glycosidic linkages may contribute (see also, Staub and Westphal, 1964).

2. O Factors with α-Glucose

As further examples of the role of an immunodominant nonreducing sugar substituent of the polysaccharide chain, its glycosidic linkage, the nature of the adjacent sugar in the main chain, the orientation of antibodies to the oligosaccharide structure, and O-antigens with factors having *α-glucosyl* side chains as immunodominant regions may be enlightening. It was found, mainly by Staub and co-workers (for review, see Lüderitz et al., 1971), that in *Salmonella* terminally α-linked glucose exerts immunodominant function in at least seven different O factors, namely 1, 12_2, 19, 34, 6, 7, and 14. In Table XXIII the structures related to these factors are given.

As can be seen from Table XXIII a disaccharide, glucosyl-α-1,6-galactose, is related to both factors 1 and 19, but in factor 1 the galactose residue in the main chain is linked α-1,2 to mannose and in factor 19 the galactosyl-mannose linkage is α-1,6. In factors 12_2 and 34 the same disaccharide of glucosyl-α-1,4-galactose is found, but again the galactosyl-mannose linkage in the main chain is α-1,2 in factor 12_2 and α-1,6 in factor 34. In rabbit anti-12_2 and anti-34 sera only very little cross-reacting antibodies are detectable which can easily be cross-absorbed to give single-specific anti-12_2 or anti-34

TABLE XXIII

Structure of Salmonella O Factors with an Immunodominant
α-Glucosyl Side Chain[a]

Group	Factor	Oligosaccharide structure	References
A, B	1	$\text{Glc (Par/Abe)} \\ \alpha \downarrow 1,6 \\ \rightarrow^3 \text{Gal} \xrightarrow{1,2} \text{Man} \xrightarrow{1,4} \text{Rha} \xrightarrow{1}{}_\alpha \rightarrow$	Stocker et al. (1960) Hellerqvist et al. (1969a,b) Dagorn and Staub (1974)
B, D	12_2	$\text{Glc (Abe/Tyv)} \\ \alpha \downarrow 1,4 \\ \rightarrow^3 \text{Gal} \xrightarrow{1,2} \text{Man} \xrightarrow{1,4} \text{Rha} \xrightarrow{1}{}_\alpha \rightarrow$	Tinelli and Staub (1960a,b) Bagdian et al. (1969) Dagorn and Staub (1974)
E_3	34	$\text{Glc} \\ \alpha \downarrow 1,4 \\ \rightarrow^3 \text{Gal} \xrightarrow{1,6} \text{Man} \xrightarrow{1,4} \text{Rha} \xrightarrow{1}{}_\beta \rightarrow$	Uchida et al. (1963, 1965)
E_4	19	$\text{Glc} \\ \alpha \downarrow 1,6 \\ \rightarrow^3 \text{Gal} \xrightarrow{1,6} \text{Man} \xrightarrow{1,4} \text{Rha} \xrightarrow{1}{}_\alpha \rightarrow$	Staub and Girard (1965) Dagorn and Staub (1974)
C_1	6, 7	$\text{Glc} \\ \alpha \downarrow 1,3 \\ \rightarrow^4 \text{Man} \xrightarrow{1,4} \text{Man} \xrightarrow{1,4} \text{Man} \xrightarrow{1,3} \text{GlcNAc-}$	Fuller and Staub (1968)
	6_2, (7), 14	$\text{Man} \xrightarrow{1,4} \text{Man} \xrightarrow{1,4} \text{Man} \xrightarrow{1,4} \overset{\text{Glc}}{\underset{\alpha \downarrow 1,3}{\text{Man}}} \xrightarrow{1,3} \text{GlcNAc-}$	Fuller et al. (1968)

[a] From Table VII in Lüderitz et al. (1971).

1. Microbial Polysaccharides

sera, respectively (Kauffmann, 1966). This was also demonstrated recently by Kleinhammer *et al.* (1973) in immunization experiments with an artificial antigen containing the trisaccharidic determinant Glc $\xrightarrow[\alpha]{1,4}$ Gal $\xrightarrow[\alpha]{1,6}$ Man.

In *Salmonella* group C_1 Staub and Girard (1965) showed that all three O factors—6, 7, and 14—had an α-glucosyl side chain with immunodominant function. This fact will be discussed under Section III,D.

3. O Factors Present in the Main Chains

According to structural analyses some O-antigens can be built up from only nonbranched oligosaccharide units, not having any monosaccharide side chain. After immunization, the elicited anticarbohydrate antibodies must, therefore, be directed against O factors present in the main chain. On the basis of serologic cross-reactions, Heidelberger (1973a) had suggested, long time ago, that such internal structures may well exert immunologic specificity. In *Salmonella* group E (see Table III) Uchida *et al.* (1963) showed that *mannose* is the immunodominant sugar of factor 3. Interestingly, the three oligosaccharides α-Gal → Man → Rha, β-Gal → Man → Rha, and Man → Rha had almost the same inhibitory power in a 3–anti-3 system. Cross-reactions, due to the common factor 3, were found by Staub and Girard (1965) to be stronger between *Salmonella* groups E_1 and E_4 (with α-bound Gal in both groups) than between E_1 and E_2 (with β-bound Gal in E_2), indicating that the whole determinant factor 3 extends from Man into the Gal region. In group D_2 the 3-specificity was designated (3) because it crossreacted only rather weakly with other 3-systems. In D_2-polysaccharides mannose is substituted by α-1,3-linked tyvelose (see Table III). Any anti-3 antibody could, therefore, only have access from the nonsubstituted side of mannose. Staub (in Lüderitz *et al.*, 1971, p. 180) suggested that the totality of anti-3 antibodies may consist of at least two different populations oriented toward the immunodominant mannose region from two different sides, as indicated in Fig. 23.

These antibodies can be designated as subpopulations anti-3a and anti-(3), respectively, which would make up the whole population of anti-3 antibodies.

For a 15–anti-15 system Uchida *et al.* (1963) found the β-Gal → Man → Rha trisaccharide to be the best inhibitor. The immunodominant sugar for factor 15 is *galactose*.

For the *Salmonella* factor 12, Kauffmann (1941a,b, 1961) found that this is in fact a complex specificity giving rise to three specific an-

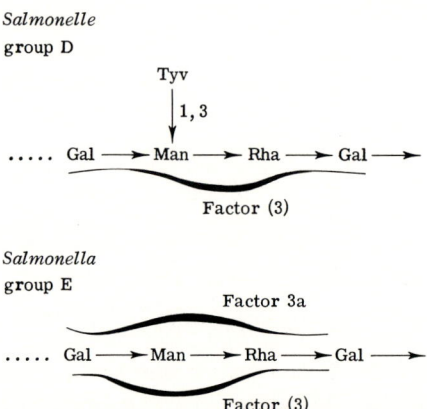

Fig. 23. Subdivision of factor 3 into factors (3) and 3a. From Lüderitz et al. (1971).

tibodies, anti-12_1, -12_2 and -12_3. In *Salmonella* group D a variant of *S. typhi* (factors 9, 12_1, 12_2, 12_3) was isolated, *S. typhi* T_2 A.S. (with factors 9, 12_1, 12_3), lacking factor 12_2 (Kauffmann, 1941a,b) and at the same time lacking the α-glucosyl side chains on the main chain (Kauffmann *et al.*, 1960). It was suggested that for 12_1 and 12_3 rhamnose or mannose, respectively, in the main chain have immunodominant function.

These facts indicate that, along the straight polysaccharide chains with Gal → Man → Rha trisaccharide units, in principle every sugar—for example mannose in factor 3, galactose in factor 15, and rhamnose or galactose in factors 12_1 or 12_3—can exert immunodominant function, and for one individual sugar even distinct substructures can be immunodominant. By the isolation of variants or mutants with slight differences in determinant structures a defined O factor (determinant) may turn out to represent several factors often with overlapping structures. As long as these (sub)factors are genetically linked, they would be recognized only as *one* factor. Therefore, the isolation of variants and mutants is of prime importance for a refined serologic analysis of polysaccharide (as well as other) antigens.

D. Significance of Mutations, Form Variations, and Lysogenic Conversions for the Immunochemical Analysis of Polysaccharide Antigens

Changes in the structure of a given O factor (oligosaccharide) will always be accompanied with changes in serologic O specificity (Lüderitz et al., 1971, p. 185). Such changes occur as a result of bacterial *mutation, form variation,* and *lysogenic conversion* (for review, see Mäkelä and Stocker, 1969; Stocker and Mäkelä, 1971).

Mutations which affect the biosynthesis of the repeating units of O-specific chains will always lead to rough strains (R forms) having no O-antigenic polysaccharide. In many *Salmonella* glucosyl or O-acetyl substitution of the O-specific polysaccharide chain occurs. Block in the transfer of these groups into sugars of the main chain does not affect LPS synthesis of the S form, but will lead to changes in the specificity of O factors involved. An example is the presence of a 2-O-acetyl group on abequose in factor 5 and its absence in factor 4. Strains having factor 5 exert also 4 specificity, probably due to incomplete acetylation. Recently, Uchida and co-workers (Uchida *et al.,* 1974; Sasaki and Uchida, 1974) showed that mutants of group D *Salmonella,* which were induced with N-methyl-N'-nitro-N-nitrosoguanidine, carried the somatic antigen of group A organisms. The mutant lost the O9 antigen factor (3,6-dideoxy-D-mannose = tyvelose) and acquired the O2 antigen factor (3,6-dideoxy-D-glucose = paratose), due to deficiency in the enzyme cytidine diphosphate paratose-2-epimerase which converts CDP-paratose to CDP-tyvelose (Matsuhashi and Strominger, 1965). This phenomenon illustrates a close biochemical relationship between non-cross-reacting structures of serologically distinct bacterial species.

The already mentioned disappearance of factor 12_2 in *Salmonella* of group D is due to a mutation connected with the disappearance of α-glucosyl side chains (Kauffmann *et al.,* 1962) bound to galactose in the parent strain (Tinelli and Staub, 1960a,b) (Fig. 24).

Factor 12_2 is subject to *form variation,* first described by Kauffmann (1940). Any culture of a strain able to synthesize an O antigen with factor 12_2 will consist of a population with cells in which factor 12_2 is well established and other cells in which 12_2 is nearly absent. Kauffmann (1940, 1961) found a rapid reversible change from the

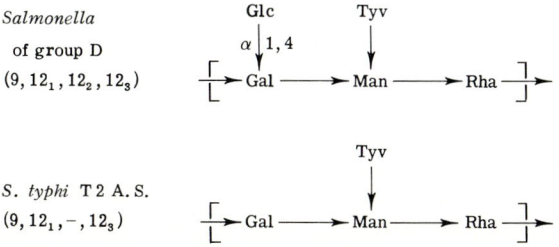

Fig. 24. Structure of the O-specific chain of *Salmonella* group D strains with and without factor 12_2.

12_2^+ to the 12_2^- state, the genetic control of which was studied by Mäkelä and Mäkelä (1966; see also Mäkelä and Stocker, 1969). Many other form variations in *Salmonella* have been described and summarized by Kauffmann (1961).

Many changes in O-antigenic specificity depend on bacteriophages which infect a given strain. This change is called *lysogenic conversion* (for review, see Lüderitz et al., 1966a, 1971). After phage infection, conversion is effected when the phage multiplies vegetatively and/or when it is present as prophage (Young et al., 1964; Zinder, 1957). As to the mechanism of phage action, it is either possible that the phage carries the structural gene for the enzyme or enzymes involved in the change of polysaccharide structure, or the phage codes for a derepressor of the relevant bacterial gene(s). According to Mäkelä and Stocker (1969) the first possibility is strongly supported by more recent work on the ϵ_{15} phage conversion system.

Phage conversions were—and are still—the subject of extended immunochemical analyses, performed hitherto mainly by Staub et al. (1959) and Robbins et al. (1965). The first more detailed structural investigation dealt with a conversion observed in *Salmonella* of groups A, B and D, brought about by phage P22 (Kauffmann, 1953; Iseki and Kashiwagi, 1953; Stocker, 1958). Its action leads to the disappearance of factor 12_2 (glucosyl $\xrightarrow[\alpha]{1,4}$ galactose) and the appearance of factor 1 (glucosyl $\xrightarrow[\alpha]{1,6}$ galactose), as shown by Stocker et al. (1960) and Staub (1961). This factor was therefore specified as I_{12} (see Table XXIV). Phage P22 provokes the appearance of a glucosyl-α-1,6-transferase. In *Salmonella* strains having factor 1 the presence of prophage P22 was demonstrated (Le Minor, 1963).

In *Salmonella* group C_1 many phage conversions of *S. cholerae suis* (O factors 6_2, 7) have been observed (Escobar and Edwards, 1964; Le Minor, 1965, 1968). Conversion by phage φ_{14} was extensively studied by Fuller and Staub (1968) and Fuller et al., (1968). The O-specific chain of *S. cholerae suis* is constituted of Man-Man-Man-Man-GlcNAc units to which an α-glucosyl substituent is attached to the third mannose residue (Table XXIV). Conversion by phage φ_{14} leads to a strain having O factors 6_2, (7), and 14, and the only structural change is a shift of the α-glucosyl substituent from the third mannose unit to the one next to N-acetylglucosamine (Table XXIV). Fuller and Staub (1968) and Fuller et al. (1968) found that for all three factors (6^2, 7, and 14) α-glucose is the immunodominant sugar. As an explanation, the authors suggested that factor 6_2 extends to the left side of glucose (Fig. 25) while factor 7 extends to its right side. After

1. Microbial Polysaccharides

TABLE XXIV

Changes in O-Specific Polysaccharides Provoked by the Action of Phages[a]

Phage conversions and changes in O Specificity	Structural changes
Salmonella Group B $4_1, 4_2, 12_2, 12_1, 12_3$	Abe Glc $\|$ $\alpha\|1,4$ $\xrightarrow{2}$ Man $\longrightarrow$ Rha $\longrightarrow$ Gal $\xrightarrow{1}$
$\downarrow$ Phage P_{22}	
$4_1, 4_2, 1_{12}, 12_1, 12_3$	Glc $\alpha\|1,6$ $\xrightarrow{2}$ Man $\longrightarrow$ Rha $\longrightarrow$ Gal $\xrightarrow{1}$
$\downarrow$ Phage φ_{27}	
$4_1, 27_B, 19, (12, 12_3)$	Glc $\downarrow$ $\xrightarrow{6}$ Man $\longrightarrow$ Rha $\longrightarrow$ Gal $\xrightarrow{1}$
Salmonella Group C_1 $6_2, 7$	Glc $\alpha\|1,3$ $\longrightarrow$ Man $\longrightarrow$ Man $\longrightarrow$ Man $\longrightarrow$ Man $\longrightarrow$ GlcNAc $\longrightarrow$
$\downarrow$ Phage φ_{14}	
$6_2, (7), 14$	Glc $\alpha\|1,3$ $\longrightarrow$ Man $\longrightarrow$ Man $\longrightarrow$ Man $\longrightarrow$ Man $\longrightarrow$ GlcNAc $\longrightarrow$
Salmonella Group E E_1 3, 10	Ac $\|$ $\longrightarrow$ Man $\longrightarrow$ Rha $\xrightarrow{\alpha}$ Gal $\longrightarrow$
$\downarrow$ Phage ϵ_{15}	
E_2 3, 15	$\longrightarrow$ Man $\longrightarrow$ Rha $\xrightarrow{\beta}$ Gal $\longrightarrow$
$\downarrow$ Phage ϵ_{34}	
E_3 3, (15), 34	Glc $\alpha\|1,4$ $\longrightarrow$ Man $\longrightarrow$ Rha $\xrightarrow{\beta}$ Gal $\longrightarrow$

[a] Only those glycosidic linkages are indicated which are altered by phage conversion.

conversion, the 6_2 specificity is retained: There is no change in the mannosyl linkages and therefore no structural change to the left of the glucosyl substituent. But on the right side the proximal mannose of the original strain is now replaced by N-acetylglucosamine, thus leading to a new specificity 14 and only some residual weakly cross-reacting factor (7), as indicated in Fig. 25.

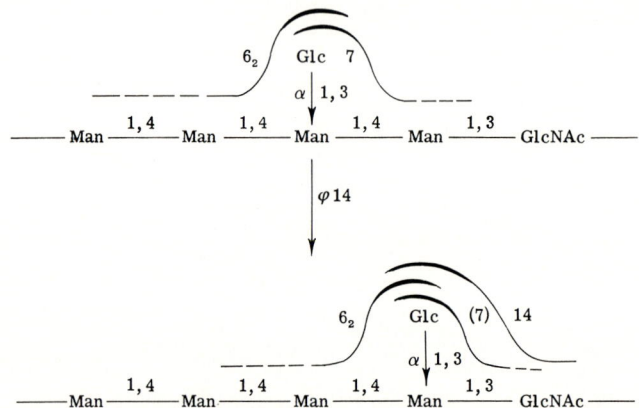

Fig. 25. Conversion of *Salmonella* Group C by Phage 14; 6_2, $7 \to 6_2(7)$, 14. From Lüderitz *et al.* (1971), after Fuller (1967).

This shows again that in the immune response to polysaccharide antigens the same immunodominant sugar, here α-glucose, can lead to different antibody populations which are differently adapted to substructures of that region.

Phage conversions in *Salmonella* group E were studied by Robbins and Uchida (1962, 1965). Strains of group E_1 with O factors 3 and 10 are converted by phage ϵ_{15} into strains of group E_2 with O factors 3 and 15, and the latter ones are converted by phage ϵ_{34} into strains of group E_3 with O factors 3, (15), and 34 (Uetake and Hagiwara, 1960). The structural changes in the respective polysaccharides are shown in Table XXIV. In group E_1 factor 10 is related to O-acetyl-α-galactose in the Man $\to$ Rha $\to$ Gal repeating unit. Phage ϵ_{15} provides different informations: change of the α-configuration into β-, and no more acetylation of galactose. After conversion with phage ϵ_{34}, an α-glucosyl substituent, attached 1,4 to β-galactose in the main chain will be found in the converted E_3 strain, giving rise to the new factor 34. Biochemical analyses of these conversions have been reviewed by Robbins and Wright (1971).

Conversions with phage φ_{27} have been observed in *Salmonella* groups A, B, and D. In Table XXIV the change by φ_{27} is exemplified in *Salmonella* group B. Staub and Forest (1963) and Staub and Bagdian (1966) showed that the mechanism of conversion by this phage in all three *Salmonella* groups is quite similar: in the main [Gal-Man-Rha] chain the -Gal $\xrightarrow[\alpha]{1,2}$ Man- linkage changes into the corre-

1. Microbial Polysaccharides

sponding -Gal $\xrightarrow[\alpha]{1,6}$ Man-linkage. In the unconverted strains glucosyl substitution of the galactose residue expresses factor 1_{12}, and substitution of the mannose residue by the 3,6-dideoxyhexoses paratose (in group A), abequose (in group B), and tyvelose (in group D) expresses the factors 2, 4, and 9, respectively. Change of the galactosyl-mannose linkage by conversion also changes all the adjacent factors, namely $12 \to 19$; $2 \to (2)$, 27A; $4 \to (4)$, 27B; and $9 \to (9)$, 27D.

On the basis of these observations, Staub proposed to subdivide the main factors 2, 4, and 9 into 2_1, 2_2; 4_1, 4_2; and 9_1, 9_2, respectively, of which factors 2_1, 4_1 and 9_1 are extending from the 3,6-dideoxyhexose region in the direction to the attached rhamnose, while 2_2, 4_2, and 9_2 are extending to the attached galactose side and therefore change with the conversion of Gal-1,2-Man into Gal-1,6-Man. The changes induced in *Salmonella* group B by conversion with phage φ_{27} are shown in Fig. 26.

It should be pointed out that all hitherto observed phage conversions, as far as they have been structurally clarified, are related (a) to the linkage between the biologic repeating units, and thus concerning the enzyme polymerase, or (b) to side chains or acyl substit-

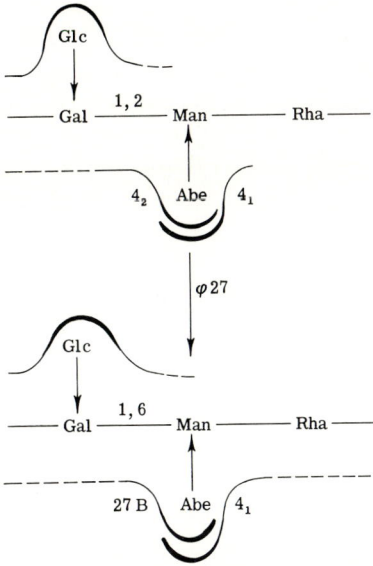

Fig. 26. Role of the galactosyl-mannose linkage adjacent to immunodominant sugars. Only those linkages are specified which are altered by the phage conversion.

uents of sugars, and thus concerning modifying enzymes. Other structural changes would probably modify the repeating units involved in such a way that polymerization to the O-specific polysaccharide chain would no longer be possible, and as a result rough strains would appear.

E. Artificial Antigens with Carbohydrate Determinants

1. MONOSPECIFIC CARBOHYDRATE DETERMINANTS

Immunochemical analyses have revealed that determinant groups in polysaccharide immunogens are generally of the size of smaller oligosaccharides.

The classic example of a disaccharide as a determinant group was the elaboration of cellobiuronic acid as the repeating unit of type III *Pneumococcus* polysaccharide by Goebel (1935, 1938, 1939, 1940). It was demonstrated that cellobiuronic acid strongly inhibited the precipitation of type III polysaccharide with type III antiserum. Goebel produced an artificial antigen which, on immunization, elicited antibodies that not only reacted with cellobiuronic acid (inhibition), but also with type III polysaccharide (precipitation) and actively protected animals against otherwise fatal infections with highly pathogenic type III organisms (Goebel, 1938, 1939).

Arakatsu *et al.* (1966) oxidized isomaltose and isomaltotriose with bromine to the corresponding aldonic acids. These were then coupled to protein by aid of isobutylchlorocarbonate, creating an amide bond between the sugar carboxyl and amino groups of the protein. The reducing terminal glucose units were altered by oxidation and coupling. Thus, from isomaltose an artificial antigen with α-glucosyl specificity and from isomaltotriose one with isomaltose specificity were obtained (Fig. 27).

Himmelspach *et al.* (1971) developed a method for the conversion of higher oligosaccharides into artificial antigens. The authors used glucooligosaccharides of the malto series (α-1,4), the isomalto series (α-1,6) and the cello series (β-1,4). The reducing terminal sugar residues were converted into the 1(*m*-aminophenyl) flavazol derivative by condensation with *o*-phenylene diamine and *m*-nitrophenyl hydrazine (Ohle and Melkonian, 1941a,b; Ohle and Liebig, 1942; Ohle and Kruyff, 1944), a reaction which has been used widely in carbohydrate chemistry (Himmelspach *et al.* 1971; Himmelspach and Wrede, 1971; Robbins *et al.*, 1965; Nordin, 1962) and which is schematized in Fig. 28.

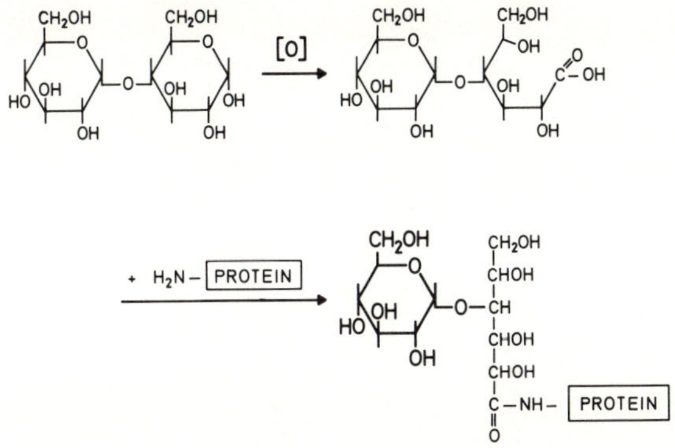

1. Microbial Polysaccharides

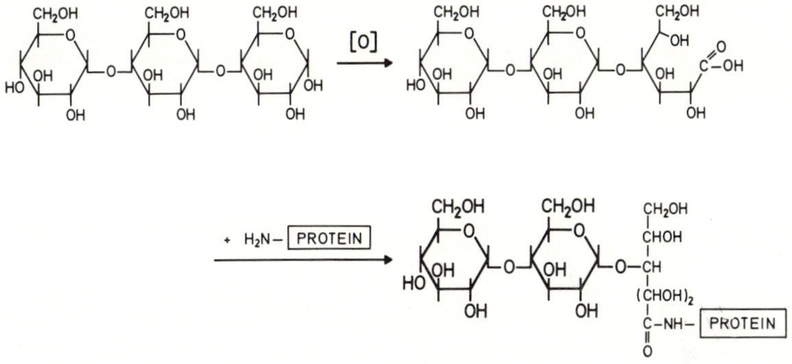

Fig. 27. Preparation of α-glucosyl-specific (a) and α-maltosyl-specific (b) artificial antigens by coupling of glucosyl- and maltosyl-substituted gluconic acids to protein. After Arakatsu et al. (1966).

The reaction requires unsubstituted hydroxyl groups on positions 2 and 3 of the reducing sugar residue. Tri- to octasaccharides were converted into the corresponding di- to heptasaccharide–aminophenyl–flavazoles which could be diazotized and coupled to protein (Fig. 28). Oligosaccharide–flavazole–phenylazoedestin conjugates were tested for immunogenicity in rabbits, and specific antioligosaccharide antibodies were obtained in all instances. On immunization with isomaltoheptaose-flavazole-phenylazoedestin (Himmelspach et al., 1971), high titers of dextran-specific antibodies were produced—in accordance with Kabat's finding that isomalto-

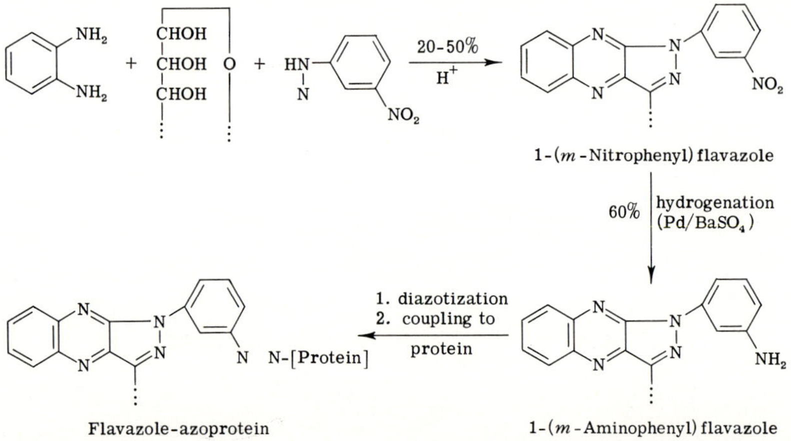

Fig. 28. Preparation of flavazole azoproteins. From Himmelspach *et al.* (1971).

hexaose maximally represents the determinant region for serologic dextran specificity (Kabat 1956, 1957).

The flavazole method was recently applied for the conversion of the tetrasaccharide repeating unit Glc $\xrightarrow[\alpha]{1,4}$ Gal $\xrightarrow[\beta]{1,6}$ Man $\xrightarrow[\alpha]{1,4}$ Rha of the O antigen of *Salmonella illinois* [group E_3 with O factors 3, (15), 34] (see Tables III and XXIV) (Kleinhammer *et al.*, 1973). In the flavazole condensation reaction (Fig. 28) the reducing rhamnose unit of the tetrasaccharide is involved and probably will no longer show the specificity it did in the original antigen. The antigen, therefore, contains the trisaccharide Glc $\xrightarrow[\alpha]{1,4}$ Gal $\xrightarrow[\beta]{1,6}$ Man $\xrightarrow[\alpha]{}$ as the determinant group (Fig. 29).

Antisera obtained after immunization of rabbits with the artificial T_{ill} antigen contained TS_{ill}-specific antibodies, as shown by agglutination of *S. illinois* bacteria (titers up to 1:2500). The specificity of these antibodies was tested by cross-agglutination with various bacterial strains having either factor 3, 15, or 34 in common. The antibodies were predominantly directed against the nonreducing end group Glc $\xrightarrow[\alpha]{1,4}$ Gal $\xrightarrow[\beta]{1,6}$ (Man), the O factor 34-specific structure of the *S. illinois* polysaccharide. Interestingly, the rabbit antibodies did not show cross-reactions with O factor 12_2 which differs from O factor 34 in the configuration of the Gal $\xrightarrow{1,6}$ Man linkage (12_2:α-glycosidic).

After these findings it is obvious that the entire antibody combining site which is complementary to more than a single sugar is

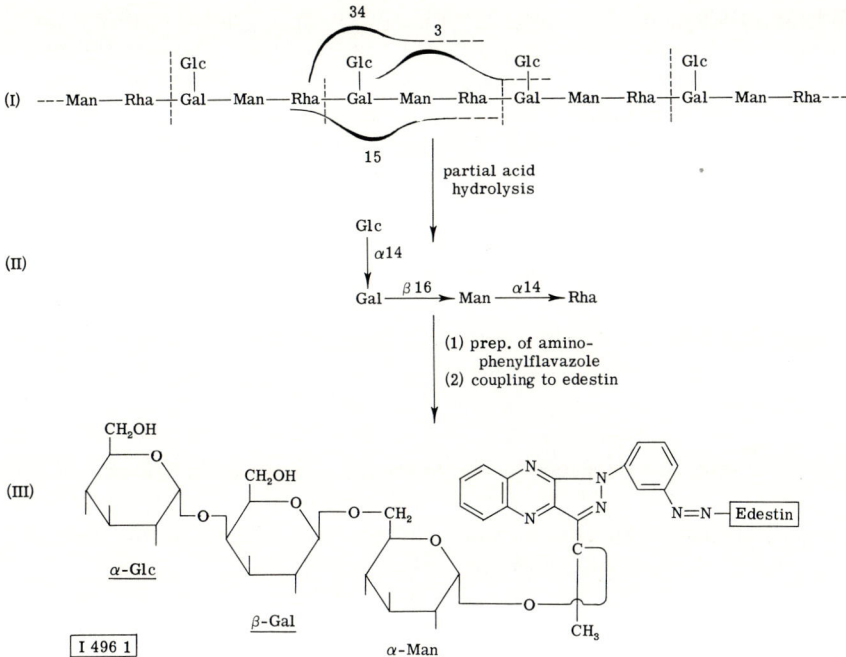

Fig. 29. Synthesis of the flavazole phenylazo edestin conjugate of a trisaccharide from *S. illinois*. From Kleinhammer *et al.* (1973).

not fully satisfied by a monosaccharide. Nevertheless, the observation that O factor/anti-O factor systems are frequently strongly inhibited by single immunodominant sugars prompted the production of artificial antigens containing the immunodominant monosaccharide linked to suitable protein carriers.

Of special interest in this context appeared 3,6-dideoxyhexoses, the immunodominant sugars of many enterobacterial, O-antigenic lipopolysaccharides (see Tables I–III, XXI, and XXIII). Inhibition studies, using *p*-nitro- or *p*-aminophenyl-α- and β-3,6-dideoxyhexopyranosides had given evidence (see Table XXII) for the α-pyranosidic configuration of the dideoxysugar side chains in enterobacterial LPS. Consequently, synthetic *p*-aminophenyl-α-glycosides of colitose, abequose, and tyvelose (Lüderitz *et al.*, 1960; Stirm *et al.*, 1966a,b) were diazotized and coupled to either egg albumin or bovine serum albumin (Lüderitz *et al.*, 1960; Staub *et al.*, 1966). Immunization of *rabbits* provided 3,6-dideoxyhexose-specific antisera which did not react with the same sugar present on the bacterial polysaccharide—in agreement with earlier findings of Goebel

(1938, 1939) and McCarty (1958, 1964) on artificial antigens with other monosaccharide determinants. One must assume that the phenylazo group attached to the sugar and even part of the protein may be involved in specificity.

When the same artificial 3,6-dideoxyhexose antigens were, however, injected into goats, the elicited goat antibodies reacted also with the corresponding bacterial polysaccharide and possessed the same properties as those obtained by immunization of goats with the respective bacterial strain (Lüderitz et al., 1960; Staub et al., 1966).

These results are in agreement with the more general findings that different polysaccharides with only the immunodominant sugar in common frequently cross-react in goat or horse sera, but not in the stringently specific rabbit sera (see Heidelberger and Kendall, 1933). This is why a serologic classification of bacterial genera, on the basis of their specific polysaccharide antigens, like the Kauffmann–White scheme of *Salmonella*, could only be elaborated with highly specific rabbit antisera, obtained after short-term immunization with the respective bacteria (Kauffmann, 1961, 1966).

With regard to immunodominant 3,6-dideoxyhexoses, abequose in O antigens of *Salmonella* group B is of special interest. Nonreducing abequose linked α-1,3 to the mannose residue of the polysaccharide chain represents the immunodominant region for O factor 4, while 2-O-acetylabequosyl-α-1,3-(Man) residues are immunodominant for factor 5 (see Table XXI). Stellner et al. (1970) have synthesized an artificial antigen by coupling p-aminophenyl-2-O-acetyl-α-abequoside to bovine serum albumin to give 2-O-acetyl-α-abequo-(pyranosido)-phenylazo-BSA (Fig. 30). This antigen, in contrast to the above mentioned corresponding antigen with nonsubstituted abequose, evoked in *rabbits* not only anti-2-O-acetylabequose antibodies, but also agglutinin titers against *Salmonella paratyphi B* (factors 4, 5, 12) which were specific for factor 5 and not cross-reacting with related strains having only factors 4 and 12 (Stellner et

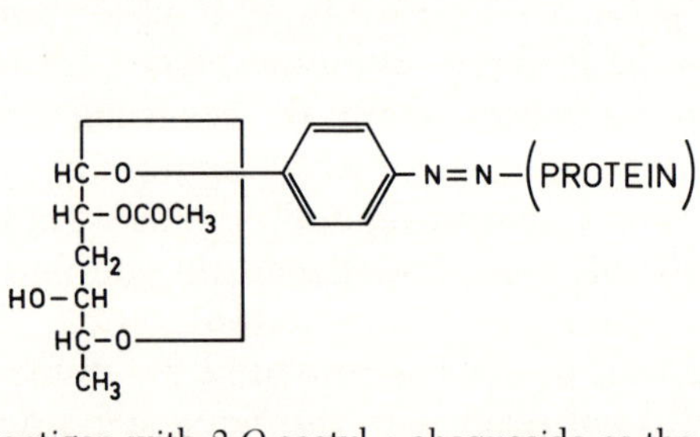

Fig. 30. Artificial antigen with 2-O-acetyl-α-abequoside as the determinant. From Stellner et al. (1970).

al., 1972), in accordance with earlier findings of Goebel *et al.* (1934a), using artificial antigens with glucose and 6-*O*-acetylglucose as the determinants. The above results are further proof for 2-*O*-acetyl abequose and not the isosteric 2-*O*-acetyl-D-galactose (Kotelko *et al.*, 1961) being the immunodeterminant sugar for O factor 5.

These results showed for the first time that it is possible to obtain in *rabbits* antibacterial antibodies with an artificial antigen having a single substituted monosaccharide determinant and demonstrated also the strong influence of a small group, like acetyl, on the specificity *and* on the conformation of the reactive site of the corresponding antibody.

2. MULTISPECIFIC CARBOHYDRATE DETERMINANTS

It is known that the immunogenicity of pure polysaccharides is dependent of the animal species used for immunization. The classic example are pneumococcal capsular polysaccharides which are nonimmunogenic for *rabbits* but are excellent immunogens for *man* (Heidelberger *et al.*, 1946, 1947; MacLeod *et al.*, 1946).

To transform polysaccharides which are haptenic for rabbits (or other species) into immunogens, Goebel and Avery (1931a,b) synthetized the *p*-aminobenzyl ether derivative of a pneumococcal polysaccharide, which was diazotized and coupled to protein, and showed that the polysaccharide–protein conjugate was immunogenic for rabbits, giving rise to anti-polysaccharide and antibacterial antibodies. More recently, 2-(4-aminophenylsulfonyl)ethyl hydrogen sulfate was introduced as a coupling agent (Himmelspach and Wrede, 1971). A disadvantage of the method is that only alkali-stable polysaccharides can be used because of the strongly alkaline reaction medium. Another method was developed by Morgan and Partridge, 1940, 1941, 1942) when they showed that the protein moiety of the endotoxic complex of Enterobacteriaceae (see Figs. 2 and 3) could be combined with many haptenic polysaccharides or mucopolysaccharides to give highly immunogenic polysaccharide conjugates.

Later, through the work of Sela and his co-workers (Sela, 1966), it was shown that not only protein but also special polypeptides may render otherwise nonimmunogenic molecules immunogenic. Sela demonstrated the important role of aromatic amino acids for immunogenicity. In connection with these findings, Sorg *et al.* (1970a) tyrosylated polysaccharides that were nonimmunogenic for rabbits, to introduce immunogenicity. When polytyrosyl chains containing 6 to 8 tyrosyl groups were introduced into nonimmunogenic dextran, the latter acquired immunogenicity in rabbits, giving rise to anti-dextran as well as anti-tyrosyl antibodies (Sorg et al., 1970b).

F. Noncarbohydrate Determinants

Polysaccharides often contain additional noncarbohydrate constituents such as acyl groups, pyruvate, or phosphate. Such substituents may function as antigenic determinants.

1. ACETYL SUBSTITUTION

O-Acetyl groups are frequently part of a determinant region. In S. *typhimurium* the O-antigenic determinant 5 is due to an acetyl substitution on position C2 of (α-linked) abequose (Hellerqvist et al., 1968; Stellner et al., 1972; see also Kotelko et al., 1961). This abequose, when not acetylated represents the O4 determinant of the same strain. Since not all abequose constituents are acetylated in the (lipo)polysaccharides of most S. *typhimurium* strains, these have the non-cross-reacting specificities 4 and 5 simultaneously. Specificity 5, which is due to acetylation, is lost upon alkali treatment (saponification) of the lipopolysaccharide.

The alkali lability of factor 10 in *Salmonella* group E_1 led to the idea that an O-acetyl sugar may also be involved in this specificity, but no acetylated oligosaccharide could be isolated. However, partial acetylation of the trisaccharide Gal $\xrightarrow{1,6}$ Man $\xrightarrow{1,4}$ Rha (see Table XXIV), in which the 6-hydroxyl group of galactose can be assumed to be the preferred position for selective acetylation, gave a serologically active inhibitor of the 10–anti-10 system (Uchida et al., 1963), suggesting that 6-*O*-acetylgalactose may be the immunodominant sugar in factor 10. Robbins et al. (1965) found an enzyme, transacetylase, responsible for O-acetylation of *Salmonella* group E_1 LPS or derived oligosaccharides, but the structure of the acetyl acceptor has not been elaborated.

Alkali lability can be taken as a general indication for participation of ester groups in a given antigenic specificity. In this way it was found that O-acetyl groups are essential for specificity of the K30 antigen of *E. coli* (Hungerer et al., 1967). In most cases the position of O-acetyl groups has not been established (see Björndal et al., 1970a). What was said for acetyl groups in principle also applies for acyl groups other than acetyl.

2. KETAL AND ACETAL SUBSTITUTION

Recently, attention focused on substituents that are linked to the carbohydrate via ketal or acetal bonds. Such compounds are familiar to the carbohydrate chemist who uses them as protecting groups in synthetic reactions. Their formation can be schematized as follows:

$$\begin{array}{c} \diagdown C\diagup OH \\ \diagup C \diagdown OH \end{array} + O=C\diagup^{R_1}_{R_2} \xrightarrow{-H_2O} \begin{array}{c} \diagdown C\diagup^{O}\diagdown \\ \diagup C\diagdown_{O}\diagup C \diagdown^{R_1}_{R_2} \end{array}$$

R_1 and R_2 may be hydrogen or any organic radical; thus the reaction product may be an acetal or a ketal.

Vicinal (1,2-)hydroxyl groups can be involved in this reaction with formation of a five-membered ring; with 1,3-positioned hydroxyl groups a six-membered ring is formed. These substituents introduce drastic changes in local conformation, which is expressed by changes of serologic specificity. The structural change which accompanies a 4,6-substitution of glucose and galactose is demonstrated in Fig. 31. It is understandable that opposite to an antibody combining site the unsubstituted saccharide is quite different from the substituted one. It would be interesting to know in ring systems such as those shown in Fig. 31 which difference there is in antibody recognition, if any, between a substituted glucose and an identically substituted mannose. These sugars differ only in the position of their hydroxyl groups at C-2. It is not known whether ketal substitution would bury and obliterate the antigenic difference between these two sugars.

In many instances the ketal-linked noncarbohydrate substituent is

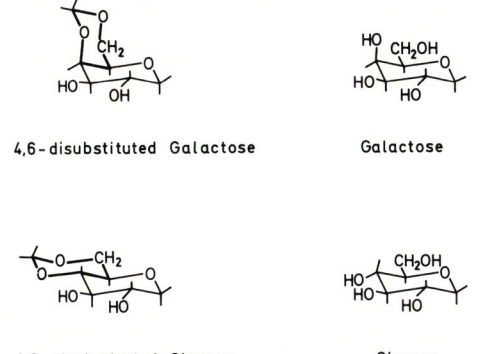

Fig. 31. Stereochemical change due to ketal substitution of glucose and galactose.

pyruvate, which introduces not only a conformational change but in addition imposes a charge on a polysaccharide. These two effects may be additive, but this has not yet been elaborated.

3. SULFATE AND PHOSPHATE SUBSTITUTION

The most common charged noncarbohydrate substituents are sulfate and phosphate ester groups. Sulfate groups are essential substituents of keratene and related compounds which play a role in immunologic disorders due to antigenic relatedness. Many polysaccharides contain phosphate. Their structures range from linear phosphomannans of the yeast *Hansenula capsulata* (Slodki, 1962) in which mannose units are joined through phosphodiester bridges and helical polyphosphoribose of *Hemophilus influenzae* (Zamenhof *et al.*, 1953) to heteropolysaccharides in which substitution by glycerol phosphate occurs, such as in SXVIII, the capsular polysaccharide of *Pneumococcus* Type XVIII (Estrada-Parra and Heidelberger, 1963; Estrada-Parra *et al.*, 1962) and the O100 antigen of *E. coli* (Jann *et al.*, 1970). From what is reported on antigenic specificity of phosphate groups no coherent picture can be drawn. In the polysaccharide SXVIII glycerol phosphate plays a minor role with regard to antigenic specificity of the polysaccharide (Estrada-Parra and Heidelberger, 1963), but in the O100-polysaccharide definite participation of the glycerol phosphate substituent was found (Jann *et al.*, 1970). In both instances serologic properties of native and alkali-treated polysaccharides were compared. Alkali treatment cleaved glycerol phosphate in both instances. All evidence taken together, it becomes obvious that phosphate is sometimes part of an antigenic determinant, but the antibody production and specificity is not necessarily directed against ionic areas of a polysaccharide. This falls in line with what is known about the role of charge in hexuronic acid and sialic acid-containing polysaccharides.

G. Cross-Reactions between Microbial Polysaccharides

A large number of cross-reactions can be observed with the O antigenic lipopolysaccharides of *Salmonella*. They were detected by bacterial cross-agglutination in antisera (Kauffmann 1954, 1961, 1966) long before the chemical nature of the reacting O antigens was known. The cross-reacting specificities were given numbers and they were termed "factors." Their chemical basis is described in Section III,C.

1. Microbial Polysaccharides

In another group of microbial polysaccharide antigens, the capsular polysaccharides of pneumococci, serologic cross-reactivity and chemical structure were studied at the same time. The elegant work of Heidelberger and his school showed that cross-reactivity can be of great help in the elucidation of polysaccharide structures (see Heidelberger, 1973a).

Studies with the cross-reacting polysaccharides SIII and SVIII from *Pneumococcus* (Pappenheimer *et al.*, 1968) may serve as an example. The structures of the two polysaccharides are shown in Table IX. In the homologous systems, i.e., SIII–anti-SIII and SVIII–anti-SVIII the best inhibitors were hexa- and octasaccharides, respectively. This indicates, quite in line with other inhibition studies (Mage and Kabat, 1963a), that in both serologic systems the antibody combining site extends beyond that of *one* oligosaccharide repeating unit. In contradistinction, the heterologous systems, i.e., SIII–anti-SVIII and SVIII–anti-SIII, can be completely inhibited by low concentrations of tetrasaccharides and even by the disaccharide cellobiuronic acid which is common to both polysaccharides and therefore the cause of cross-reactivity. Thus, cross-reactions involve only parts of those determinants which function in the respective homologous systems.

When the structure of the common determinant is known, one can isolate it from the polysaccharide(s) by partial hydrolysis (acidic or enzymatic) and couple it to a protein, using techniques described in Section III,E. The resulting conjugate is immunogenic, and can be used to raise antibodies directed against the common determinant. The extent of cross-reactivity can then be studied by testing both polysaccharides in this serum. Cross-reactions which involve larger oligosaccharides are more pronounced than those involving smaller oligosaccharides. With larger regions of identity greater amounts of antibody are precipitated by a cross-reacting antigen. This is understandable because in such cases cross-reactivity comes close to homologous reactivity.

Cross-reactions often cause difficulties in serologic classifications. Once this has been realized, the situation becomes more straightforward and cross-reactivity may be put to use in more detailed studies. In early investigations many atypical strains of pneumococci were found, for instance in types II and III (Avery, 1915; Sugg *et al.*, 1928), which reacted only weakly and incompletely in the respective original anti-pneumococcal antisera. Later, it was discovered that these strains represent independent types and IIA became type V and IIIA became type VIII. On the basis of quantitative precipitation, Heidelberger and Kendall (1929) studied the immunochemistry of isolated pneumococcal polysaccharides, which opened a new field of thought and methodology in immunochemistry. The analysis of a very great number of cross-reactions between polysaccharides of pneumococci and of other origin allowed the characterization of antibodies reacting with partial structures of these polysaccharides (Heidelberger, 1960; How et al., 1964). In these studies the amount of antibody precipitated with the cross-reacting antigen is compared with that precipitated by the homologous antigen. In the course of such studies the specificities of anti-SII and anti-SV antibodies could be elaborated. They are listed in Table XXV. The chemical basis of the cross-reactivity between SII and SV, which was the cause of the original difficulties in the classification of pneumococci of type II, is centered around the glucuronic acid constituent of both polysaccharides. However, in SII this is at terminal positions and in SV it is in 1,2 links within the polysaccharide chain. The antibody which is directed against terminal glucuronic acid can obviously also recognize an internal glucuronic acid substituted at C-2. With regard to the respective conformations this is quite understandable (Fig. 32). By a 1,2 bond a polysaccharide chain is buckled up so that the 2-substituted sugar ring is practically as exposed as if it were terminal. Therefore, one may say that a 1,2-linked sugar component is the immunologic equivalent of the same sugar in terminal position. The same conformational relation with galactose as the immunodominant sugar was found in the *Pneumococcus* type VI system (Heidelberger and Rebers, 1960; Rebers *et al.*, 1961). In most cases cross-reactions are based on identities of partial structures. This is the case with the cross-reacting pneumococcal polysaccharides SIII and SVIII. It was shown by Heidelberger and Rebers (1957, 1958) that cross-reactivity is due to the presence of cellobiuronic acid which is the structural repeating unit of SIII and part of that of SVIII (see Table IX). There

TABLE XXV

Specificities of Antibodies Directed against the Capsular Polysaccharides SII and SV of Pneumococcus Types II and V

Antibodies against	Determinant	Reference
SII	GlcUA-1 (terminal)	Heidelberger (1960)
	4,6-Glc-1 (branch point)	
	3-Rha-1 (chain)	
SV	2-GlcUA-1 (chain)	Heidelberger (1960)

1. Microbial Polysaccharides

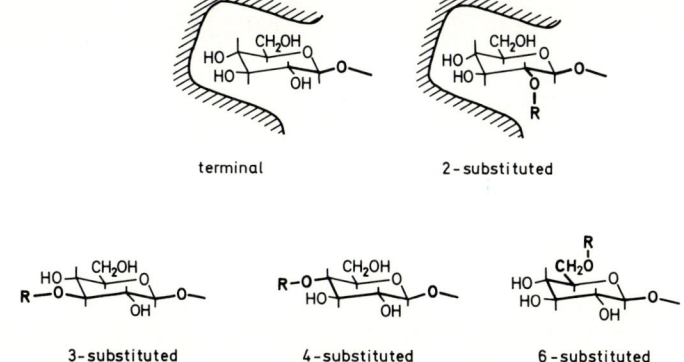

Fig. 32. Steric comparison of terminal 2-, 3-, 4-, and 6-substituted D-glucosides in their reaction with antibody. The hatched profile represents the antibody combining site.

are two major determinants conceivable for SIII: GlcUA $\xrightarrow[\beta]{1,4}$ Glc and Glc $\xrightarrow[\beta]{1,3}$ GlcUA, because both may be taken as repeating unit. Of these only the disaccharidic unit $\xrightarrow{3}$ GlcUA $\xrightarrow{1,4}$ Glc is also present in SVIII. Therefore cross-reactivity is due to this partial structure and antibodies against it react with SIII and SVIII. Out of many other cross-reactions in which SVIII takes part only those with glucan from oat and barley (Heidelberger, 1960) and with the K87 antigen of *E. coli* (Heidelberger and Jann, unpublished) in the respective horse antisera shall be mentioned. The region of structural identity with the glucans is the disaccharide unit Glc $\xrightarrow[\beta]{1,4}$ Glc (cellobiose). In this the nonreducing glucose moiety is the same as the reducing moiety in the disaccharidic determinant GlcUA $\xrightarrow[\beta]{1,4}$ Glc which cross-reacts with SIII. The partial structure common to SVIII and the K87 antigen of *E. coli* is Gal $\xrightarrow{1,4}$ GlcUA. The substructures responsible for these cross-reactions are shown in Fig. 33. These are schematized so that the specificities are arbitrarily termed SVIII, SVIIIb, and SVIIIc, using the symbols that were introduced by Staub in the course of immunochemical studies of the O-antigenic (lipo)polysaccharides of *Salmonella* (Lüderitz *et al.*, 1966a). Their cross-reactivities are indicated by arrows (Fig. 33).

The comparative immunochemistry of SIII, SVIII, oat glucan, and the K87 antigen indicates the value that the recognition of polysaccharides as antigens lends to polysaccharide chemistry. In fact, the phenomenon of cross-reactivity has become a useful tool in the structural elucidation of polysaccharides (Heidelberger, 1960; Lüderitz

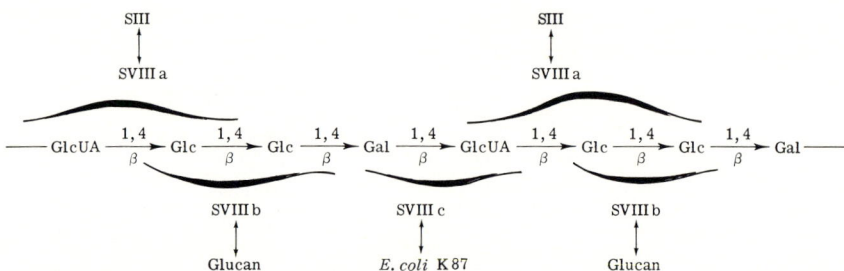

Fig. 33. Specificities of the capsular polysaccharide from *Pneumococcus* type VIII, expressed as SVIII a, b, and c. Cross-reacting antigens that show the respective substructure with SVIII are indicated by arrows. SIII, capsular polysaccharide of *Pneumococcus* type III; *E. coli* K87, capsular polysaccharide of *E. coli* O8:K87; Glucan, glucan from oat.

et al., 1966a). Usually, antibody against a known structure is used as probe for unknown polysaccharide structures. Alternatively, oligosaccharides of known structure may be used as inhibitors of serologic reactions with polysaccharides the structures of which are only imperfectly known. Even if the informations obtained through cross-reactions are circumstantial, they are often a great help in differentiating between alternative structural formulations. Thus, the K30-specific capsular polysaccharide of *E. coli* O9:K30 contains in its chain glucuronic acid which is linked either through C-2 or C-4 (see Table XIV). Its serologic reactivity in a great number of antipneumococcal antisera was tested with the result that it cross-reacted only in anti-SII and anti-SV (Heidelberger *et al.*, 1968). With the known specificities of these antisera (see Table XXV) and the structural information of the K30 polysaccharide at hand, these cross-reactions are a strong indication that substitution of the glucuronic acid constituent in the K30-polysaccharide is at C-2 and not at C-4.

With multiple cross-reactions chemical similarities could be detected between the teichoic acid of *Streptococcus* group N, an acetylphosphogalactan from *Sporoblomyces* and the capsular polysaccharides from *Pneumococcus* types VI, XVI, XVIII, and XXVII (Heidelberger and Elliot, 1966; Heidelberger and Slodki, 1968). The teichoic acid cross-reacted with SVI, SXVI, and SXXVII and with the acetylphosphogalactan. All these polysaccharides contain galactose or galactose phosphate. Later it was found that of all these polysaccharides only the acetylphosphogalactan also cross-reacts with SXVIII. The cross-reaction between the teichoic acid and the acetylphosphogalactan on the one hand and SVI, SXVI, and SXXVII on

1. Microbial Polysaccharides

the other was not reduced after removal of acetyl groups, whereas that between the acetylphosphogalactan and SXVIII was abolished after deacetylation. It was already known (Estrada-Parra and Heidelberger, 1963) that SXVIII contains an immunodominant acetyl group, possibly on the galactose residue of the repeating unit (see Table IX). Therefore, these results can be interpreted as follows: The cross-reactions between the teichoic acid, the acetylphosphogalactan, SVI, SXVI and SXXVII are due to galactose, and the cross-reaction between the acetylphosphogalactan and SXVIII is due to acetylgalactose. Further structural specifications are possible if the structures of SXVIII (see Table IX) and the acetylphosphogalactan are compared. The latter was proposed by Slodki (1966) as shown in Formula I. This polysaccharide contains one O-acetyl group per repeating unit. With these data it is clear that the galactose moiety that cross-reacts with SXVIII must be acetylated and 1,3-linked as in SXVIII. Therefore, we can postulate that Formula II depicts the ace-

$$\xrightarrow{6} Gal \xrightarrow{(1,3)} Gal \xrightarrow{1} \underset{\underset{OH}{|}}{\overset{\overset{O}{\|}}{P}} \xrightarrow{}_n \qquad \xrightarrow{6} Gal \xrightarrow{1,3} \underset{\underset{O-Ac}{|}}{Gal} \xrightarrow{1} \underset{\underset{OH}{|}}{\overset{\overset{O}{\|}}{P}} \xrightarrow{}_n$$

(I)   (II)

tylphosphogalactan of *Sporoblomyces*. If the cross-reactions of the phosphogalactan with the teichoic acid, SVI, SXVII, and SXXVII are due to the unacetylated galactose, this sugar must be 1,6-linked in all polysaccharides mentioned.

When polysaccharides are altered chemically, through enzyme action, or by mutation of the cell synthesizing them, their serologic specificities are also changed. If the immunochemical characteristics of polysaccharides are changed then, as a logical consequence, their cross-reactivities are also changed. This shall be demonstrated by two examples.

The specific polysaccharide of *Streptococcus* group A cross-reacts weakly with SII and strongly with the polysaccharide of *Streptococcus* group L. It is known that the group A polysaccharide contains immunodominant N-acetylglucosamine (Araujo and Krause, 1963) and so does the group L polysaccharide (Karakawa et al., 1971). This explains the cross-reactivity of the two polysaccharides. SII does not contain N-acetylglucosamine but, like the group A polysaccharide, it contains rhamnose which is in part 1,3-linked. This explains the cross-reactivity of the group A polysaccharide with SII. Because this latter cross-reaction is only weak, one must conclude that either only few 1,3-rhamnosyl groups are present in the group A polysaccharide, or otherwise that these groups are masked. As shown in Section II,D,1 *Streptococcus* group A strains can mutate to serologically distinct strains which were termed A-variant. Moreover, the group A polysaccharide can be transformed to group A-variant polysaccharide through the action of an enzyme. The A-variant polysaccharide reacts with SII and with group L polysaccharide in the opposite way as the parent group A polysaccharide. There is practically no cross-reaction with the L polysaccharide and a very strong cross-reaction with SII. These results are in full agreement with the chemical alterations (see Table XIX). Change from A to A-variant is accompanied by loss of practically all the N-acetylglucosamine residues. This is not only proof that this sugar constituent is responsible for cross-reactivity between the group A and L polysaccharides of *Streptococcus* but also an indication that lack of cross-reactivity between group A polysaccharide and SII was indeed caused by masking of the 1,3-rhamnosyl groups with N-acetylglucosamine (Karakawa et al., 1971).

As shown in Fig. 31, pyruvate substitution imposes a characteristic conformation on the polysaccharide. Since it is bound through a ketal linkage and this is more acid-labile than an ordinary glycosidic bond, it can be preferentially removed by mild acid hydrolysis under conditions that leave the polysaccharide chain intact. This situation should be ideally suited for comparative study of cross-reactivities. This was recently done by Heidelberger and associates (Higginbotham et al., 1972; Heidelberger and Nimmich, 1972; Heidelberger et al., 1970) with pyruvate-containing polysaccharides of *Rhizobium* using anti-pneumococcal antisera. It was known that SIV and SXXVII contain pyruvate, and thus cross-reactivity of the *Rhizobium* polysaccharides with SIV and SXXVII was expected. After depyruvylation the two polysaccharides did not cross-react in the anti-pneumococcal antisera SIV and SXXVII, and showed a great variety of cross-reactions with other pneumococcal polysaccharides. This is indicated in Table XXVI with the polysaccharides from *R. trifolii* TA1 and *R. radicicolum*. The cross-reactions that appear after depyruvylation are due to similarity or partial identity with respect to saccharide constituents and linkages. Thus, cross-reactions with SVIII seem to be due to cellubiuronic acid and those with SXIV to terminal galactose (Heidelberger et al., 1970; Dudman and Heidelberger, 1969). Upon depyruvylation (Heidelberger et al., 1972), SIV, which is known to be one of the most stringently type-specific pneumococcal polysaccharide antigens, lost this characteristic and became much like the group-specific C polysaccharide. It not only

TABLE XXVI

Cross-Reactivities of Two Representative Polysaccharides from
Rhizobium before and after Depyruvylation[a]

Polysaccharide	IV	VI	VIII	IX	XIV	XIX	XXVII	XXIX
R. trifolii	+	−	−	−	−	−	+	−
R. radicicolum	+	−	−	−	−	−	+	−
(R. trifolii)dp[b]	−	+	+	+	+	+	−	+
(R. radicicolum)dp[b]	−	−	+	+	+	+	−	+

[a] Adapted from Heidelberger et al. (1970).
[b] Depyruvylated polysaccharide.

cross-reacted with C polysaccharide but also, like C-polysaccharide, precipitated C-reactive protein of human serum. In addition to pyruvate, SIV contains galactose, N-acetylgalactosamine, N-acetylmannosamine, and N-acetyl-L-fucosamine (Brundish and Baddiley, 1968). Of these components only N-acetylgalactosamine is also present in the C polysaccharide (see Fig. 10). Therefore, this sugar must be responsible for cross-reactivity of the depyruvylated SIV and the C polysaccharide. In the original SIV, N-acetylgalactosamine is supposed to be masked by a proximal galactose, bearing a pyruvate substituent.

Cross-reactions between polysaccharides of bacterial and mammalian cells will be mentioned in Section IV,D.

IV. Immunobiology of Microbial Polysaccharide Antigens

A. Parameters of Immunogenicity

The immunogenicity of polysaccharides, i.e., their capacity to stimulate the formation of specific antibodies in animals or man, depends on the interplay of many parameters. Some of these concern the antigen, such as physical state of the polysaccharide (free or bound to carrier), molecular size, or resistance to enzymatic degradation in the animal. Other prerequisites for immunogenicity are posed by the animal—species, age, and genetic control. Finally, the dose in which the polysaccharide is administered is of great importance with respect to the animal's response. Changes in the dose given may drastically alter the response from immunity to immunologic paralysis (tolerance). More recently, it was found that, depending on the nature of the polysaccharide, different populations of immune cells are involved in the response.

1. MOLECULAR WEIGHT

Natural polysaccharides have molecular weights that are in the same range as those of proteins but, in contradistinction to proteins, they have a rather simple composition and conformation. One of the major factors determining the immunogenicity of a polysaccharide is its molecular weight. After it had been demonstrated by Heidelberger and his colleagues (Heidelberger and MacPherson, 1943a,b; MacLeod et al., 1946; Heidelberger et al., 1946, 1947) that pneumococcal polysaccharides are immunogenic in man, Kabat (Kabat and Berg, 1952, 1953; Kabat and Bezer, 1958) and Maurer (1953) showed that native dextrans that have molecular weights of several millions also evoke antibody production in man. Injection of 1 mg of native dextran gives rise to precipitating antibody and to skin sensitivity. The same is true for levans (Allan and Kabat, 1957). Teichoic acids (Torii et al., 1964) and group A and C polysaccharides of *Meningococcus* (Gotschlich et al., 1969) are also immunogenic. It was of interest to study the correlation between the mean molecular weight of a polysaccharide preparation and its immunogenicity under comparable conditions. This was done *inter alia* by Kabat and Bezer (1958) with dextrans in humans and by Howard et al. (1971a,b,c) with pneumococcal polysaccharides in mice.

Kabat's study on dextrans pertained to theoretical and clinical aspects at the same time. From native dextrans of *Leuconostoc* the clinical dextrans were obtained by partial hydrolysis and fractional precipitation with ethanol according to molecular weight ranges. These clinical dextrans were used as plasma volume expanders (Gronwall and Ingelman, 1944). In extensive studies Kabat and Bezer (1958) compared the immunogenicity of the various fractions. The results are shown in Table XXVII. The data indicate that dextrans with a mean molecular weight of 90,000 and above are good immunogens for man, and dextrans having an average molecular weight of 50,000 and below are not immunogenic. The results may help to explain the occurrence of systemic and local allergic reactions — especially since dextrans are found in food and can be produced by certain microorganisms in the digestive tract.

The work of Howard et al. (1971a–c) was initiated by contradicting reports concerning the dose response of mice to the type-specific polysaccharide of *Pneumococcus* type III (SIII). The native polysac-

TABLE XXVII

Response of Humans to Immunization with Various Dextran Fractions[a]

Average molecular weight	Antibody response[b] tested with	
	Dextran used for immunization	Native dextran
194,900	4/6	5/5
135,000	3/6	3/6
91,700	3/6	4/6
51,000	0/11	2/11
35,000	1/12	1/12
10,000	0/6	0/6

[a] Taken from Kabat and Bezer (1958).
[b] Expressed as fraction of individuals showing a rise of 2.0 µg of antibody N/ml or more when immune sera are compared with preimmune sera.

charide SIII (free acidic form), which has an average molecular weight of 220,000, was degraded by heating in aqueous solution. This reaction is frequently used as a mild autodegradation procedure for acidic polysaccharides. According to the duration of heating, degradation products are obtained ranging in size from polysaccharide to small oligosaccharides. Howard used fractions of molecular weights of 121,000, 31,000, and 4000 in comparison to native SIII. Whereas Kabat measured serum antibody titers, Howard monitored the number of plaque-forming cells (PFC) per spleen in the direct assay (Howard *et al.*, 1971a; see also Jerne and Nordin, 1963). The data shown in Table XXVIII indicate a steady drop in immunogenicity with reduction in size. With SIII smaller fragments than those of clinical dextrans are still immunogenic in mice, but the data are not directly comparable since dextran is a neutral polysaccharide with random structure and SIII is a highly charged polysaccharide with a regular structure made up by structural repeating units (see Section II,C,1). Differences also exist with respect to immune response *versus* dose.

Pure O-antigenic polysaccharides of gram-negative organisms which are obtained only after dissociation of the whole protein–lipid–polysaccharide complex (see Figs. 1–3) have molecular weights on the order of 10,000–20,000 and are nonimmunogenic. They exert immunogenicity when bound to lipid (lipid A) in the form of lipopolysaccharide and/or to protein (Boivin-type O antigen).

TABLE XXVIII

Effect of Reduction in Molecular Weight of SIII on the Direct PFC Response in the Spleen of Adult CBA Mice[a]

Average molecular weight	Direct PFC per spleen[b]		
	day 3	day 6	day 9
220,000	138,200	65,120	51,500
121,000	16,110	11,110	1,858
31,000	2,896	1,869	577
4,000	1,020	1,104	756

[a] Adapted from Howard et al. (1971a).
[b] Injected dose (i.v.) was 5 mg per animal (5 g of weight).

The lipopolysaccharides tend to aggregate, especially in the presence of divalent cations, to form particle sizes in the order of several millions (Schramm et al., 1952). Neter et al. (1973) demonstrated that the immune response of rabbits largely depends on the degree of aggregation. Heating of LPS solutions to 100°C for 1 hour, which causes dissociation, reduces immunogenicity, measured by passive hemagglutination, by more than 95%. Freezing at −20°C and thawing of heated solutions restores immunogenicity to a large extent. However, the heated LPS preparations were able to prime rabbits for specific secondary anti-polysaccharide response to a much higher degree than nonprimed rabbits. Rudbach (1971) and Reed et al. (1973) have shown that a few molecules of *E. coli* O111 and O113 lipopolysaccharide will suffice to sensitize mice for a heightened specific anti-polysaccharide response, thus demonstrating the high immunogenicity of protein-free LPS in suitable animals.

2. Dose and Persistence

In early experiments during the 1920's concerned with studies of pneumonia and its possible prevention by active immunization, Perlzweig and Steffen (1923) found that mice were rendered immunologically nonresponsive (i.e., could not be protected against *Pneumococcus* infection) by relatively large doses of a "non protein-non lipid fraction" from pneumococci. These results were verified soon afterwards by Schiemann and Casper (1927). At about the same time Felton and his associates studied the immune response of pneumococcal polysaccharides SI, SII, and SIII in mice. This was monitored by challenge of immunized mice and observation of the rate of specific protection. Dose response studies showed that injection of relatively large amounts of polysaccharide (about 500 µg) rendered mice unresponsive, whereas relatively small doses (about 0.5–1 µg) protected mice effectively against subsequent challenge with the bacteria from which the polysaccharides were derived. A single injection of about 500 µg polysaccharide abrogated the immunologic potency, so that a subsequent injection of an immunizing dose did no more elicit protection of mice against pneumococci of the same type. This phenomenon was termed "immunological paralysis" by Felton and Ottinger (1942) and defined as the condition produced in the host by an antigen given in such an amount that a subsequent immunizing dose of the same antigen fails to specifically stimulate active immunity. The paralysis with pneumococcal polysaccharides is type-specific and persists in mice for at least 15 months. Felton suggested that the polysaccharide antigen might not be degraded by the enzymes of the higher organism. Thus, it would persist in cells and in the circulation and continuously neutralize the homologous antibody which thus escapes detection. As a proof Felton isolated specific pneumococcal polysaccharides from liver and spleen of paralyzed mice (Felton, 1949; Felton et al., 1947, 1955) even months after administration. This situation, which was later described as "treadmill effect" (Dixon et al., 1955), is now known to be one of the effects observed upon the injection of large doses of some polysaccharides. Mice and rabbits seem to be especially prone to immune paralysis. Because the genetics of mice are well studied and inbred strains can be kept pure for many generations, most of the studies pertaining to this phenomenon were performed on mice. Quantitative studies by Howard et al. (1971a, 1969, 1972), Baker et al. (1971a,b), Halliday (Kearney and Halliday, 1970a,b,c; Halliday, 1971), and many others showed an unusual dose response curve obtained with pneumococcal polysaccharides and with the O-specific lipopolysaccharides of gram-negative bacteria. As shown in Fig. 34, the antibody titer (expressed as serum titer and number of spleen PFC) rises with the amount of polysaccharide given, reaches a sharp peak, and then drops again. This is quite distinct from a response curve obtained with erythrocytes as immunogens where finally a plateau is reached (Fig. 35). The polysaccharides used in these studies consist of structural repeating units (see Table IX), which are not found in polysaccharides such as amylose or dextran. Furthermore, they are not degraded by enzymes of the host.

Persistence of pneumococcal polysaccharide antigens and their

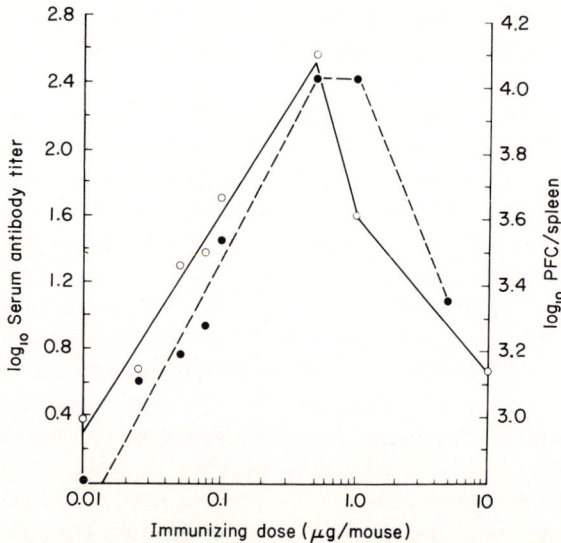

Fig. 34. Maximal serum antibody levels and maximal numbers of direct plaque-forming cells (PFC) obtained from mice immunized with various amounts of the capsular polysaccharide (SIII) of *Pneumococcus* type III. From Baker *et al.* (1971a).

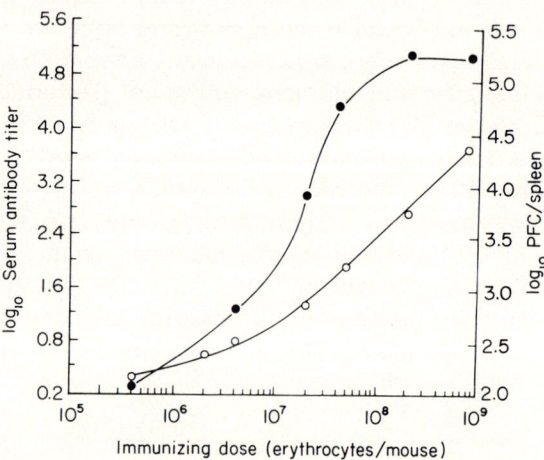

Fig. 35. Maximal serum antibody levels and maximal numbers of direct plaque-forming cells (PFC) obtained from mice immunized with various amounts of sheep erythrocytes. From Rebers *et al.* (1961).

stability to host enzymes was repeatedly confirmed in mice—for instance by blood clearing of ^{141}I-labeled SIII (Siskind et al., 1967) or ^{14}C-labeled SIII (Howard et al., 1970a,b, 1972). The cellular location of injected SII and SIII was examined by Kaplan et al. (1950) using immunofluorescence methods. Small doses were found predominantly in spleen macrophages. Large doses were initially distributed among many different cells, but after longer periods of time the main residual amount was again found in spleen macrophages. These and other studies led Howard and his colleagues to postulate that the pneumococcal polysaccharide antigens initially induce antibody formation. The polysaccharides will bind antibody, and are then phagocytized as antigen–antibody complexes. Whereas antibody is degraded within the macrophages, the polysaccharides remain intact and are eventually excreted back into the circulation. There they may stimulate the production of antibody again and the whole process is repeating (treadmill effect).

Confirmation of this explanation comes also from experiments of Brooke (1964, 1966a,b) who used a specific enzyme from *Bacillus palustris* which degrades SIII to mainly hexasaccharides (Dubos and Avery, 1931; Campbell and Pappenheimer, 1966, 1967). When SIII was incubated with the enzyme prior to injection into mice, no paralysis was observed with amounts of SIII which, when undegraded, would clearly have resulted in paralysis. However, the degraded polysaccharide had also lost its ability to induce immunogenicity. When SIII was injected first, followed by administration of the enzyme several hours later, the animals showed an immune response. These results showed that (1) the persistence of the polysaccharide is necessary for immune paralysis and the presence of material with a relatively high molecular weight is needed for an immune response, and (2) the immune response is initiated by the animal within hours after the injection of the polysaccharide antigen. Obviously, animals that have already started on the route to immunity can still be paralyzed, an interpretation that is also substantiated by other results (Felton et al., 1955; Brooke and Karnovsky, 1961).

3. IMMUNOGENICITY VERSUS TOLEROGENICITY

With some protein antigens immunologic tolerance is observed not only with high doses (high zone tolerance); also with very low doses (low zone tolerance) animals can be rendered immunologically unresponsive (Dresser and Mitchison, 1968; Mitchison, 1968a,b; Shellam and Nossal, 1968; Parish and Ada, 1969). Between these limiting concentrations the proteins are immunogenic. For a long time the phenomenon of low zone tolerance has not been observed with polysaccharide antigens such as pneumococcal polysaccharides or lipopolysaccharides of gram-negative bacteria; it was only recently demonstrated in mice with the capsular polysaccharide of *Pneumococcus* type III (Baker *et al.*, 1971a, 1974). The phenomenon of high zone tolerance was examined more closely by Howard *et al.* (1970b) who compared the kinetics of humoral and cellular immune response in mice. Data, like those shown in Fig. 36 demonstrated that higher concentrations of polysaccharide antigens induce two independent types of response. Using SIII, it was found that doses of 2–50 μg evoked the formation of antibody forming cells (PFC) in the spleen without detectable serum antibody. This represents the "treadmill" effect, first discussed by Felton and his associates (Felton, 1949; Felton and Ottinger, 1942; Felton *et al.*, 1947, 1955). At concentrations in excess of 50 μg the number of PFC per spleen falls off rapidly until there is practically no antibody forming cell left. Thus, high zone tolerance induced with nondegradable polysaccharides can be divided into treadmill neutralization of produced antibody

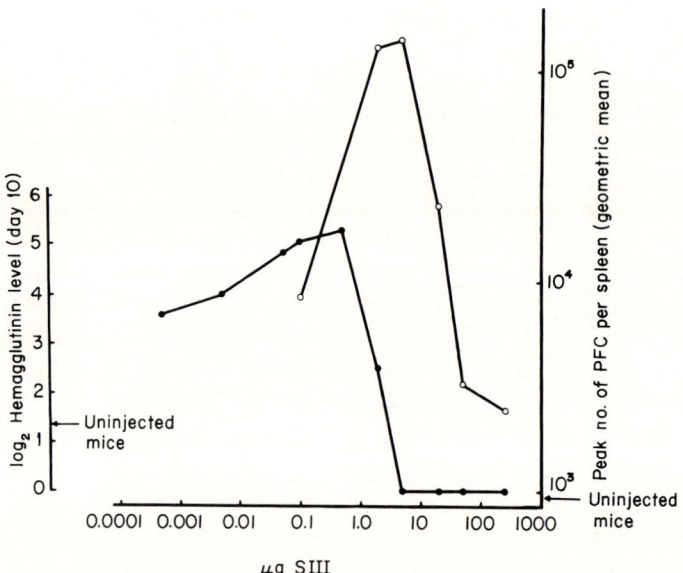

Fig. 36. Maximal serum antibody levels and maximal numbers of direct plaque-forming cells (PFC) obtained from mice immunized with various amounts of the capsular polysaccharide (SIII) of *Pneumococcus* type III. From Howard *et al.* (1970a).

1. Microbial Polysaccharides

and, with still higher doses, actual paralysis of the antibody forming system. These phenomena were termed peripheral inhibition and central inhibition, respectively (Parish and Ada, 1969). Recently, Howard and Courtenay (1974) showed that tolerance to levan and SIII pneumococcal polysaccharide can be induced in mice, if these antigens are injected in very small amounts (100 ng) together with cyclophosphamide (150 mg/kg).

Since it was shown that with decreasing size of a polysaccharide its immunogenicity also decreases (Kabat and Bezer, 1958; Howard et al., 1971a,b,c), it was of interest to examine the influence of molecular weight also on the tolerogenicity of a polysaccharide. This was done by Howard et al. (1970b) with SIII. Contrary to expectation, based on results with proteins (Dresser and Mitchison, 1968; Parish and Ada, 1969) and synthetic polypeptides (Janeway and Sela, 1967; Medlin et al., 1970), it was found that with decreasing molecular weight not only the immunogenicity of SIII but also its paralyzing effect decreased. This is shown in Table XXIX. The ability of depolymerized SIII to inhibit plaque-forming spleen cells (PFC) by antibody neutralization was also tested. This can be achieved by incorporation of the antigen or hapten into the agar when plaque assays are performed (Howard et al., 1971a,b,c). With the same preparation as used to examine immunogenicity and to-

TABLE XXIX

The Effect of Previous Injections of 250 µg Hydrolyzed SIII with Different Molecular Weights on the Spleenic PFC Response to 5 µg SIII[a]

Molecular weight of hydrolyzed SIII	Material injected		PFC's per spleen (day 14)
	250 µg hydrolyzed SIII (day 0)	5 µg native SIII (day 10)	
121,000	+	−	3,956
	+	+	368
	−	+	143,520
31,000	+	−	4,905
	+	+	31,470
	−	+	173,620
4,000	+	−	3,480
	+	+	38,720
	−	+	86,620

[a] From Howard et al. (1971a).

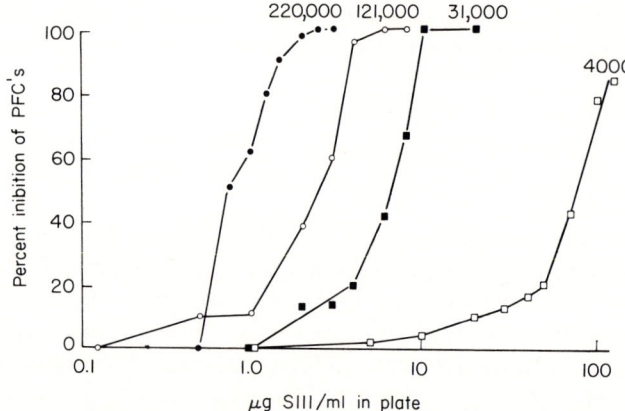

Fig. 37. Comparison of the inhibitory capacity of native and depolymerized capsular polysaccharide (SIII) from *Pneumococcus* type III against spleenic plaque-forming cells (PFC) from mice immunized with various amounts of SIII. From Howard *et al.* (1971a).

lerogenicity, it was found that also antibody-neutralizing capacity decreased, as shown in Fig. 37. The result was surprising, especially since the preparation of smallest size which did only very ineffectively neutralize antibodies still contained about 10 repeating units and thus should carry enough antigenic determinants for reaction with antibody.

In summary, with respect to pneumococcal polysaccharide immunogens and O-specific lipopolysaccharide immunogens of gram-negative bacteria (Friedman, 1966a,b; 1968; Allen and Friedman, 1970; Britton and Möller, 1968; Britton, 1969a,b), a number of typical phenomena have been observed. As worked out predominantly with pneumococcal polysaccharides, these are the following: Immunogenicity is dependent on high molecular weight and is initiated only with low or moderate doses; there is high zone tolerance but the phenomenon of low zone tolerance was observed only in one case. Baker *et al.* (1971a, 1974) presented evidence for the existence in mice of low zone tolerance to SIII. This was achieved by priming with subimmunogenic or marginally immunogenic doses of SIII. Not only immunogenicity but also tolerogenicity and antibody neutralizing capacity are abrogated on degradation of the polysaccharide antigen. Some, if not all of these properties are found also with polymers of D-amino acids and polyvinyl compounds (Mozes and Shearer, 1971; Shearer *et al.*, 1972; Lichtenberg *et al.*, 1972; Sela *et al.*, 1972; Howard, 1972; Andersson, 1969, 1971; Andersson and

Blomgren, 1971). These antigens have in common that they are not degraded by enzymes of the host and thus persist and, further, that all these polymers have regular structures expressing the same determinant(s) many times in sequence.

4. IMMUNOLOGIC MECHANISMS

Recent developments in immunology offer an explanation for the uncommon properties of these antigens. It is postulated that for the production of antibodies to a given immunogen certain cells of the immune system must cooperate (for a review, see Feldmann and Nossal, 1972, and Volume I of *Transplantation Reviews*, 1969; for more recent hypotheses, see Bretscher, 1974). These are the T lymphocytes (thymus derived) which recognize and concentrate the antigen, and present it to the B lymphocytes (bone marrow derived) which, after further differentiation, produce antibody molecules. Macrophages also play a role in the presentation of the antigen. It is not attempted here to describe the various theories of antibody formation in which the presence of mediator substances produced by T lymphocytes and/or cell–cell contact between T lymphocytes, B lymphocytes, and macrophages are postulated. In context with these considerations it is interesting to note that the only antigens found until now which do not need T lymphocytes for the production of humoral antibody are pneumococcal polysaccharides, enterobacterial lipopolysaccharides, poly-D-amino acids, and polyvinyl compounds (Baker *et al.*, 1971a; Anderson and Blomgren, 1971; Howard *et al.*, 1971a,b,c; Andersson *et al.*, 1972; Howard, 1972; Manning *et al.*, 1972; Coutinho and Möller, 1974). It has been shown for lipopolysaccharides that, when bound to T lymphocyte-dependent carriers, they confer T lymphocyte independence to the latter (Möller *et al.*, 1972; Manning *et al.*, 1972). Furthermore, it was found that all these give rise exclusively to macroimmunoglobulins (Howard *et al.*, 1971a,b,c; Kearney and Halliday, 1970a–c; Andersson *et al.*, 1972). These require a larger number of antigenic determinants for neutralization than do IgG molecules (Torii *et al.*, 1964) which might explain the decrease in antibody neutralizing capacity of SIII upon degradation, especially in antibody binding tests (Neumüller, 1945; Goebel *et al.*, 1934a,b; Arakatsu *et al.*, 1966; Himmelspach *et al.*, 1971; Himmelspach and Wrede, 1971; Harrisdangkul and Kabat, 1972).

It has been postulated that immune paralysis by large doses of antigen (high zone tolerance) may set in at the level of B lymphocytes (Mitchison, 1968a,b; Howard *et al.*, 1971a,b,c; Andersson *et al.*, 1972).

Normally, an antigen is thought to be bound to receptors of T lymphocytes and then offered in a spatially concentrated form to B lymphocytes. On the latter ones the antigens are then cross-linked or arranged in such a way that the membrane of the B lymphocyte is altered, which induces a signal for the transformation of B lymphocytes followed by production of antibody. If the concentration of the antigen on the surface of the B lymphocyte becomes too high, membrane alterations would be impaired and (high zone) tolerance would ensue. Polysaccharides which are T lymphocyte-independent antigens may be so because the determinants of their repetitive structure are already close enough to each other and in the macromolecule also numerous enough to react effectively with B lymphocytes. With larger amounts of polysaccharide the concentration of antigenic determinants per cell surface may become so high that the necessary membrane alterations can no longer be induced. This would then result in high zone tolerance to these polysaccharides. Reduction in size of a T lymphocyte-independent polysaccharide would result in reduction of the cell surface area which is densely covered with antigenic determinants. This would explain the parallel reduction of immunogenicity and tolerogenicity with reduction of molecular size.

Low zone tolerance is assumed to occur on T lymphocytes (Howard et al., 1971a,b,c; Mitchison, 1968a,b; Chiller et al., 1971). Since T lymphocytes seem to play no role in the immune response to regularly built polysaccharides, low zone tolerance with these antigens should not be expected—and hitherto has not been encountered.

5. Genetic Control of the Immune Response

The immune response to an antigen depends not only on its physical and chemical structure but also on the genetic constitution of the individual into which the antigen is injected. This has been studied mainly in the mouse, using inbred strains.

The immune response to a number of synthetic polypeptides and proteins such as bovine γ-globulin or ovalbumin in low doses—all of which are T cell-independent—is linked to the histocompatibility gene (H-2 gene in the mouse). For a review, see, e.g., Benacerraf and McDevitt (1972), McDevitt and Landy (1972), Hämmerling and McDevitt (1973), and Marchalonis et al. (1974).

With α-1,3-dextran the immune response is linked to the allotypes of the heavy chain constant region (Blomberg et al., 1972). This probably means a direct control of the antibody combining site.

Amsbaugh et al. (1972, 1974) demonstrated another type of genetic linkage. In mice the responsiveness to the capsular polysaccharide of

Pneumococcus type III (SIII) is governed by at least two types of genetic control. One influences the response in an "all-or-nothing" manner. This gene is carried on the X chromosome (it is X-linked). A second, probably autosomal gene (not linked to the H-2 gene) regulates the magnitude of the antibody response. The X-linked gene influences the *specific* IgM response directly. However, this control is not exerted on the production of normal IgM produced by unspecific stimulation with B-cell mitogens like lipopolysaccharide or lipid A (Amsbaugh *et al.*, 1974). In this context the fact should be mentioned that in humans the level of serum IgM is also controlled by an X-linked gene (Grundbacher, 1972).

In short, the immune response to a polysaccharide antigen may be allotype-linked or X-linked; in autosomal control no linkage to histocompatibility genes could be found.

B. *Polysaccharide Antibodies with Restricted Heterogeneity*

1. Induction and Genetic Aspects

For the study of cross-reactivity and for the examination of antibody combining sites it is ideal to have specific antibodies with molecular homogeneity or restricted heterogeneity. For a long time this seemed to be an unattainable goal, since all immunizations—also with respect to a single determinant—led to antisera with complex populations of antibodies. Therefore, the observation of Kunkel *et al.* (1962), Krause (1970), and Haber (1970) that very intensive immunizations of rabbits with bacteria may result in the production of antibodies with restricted heterogeneity, was of great importance. In these studies killed streptococci and pneumococci were used. With pneumococci the immune response is directed practically entirely against the capsular polysaccharide. With streptococci this is not the case, and antibodies are directed to a large extent against the outermost hyaluronic acid and protein antigens of the bacterial cells. However, when these are removed by repeated washing and with proteases, the underlaying polysaccharide antigens are exposed and then dominate the immune response (Krause, 1970). The antibodies considered here are all directed against bacterial polysaccharides that have been presented to the animals on the bacterial cells as carriers. As shown in Table IX, the pneumococcal polysaccharides SIII and SVIII have regular structures consisting of repeating di- and tetrasaccharides, respectively. The specific structure of SIII is also present in SVIII. This monotonous regularity of structure is often thought to be the reason for the restricted response. This is hard to maintain with the polysaccharide antigens of *Streptococcus*, because they do not fit the concept of a simple structure (Krause, 1963).

From the pneumococcal polysaccharides SIII and SVIII a number of oligosaccharides with the length of 1–4 repeating units were isolated, labeled by reduction with sodium borotritiate, and studied in equilibrium dialysis with rabbit antibodies of restricted heterogeneity (Haber, 1970; Katz and Pappenheimer, 1969; Pappenheimer *et al.*, 1968; see also Campbell and Pappenheimer, 1966). The results indicated homogeneity in binding. Uniform binding properties, however, are not unambiguous proof of homogeneity of an antibody population. It had been shown (Pincus *et al.*, 1968) that antibodies against pneumococcal polysaccharides that were polydisperse in electrophoresis can also show uniform binding. Therefore, uniformity of antibody response was defined on the basis of (1) pattern of electropherograms of whole serum on cellulose acetate, (2) isoelectric focusing (Rodkey *et al.*, 1970), and (3) pattern of polyacrylamide gel electrophoresis of the fully reduced and alkylated light chains of the antibodies (Jaton *et al.*, 1970; Haber, 1970; Reisfeld and Small, 1966). An important proof of molecular homogeneity was the recent finding that the N-terminus of the respective light chain of the antibodies under study had homogeneous sequences (Jaton *et al.*, 1970; Eichmann *et al.*, 1970; Kindt *et al.*, 1970).

The amounts of antibody produced in rabbits was often amazing, and in some instances even exceeded 60 mg/ml. This, and the fact that in some sera the immune electrophoretic pattern very much resembled that of human myeloma sera, raised the question whether malignant transformation may have been induced by these hyperimmunizations, and whether the antibodies with restricted heterogeneity may be the products of myeloma tumors. However, it could be shown that this is not the case. Restricted heterogeneity which is established during hyperimmunization vanishes and gives way to normal heterogeneity when the immunization is discontinued. Further, histological studies at the height of the "restricted immune response" did not reveal any sign of malignancy (Haber, 1970).

In a search for possible genetic factors influencing the immune response, large numbers of rabbits were studied (Braun *et al.*, 1969; Eichmann *et al.*, 1971; Jaton *et al.*, 1970). The animals could be grouped into low and high responders, with respect to antibody concentration in their sera. The high responders consistently produced antibodies with restricted heterogeneity. Breeding experiments showed that a line of progeny can be established which inherited the trait of a restricted immune response. This is an indication that the type of immune response to which an animal is capable is fixed genetically. This concept does not go without contradiction (Kimball *et al.*, 1971; Chen *et al.*, 1973). In a comparative study Chen *et al.* (1973) showed that more than 90% of outbred rabbits responded to *Pneumococcus* types III and VIII at any one time with the production of the respective anti-polysaccharide antibodies with restricted heterogeneity. A correlation between antibody concentration and degree of heterogeneity was not seen. These results cannot be fully reconciled with any of the existing attempts to interpret the phenomenon of "restricted immune response" to polysaccharide antigens.

Some antibodies with restricted heterogeneity, together with their homologous antigens and serologic specificities, are listed in Table XXX. With respect to the induction of homogeneous antibodies and to their value as probes for the antibody problem, the reader is referred to a recent review by Braun and Jaton (1974).

2. STUDY OF CROSS-REACTIONS

Antibodies with restricted heterogeneity are a useful tool for the study of cross-reactions. This has been used with the pneumococcal capsular polysaccharides SIII and SVIII. Hyperimmunization resulted in antisera which had 1–2 bands (anti-SIII) and 3 bands (anti-SVIII), as judged by electrophoresis on cellulose acetate (Pincus *et al.*, 1970a,b, Jaton *et al.*, 1970). From these sera the specific antibodies were precipitated almost quantitatively by the homologous polysaccharide antigens. When anti-SVIII was passed through a SIII-immune absorbent column (Cheng and Haber, 1971) one of the 3 original bands was missing on subsequent paper electrophoresis. Elution of the retained antibody led to a preparation that was electrophoretically homogeneous and corresponded to the missing band in the depleted antiserum. This antibody reacted with SIII and SVIII, in contradistinction to the depleted anti-SVIII which did not react with SIII. The specificity of the isolated homogeneous anti-SIII portion of the anti-SVIII antiserum was directed against the cellubiuronic acid determinant. These results show that antibodies with restricted heterogeneity of more than one specificity may be induced by hyperimmunization. Partial structural identity of SVIII with SIII is fully reflected in the homogeneous antibodies.

More recently, the main band that appeared on cellulose acetate chromatography of anti-SIII hyperimmune serum of one individual rabbit was studied in more detail (Holowka *et al.*, 1972). The homo-

TABLE XXX

Rabbit Antibodies with Restricted Heterogeneity Provoked with Bacterial Vaccines[a]

Bacteria	Antigen	Determinant	References
Streptococcus			
A	Polysaccharide	GlcNAc	Eichmann and Krause, 1969
A variant	Polysaccharide	L-Rha ⟶ L-Rha	Osterland et al., 1966; Fleischmann et al., 1968
B	Polysaccharide	L-Rha	Davie et al., 1967
C	Polysaccharide	GalNAc	Miller et al., 1967
Pneumococcus			
III	Polysaccharide	GlcUA $\xrightarrow[\beta]{1,4}$ Glc	Pincus et al., 1970a,b; Jaton et al., 1970
VIII	Polysaccharide	GlcUA $\xrightarrow[\beta]{1,4}$ Glc $\xrightarrow[\beta]{1,4}$ Glc $\xrightarrow[\beta]{1,4}$ Gal[b]	Pincus et al., 1970a,b; Jaton et al., 1970
Meningococcus A	Polysaccharide	ManNAc(OAc)P	Cited in Haber, 1970
S. typhi	Lipopolysaccharide	?	Dudin and Michel, 1963

[a] Adapted from Krause (1970).
[b] Also substructures like GlcUA $\xrightarrow[\beta]{1,4}$ Glc.

geneous fraction was isolated on an immune absorbent column and then fractionated by isoelectric focusing into 3 bands. This method is known to separate more minutely than paper electrophoresis. The 3 corresponding antibody fractions were homogeneous and all reacted with polysaccharide antigen SIII. Their binding of the trimer of the SIII-repeating unit ($\xrightarrow{3}$ GlcUA $\xrightarrow[\beta]{1,4}$ Glc $\xrightarrow[\beta]{1}$)$_3$ was uniform. Difference circular dichroic spectrometry indicated that all 3 antibody fractions reacted similarly but not identically. The results, based mainly on the dichroism of tryptophan residues, permit the interpretation that conformational changes outside the Fab region of the immunoglobulin occurred when the oligosaccharide hapten was bound. Such a phenomenon had been described before with lysozyme (Glazer and Simmons, 1966; Johnson and Phillips, 1965; Teichberg and Sharon, 1971) but not with antibody. Previous failure to detect this with antibody molecules may be due to the heterogeneity of normal antibody populations but also to the fact that haptens were used which also absorbed in the spectral region studied. This indicates the advantage not only of homogeneous antibodies but also of polysaccharide antigens and oligosaccharide haptens for such quantitative studies. On the basis of these results one might assume that specific binding of small ligands to proteins may generally result in conformational change of the protein. The fact that 3 homogeneous but physically distinct antibodies with practically identical hapten recognition are formed in one individual is striking. It may be taken as an indication that the immune response is degenerate. Possible biologic advantages of such a degeneracy are not known.

C. Myeloma Proteins with Anti-polysaccharide Specificity

1. General Considerations

Myeloma proteins of human (Waldenström proteins) and murine origin have been studied extensively (Cohn, 1967; Cohen and Milstein, 1967; Potter, 1967). Only myeloma proteins of the mouse will be considered here. These can be induced by intraperitoneal application of mineral oil or bacteriophage mainly in BALB/c mice and their hybrids (Cohn, 1967; Potter and Liebermann, 1967). These proteins have the characteristics of γ-globulins and most of them belong to the IgA class (Cohn, 1967; Potter, 1970). In extended screening experiments using gel precipitation it was found that many of them reacted specifically with polysaccharides of microbial origin. As shown in Table XXXI these polysaccharides are a heterogeneous

TABLE XXXI

Specificity of Some Myeloma Globulins

Myeloma globulin				
From tumor	Ig class	Antigen	Antigenic determinant	Reference
MOPC 167	A	*Pneumococcus* C polysaccharide (β-lipoprotein)	Phosphorylcholine	Potter and Leon, 1968; Leon and Young, 1971; Cohn et al., 1969
MOPC 299				
MOPC 603				
S 63				
S 107				
TEPC 15				
MOPC 104E	M	Dextran B1355l, 3	$\xrightarrow{3} Glc \xrightarrow{1}_{\alpha} 3$	Leon et al., 1970; Young et al., 1971
J558	A	Dextran B1498S	$\xrightarrow{3} Glc \xrightarrow{1}_{\alpha} 5$	Ghanta et al., 1972; Lundblad et al., 1970
S117	A	β-Teichoic acid	$GlcNAc \xrightarrow{1}_{\beta}$ (terminal)	Vicari et al., 1970
		Streptococcus A polysaccharide		
J606	G3	Levan (inulin)	$\xrightarrow{6} Fru \xrightarrow{2}_{\beta} n$ $\xrightarrow{1} Fru \xrightarrow{2}_{\beta} n$	Grey et al., 1971
MOPC 252	A	*S. worthington* (G) LPS	$Gal \xrightarrow{1,3}_{\beta} GalNAc$	Rovis et al., 1972
MOPC 406	A	*S. weslaco* LPS		Rovis et al., 1972
		S. kampele LPS	$ManNAc \xrightarrow{1}$ (terminal)	Potter, 1970
		E. coli O31 LPS		
MOPC 384	A	*S. illinois* (E3) LPS	$Gal \xrightarrow{1}_{\alpha}$ (terminal)	Rovis et al., 1972

1. Microbial Polysaccharides

group comprising enterobacterial lipopolysaccharides, teichoic acid, and dextrans. It had to be established that the reaction myeloma globulin–bacterial polysaccharide is indeed a specific antibody–antigen reaction. With myeloma globulins of the IgA class it was demonstrated that the reaction involved the Fab piece and not the Fc piece (Potter and Leon, 1968; Leon and Young, 1971; Cohn et al., 1969). There was no unspecific binding to hydrophobic regions of the Fab piece, as is known to occur with 8-anilino-1-naphthalenesulfonic acid (Parker and Osterland, 1970). Although myeloma globulins are known which react with the dinitrophenyl and trinitrophenyl haptens, this was not the case with those myeloma globulines that reacted with the pneumococcal C polysaccharide. Immune precipitations involving IgA antibodies are often hampered by the fact that a serum may contain monomeric and oligomeric IgA molecules in varying concentrations and monomeric IgA will bind antigen without formation of a precipitate (Tomasi and Grey, 1972). The same was shown to be the case with IgA myeloma proteins (Potter and Leon, 1968; Cohn et al. 1969). After reductive alkylation the monomers did not precipitate with the polysaccharide antigen but inhibited completely the precipitation of polysaccharide with the oligomeric IgA myeloma protein.

It is unknown how these polysaccharide specific myeloma globulins originate. However, in this context some observations should be mentioned which might help in understanding the phenomenon. The lipopolysaccharides that react specifically with the induced myeloma globulins are surface antigens of bacteria most of which are inhabitants of the mouse intestine. Some helminths that infest rodents have surface antigens closely resembling the pneumococcal C polysaccharide (cited in Potter, 1970). Bacteria and yeasts found in the mouth flora synthesize extracellular α-1,3-dextrans (Johnston, 1965; Bacon et al., 1968). This lends itself to the speculation (Potter, 1970) that silent infections or interaction with such microorganisms may stimulate precursors of IgA producing plasma cells. Intraperitoneal application of mineral oil might induce neoplasia (uncontrolled clonal expansion) of antibody producing cells which do not lose their synthetic capacity in the process. Such an assumption is sustained by the finding (McIntire and Princler, 1969) that no incidence of myeloma globulins with anti-polysaccharide specificity was found in germfree BALB/c mice. It is interesting to speculate on the possibility of inducing myeloma tumors in animals that were previously exposed to bacteria. It might thus be possible to induce polysaccharide specific myelomas at will.

2. Specificity

In most cases the specificity of myeloma globulins has been worked out (see Table XXXI). This shall be discussed in a few examples.

The *C polysaccharide* of *Pneumococcus* is an antigen for some myeloma proteins of the IgA class (see Table XXXI), yet some type specific pneumococcal polysaccharides (SI, SII, SVI, SX) also reacted with these proteins. It was shown that this was due to contamination of these specific polysaccharides with C polysaccharide and after removal of the latter the purified specific polysaccharides did not react. C polysaccharide contains ribitol, galactosamine, a diamino sugar, choline, and phosphate. Its repeating unit is shown in Fig. 10. Inhibition studies showed that phosphorylcholine is the immunodominant residue that is recognized by the myeloma proteins. Choline itself does not inhibit the reaction. Both compounds differ in charge. Therefore, the difference in binding must be due to this charge difference, and it has been suggested (Leon and Young, 1971) that binding of phosphoryl choline might be a two-step process, with the phosphate group interacting first. This could lead to a conformational change in the binding site of the myeloma protein, necessary for additional binding of the choline residue. There are a number of examples in which binding results in change of conformation (Holowka *et al.*, 1972; Harrisdangkul *et al.*, 1972; Leon and Takahashi, 1970; Parkhouse and Askonas, 1969) Phosphoryl choline is found in many phospholipids and in various lipoproteins. In accord with this, *sn*-glycero-3-phosphoryl choline is also a good inhibitor of the reaction of these myeloma globulins with pneumococcal C polysaccharide. The myeloma globulins also react with β-lipoproteins. Since lipoproteins are components of cell membranes, it was of interest to see whether these myeloma globulins would also react with cell membranes. Using the incorporation of tritiated thymidine, it was found (Leon and Takahashi, 1970) that the myeloma globulins which are reactive against pneumococcal C polysaccharide will transform lymphocytes. Whether they are B cell or T cell mitogens or both is not yet known.

One IgA myeloma globulin (S117) reacts with β-*teichoic acid*, group A polysaccharide of *Streptococcus*, and also with *blood group H substance* after Smith degradations (Vicari *et al.*, 1970). From this it was concluded that the immunodominant group must be *terminally β-linked N-acetylglucosamine*. This was verified by inhibition studies and by serologic reactions with proteins to which β-N-acetylglucosaminyl residues were linked.

A mouse myeloma globulin of the IgM class (MOPC 104E) has been studied extensively (Leon et al., 1970; Young et al., 1971, Ghanta et al., 1972). It is synthesized by myeloma tumor cells which were used during the investigation of IgM biosynthesis (Parkhouse and Askonas, 1969). This macroglobulin is an antibody against dextrans with a high proportion of α-1,3 bonds. Its combining site has the size of a trisaccharide which is about half the maximum size found with human anti-dextran antibodies (Leon et al., 1970; Young et al., 1971). This was established through inhibition of immune precipitation and equilibrium dialysis with tritiated oligosaccharides. Nigerose (Glc $\xrightarrow[\alpha]{1,3}$ Glc $\xrightarrow[\alpha]{1,3}$ Glc) and the hexasaccharides (Nigerose) $\xrightarrow[\alpha]{1,3}$ (Nigerose) and (Nigerose) $\xrightarrow[\alpha]{1,4}$ (Nigerose) react equally well. The protein was studied in electron microscopy and 10 subunits were demonstrable. A plaque technique was elaborated in which periodate oxidized dextran was chemically coupled to sheep red blood cells (Ghanta et al., 1972), which were then used as antigen-modified indicator cells. Myeloma cells producing IgM antibody against the dextran can thus be detected and quantitated, which is helpful in studying myeloma transplantation and in studies of IgM biosynthesis.

D. Polysaccharides in Infection

The fate of a host which is invaded by microorganisms depends on the effectiveness of its defense reactions. To a large measure these are directed against the surface of the microorganisms and, since in many cases polysaccharides are prominent microbial surface antigens, it is just to say that microbial polysaccharide antigens play an important role in many host–parasite interactions. They may inhibit host defenses and thus enable the microorganisms to multiply to such an extent as to eventually damage or kill the host. This phenomenon is called virulence. It describes the overall effect of microorganisms on a host, and is measured as the number of bacteria which upon inoculation will kill half the number of the animal population studied (LD_{50}).

It was found—especially with *Pneumococcus* and *E. coli* (Wood et al., 1956; Knecht et al., 1970; Howard and Glynn, 1971; Howard et al., 1971a,b,c)—that polysaccharide capsules tend to increase bacterial virulence. *E. coli* strains isolated from renal involvements, peritonitis, appendicitis, and urinary tract infections frequently have large capsules (Vahlne, 1945; Sjöstedt, 1946; Kaijser and Olling, 1973; see also Glynn, 1972). The Vi antigen of *S. typhi* was held responsible for the virulence of this bacterium (Felix and Pitt, 1934a,b), although its role in infection has not yet been clearly established.

Not only capsular polysaccharides but also the somatic (lipo)polysaccharides seem to play a role in bacterial virulence. When gram-negative enterobacteria undergo S→R mutation they lose the ability to synthesize the O-specific polysaccharide moiety of their somatic lipopolysaccharides (see Section II,B,3). Concomitantly, the virulence of the wild (S) strains is lost (for references, see Lüderitz *et al.*, 1966a; Roantree, 1967). The role of microbial polysaccharide antigens in virulence may be studied by comparing the LD_{50} of bacterial wild-types with those of mutants or recombinants which have altered polysaccharide structures or lack certain polysaccharides. From different strains recombinants have been prepared which differ in amount and/or nature of their O-specific somatic polysaccharide (Valtonen, 1970; Valtonen and Mäkelä, 1971; Valtonen *et al.*, 1971a,b; Mäkelä *et al.*, 1973).

The influence of bacteriophage conversion (see Section III,D)— which alters the structure of the O-specific polysaccharide — on virulence was studied more recently (Smith and Parsell, 1974). The results of all these studies supported the view that not only the amount but also the fine structure of the somatic (lipo)polysaccharides influence the virulence of the respective bacteria.

Because virulence can be regarded as the result of an effective inhibition of host defense reactions by microorganisms in which microbial polysaccharide antigens play a role, we shall sum up briefly what is known about these processes. The best understood defense reactions with which microbial polysaccharides are known to interact are those which involve primarily circulating antibody and the complement system, viz., the bactericidal reaction and phagocytosis. Both have been reviewed (Mudd, 1970; Smith, 1968; Smith and Path, 1969; Glynn, 1972).

In the *bactericidal reaction* the interaction of serum antibody with its antigenic determinant activates the complement system (Mudd, 1970; Muschell and Treffers, 1956; Glynn and Howard, 1970). A bacterium resistant against the bactericidal reaction is therefore termed complement-resistant. Polysaccharide capsules like those of *E. coli* (K antigens), *S. typhi* (Vi antigen) or *Pneumococcus* (type specific antigens) render the strain complement-resistant (Bhatnagar *et al.*, 1938; Knecht *et al.*, 1970; Glynn, 1969, 1972). Practically all capsular polysaccharides are acidic (Lüderitz *et al.*, 1968a) and they inactivate complement, probably through their charge (Glynn, 1972). Glynn and Howard (1970) attempted to quantitate the protection which capsular polysaccharides provide to bacteria against the complement action. They measured the adsorption of the basic protein lysozyme to encapsulated *E. coli* and found that the degree of complement resistance parallels the amount of ^{125}I-labeled lysozyme adsorbed. It was also found that charged capsular polysaccharides (from complement resistant bacteria) inhibited red cell agglutination and also hemolysis by hemolysin and complement (Ceppellini and Landy, 1963; Glynn and Howard, 1970). Complement resistance of encapsulated bacteria cannot be overcome with antibodies against the capsular polysaccharides. From these facts it can be concluded that the polysaccharide–antibody reaction activates complement too far away from the bacterial cell wall for this reaction to be harmful. Thus, thickness of the capsule as well as surface charge seem to play a role in complement resistance.

A part of the complement system is also involved in *phagocytosis*, the engulfment and killing of bacteria by macrophages and leukocytes (Mudd, 1970). Again, the capsular material provides a protective coat for the bacterial cell. In contrast to the bactericidal reaction, antibodies (opsonins) against the capsular polysaccharides enhance phagocytosis. The antiphagocytic effect of capsular polysaccharides is probably not specific, charge and viscosity of the capsular material being prerequisites. (see Schwarzmann and Boring, 1971). This would be in accord with the already mentioned observation that mucins generally enhance virulence of bacteria injected intraperitoneally. While the role of charged capsular polysaccharides in the bactericidal reaction and phagocytosis is relatively easy to circumscribe, this is not so with the somatic (lipo)polysaccharides. Clearly, also here the reaction of homologous antibody with a determinant activates complement, and the antibacterial reaction might follow. However, in many cases the somatic polysaccharides, which provide the specific point of attack by an antibody, protect a microorganism against the ensuing consequences. Possibly, like with capsular polysaccharides, the layer of somatic (lipo)polysaccharides sometimes exceeds a critical thickness. R mutants which do not have the polysaccharide moiety of the lipopolysaccharides (region I in Fig. 1) are all complement-sensitive in the presence of anti-R antibody and are readily phagocytized. Therefore, the sensitivity of some enterobacterial wild strains could be interpreted to the effect that their underlying R structures are partly exposed. That the latter is true in principle was demonstrated by Schlecht *et al.* (1971) who showed that S strains react with R antibody, and that immunization with S forms may give rise to low, but definite, titers against underlying R determinants (Schlecht et al., 1971; see, also, McCabe, 1972; McCabe et al., 1973).

It has been shown that anti-polysaccharide antibodies are protective against certain infections. Parenteral *vaccination* may be performed with whole bacteria, but in some cases the purified microbial polysaccharides were used successfully. Heidelberger (Heidelberger and MacPherson, 1943a,b; Heidelberger et al., 1951; Heidelberger, 1957; MacLeod et al., 1946) immunized humans with pneumococcal polysaccharides and found that the antibodies persisted for a long time. Immunization with four polysaccharides (from types I, II, V, and VII) provided a significant degree of protection in an epidemic in which the corresponding pneumococci were involved. Protective antibodies against pneumococci were also successfully induced in pregnant cattle (Hammer, 1961a,b). Passive transfer of all these antibodies to mice protected the animals against lethal challenges with homologous pneumococci.

Ever since Felix and Pitt (1934a,b) pointed out a correlation between the Vi antigen and the virulence of *S. typhi*, the protective role of the Vi antigen in anti-typhoid vaccines was an issue of controversy (Spaun and Uemura, 1964). It has been shown that the Vi antigen is protective in mice (Spaun and Uemura, 1964; Wong et al., 1972). In a recent study the protective activity of *Citrobacter* and *S. typhi* vaccines before and after treatment with a Vi degrading enzyme (Baker and White, 1965) was studied in mice which were then challenged with *S. typhi*. The protective effect of the *Citrobacter* vaccine was solely due to the Vi antigen, whereas that of the homologous *S. typhi* vaccine was only in part due to this polysaccharide (Wong et al., 1972).

While the efficiency of anti-polysaccharide antibodies against infection with gram-positive organisms, such as *Pneumococcus* (Heidelberger et al., 1946, 1947), or encapsulated forms of gram-negative organisms, such as *E. coli* K^+ strains (Wolberg and de Witt, 1969), is well established, the role of O antibodies in many gram-negative infections needs still further clarification.

Often no correlation can be found between O antibody titers and relative protective efficiency. Recurrence of urinary tract infections with enterobacterial strains seems to be independent of the amount of circulaing antibacterial (anti-polysaccharide) antibody (Vosti et al., 1965).

Immunization with somatic antigens (protein–lipopolysaccharide complexes) from a variety of gram-negative bacilli gave evidence for the elicitation of specific protection against subsequent infection (Sanford *et al.*, 1961; Markley and Smallmann, 1968; McCabe, 1972; Kaijser and Olling, 1973). But even in these protective experiments the specific role of the polysaccharide moiety in the respective immunogen (vaccine) was not clearly established (see Vosti *et al.*, 1965; McCabe *et al.*, 1973).

There is, of course, another possible reason for the apparent lack of correlation between protection and anti-somatic antibody levels, which is related to the site of infection. Most infections with gram-negative organisms occur at secretory surfaces, in the urinary or intestinal tracts, and antibody levels have invariably been measured in the serum due to its convenience. It now seems probable that one should be concerned with antibody levels in secretory fluids, and that these may correlate with protection (see Chaicumpa and Rowley, 1972).

Protective immunizations in which anti-polysaccharide antibodies play a role may be not only performed with bacterial vaccines and isolated polysaccharides but also with artificial antigens (see Section III,E). The advantage of using polysaccharides or artificial antigens with polysaccharide or oligosaccharide specificity would be that unspecific toxic effects of bacteria could thus be avoided. Such studies will be only promising with infections in which humoral events are prominent. The role of polysaccharides in cellular events (activation of macrophages by antigenically stimulated lymphocytes) in infection immunity is not clear. It has been reported that cellular responses to dextran and SII can be seen in delayed hypersensitivity with mice and guinea pigs (Crowle and Hu, 1967; Battisto *et al.*, 1968; Gerety *et al.*, 1970). The situation is complicated insofar as considerable controversy still exists concerning the relative importance of humoral and cell-mediated resistance to bacterial infections (Jenkin and Rowley, 1963; Rowley *et al.*, 1964; Mackaness *et al.*, 1966; Blanden *et al.*, 1966; Mackaness, 1970, 1971; World Health Organization, 1973). The possible role of polysaccharides in infection immunity should therefore be emphasized in further studies—especially since our knowledge of the chemistry and immunology of these antigens is so much advanced.

More recently, cross-reactions between partial structures of microbial polysaccharide antigens and components of mammalian cells were reported. Antigenic relatedness between man and microbe include those between blood group substances and bacterial (lipo)polysaccharides (Springer and Horton, 1969; Springer, 1970, 1971; Drach *et al.*, 1972, 1973), between cardiac tissue and streptococcal antigens in which polysaccharides were implicated (Nakla and Glynn, 1967), and between kidney tissue and lipopolysaccharides of *E. coli*—especially the O2 antigen (Holmgren *et al.*, 1971; Drach *et al.*, 1971). Cross-reactions exist also between human histocompatibility antigens (HL-A antigens) (Springer *et al.*, 1973; Hirata and Terasaki, 1970; Mittal *et al.*, 1973) and bacterial lipopolysaccharides and the Vi antigen of *S. typhi*. The importance of these cross-reactions is not clear yet. They may play a role as a pathogenic factor in tissue damage through autologous antibody. They may also render a host unresponsive and therewith sensitive to infection with cross-reacting bacteria, as has been discussed by Rowley and Jenkins (1962) during their study of infection of mice with *S. typhimurium*. Unresponsiveness may also ensue from antigenic relatedness between microbial polysaccharide antigens and HL-A antigens. However, interesting as these phenomena and speculations are, much has to be done to shed light on this fascinating area.

V. Summary and Conclusions

With modern analytic techniques, the elucidation of a polysaccharide structure has become much less of a problem than it used to be a decade or so ago. The structures of very many microbial polysaccharides are known and their number is rapidly increasing. New and exotic sugars were found as constituents of polysaccharides and, certainly, many more are in store for the natural products chemist. Groups of structurally closely related polysaccharides are built by different members of a bacterial species. Comparison of those within one bacterial species, and between different species, has revealed a common structural feature; it was found that they are made up from oligosaccharide repeating units. These findings stimulated greatly research work in the field of bacterial genetics and in biochemistry. As a result we have today a quite clear picture of how information for the synthesis of these polysaccharides is determined on the bacterial chromosome, and how they are synthesized by complex systems. Our understanding of genetic changes by mutation and lysogenic conversion by bacteriophages, and their influence on the structure of microbial polysaccharides, has considerably grown. All this will help us to understand the play of nature in the many variations, and will allow considerations about evolution, variation, adaptation, etc. Much of our knowledge gained with microbial polysaccharides can be put to use in the study of carbohydrate structures of mammalian cells and with such problems as cell transformation by oncogenic viruses and concomitant changes in the cell surface carbohydrates. Many phenomena observed first with microorganisms find their parallel in mammalian cells.

The microbial polysaccharides dealt with in this article are prominent surface structures of the microbial cells. They are either components of the outer membrane, such as the lipopolysaccharides, or they surround the cells as polysaccharide capsules. In animal and man they induce the formation of antibodies—they are antigens. The antibodies formed react specifically with the homologous polysaccharide antigens. This interaction involves partial structures of the polysaccharides ranging in size from a monosaccharide to about a hexasaccharide. These serologically important substructures were termed antigenic determinants and the sugar constituent that is primarily involved in antibody binding is called the immunodominant sugar. One and the same antigenic determinant may be present in several polysaccharide antigens which, in consequence, cross-react serologically. Cross-reactions have been used since a long time for the immunochemical analysis of polysaccharides. Comparison of immunochemical data with structural, biochemical, and genetic information is certain to deepen our understanding of the microbial world. Furthermore, antisera are of great importance in the serologic classification and rapid diagnosis of bacteria—especially so in epidemics.

Microbial polysaccharides have helped in our understanding of the immune response. Many polysaccharides are not degraded by host enzymes, and thus persist for a long time in circulation and/or tissue. They have provided the immunologist with a stable antigenic model in which cellular events in the immune response and the problem of tolerance and immune paralysis can be studied. The phenomenon of the treadmill effect was described on microbial polysaccharides. More recently, the role of (lipo)polysaccharides as mitogens has come to light. This will doubtless stimulate further work on the immune response and on receptor problems.

The significance of microbial polysaccharides in many infections, although not clearly defined yet, is beyond doubt. It is known that polysaccharides, especially the charged capsular ones, inhibit host defense reactions. This classifies them as parameters of microbial virulence. It is conceivable that also in this context the persistence of polysaccharide antigens in the host plays an important role.

Far as our knowledge of microbial polysaccharides is advanced, many problems remain to be solved. Microbial polysaccharides provide a valuable model for studying evolutionary events; a comprehensive analysis is very desirable and appears to be worthwhile. Our present knowledge about the immunologic response, its genetics, the involvement of B and T lymphocytes and macrophages, in relation to the structure and physicochemical makeup of the immunogen under investigation, appears to be advanced enough that efforts to manufacture "tailor-made" (see Sela, 1973, 1974) artificial polysaccharide vaccines should be stimulated. This could prove—and verify—or disprove their significance as means in the fight of medicine against infectious diseases. This is very important in the face of growing epidemic outbursts of bacteria-borne diseases such as *Salmonella*, *Shigella*, and *Cholera* infections as well as chronic *E. coli* infections of the urinary tract. Finally, the antigenic relation between man and microbe should be mentioned in which common carbohydrate structures play a role. This will help us to understand pathogenic processes in which autologous antibodies are involved and has, in some instances, already been offered as an explanation. Furthermore, regulatory phenomena and evolutionary stimuli involving host–parasite relationships may be revealed by such studies.

Acknowledgments

The authors are grateful to Drs. Elvin A. Kabat, New York, and Otto Lüderitz, Freiburg, for reading the manuscript and for valuable suggestions. They also wish to thank Professor Derrick Rowley, Adelaide, for suggestions with regard to Section IV,D. The great help and patience of Mrs. Liselotte ter Haak in the preparation of the manuscript is gratefully acknowledged.

References

Abdel-Akher, M., Hamilton, J. K., and Smith, F. (1951). *J. Amer. Chem. Soc.* **73**, 4691.
Adams, M. H., Reeves, R. E., and Goebel, W. F. (1941). *J. Biol. Chem.* **140**, 653.
Allan, P. Z., and Kabat, E. A. (1957). *J. Exp. Med.* **105**, 383.
Allan, P. Z., Gleich, G. J., and Perlin, A. D. (1965). *Immunochemistry* **2**, 433.
Allen, J. L., and Friedman, H. (1970). *Immunology* **105**, 1001.
Amsbaugh, D. F., Hansen, C. T., Prescott, B., Stashak, P. W., Barthold, D. R., and Baker, P. J. (1972). *J. Exp. Med.* **136**, 931.
Amsbaugh, D. F., Hansen, C. T., Prescott, B., Stashak, P. W., Asofsky, R., and Baker, P. J. (1974). *J. Exp. Med.* **139**, 1499.
Anderson, E. S. (1961). *Nature (London)* **190**, 284.

1. Microbial Polysaccharides 111

Anderson, E S., and Rogers, A H. (1963). *Nature (London)* **198,** 714.
Andersson, B. (1969). *J. Immunol.* **102,** 1309.
Andersson, B. (1971). *In* "Cell Interactions and Receptor Antibodies in Immune Responses" (O. Mäkelä, A. Cross, and T. U. Kosunen, eds.), p. 435. Academic Press, New York.
Andersson, B., and Blomgren, H. (1971). *Cell. Immunol.* **2,** 411.
Andersson, J. Sjöberg, O., and Möller, G. (1972). *Eur. J. Immunol.* **2,** 349.
Arakatsu, Y., Ashwell, G., and Kabat, E. A. (1966). *J. Immunol.* **97,** 858.
Araujo, P., and Krause, R. M. (1963). *J. Exp. Med.* **118,** 1059.
Archibald, A. R., Baddiley, J., and Dutton, D. (1965). *Biochem. J.* **95,** 8c.
Archibald, W. J. (1947). *J. Phys. Colloid Chem.* **51,** 1204.
Ashwell, G., and Hickman, J. (1971). *In* "Microbial Toxins" (G. Weinbaum, S. Kadis, and S. J. Ajl, eds.), Vol. IV, pp. 235-266. Academic Press, New York. London.
Avery, O. T. (1915). *J. Exp. Med.* **22,** 804.
Bacon, J. S. D., Jones, D., Farmer, V. C., and Webley, D. M. (1968). *Biochim. Biophys. Acta* **158,** 313.
Baddiley, J. (1962). *Fed. Proc., Fed. Amer. Soc. Exp. Biol.* **21,** 1084.
Baddiley, J. (1968). *Proc. Roy. Soc. Ser., B* **170,** 331.
Baddiley, J., Buchanan, J. G., Martin, R. O., and Rajbhandary, U. L. (1962). *Biochem. J.* **85,** 49.
Bagdian, G., Lüderitz, O., and Staub, A. M. (1966). *Ann. N. Y. Acad. Sci.* **133,** 405.
Bagdian, G., Etiévant, M., and Staub, A. M. (1969). *In* "Structure et effets biologiques des produits bactériens provenant des germes gram négatifs," p. 161. CNRS, Paris.
Baker, E. E., and White, R. E. (1965). *J. Bacteriol.* **89,** 1217.
Baker, P. J., Stashak, P. W., and Prescott, B. (1969). *Appl. Microbiol.* **17,** 422.
Baker, P. J., Stashak, P. W., Amsbaugh, D. F., and Prescott, B. (1971a). *Immunology* **20,** 469.
Baker, P. J., Stashak, P. W., Amsbaugh, D. F., and Prescott, B. (1971b). *Immunology* **20,** 481.
Baker, P. J., Stashak, P. W., Amsbaugh, D. F., and Prescott, B. (1974). *J. Immunol.* **112,** 2020.
Ballou, C. E. (1970). *J. Biol. Chem.* **245,** 1187.
Ballou, C. E., Lipke, P. N., and Raschke, W. C. (1974). *J. Bacteriol.* **117,** 461.
Barker, S. A., Foster, A. B., Siddiqui, I. R., and Stacey, M. (1958). *Nature (London)* **181,** 999.
Barker, S. A., Brimacombe, J. S., Eriksen, J. L., and Stacey, M. (1963). *Nature (London)* **197,** 899.
Barker, S. A., Bick, S. M., Brimacombe, J. S., and Somers, P. J. (1966a). *Carbohyd. Res.* **1,** 393.
Barker, S. A., Bick, S. M., Brimacombe, J. S., How, M. J., and Stacey, M. (1966b). *Carbohyd. Res.* **2,** 224.
Barker, S. A., Somers, P. J., and Stacey, M. (1967). *Carbohyd. Res.* **3,** 261.
Battisto, J. R., Chiappetta, G., and Hixon, R. (1968). *J. Immunol.* **101,** 203.
Benacerraf, B., and McDevitt, H. O. (1972). *Science* **175,** 273.
Berst, M., Hellerqvist, C. G., Lindberg, B., Lüderitz, O., Svensson, S., and Westphal, O. (1969). *Eur. J. Biochem.* **11,** 353.
Bhatnagar, S. S., Speechley, C. G. J., and Singh, M. (1938). *J. Hyg.* **38,** 663.
Björndal, H., Hellerqvist, C. G., Lindberg, B., and Svensson, S. (1970a). *Angew. Chem., Int. Ed. Engl.* **9,** 610.

Björndal, H., Lindberg, B., and Nimmich, W. (1970b). *Acta Chem. Scand.* **24**, 3414.
Björndal, H., Lindberg, B., and Nimmich, W. (1971). *Acta Chem. Scand.* **25**, 750.
Björndal, H., Lindberg, B., Lönngren, J., Nilsson, K., and Nimmich, W. (1972). *Acta Chem. Scand.* **26**, 1269.
Björndal, H., Lindberg, B., Lönngren, J., Rosell, K. G., and Nimmich, W., (1973). *Carbohyd. Res.* **27**, 373.
Blanden, R. V., Mackaness, G. B., and Collins, F. M. (1966). *J. Exp. Med.* **124**, 585.
Bleiweis, A. S., and Krause, R. M. (1965). *J. Exp. Med.* **122**, 237.
Blomberg, B., Geckeler, W. R., and Weigert, M. (1972). *Science* **177**, 178.
Boivin, A., and Mesrobeanu, L. (1935). *Rev. Immunol.* **1**, 553.
Bott, E. M., Bonynge, C. W., and Joyce, R. L. (1936). *J. Infec. Dis.* **18**, 5.
Braun, D. G., Eichmann, K., and Krause, R. M. (1969). *J. Exp. Med.* **129**, 809.
Braun, D., and Jaton, J. C. (1974). *Curr. Top. Microbiol. Immunol.* **66**, 29.
Bretscher, P. A. (1974). *Cell. Immunol.* **13**, 171.
Britton, S. (1969a). *Immunology* **16**, 513.
Britton, S. (1969b). *Immunology* **16**, 527.
Britton, S., and Möller, G. (1968). *Immunology* **100**, 1320.
Brooke, M. S. (1964). *Nature (London)* **204**, 1319.
Brooke, M. S. (1966a). *J. Immunol.* **96**, 358.
Brooke, M. S. (1966b). *J. Immunol.* **96**, 364.
Brooke, M. S., and Karnovsky, M. J. (1961). *J. Immunol.* **87**, 205.
Brundish, D. E., and Baddiley, J. (1968). *Biochem. J.* **110**, 573.
Campbell, J. H., and Pappenheimer, A. M., Jr. (1966). *Immunochemistry* **3**, 195.
Campbell, J. H., and Pappenheimer, A. M., Jr. (1967). *Annu. Rev. N. Y. Acad. Sci.* **103**, 1014.
Ceppellini, R., and Landy, M. (1963). *J. Exp. Med.* **117**, 321.
Chaicumpa, W., and Rowley, D. (1972). *J. Infec. Dis.* **125**, 480.
Chen, F. W., Strosberg, A. D., and Haber, E. (1973). *J. Immunol.* **110**, 98.
Cheng, W. C., and Haber, E. (1971). *Fed. Proc., Fed. Amer. Soc. Exp. Biol.* **30**, 527.
Chiller, J. M., Habicht, G. S., and Weigle, W. O. (1971). *Science* **171**, 183.
Chionglo, T. D., and Hayashi, J. A. (1969). *Arch. Biochem. Biophys.* **130**, 39.
Chittenden, G. J. F., Roberts, W. K., Buchanan, J. G., and Baddiley, J. (1968). *Biochem. J.* **109**, 597.
Choy, Y. M., and Dutton, G. G. S. (1972). *J. Bacteriol.* **112**, 635.
Choy, Y. M., and Dutton, G. G. S. (1973). *Can. J. Chem.* **51**, 198.
Clark, W. R., McLaughlin, J., and Webster, M. E. (1958). *J. Biol. Chem.* **230**, 81.
Claus, D. (1965). *Biochem. Biophys. Res. Commun.* **20**, 745.
Cohen, S., and Milstein, C. (1967). *Advan. Immunol.* **7**, 1.
Cohn, M. (1967). *Cold Spring Harbor Symp. Quant. Biol.* **32**, 211.
Cohn, M., Notani, G., and Rice, S. A. (1969). *Immunochemistry* **6**, 111.
Conrad, H. E., Bamburg, J. R., Epley, J. D., and Kindt, T. J. (1966). *Biochemistry* **5**, 2808.
Coutinho, A., and Möller, G. (1973). *Eur. J. Immunol.* **3**, 608.
Coutinho, A. and Möller, G. (1974). *Scand. J. Immunol.* **3**, 133.
Cramer, M., and Braun, D. G. (1973). *J. Exp. Med.* **138**, 1533.
Crowle, A. J., and Hu, C. C. (1967). *Int. Arch. Allergy Appl. Immunol.* **31**, 123.
Curtis, S. N., and Krause, M. D. (1964). *J. Exp. Med.* **120**, 629.
Curvall, M., Lindberg, B., Lönngren, J., and Nimmich, W. (1973a). *Acta Chem. Scand.* **27**, 2645.
Curvall, M., Lindberg, B., Lönngren, J., Ruden, U., and Nimmich, W. (1973b). *Acta Chem. Scand.* **27**, 4019.

Dagorn, M. B., and Staub, A. M. (1974). *Ann. Inst. Pasteur, Paris* (in press).
Das, A., Higginbotham, J. D., and Heidelberger, M. (1972). *Biochem. J.* **126**, 233.
Davie, J. M., Osterland, C. K., Miller, E. J., and Krause, R. M. (1967). *J. Immunol.* **98**, 710.
Dhir, S. P., Hakomori, S., Kenny, G. E., and Grayston, J. T. (1972). *J. Immunol.* **109**, 116.
Dixon, F. J., Maurer, P. H., and Weigle, W. O. (1955). *J. Immunol.* **74**, 188.
Dixon, R. J., Buchanan, J. G., and Baddiley, J. (1966). *Biochem. J.* **100**, 507.
Drach, G. W., Reed, W. P., and Williams, R. C. (1971). *J. Lab. Clin. Med.* **78**, 725.
Drach, G. W., Reed, W. P., and Williams, R. C. (1972). *J. Lab. Clin. Med.* **79**, 38.
Drach, G. W., Reed, W. P., and Williams, R. C. (1973). *J. Lab. Clin. Med.* **81**, 919.
Dresser, D. W., and Mitchison, N. A. (1968). *Advan. Immunol.* **8**, 129.
Dubos, R. J., and Avery, O. T. (1931). *J. Exp. Med.* **54**, 51.
Dudin, J., and Michel, M. (1963). *C. R. Acad. Sci.* **257**, 805.
Dudman, W. F., and Heidelberger, M. (1969). *Science* **164**, 954.
Dudman, W. F., and Wilkinson, J. F. (1956). *Biochem. J.* **62**, 289.
Dutton, G. G. S., and Yang, Y. (1972). *Can. J. Chem.* **50**, 2382.
Dutton, G. G. S., and Choy, Y. M. (1972). *Carbohyd. Res.* **21**, 169.
Edstrom, R. D., and Heath, E. C. (1965). *Biochem. Biophys. Res. Commun.* **21**, 638.
Eichenberger, E., Schmidhauser-Kopp, M., Hurni, H., Fricsay, M., and Westphal, O. (1955). *Schweiz. Med. Wochenschr.* **85**, 1190 and 1213.
Eichmann, K., and Krause, R. W. (1969). *Fed. Proc., Fed. Amer. Soc. Exp. Biol.* **28**, 695.
Eichmann, K., Lackland, H., Hood, L., and Krause, R. M. (1970). *J. Exp. Med.* **131**, 207.
Eichmann, K., Brown, D. G., and Krause, R. M. (1971). *J. Exp. Med.* **134**, 48.
Eriksen, J. (1963). *Acta Pathol. Microbiol. Scand.* **58**, 245.
Eriksen, J., and Henriksen, S. D. (1963). *Acta Pathol. Microbiol. Scand.* **58**, 245.
Escobar, M. R., and Edwards, P. R. (1964). *Bacteriol. Proc.* p. 146.
Estrada-Parra, S., and Gomez, I. (1972). *Immunochemistry* **9**, 1095.
Estrada-Parra, S., and Heidelberger, M. (1963). *Biochemistry* **2**, 1288.
Estrada-Parra, S., Rebers, P. A., and Heidelberger, M. (1962). *Biochemistry* **1**, 1175.
Fehmel, F. (1972). Dissertation, University Freiburg.
Feldmann, M., and Nossal, E. T. V. (1972). *Quart. Rev. Biol.* **47**, 269–302.
Felix, A., and Pitt, R. M. (1934a). *J. Pathol. Bacteriol.* **38**, 409.
Felix, A., and Pitt, R. M. (1934b). *Lancet* **227**, 186.
Felton, L. D. (1949). *J. Immunol.* **61**, 107.
Felton, L. D., and Ottinger, B. (1942). *J. Bacteriol.* **43**, 94.
Felton, L. D., Prescott, B., Kauffmann, G., and Ottinger, B. (1947). *Fed. Proc., Fed. Amer. Soc. Exp. Biol.* **6**, 427.
Felton, L. D., Kauffmann, G., Prescott, B., and Ottinger, B. (1955). *J. Immunol.* **74**, 17.
Fisher, M. W. (1959). *Nature (London)* **183**, 1692.
Fisher, M. W., Delvin, H. B., and Erlandson, A. L. (1963). *Nature (London)* **199**, 1074.
Fleischmann, J. G., Braun, D. G., and Krause, R. M. (1968). *Proc. Nat. Acad. Sci. U. S.* **60**, 134.
Freeman, G. G. (1942). *Biochem. J.* **36**, 340.
Friedman, H. (1966a). *J. Bacteriol. Fed. Amer. Soc. Exp. Biol.* **92**, 820.
Friedman, H. (1966b). *J. Immunol.* **96**, 289.
Friedman, H. (1968). *J. Bacteriol.* **96**, 1124.
Fuller, N. A. (1967). Thesis, University of Paris.
Fuller, N. A., and Staub, A. M. (1968). *Eur. J. Biochem.* **4**, 286.
Fuller, N. A., Etiévant, M., and Staub, A. M. (1968). *Eur. J. Biochem.* **6**, 525.

Gahan, L. C., Sandford, P. A., and Conrad, H. E. (1967). *Biochemistry* **6**, 2755.
Galanos, C., Lüderitz, O., and Himmelspach, K. (1969a). *Eur. J. Biochem.* **8**, 332.
Galanos, C., Lüderitz, O., and Westphal, O. (1969b). *Eur. J. Biochem.* **9**, 245.
Galanos, C., Rietschel, E. T., Lüderitz, O., and Westphal, O. (1971a). *Eur. J. Biochem.* **19**, 143.
Galanos, C., Lüderitz, O., and Westphal, O. (1971b). *Eur. J. Biochem.* **24**, 116.
Garegg, P. J., Lindberg, B., Onn, T., and Holme, T. (1971a). *Acta Chem. Scand.* **25**, 1185.
Garegg, P. J., Lindberg, B., Onn, T., and Sutherland, I. W. (1971b). *Acta Chem. Scand.* **25**, 2103.
Gelzer, J., and Kabat, E. A. (1964). *Immunochemistry* **1**, 303.
Gerety, R. J., Ferraresi, R. W., and Raffel, S. (1970). *J. Exp. Med.* **131**, 189.
Ghanta, V. K., Hamlin, N. M., Pretlow, T. G., and Hiramoto, R. N. (1972). *J. Immunol.* **109**, 810.
Girard, R., and Staub, A. M. (1974). *Carbohydr. Res.* **37**, 127.
Glazer, A. N., and Simmons, N. S. (1966). *J. Amer. Chem. Soc.* **88**, 2335.
Gleich, G. J., and Allan, P. Z. (1965). *Immunochemistry* **2**, 417.
Glynn, A. A. (1969). *Immunology* **16**, 463.
Glynn, A. A. (1972). "Microbial Pathogenicity in Man and Animals," p. 75. Cambridge Univ. Press, London and New York.
Glynn, A. A., and Howard, C. J. (1970). *Immunology* **18**, 331.
Gmeiner, J., Lüderitz, O., and Westphal, O. (1969). *Eur. J. Biochem.* **7**, 370.
Goebel, W. F. (1935). *J. Biol. Chem.* **110**, 391.
Goebel, W. F. (1938). *J. Exp. Med.* **68**, 469.
Goebel, W. F. (1939). *Nature (London)* **143**, 77.
Goebel, W. F. (1940). *J. Exp. Med.* **72**, 33.
Goebel, W. F. (1965). *Proc. Nat. Acad. Sci. U. S.* **49**, 464.
Goebel, W. F., and Avery, O. T. (1931a). *J. Exp. Med.* **54**, 431.
Goebel, W. F., and Avery, O. T. (1931b). *J. Exp. Med.* **54**, 457.
Goebel, W. F., Babers, F. H., and Avery, O. T. (1934a). *J. Exp. Med.* **60**, 85.
Goebel, W. F., Avery, O. T., and Babers, F. H. (1934b). *J. Exp. Med.* **60**, 599.
Goldstein, I. J., Hay, G. W., Lewis, B. A., and Smith, F. (1959). *Abstr. Pap. 135th Meet., Amer. Chem. Soc.* Paper No. 3D.
Goldstein, I. J., Hay, G. W., Lewis, B. A., and Smith, F. (1965). *Methods Carbohyd. Chem.* **5**, 361.
Gormus, B. J., and Wheat, R. W. (1971). *J. Bacteriol.* **108**, 1304.
Gormus, B. J., Wheat, R. W., and Porter, J. F. (1971). *J. Bacteriol.* **107**, 150.
Gotschlich, E. C., Goldschneider, I., and Artenstein, M. S. (1969). *J. Exp. Med.* **129**, 1367.
Grey, H. M., Hirst, J. W., and Cohn, M. (1971). *J. Exp. Med.* **133**, 289.
Gronwall, A., and Ingelman, B. (1944). *Acta Physiol. Scand.* **7**, 97.
Grundbacher, F. J. (1972). *Science* **176**, 311.
Guy, R. C. E., How, M. J., Stacey, M., and Heidelberger, M. (1967). *J. Biol. Chem.* **242**, 5106.
Haber, E. (1970). *Fed. Proc., Fed. Amer. Soc. Exp. Biol.* **29**, 66.
Hakomori, S. (1964). *J. Biochem. (Tokyo)* **55**, 205.
Halliday, W. J. (1971). *Bacteriol. Rev.* **35**, 267.
Hammer, D. (1961a). *Zentralbl. Veterinaermed.* **4**, 369.
Hammer, D. (1961b). *Zentralbl. Veterinaermed.* **5**, 405.
Hämmerling, G. J., and McDevitt, H. O. (1973). *Behring Res. Comm.* **53**, 28.

Hämmerling, G., Lüderitz, O., and Westphal, O. (1970). *Eur. J. Biochem.* **15**, 48.
Hämmerling, G., Lüderitz, O., Westphal, O., and Mäkelä, P. H. (1971). *Eur. J. Biochem.* **22**, 331.
Hämmerling, U., and Westphal, O. (1967). *Eur. J. Biochem.* **1**, 46.
Hanessian, S., and Haskell, T. (1964). *J. Biol. Chem.* **239**, 2758.
Hanson, L. Å. (1959). *Int. Arch. Allergy Appl. Immunol.* **14**, 279.
Harrisdangkul, V., and Kabat, E. A. (1972). *J. Immunol.* **108**, 1232.
Harrisdangkul, V., Kabat, E. A., McDonough, D. J., and Sigel, M. M. (1972). *J. Immunol.* **108**, 1259.
Hasenclever, H. F., and Mitchell, W. D. (1964). *J. Immunol.* **93**, 763.
Hay, G. W., Lewis, B. A., and Smith, F. (1965). *Methods Carbohyd. Chem.* **5**, 357.
Heidelberger, M. (1957). *Proc. Nat. Acad. Sci. U. S.* **43**, 883.
Heidelberger, M. (1960). *Fortschr. Chem. Org. Naturst.* **18**, 503.
Heidelberger, M. (1961). *Cancer Res.* **21**, 1524.
Heidelberger, M. (1962). *Arch. Biochem. Biophys. Suppl.* **1**, 169.
Heidelberger, M. (1963). *J. Immunol.* **91**, 735.
Heidelberger, M. (1967). *Annu. Rev. Biochem.* **36**, 1.
Heidelberger, M. (1973a). *Res. Immunochem. Immunobiol.* **3**, 1.
Heidelberger, M. (1973b). *In* "Immunologie" (P. Bordet, ed.), Suppl. Flammarion médecine-sciences, Paris.
Heidelberger, M., and Avery, O. T. (1923). *J. Exp. Med.* **38**, 73.
Heidelberger, M., and Avery, O. T. (1924). *J. Exp. Med.* **40**, 301.
Heidelberger, M., and Elliot, S. (1966). *J. Bacteriol.* **92**, 281.
Heidelberger, M., and Kendall, F. G. (1929). *J. Exp. Med.* **50**, 809.
Heidelberger, M., and Kendall, F. G. (1933). *J. Exp. Med.* **57**, 373.
Heidelberger, M., and MacPherson, C. F. C. (1943a). *Science* **97**, 405.
Heidelberger, M., and MacPherson, C. F. C. (1943b). *Science* **98**, 63.
Heidelberger, M., and Nimmich, W. (1972). *J. Immunol.* **109**, 1337.
Heidelberger, M., and Rebers, P. A. (1957). *Fed. Proc., Fed. Amer. Soc. Exp. Biol.* **16**, 194.
Heidelberger, M., and Rebers, P. A. (1958). *J. Amer. Chem. Soc.* **86**, 116.
Heidelberger, M., and Rebers, P. A. (1960). *J. Bacteriol.* **80**, 145.
Heidelberger, M., and Slodki, M. E. (1968). *J. Exp. Med.* **128**, 189.
Heidelberger, M., Kendall, F. G., and Scherp, H. W. (1936). *J. Exp. Med.* **64**, 559.
Heidelberger, M., MacLeod, C. M., Kaiser, S. J., and Robinson, B. (1946). *J. Exp. Med.* **83**, 303.
Heidelberger, M., MacLeod, C. M., Hodges, R. G., Bernhard, W. G., and diLapi, M. M. (1947). *J. Exp. Med.* **85**, 227.
Heidelberger, M., MacLeod, C. M., and DiLapi, M. M. (1951). *J. Immunol.* **66**, 145.
Heidelberger, M., Jann, K., Jann, B., Ørskov, F., Ørskov, I., and Westphal, O. (1968). *J. Immunol.* **95**, 2415.
Heidelberger, M., Roy, N., and Claudemans, C. P. J. (1969). *Biochemistry* **8**, 4822.
Heidelberger, M., Dudman, W. F., and Nimmich, W. (1970). *J. Immunol.* **104**, 1321.
Heidelberger, M., Gotschlich, E. C., and Higginbotham, J. D. (1972). *Carbohyd. Res.* **22**, 1.
Hellerqvist, C. G., Lindberg, B., Svensson, S., Holme, T., and Lindberg, A. A. (1968). *Carbohyd. Res.* **8**, 43.
Hellerqvist, C. G., Lindberg, B., Svensson, S., Holme, T., and Lindberg, A. A. (1969a). *Carbohyd. Res.* **9**, 237.

Hellerqvist, C. G., Lindberg, B., Svensson, S., Holme, T., and Lindberg, A. A. (1969b). *Acta Chem. Scand.* **23,** 1588.
Hellerqvist, C. G., Larm, O., Lindberg, B., Holme, T., and Lindberg, A. A. (1969c). *Acta Chem. Scand.* **23,** 2217.
Hellerqvist, C. G., Lindberg, B., Lönngren, J., and Lindberg, A. A. (1971a). *Carbohyd. Res.* **16,** 289.
Hellerqvist, C. G., Lindberg, B., Samuelson, K., and Lindberg, A. A. (1971b). *Acta Chem. Scand.* **25,** 955.
Hellerqvist, C. G., Lindberg, B., Pilotti, A., and Lindberg, A. A. (1971c). *Carbohyd. Res.* **16,** 297.
Hellerqvist, C. G., Lindberg, B., Samuelson, K., and Brubaker, R. R. (1972). *Acta Chem. Scand.* **26,** 1389.
Henriksen, S. D., Eriksen, J. (1962). *Acta Pathol. Microbiol. Scand.* **54,** 387.
Henriksen, S. D., Eriksen, J., and Maini, V. (1961). *Acta Pathol. Microbiol. Scand.* **51,** 259.
Heyns, K., and Kiessling, G. (1967). *Carbohyd. Res.* **3,** 340.
Higginbotham, J. D., and Heidelberger, M. (1972). *Carbohyd. Res.* **23,** 165.
Higginbotham, J. D., Das, A., and Heidelberger, M. (1972). *Biochem. J.* **126,** 225.
Himmelspach, K., and Wrede, J. (1971). *FEBS (Fed. Eur. Biochem. Soc.) Lett.* **18,** 118.
Himmelspach, K., Westphal, O., and Teichmann, B. (1971). *Eur. J. Immunol.* **1,** 106.
Hirase, S. (1957). *Bull. Chem. Soc. Jap.* **30,** 75.
Hirata, A. A., and Terasaki, P. I. (1970). *Science* **168,** 1095.
Holmgren, J., Eggersten, G., Hanson, L. Å., and Lincoln, K. (1969). *Acta Pathol. Microbiol. Scand.* **76,** 304.
Holmgren, J., Hanson, L. Å., Holm, S. E., and Kaijser, B. (1971). *Int. Arch. Allergy Appl. Immunol.* **41,** 463.
Holowka, D. A., Strosberg, A. D., Kimball, J. W., Haber, E., and Cathou, R. E. (1972). *Proc. Nat. Acad. Sci. U. S.* **69,** 3399.
How, M. J., Brimacombe, J. S., and Stacey, M. (1964). *Advan. Carbohyd. Chem.* **19,** 303.
Howard, C. J., and Glynn, A. A. (1971). *Immunology* **20,** 767.
Howard, J. G. (1972). *Transplant. Rev.* **8,** 50.
Howard, J. G., Elson, J., Christie, G. H., and Kinski, R. G. (1969). *Clin. Exp. Immunol.* **4,** 41.
Howard, J. G., Christie, G. H., and Courtenay, B. M. (1970a). *Transplantation* **10,** 351.
Howard, J. G., Christie, G. H., Jacob, M. J., and Elson, J. (1970b). *Clin. Exp. Immunol.* **7,** 583.
Howard, J. G., Zola, H., Christie, G. H., and Courtenay, B. M. (1971a). *J. Immunol.* **21,** 535.
Howard, J. G., Christie, G. H., and Courtenay, B. M. (1971b). *Proc. Roy. Soc., Ser. B* **178,** 417.
Howard, J. G., Christie, G. H., Courtenay, B. M., Leuchars, E., and Davies, A. J. S. (1971c). *Cell. Immunol.* **2,** 614.
Howard, J. G., Christie, G. H., Courtenay, B. M., and Biozzi, G. (1972). *Eur. J. Immunol.* **2,** 269.
Howard, J. G., and Courtenay, B. M. (1974). *Eur. J. Immunol.* **4,** 603.
Hungerer, D., Jann, K., Jann, B., Ørskov, F., and Ørskov, I. (1967). *Eur. J. Biochem.* **2,** 115.
Isbell, H. S. (1951). *Science* **113,** 532.

1. Microbial Polysaccharides 117

Iseki, S., and Kashiwagi, K. (1953). *Proc. Jap. Acad.* **31**, 558.
Iseki, S., and Sakai, T. (1953). *Proc. Jap. Acad.* **29**, 127.
Janeway, C. A., Jr., and Sela, M. (1967). *Immunology* **13**, 29.
Jann, B., and Jann, K. (1975). In preparation.
Jann, B., Jann, K., Schmidt, G., Ørskov, I., and Ørskov, F. (1970). *Eur. J. Biochem.* **15**, 29.
Jann, B., Jann, K., Schmidt, G., Ørskov, I. (1972). *Eur. J. Biochem.* **23**, 515.
Jann, K., Jann, B, Ørskov, F., Ørskov, I., and Westphal, O. (1965). *Biochem. Z.* **342**, 1.
Jann, K., Jann, B., and Schneider, K. F. (1968). *Eur. J. Biochem.* **5**, 456.
Jann, K., Jann, B., Ørskov, F., and Ørskov, I. (1971). *Biochem. Z.* **346**, 368.
Jaton, J. C., Waterfield, M. D., Margolies, M. N., and Haber, E. (1970). *Proc. Nat. Acad. Sci. U. S.* **66**, 959.
Jenkin, C. R., and Rowley, D. (1963). *Bacteriol. Rev.* **27**, 391.
Jerne, N. K., and Nordin, A. A. (1963). *Science* **140**, 405.
Johnson, C. N., and Phillips, D. C. (1965). *Nature (London)* **206**, 761.
Johnston, I. R. (1965). *Biochem. J.* **96**, 689.
Johnston, J. H., Johnston, R. J., and Simmons, D. A. R. (1968). *Arch. Immunol. Ther. Exp.* **16**, 252.
Jones, G. H., and Ballou, C. E. (1969a). *J. Biol. Chem.* **244**, 1043.
Jones, G. H., and Ballou, C. E. (1969b). *J. Biol. Chem.* **244**, 1052.
Jones, J. K. N., and Perry, M. B. (1957). *J. Amer. Chem. Soc.* **79**, 2787.
Kabat, E. A. (1956). *J. Immunol.* **77**, 377.
Kabat, E. A. (1957). *Rev. Hematol.* **12**, 606.
Kabat, E. A. (1960). *J. Immunol.* **84**, 82.
Kabat, E. A. (1966). *J. Immunol.* **97**, 1.
Kabat, E. A. (1968). "Structural Concepts in Immunology and Immunochemistry." Holt, New York.
Kabat, E. A., and Berg, D. (1952). *Ann. N. Y. Acad. Sci.* **55**, 471.
Kabat, E. A., and Berg, D. (1953). *J. Immunol.* **70**, 514.
Kabat, E. A., and Bezer, A. E. (1958). *Arch. Biochem. Biophys.* **78**, 306.
Kabat, E. A., and Mayer, M. M. (1961). "Experimental Immunochemistry," 2nd ed. Thomas, Springfield, Illinois.
Kaijser, B., and Olling, S. (1973). *J. Infec. Dis.* **128**, 41.
Kang, S., and Markovitz, A. (1966). *Fed. Proc., Fed. Amer. Soc. Exp. Biol.* **25**, 836.
Kaplan, M. H., Coons, A. H., and Deane, H. W. (1950). *J. Exp. Med.* **91**, 15.
Karakawa, W. W., Wagner, J. E., and Pazur, J. H. (1971). *J. Immunol.* **107**, 554.
Kärkäinen, J. (1970). *Carbohyd. Res.* **14**, 27.
Katz, M., and Pappenheimer, A. M. R. (1969). *J. Immunol.* **103**, 491.
Kauffmann, F. (1940). *Acta Pathol. Microbiol. Scand.* **17**, 134.
Kauffmann, F. (1941a). *J. Bacteriol.* **41**, 127.
Kauffmann, F. (1941b). *Acta Pathol. Microbiol. Scand.* **18**, 225.
Kauffmann, F. (1953). *Acta Pathol. Microbiol. Scand.* **33**, 409.
Kauffmann, F. (1954). "Enterobacteriaceae," Munksgaard, Copenhagen.
Kauffmann, F. (1956). *Acta Pathol. Microbiol. Scand.* **39**, 299.
Kauffmann, F. (1957). *Acta Pathol. Microbiol. Scand.* **40**, 343.
Kauffmann, F. (1961). "Die Bakteriologie der Salmonella Species." Munksgaard, Copenhagen.
Kauffmann, F. (1966). "The Bacteriology of Enterobacteriaceae." Munksgaard, Copenhagen.

Kauffmann, F., Lüderitz, O., Stierlin, H., and Westphal, O. (1960). *Zentralbl. Bakteriol., Parasitenk., Infektionskr. Hyg., Abt. 1: Orig.* **178**, 442.
Kauffmann, F., Jann, B., Krüger, L., Lüderitz, O., and Westphal, O. (1962). *Zentralbl. Bakteriol., Parasitenk., Infektionskr. Hyg., Abt. 1: Orig.* **186**, 509.
Kearney, R., and Halliday, W. J. (1970a). *Immunology* **19**, 551.
Kearney, R., and Halliday, W. J. (1970b). *Aust. J. Exp. Med. Sci.* **48**, 215.
Kearney, R., and Halliday, W. J. (1970c). *Aust. J. Exp. Med. Sci.* **48**, 227.
Keleti, J., Mayer, H., Fromme, I., and Lüderitz, O. (1970). *Eur. J. Biochem.* **16**, 284.
Kennedy, D. A., Buchanan, J. G., and Baddiley, J. (1969). *Biochem. J.* **115**, 37.
Kimball, J. W., Pappenheimer, A. M., Jr., and Jaton, J. C. (1971). *J. Immunol.* **106**, 1177.
Kindt, T. J., Todd, D. V., Eichmann, K., and Krause, R. M. (1970). *J. Exp. Med.* **131**, 343.
Kleinhammer, G., Himmelspach, K., and Westphal, O. (1973). *Eur. J. Immunol.* **3**, 834.
Knecht, J. C., Schiffman, G., and Austrian, R. (1970). *J. Exp. Med.* **132**, 475.
Kocourek, J., and Ballou, C. E. (1969). *J. Bacteriol.* **100**, 1175.
Kotelko, K., Staub, A. M., and Tinelli, R. (1961). *Ann. Inst. Pasteur, Paris* **100**, 618.
Krause, R. M. (1963). *Bacteriol. Rev.* **27**, 369.
Krause, R. M. (1970). *Fed. Proc., Fed. Amer. Soc. Exp. Biol.* **29**, 59.
Krause, R. M., and McCarty, M. C. (1962). *J. Exp. Med.* **116**, 131.
Kunkel, H. G., Mannik, M., and Williams, R. C. (1962). *Science* **140**, 1218.
Lancefield, R. C. (1933). *J. Exp. Med.* **57**, 571.
Lancefield, R. C. (1940). *Harvey Lect.* **36**, 251.
Larm, O., Lindberg, B., Svensson, S., and Kabat, E. A. (1972). *Carbohyd. Res.* **22**, 391.
Lawson, C. J., McCleary, C. W., Nakada, H. I., Rees, D. A., Sutherland, I. W., and Wilkinson, J. F. (1969). *Biochem. J.* **115**, 947.
Le-Ba Nhan, Jann, K., Jann, B., Ørskov, F., and Ørskov, I. (1971). *Eur. J. Biochem.* **21**, 226.
Lee, Y. C., and Ballou, C. E. (1965). *Biochemistry* **4**, 257.
Le Minor, L. (1963). *Ann. Inst. Pasteur, Paris* **105**, 879.
Le Minor, L. (1965). *Ann. Inst. Pasteur, Paris* **109**, 505.
Le Minor, L. (1968). *Ann. Inst. Pasteur, Paris,* **115**, 62.
Leon, M. A., and Takahashi, I. (1970). *In* "Proceedings of the Fifth Leukocyte Culture Conference" (J. E. Harris, ed.), p. 299. Academic Press, New York.
Leon, M. A., and Young, N. M. (1971). *Biochemistry* **10**, 1424.
Leon, M. A., Young, N. M., and MacIntire, K. R. (1970). *Biochemistry* **9**, 1023.
Lichtenberg, L., Shearer, G. M., Mozes, E., and Sela, M. (1972). *Isr. J. Med. Sci.* **8**, 149.
Lindberg, A. A. (1973). *Annu. Rev. Microbiol.* **23**, 205.
Lindberg, B., Lönngren, J., and Nimmich, W. (1972a). *Carbohyd. Res.* **23**, 47.
Lindberg, B., Lönngren, J., and Nimmich, W. (1972b). *Acta Chem. Scand.* **26**, 2231.
Lindberg, B., Lönngren, J., Thompson, J. L., and Nimmich, W. (1972c). *Carbohyd. Res.* **25**, 49.
Lindberg, B., Lönngren, J., Ruden, U., and Simmons, D. A. R. (1973a). *Eur. J. Biochem.* **32**, 15.
Lindberg, B., Samuelson, K., and Nimmich, W. (1973b). *Carbohyd. Res.* **30**, 63.
Lindberg, B., Lönngren, J., Nimmich, W., and Ruden, U. (1973c). *Acta Chem. Scand.* **27**, 3787.
Lipke, P. N., Raschke, W. C., and Ballou, C. E. (1974). *Carbohydr. Res.* **37**, 23.
Losick, R., and Robbins, P. W. (1967). *J. Mol. Biol.* **30**, 445.
Lüderitz, O. (1970). *Angew. Chem., Int. Ed. Engl.* **9**, 649.
Lüderitz, O., and Westphal, O. (1966). *Angew. Chem.* **78**, 172.

Lüderitz, O., Westphal, O., Sievers, K., Kröger, E., Neter, E., and Braun, O. H. (1957). *Biochem. Z.* **330**, 21.
Lüderitz, O., Staub, A. M., Stirm, S., and Westphal, O. (1958). *Biochem. Z.* **330**, 193.
Lüderitz, O., Westphal, O., Staub, A. M., and Le Minor, L. (1960). *Nature (London)* **188**, 556.
Lüderitz, O., Staub, A. M., and Westphal, O. (1966a). *Bacteriol. Rev.* **30**, 192.
Lüderitz, O., Galanos, C., Risse, H. J., Ruschmann, E., Schlecht, S., Schmidt, G., Schulte-Holthausen, H., Wheat, R., Westphal, O., and Schlosshardt, J. (1966b). *Ann. N. Y. Acad. Sci.* **133**, 349.
Lüderitz, O., Ruschmann, E., Westphal, O., Raff, R., and Wheat, R. (1967). *J. Bacteriol.* **93**, 1681.
Lüderitz, O., Jann, K., and Wheat, R. (1968a). *Compr. Biochem.* **26A**, 105.
Lüderitz, O., Gmeiner, J., Kickhöfen, B., Mayer, H., Westphal, O., and Wheat, R. (1968b). *J. Bacteriol.* **95**, 490.
Lüderitz, O., Westphal, O., Staub, A. M., and Nikaido, H. (1971). *In* "Microbial Toxins" (G. Weinbaum, S. Kadis, and S. J. Ajl, eds.), Vol. IV, p. 145. Academic Press, New York.
Lüderitz, O., Galanos, C., Lehmann, V., Nurminen, M., Rietschel, E. T., Rosenfelder, G., Simon, M., and Westphal, O. (1973). *In* "Bacterial Lipopolysaccharides" (K. Kass and S. M. Wolff, eds.), pp. 9–21. Univ. of Chicago Press, Chicago, Illinois.
Lundblad, A., Steller, R., Kabat, E. A., Hirst, J. W., Weigert, M. G., and Cohn, M. (1970). *Immunochemistry* **9**, 535.
McCabe, W. R. (1972). *J. Immunol.* **108**, 601.
McCabe, W. R., Greely, A., DiGenio, T., and Johns, M. A. (1973). *In* "Bacterial Lipopolysaccharides" (E. H. Kass and S. M. Wolff, eds.), p. 276–81. Univ. of Chicago Press, Chicago, Illinois.
McCarty, M. C. (1956). *J. Exp. Med.* **104**, 629.
McCarty, M. C. (1958). *J. Exp. Med.* **108**, 311.
McCarty, M. C. (1964). *Proc. Nat. Acad. Sci. U. S.* **51**, 259.
McCarty, M. C., and Lancefield, R. C. (1955). *J. Exp. Med.* **102**, 11.
McDevitt, H. O. and Landy, M., eds. (1972). "Genetic Control of Immune Responsiveness." Academic Press, New York.
McIntire, K. R., and Princler, G. (1969). *Immunology* **17**, 481.
Mackaness, G. B. (1970). *In* "Infectious Agents, and Host Reactions" (S. Mudd, ed.), p. 22 Saunders, Philadelphia, Pennsylvania.
Mackaness, G. B. (1971). *In* "Cell Mediated Immunity: Cellular Interactions in the Immune Response," 2nd Int. Convoc. Immunol., 1970, p. 241. Karger, Basel.
Mackaness, G. B., Blanden, R. V., and Collins, F. M. (1966). *J. Exp. Med.* **124**, 573.
MacLeod, C. M. (1970). *In* "Infectious Agents and Host Reactions" (S. Mudd, ed.), p. 165. Saunders, Philadelphia, Pennsylvania.
MacLeod, C. M., Hodges, R. G., Heidelberger, M., and Robinson, B. (1946). *J. Exp. Med.* **83**, 303.
Mage, R. G., and Kabat, E. A. (1963a). *Biochemistry* **2**, 1278.
Mage, R. G., and Kabat, E. A. (1963b). *J. Immunol.* **91**, 633.
Mäkelä, P. H. (1966). *J. Bacteriol.* **92**, 518.
Mäkelä, P. H., and Mäkelä, O. (1966). *Ann. Med. Exp. Biol. Fenn.* **44**, 310.
Mäkelä, P. H., and Sarvas, M. (1969). *In* "Structure et effets biòlogiques des produits bactériens provenant des germes Gram négatifs," p. 201. CNRS, Paris.
Mäkelä, P. H., and Stocker, B.A. D. (1969). *Annu. Rev. Genet.* **3**, 309.
Mäkelä, P. H., Valtonen, V. V., and Valtonen, M. (1973). *J. Infec. Dis.* **128**, 81.

Manning, J. K., Reed, N. D., and Jutila, J. W. (1972). *J. Immunol.* **108**, 1470.
Marchalonis, J. J., Morris, P. J., and Harris, A. W. (1974). *J. Immunogenetics* **1**, 63.
Markley, S., and Smallmann, E. (1968). *J. Bacteriol.* **96**, 867.
Markovitz, A. (1964). *Proc. Nat. Acad. Sci. U. S.* **51**, 239.
Markovitz, A., and Rosenbaum, N. (1965). *Proc. Nat. Acad. Sci. U. S.* **54**, 1084.
Matsuhashi, S., and Strominger, J. L. (1965). *Biochem. Biophys. Res. Comm.* **20**, 169.
Maurer, P. H. (1953). *Proc. Soc. Exp. Biol. Med.* **83**, 879.
Mayer, H., Framberg, K., and Weckesser, J. (1974). *Eur. J. Biochem.* **44**, 181.
Medlin, J., Humphrey, J. H., and Sela M. (1970). *Folia Biol. (Prague)* **16**, 145.
Michel, M. F., and Krause, R. M. (1967). *J. Exp. Med.* **125**, 1075.
Mill, P. (1966). *J. Can. Microbiol.* **44**, 329.
Miller, E. C., Osterland, C. K., Davie, J. M., and Krause, R. M. (1967). *J. Immunol.* **98**, 710.
Mills, G. T., and Smith, E. E. B. (1962). *Fed. Proc., Fed. Amer. Soc. Exp. Biol.* **21**, 1089.
Minden, P., and Farr, S. R. (1973). *In* "Handbook of Experimental Immunology" (D. M. Weir, ed.), 2nd ed., 15.1. Blackwell, Oxford.
Minden, P., Anthony, B. F., and Farr, R. S. (1969). *J. Immunol.* **102**, 832.
Mitchell, W. D., and Hasenclever, H. F. (1970). *Infec. Immunity* **1**, 61.
Mitchison, N. A. (1968a). *Immunology* **15**, 531.
Mitchison, N. A. (1968b). *Immunology* **16**, 1.
Mittal, K. K., Terasaki, P. I., Springer, G. F., Desai, P. R., McIntire, F. C., and Hirata, A. A. (1973). *Transplant. Proc.* **5**, 499.
Miyuzaki, T., and Jones, J. K. N. (1969). *Chem. Pharm. Bull.* **17**, 1531.
Miyuzaki, T., and Yadomae, T. (1971). *Carbohyd. Res.* **16**, 153.
Möller, G., Andersson, J., and Sjöberg, O. (1972). *Cell. Immunol.* **4**, 416.
Morgan, W. T. J., and Partridge, S. M. (1940). *Biochem. J.* **34**, 169.
Morgan, W. T. J., and Partridge, S. M. (1941). *Biochem. J.* **35**, 1140.
Morgan, W. T. J., and Partridge, S. M. (1942). *Brit. J. Exp. Pathol.* **23**, 151.
Moyer, J. D., and Isbell, H. S. (1958). *Anal. Chem.* **30**, 1975.
Mozes, E., and Shearer, G. M. (1971). *J. Exp. Med.* **134**, 141.
Mudd, S. ed. (1970). "Infectious Agents and Host Reactions." Saunders, Philadelphia, Pennsylvania.
Müller-Seitz, E., Jann, B., and Jann, K. (1968). *FEBS (Fed. Eur. Biochem. Soc.) Lett.* **1**, 311.
Muschel, L. H., and Treffers, H. P. (1956). *Immunology* **76**, 1.
Naide, Y., Nikaido, H., Mäkelä, P. H., Wilkinson, R. G., and Stocker, B. A. D. (1965). *Proc. Nat. Acad. Sci. U. S.* **53**, 147.
Nakla, L. S., and Glynn, L. E. (1967). *Immunology* **13**, 209.
Neter, E. (1956). *Bacteriol. Rev.* **20**, 166.
Neter, E. (1962). *Nature (London)* **194**, 1256.
Neter, E., Westphal, O., Lüderitz, O., Borzynski, E. A., and Eichenberger, E. (1956). *J. Immunol.* **76**, 377.
Neter, E., Whang, H. Y., and Mayer, H. (1973). *In* "Bacterial Lipopolysaccharides" (E. H. Kass and S. M. Wolff, eds.), Univ. of Chicago Press, p. 48. Chicago, Illinois.
Neufeld, F. (1902). *Z. Hyg.* **11**, 54.
Neumüller, G. (1945). *Ark. Kemi* **21A**, 1.
Nghiem, H. O., Bagdian, G., and Staub, A. M. (1967). *Eur. J. Biochem.* **2**, 392.
Nikaido, H. (1968). *Advan. Enzymol.* **31**, 77.
Nikaido, H. (1974). *In* "Bacterial Membranes and Walls" (L. Leive, ed.), Microbiol. Ser., Vol. 1, p. 131. Dekker, New York.

Nikaido, H., Naide, Y., and Mäkelä, P. H. (1966). *Ann. N. Y. Acad. Sci.* **133**, 299.
Nimmich, W. (1968). *Z. Med. Mikrobiol. Immunol.* **154**, 117.
Nimmich, W. (1969). *Acta Biol. Med. Germ.* **22**, 191.
Nimmich, W. (1971). *Acta Biol. Med. Germ.* **26**, 397.
Nordin, P. (1962). *Methods Carbohyd. Chem.* **2**, 136.
Northcote, D. H., and Horne, R. W. (1952). *Biochem. J.* **51**, 232.
Ohle, H., and Kruyff, J. J. (1944). *Ber. Deut. Chem. Ges.* **77**, 507.
Ohle, H., and Liebig, R. (1942). *Ber. Deut. Chem. Ges.* **75**, 1536.
Ohle, H., and Melkonian, G. A. (1941a). *Ber. Deut. Chem. Ges.* **74**, 279.
Ohle, H., and Melkonian, G. A. (1941b). *Ber. Deut. Chem. Ges.* **74**, 398.
Orentas, D. G., Sloneker, J. H., and Jeanes, A. (1965). *Can. J. Microbiol.* **9**, 427.
Ørskov, F., Ørskov, I., Jann, B., Jann, K., Müller-Seitz, E., and Westphal, O. (1967). *Acta Pathol. Microbiol. Scand.* **71**, 339.
Ørskov, F., Ørskov, I., Jann, B., and Jann, K. (1971). *Acta Pathol. Microbiol. Scand.* **79**, 142.
Ørskov, I., Ørskov, F., Jann, B. and Jann, K. (1963). *Nature (London)* **200**, 144.
Osborn, M. J. (1969). *Annu. Rev. Biochem.* **38**, 501.
Osterland, C. K., Miller, E. J., Karakawa, W. W., and Krause, R. M. (1966). *J. Exp. Med.* **123**, 599.
Ouchterlony, Ö. (1958). *Progr. Allergy* **5**, 1.
Painter, T. J. (1960). *Chem. Ind. (London)* p. 1214.
Painter, T. J., and Morgan, W. T. J. (1961). *Chem. Ind. (London)* p. 437.
Pappenheimer, A. M., Jr., Reed, W. D., and Brown, J. (1968). *J. Immunol.* **100**, 1237.
Parish, C. R., and Ada, G. L. (1969). *Immunology* **17**, 153.
Parker, C. W., and Osterland, C. K. (1970). *Biochemistry* **9**, 1074.
Parkhouse, R. M. E., and Askonas, B. A. (1969). *Biochem. J.* **115**, 163.
Pavlovskis, O. R., and Slade, H. D. (1971). *Int. Arch. Allergy Appl. Immunol.* **40**, 820.
Perlzweig, W. A., and Steffen, G. I. (1923). *J. Exp. Med.* **38**, 163.
Pinckard, R. N., and Weir, D. M. (1973). *In* "Handbook of Experimental Immunology" (D. M. Weir, ed.), 2nd ed., 16.1. Blackwell, Oxford.
Pincus, J. H., Haber, E., and Katz, M. (1968). *Science* **162**, 667.
Pincus, J. H., Jaton, J. C., Bloch, K. J., and Haber, E. (1970a). *J. Immunol.* **104**, 1143.
Pincus, J. H., Jaton, J. C., Bloch, K. J., and Haber, E. (1970b). *J. Immunol.* **104**, 1149.
Potter, M. (1967). *Methods Cancer Res.* **2**, 105.
Potter, M. (1970). *Fed. Proc., Fed. Amer. Soc. Exp. Biol.* **29**, 85.
Potter, M., and Leon, M. A. (1968). *Science* **162**, 369.
Potter, M., and Liebermann, R. (1967). *Cold Spring Harbor Symp. Quant. Biol.* **32**, 187.
Prehm, P. (1974). Dissertation, University of Freiburg.
Prehm, P., Jann, B., Stirm, S., and Jann, K. (1975). *Eur. J. Biochem.* (in press).
Rao, C. V. N., and Heidelberger, M. (1966). *J. Exp. Med.* **123**, 913.
Raschke, W. C., and Ballou, C. E. (1971). *Biochemistry* **10**, 4130.
Raschke, W. C., and Ballou, C. E. (1972). *Biochemistry* **11**, 3807.
Rebers, P. A., and Heidelberger, M. (1959). *J. Amer. Chem. Soc.* **81**, 2415.
Rebers, P. A., and Heidelberger, M. (1961). *J. Amer. Chem. Soc.* **83**, 3056.
Rebers, P. A., Hurwitz, E., and Heidelberger, M. (1961). *J. Bacteriol.* **82**, 920.
Reed, N. D., Manning, J. K., and Rudbach, J. A. (1973). *In* "Bacterial Lipopolysaccharides" (E. H. Kass and S. M. Wolff, eds.), p. 62. Univ. of Chicago Press, Chicago, Illinois.
Rees, D. A. (1969). *J. Chem. Soc., London* p. 217.
Rees, D. A. (1972). *Biochem. J.* **126**, 257.

Reeves, R. E., and Goebel, W. F. (1941). *J. Biol. Chem.* **19**, 511.
Reisfeld, R. A., and Small, P. A., Jr. (1966). *Science* **152**, 1253.
Reske, K., and Jann, K. (1972). *Eur. J. Biochem.* **31**, 320.
Reske, K., Wallenfels, B., and Jann, K. (1973). *Eur. J. Biochem.* **36**, 167.
Ribi, E., Anacker, R. L., Brown, R., Haskins, W. T., Malmgren, B., Milner, K. C., and Rudbach, J. A. (1966). *J. Bacteriol.* **92**, 1493.
Rietschel, E. T., Galanos, C., Tanaka, A., Ruschmann, E., Lüderitz, O., and Westphal, O. (1971). *Eur. J. Biochem.* **22**, 218.
Roantree, R. J. (1967). *Annu. Rev. Microbiol.* **21**, 443.
Robbins, P. W., and Uchida, T. (1962). *Biochemistry* **1**, 323.
Robbins, P. W., and Uchida, T. (1965). *J. Biol. Chem.* **240**, 375.
Robbins, P. W., and Wright, A. (1971). *In* "Microbial Toxins" (G. Weinbaum, S. Kadis, and J. S. Ajl, eds.), Vol. IV, p. 351. Academic Press, New York.
Robbins, P. W., Keller, J. M., Wright, A., and Bernstein, R. L. (1965). *J. Biol. Chem.* **240**, 384.
Rodkey, L. S., Choi, T. K., and Nisonoff, A. (1970). *J. Immunol.* **104**, 63.
Romeo, D., Girard, A., and Rothfield, L. (1970). *J. Mol. Biol.* **53**, 475.
Rosenberg, E., Leidy, G., Jaffee, I., and Zamenhof, S. (1961). *J. Biol. Chem.* **236**, 2845.
Rothfield, L., and Romeo, D. (1971). *Bacteriol. Rev.* **35**, 14.
Rovis, L., Kabat, E. A., and Potter, M. (1972). *Carbohyd. Res.* **23**, 223.
Rowley, D., and Jenkin, C. R. (1962). *Nature (London)* **193**, 151.
Rowley, D., Turner, K. J., and Jenkin, C. R. (1964). *Aust. J. Exp. Biol. Med. Sci.* **42**, 237.
Roy, N., Carroll, W. R., and Glaudemans, C. P. J. (1970). *Carbohyd. Res.* **12**, 89.
Rudbach, J. A. (1971). *J. Immunol.* **106**, 993.
Russell, H., and Norcross, N. L. (1972). *J. Immunol.* **109**, 90.
Samuelson, K., Lindberg, B., and Brubaker, R. R. (1974). *J. Bacteriol.* **117**, 1010.
Sandford, P. A., and Conrad, H. E. (1966). *Biochemistry* **5**, 1508.
Sanford, J. P., Hunter, B. M., and Souda, L. L. (1961). *J. Exp. Med.* **115**, 383.
Sasaki, T., and Uchida, T. (1974). *J. Bacteriol.* **117**, 13.
Sawardeker, J. S., Sloneker, J. H., and Jeanes, A. (1967). *Anal. Chem.* **37**, 1602.
Schachman, H. K. (1959). "Ultracentrifugation in Biochemistry." Academic Press, New York.
Schalch, D. S., and Parker, M. I. (1964). *Nature (London)* **203**, 1241.
Scher, M., Kramer, K., and Lennartz (1967). *Abstr. Pap., 154th Nat. Meet. Amer. Chem. Soc. Abstract, D43.*
Schiemann, O., and Casper, W. (1927). *Z. Hyg.* **108**, 220.
Schlecht, S., and Westphal, O. (1970). *Zentralbl. Bakteriol., Parasitenk., Infektionskr. Hyg., Abt. 1: Orig.* **213**, 356.
Schlecht, S., Böhlck, I., and Westphal, O. (1971). *Zentralbl. Bakteriol., Parasitenk., Infektionskr. Hyg., Abt. 1: Orig.* **216**, 472.
Schlosshardt, J. (1960). *Zentralbl. Bakteriol., Parasitenk., Infektionskr. Hyg., Abt. 1: Orig.* **177**, 176.
Schlosshardt, J. (1964). *Zentralbl. Bakteriol., Parasitenk., Infektionskr. Hyg., Abt. 1: Orig.* **192**, 54.
Schlossman, S. F., and Kabat, E. A. (1962). *J. Exp. Med.* **116**, 535.
Schmidt, G. (1973). *J. Gen. Microbiol.* **77**, 151.
Schmidt, G., Jann, B., and Jann, K. (1969). *Eur. J. Biochem.* **10**, 501.
Schmidt, G., Fromme, I., and Mayer, H. (1970a). *Eur. J. Biochem.* **14**, 357.
Schmidt, G., Jann, B., and Jann, K. (1970b). *Eur. J. Biochem.* **16**, 382.

1. Microbial Polysaccharides

Schmidt, G., Jann, B., and Jann, K. (1974). *Eur. J. Biochem.* **42**, 303.
Schmidt, W. C. (1952). *J. Exp. Med.* **95**, 105.
Schramm, G., Westphal, O., and Lüderitz, O. (1952). *Z. Naturforsch.* **7b**, 594.
Schwarzman, S., and Boring, J. R., III. (1971). *Infect. Immun.* **3**, 762.
Schwarzmüller, E. (1972). Dissertation, University of Freiburg.
Scott, J. E. (1960). *Methods Biochem. Anal.* **8**, 145.
Sela, M. (1966). *Advan. Immunol.* **5**, 29.
Sela, M. (1973). *Harvey Lect.* **67**, 213.
Sela, M. (1974). *Bull. Inst. Pasteur*, **72**, 73.
Sela, M., Mozes, E., and Shearer, G. M. (1972). *Proc. Nat. Acad. Sci. U. S.* **69**, 2696.
Sela, M., Schechter, T., Schechter, B., and Borek, F. (1967). *Cold Spring Harbor Symp. Quant. Biol.* **32**, 537.
Seltmann, G. (1968). *Arch. Immunol. Ther. Exp.* **16**, 367.
Seltmann, G., and Hofmann, S. (1966). *Zentralbl. Bakteriol., Parasitenk., Infektionskr. Hyg., Abt. 1: Orig.* **199**, 497.
Shabarova, Z. A., Buchanan, J. G., and Baddiley, J. (1962). *Biochim. Biophys. Acta* **57**, 146.
Shaw, N., and Baddiley, J. (1964). *Biochem. J.* **93**, 317.
Shearer, G. M., Mozes, E., and Sela, M. (1972). *J. Exp. Med.* **135**, 1009.
Shellam, G. R., and Nossal, G. J. V. (1968). *Immunology* **14**, 273.
Simmons, D. A. R. (1957). *J. Gen. Microbiol.* **17**, 650.
Simmons, D. A. R. (1962). *Biochem. J.* **84**, 353.
Simmons, D. A. R. (1966). *Biochem. J.* **98**, 903.
Simmons, D. A. R., Lüderitz, O., and Westphal, O. (1965a). *Biochem. J.* **97**, 807.
Simmons, D. A. R., Lüderitz, O., and Westphal, O. (1965b). *Biochem. J.* **97**, 815.
Simmons, D. A. R., Lüderitz, O., and Westphal, O. (1965c). *Biochem. J.* **97**, 820.
Siskind, G. W., Paul, W. E., and Benacerraf, B. (1967). *Immunochemistry* **4**, 455.
Sjöstedt, S. S. (1946). *Acta Pathol. Microbiol. Scand.* **63**, *Suppl.*, 1.
Slade, H. D., and Hämmerling, U. (1968). *J. Bacteriol.* **95**, 1572.
Slodki, M. E. (1962). *Biochim. Biophys. Acta* **57**, 525.
Slodki, M. E. (1966). *J. Biol. Chem.* **241**, 2700.
Sloneker, J. H., and Orentas, D. G. (1962). *Can. J. Chem.* **40**, 2188.
Smith, F., and Montgomery, R. (1956). *Methods Biochem. Anal.* **3**, 153.
Smith, H. (1968). *Bacteriol. Rev.* **32**, 164.
Smith, H., and Path, F. C. (1969). *Brit. Med. Bull.* **25**, 126.
Smith, H. W., and Parsell, Z. (1974). *J. Gen. Microbiol.* **81**, 217.
Soprey, P., and Slade, H. D. (1971). *Infec. Immunity* **3**, 653.
Soprey, P., and Slade, H. D. (1972). *Infec. Immunity* **5**, 91.
Sorg, C., Rüde, E., and Westphal, O. (1970a). *Justus Liebigs Ann. Chem.* **734**, 180.
Sorg, C., Rüde, E., and Westphal, O. (1970b). *Eur. J. Biochem.* **17**, 85.
Spaun, J., and Uemura, K. (1964). *Bull. WHO* **31**, 761.
Springer, E. L., and Roth, I. L. (1973). *J. Gen. Microbiol.* **74**, 21.
Springer, G. F. (1970). *Ann. N. Y. Acad. Sci.* **169**, 134.
Springer, G. F. (1971). *Progr. Allergy* **15**, 9.
Springer, G. F., and Horton, R. E. (1969). *J. Clin. Invest.* **48**, 1280.
Springer, G. F., and Williamson, P. (1962). *Biochem. J.* **85**, 282.
Springer, G. F., Mittal, K. K., Terasaki, P. I., Desai, P. R., McIntire, F. C., and Hirata, A. A. (1973). *Z. Immunitaetsforsch., Exp. Klin. Immunol.* **145**, 166.
Staub, A. M. (1961). *Pathol. Microbiol.* **24**, 890.
Staub, A. M. (1965). *Methods Carbohyd. Res.* **5**, 92.

Staub, A. M., and Bagdian, G. (1966). *Ann. Inst. Pasteur, Paris* **110**, 849.
Staub, A. M., and Forest, N. (1963). *Ann. Inst. Pasteur, Paris* **104**, 371.
Staub, A. M., and Girard, R. (1965). *Bull. Soc. Chim. Biol.* **47**, 1245.
Staub, A. M., and Tinelli, R. (1957). *Bull. Soc. Chim. Biol.* **39**, Suppl. 1, 65.
Staub, A. M., and Westphal, O. (1964). *Bull. Soc. Chim. Biol.* **46**, 1647.
Staub, A. M., Tinelli, R., Lüderitz, O., and Westphal, O. (1959). *Ann. Inst. Pasteur, Paris* **96**, 303.
Staub, A. M., Stirm, S., Le Minor, L., Lüderitz, O., and Westphal, O. (1966). *Ann. Inst. Pasteur, Paris* **111**, 47.
Stellner, K., Westphal, O., and Mayer, H. (1970). *Justus Liebigs Ann. Chem.* **738**, 179.
Stellner, K., Lüderitz, O., Westphal, O., Staub, A. M., LeLuc, B., Coynault, C., and Le Minor, L. (1972). *Ann. Inst. Pasteur, Paris* **123**, 43.
Steward, T. S., Mendershausen, P. B., and Ballou, C. E. (1969). *Biochemistry* **7**, 1843.
Stirm, S., Lüderitz, O., and Westphal, O. (1966a). *Justus Liebigs Ann. Chem.* **696**, 180.
Stirm, S., Staub, A. M., LeLuc, B., Mayer, H., Lüderitz, O., and Westphal, O. (1966b). *Biochem. Z.* **344**, 401.
Stocker, B. A. D. (1958). *J. Gen. Microbiol.* **18**, IX.
Stocker, B. A. D., and Mäkelä, P. H. (1971). In "Microbial Toxins" (G. Weinbaum, S. Kadis, and S. J. Ajl, eds.), Vol. IV, p. 369. Academic Press, New York.
Stocker, B. A. D., Staub, A. M., Tinelli, R., and Kopacka, B. (1960). *Ann. Inst. Pasteur, Paris* **98**, 505.
Sugg, J. Y., Caspari, E. L., Fleming, W. L., and Neill, J. M. (1928). *J. Exp. Med.* **47**, 91.
Summers, D. F., Grollmann, A. P., and Hasenclever, H. F. (1964). *J. Immunol.* **92**, 491.
Sutherland, I. W. (1969). *Biochem. J.* **115**, 935.
Sutherland, I. W. (1970). *Biochemistry* **9**, 2180.
Sutherland, I. W. (1971a). *J. Gen. Microbiol.* **65**, v.
Sutherland, I. W. (1971b). *J. Gen. Microbiol.* **70**, 331.
Sutherland, I. W., and Wilkinson, J. F. (1968). *Biochem. J.* **110**, 749.
Suzuki, S., and Sunayama, H. (1968). *Jap. J. Microbiol.* **12**, 413.
Suzuki, S., and Sunayama, H. (1969). *Jap. J. Microbiol.* **13**, 95.
Suzuki, S., Sunayama, H., and Saito, T. (1968). *Jap. J. Microbiol.* **12**, 19.
Svedberg, T., and Pedersen, K. O. (1940). "The Ultracentrifuge." Oxford Univ. Press (Clarendon), London and New York.
Tarcsay, L., Jann, B., and Jann, K. (1971). *Eur. J. Biochem.* **23**, 505.
Teichberg, I., and Sharon, N. (1971). *FEBS (Fed. Eur. Biochem. Soc.) Lett.* **1**, 171.
Thieme, T. R., and Ballou, C. E. (1971). *Biochemistry* **10**, 4121.
Thurow, H. D. (1973). Dissertation, University of Freiburg.
Tinelli, R., and Staub, A. M. (1960a). *Bull. Soc. Chim. Biol.* **42**, 583.
Tinelli, R., and Staub, A. M. (1960b). *Bull. Soc. Chim. Biol.* **42**, 601.
Tomasi, T. B., and Grey, H. M. (1972). *Progr. Allergy* **16**, 81.
Tomasz, A. (1967). *Science* **17**, 694.
Tomasz, A. (1968). *Proc. Nat. Acad. Sci. U. S.* **59**, 86.
Torii, M., Kabat, E. A., and Bezer, A. E. (1964). *J. Exp. Med.* **120**, 13.
Tyler, J. M., and Heidelberger, M. (1968). *Biochemistry* **7**, 1384.
Uchida, T., Robbins, P. W., and Luria, S. E. (1963). *Biochemistry* **2**, 663.
Uchida, T., Makino, T., Kurahashi, K., and Uetake, H. (1965). *Biochem. Biophys. Res. Commun.* **21**, 354.
Uchida, T., Matsumozo, T., and Sasaki, T. (1974). *J. Bacteriol.* **117**, 8.
Uetake, H., and Hagiwara, S. (1960). *Nature (London)* **186**, 261.
Unrau, A. M., and Smith, F. (1957). *Chem. Ind. (London)* p. 330.

1. Microbial Polysaccharides

Vahlne, G. (1945). *Acta Pathol. Microbiol. Scand.* 62, Suppl., 1
Valtonen, V. V. (1970). *J. Gen. Microbiol.* **64**, 255.
Valtonen, V. V., and Mäkelä, P. H. (1971). *J. Gen. Microbiol.* **69**, 107.
Valtonen, V. V., Sarvas, M., and Mäkelä, P. H. (1971a). *J. Gen. Microbiol.* **69**, 99.
Valtonen, V. V., Aird, J., Valtonen, M., Mäkelä, O., and Mäkelä, P. H. (1971b). *Acta Pathol. Microbiol. Scand.* **79**, 715.
Vicari, G., Sher, A., Cohn, M., and Kabat, E. A. (1970). *Immunochemistry* **7**, 829.
Vosti, K. L., Monto, A. S., and Rantz, A. L. (1965). *J. Lab. Clin. Med.* **66**, 613.
Wasserman, E., and Levine, L. (1961). *J. Immunol.* **87**, 290.
Watson, M. J., Tyler, J. M., Buchanan, J. G., and Baddiley, J. (1972). *Biochem. J.* **130**, 45.
Webster, M. E., Sagin, F. J., Anderson, P. R., Breese, S. S., Freeman, M. E., and Landy, M. (1954). *J. Immunol.* **73**, 16.
Westphal, O., and Jann, K. (1965). *Methods Carbohyd. Res.* **5**, 83.
Westphal, O., and Lüderitz, O. (1960). *Angew. Chem.* **72**, 881.
Westphal, O., and Lüderitz, O. (1961). *Pathol. Microbiol.* **24**, 875.
Westphal, O., Lüderitz, O., and Bister, F. (1952a). *Z. Naturforsch.* **7b**, 148.
Westphal, O., Lüderitz, O., Eichenberger, E., and Keiderling, W. (1952b). *Z. Naturforsch.* **7b**, 536.
Westphal, O., Kauffmann, F., Lüderitz, O., and Stierlin, H. (1960). *Zentralbl. Bakteriol., Parasitenk. Infektionskr Hyg. Abt. 1: Orig.* **179**, 336.
Whang, H. Y., Mayer, H., and Neter, E. (1971). *J. Immunol.* **106**, 1552.
Willers, J. M. N., Michel, M. F., Sysma, M. J., and Winkler, K. C. (1964). *J. Gen. Microbiol.* **36**, 95.
Williamson, A. R., and Zamenhof, S. (1963a). *J. Biol. Chem.* **238**, 2255.
Williamson, A. R., and Zamenhof, S. (1963b). *Fed. Proc., Fed. Amer. Soc. Exp. Biol.* **22**, 239.
Williamson, A. R., and Zamenhof, S. (1964). *J. Biol. Chem.* **239**, 963.
Wolberg, G., and de Witt, C. (1969). *J. Bacteriol.* **100**, 730.
Wong, K. H., Feeley, J. C., and Pittman, M. (1972). *J. Infec. Dis.* **125**, 360.
Wood, W. B., Jr., Smit, M. R., and Watson, B. (1956). *J. Exp. Med.* **84**, 387.
World Health Organization. (1973). *World Health Organ., Tech. Rep. Ser.* **519**.
Young, B. G., Fukazawa, Y., and Hartmann, P. E. (1964). *Virology* **23**, 279.
Young, N. M., Jocius, I. B., and Leon, M. A. (1971). *Biochemistry* **10**, 3457.
Yphantis, D. A. (1960). *Ann. N. Y. Acad. Sci.* **88**, 586.
Yurewicz, E. G., Ghalambor, M. A., and Heath, E. C. (1971). *J. Biol. Chem.* **246**, 5596.
Zamenhof, S., and Leidy, G. (1954). *Fed. Proc., Fed. Amer. Soc. Exp. Biol.* **13**, 327.
Zamenhof, S., Leidy, G., Fitzgerald, P. L., Alexander, H. E., and Chargaff, E. (1953). *J. Biol. Chem.* **203**, 695.
Zinder, N. D. (1957). *Science* **126**, 1237.

CHAPTER 2

Antigenic Determinants and Antibody Combining Sites

Joel W. Goodman

I. Introduction	127
II. The Structural Specificity of Hapten–Antibody Interactions	129
III. Antigenic Determinants	133
A. Approaches to Identification	133
B. Size of the Antigenic Determinant	136
C. Factors in Selection of Antigenic Determinants	141
D. Factors Determining Immunodominance	145
IV. The Antibody Combining Site	153
A. The Concept of Complementarity	153
B. The Structure of Immunoglobulin Molecules	155
C. The Location of the Antibody Combining Site	158
V. Immunogenic Determinants	162
A. Haptens and Immunogens	162
B. Dichotomy of Humoral and Cellular Immunity	164
C. The Specificity of Humoral and Cellular Immunity	165
D. Cell Cooperation in the Immune Response	170
E. Carrier Activity of Determinants That Induce Cellular Immunity	172
F. The Libraries of Haptenic and Immunogenic Determinants	175
VI. Concluding Remarks	179
References	183

I. Introduction

An enormous variety of natural and synthetic substances is capable of eliciting an immune response in mammals, underscoring the awesome diversity and survival value of the immune mechanism, as well as its unappealing profile: allergy, graft rejection, and autoimmunity. Most, and indeed the most potent, antigens are complex macromolecules, and little was understood about the specificity of antibodies until such molecules were chemically modified. Earlier, Wells and Osborne (1913) provided glimpses into the fundamental importance of the chemical structure of the antigen in immune reactions. Their investigation of the antigenic specificity and cross-reactivity of a variety of purified plant proteins led them to infer that the specificity of the induced antibodies was dependent on the chemical structure of portions of the antigen molecule. Then a landmark development took place when Karl Landsteiner and his associates introduced small substituents of known structure into macromolecules and showed that the low molecular weight substituents, or haptens, could themselves bind antibody elicited by the conjugates (Landsteiner, 1945). Thus began a rational exploration of the exquisite structural specificity of antigen–antibody reactions, a movement that burgeoned during the succeeding decades with the development of quantitative methods for assaying antigens and antibodies by Heidelberger (1956) and others.

In what follows, we will attempt to comprehensively review what is known about antigenic determinants, which are defined as the structural components of antigen molecules against which the specificity of antibodies is directed, as well as what is known about the combining sites of the antibodies themselves. It is believed that antigenic determinants and antibody combining sites possess a configurational complementarity which may be figuratively envisioned as a "lock-and-key" arrangement (Fig. 1), although this is clearly an oversimplification. In place of notches and grooves, hydrogen, hydro-

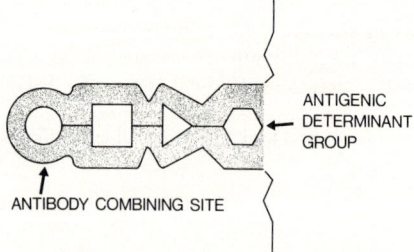

Fig. 1. A schematic view of the "lock-and-key" complementarity between an antigenic determinant group and an antibody combining site. The determinant can be considered to be composed of discrete subunits, which may be amino acids in a peptide chain or sugars in a saccharide chain. The antibody combining site is then composed of subsites, each of which can accommodate a discrete subunit of the antigenic determinant.

2. Antigenic Determinants and Antibody Combining Sites

phobic, and ionic bonds, as well as van der Waals forces, should be substituted.

The structural features of antigens that determine specificity can be considered separately from those that confer immunogenicity, which we define as the capacity of a molecule to induce an immune response of any kind: cellular, humoral, or, most commonly, both. The structural components of macromolecular antigens which confer immunogenicity have thus far eluded precise delineation, although it has been possible to demonstrate with synthetic antigens that immunogenicity is strongly enhanced by the incorporation of aromatic amino acids into an otherwise weak antigen such as gelatin (Sela, 1969). In a few instances, molecules the size of antigenic determinants or haptens have themselves induced immune responses and served as carriers for haptens (Alkan et al., 1972). Such molecules will be designated "immunogenic determinants" to distinguish them from antigenic or haptenic determinants, which can react with antibody but are unable to induce its formation. Findings concerning immunogenic determinants and what they have revealed about the process of antigen recognition will also be considered, but other aspects of immunogenicity lie outside the province of this review.

II. The Structural Specificity of Hapten–Antibody Interactions

Before proceeding to a consideration of the nature of antigenic determinants, it might profit us to briefly review the insights into immunochemical specificity which have been provided by the use of haptens. Literally hundreds of haptens have been applied to this subject, which has been treated very thoroughly by Pressman and Grossberg (1968). Hence, a few outstanding examples to illustrate specific points will suffice here. These are listed in Table I and most were originally used by Landsteiner in his classic studies. Later, when quantitative methods were developed, it became possible to express the reactions between antibody and a series of related ligands in precise terms, and consequently to define the contribution of particular structural features to the total binding energy. Such experiments brought the exquisite structural specificity of antibodies into sharp focus.

The maleate–fumarate reciprocal system dramatically highlights antibody specificity for a cis or trans configuration of the hapten (Table I). The maleate ion can only assume a cis configuration, while the fumarate ion exists only in the trans configuration. Landsteiner

TABLE I
Structural Specificity of Selected Hapten–Antibody Reactions

Haptens		Antibody specific for	K_{rel}^a	ΔF_{rel}^b
Maleanilate		Fumaranilate Succinanilate	0.00 0.11–0.25	>4000 770–1200
Fumaranilate		Maleanilate Succinanilate	0.00 0.01	>4000 2600
Succinanilate		Maleanilate Fumaranilate	0.016 0.14	2300 1100
o-Chlorobenzoate		m-Azobenzoate p-Azobenzoate	0.16 0.07	1000 1500
m-Chlorobenzoate		o-Azobenzoate p-Azobenzoate	0.35 0.64	600 250

Hapten structure reference	Hapten	K_{rel}[a]	ΔF_{rel}[b]
p-Chlorobenzoate	o-Azobenzoate	0.14	1000
	m-Azobenzoate	0.24	800
D-Phenyl-(p-nitrobenzoyl-amino)acetate	L-Phenyl-(p-azobenzoyl-amino)acetate	0.009	2600
L-Phenyl-(p-nitrobenzoyl-amino)acetate	D-Phenyl-(p-azobenzoyl-amino)acetate	0.006	2800
Lactose	p-Azophenyllactoside	1.00	0
Cellobiose	p-Azophenyllactoside	0.0025	3600

[a] $K_{rel} = \dfrac{K_{hapten}}{K_{reference\ (homologous)\ hapten}} = \dfrac{\text{concentration of reference hapten giving 50\% inhibition}}{\text{concentration of hapten giving 50\% inhibition}}$.

[b] $\Delta F_{rel} = -RT \ln K_{rel}$.

and van der Scheer (1934) demonstrated the absence of cross-reactivity between these haptens and further showed that antibody to the succinate group, which can assume a cis configuration, combines more strongly with maleate than with fumarate. These findings were confirmed and extended by Pressman and his colleagues (reviewed in Pressman and Grossberg, 1968), who quantitatively compared the binding of heterologous haptens to that of the homologous, or reference, hapten, deriving relative equilibrium constants and free energies for the reactions (Table I). The data in Table I also show that although anti-succinate antibody sites can accommodate the maleate group reasonably well ($\Delta F_{rel} = 770$–1200 calories), the converse is not true ($\Delta F_{rel} = 2300$ calories), indicating that the anti-maleate site is so closely complementary to the flat maleate group that it cannot easily accommodate the bulkier methylene groups of succinate, despite the ability of the latter to assume a cis configuration.

There have been many detailed analyses of aromatic hapten specificity, two noteworthy examples of which are the dinitro- and trinitrophenyl groups (Little and Eisen, 1965) and the *o*-, *m*-, and *p*-azobenzoates (Landsteiner and van der Scheer, 1931; Pressman *et al.*, 1954). The antibodies directed against the azobenzoates react as though they are closely complementary to the van der Waals outlines of these molecules. All three types of antibody combine well with the benzoate ion but differ markedly in their reactivity with the *o*-, *m*-, and *p*-chlorobenzoates (Table I). Each antibody combines best with the chlorobenzoate in which the chlorine atom is in the position occupied by the azo group of the homologous haptenic determinant. In that position, the chlorine atom contributes to the binding by interacting with the region of the antibody combining site which is directed against and complementary to the azo group. However, in any other position it decreases binding by sterically interfering with the region of the antibody combining site specific for the smaller hydrogen atom. Consequently, the antibodies can readily distinguish between the *o*-, *m*-, and *p*-substituted compounds.

The ability of antibodies to discriminate very sharply between optical antipodes surfaced in Landsteiner and van der Scheer's comparison of L-, D-, and *m*-tartaric acids and D- and L-phenyl-(*p*-nitrobenzoylamino)acetate (Landsteiner, 1945). Antibodies directed against one of the isomers reacted poorly with the opposite antipode. Karush (1956) studied the phenyl-(*p*-nitrobenzoylamino)acetate system quantitatively by competitive binding and found a better than 100-fold difference in the relative binding of the homologous and heterologous optical isomers by each antibody population (Table I).

2. Antigenic Determinants and Antibody Combining Sites 133

These and similar studies established the now axiomatic stereo-specificity of immunochemical reactions.

This subject should not be left without touching upon glycosidic haptens, for which the same order of structural specificity has been demonstrated. Avery and Goebel (1929) pioneered this area by converting simple sugars such as galactose and glucose into the corresponding p-aminophenyl-β-glycosides, which were then diazotized and coupled to proteins for use as antigens. The antibodies formed against the haptenic determinants showed a marked degree of structural specificity and reacted with many naturally occurring polysaccharides.

These early studies provided no quantitative information, but Karush (1957) later explored the binding of antibody against the p-azophenyl-β-lactoside hapten with various sugars by competitive equilibrium dialysis. The association of antibody with lactose was about 400 times greater than with cellobiose (Table I). These disaccharides differ in the replacement of galactose by glucose in cellobiose, the only structural difference being the configuration of the hydrogen and hydroxyl groups around the fourth carbon atom in the sugars.

These few examples, drawn from many, serve to illustrate the remarkable discriminatory power of antibody molecules.

III. Antigenic Determinants

A. Approaches to Identification

Information about the composition, structure and size of antigenic determinants has been derived from three general approaches. A limited amount of information about composition can be obtained from cross-reactions of antibodies to undefined antigens with heterologous antigens of defined composition, or vice versa. Thus, it was predicted that a lung galactan thought to be composed only of galactose also contained glucose on the basis of its cross-reactivity with horse antiserum against type III pneumococcus polysaccharide (Heidelberger, 1956). The latter is composed only of glucose and glucuronic acid. A more sensitive analysis of the galactan bore this out.

Another example serves to illustrate the heterogeneity of antibodies usually found in antisera to even relatively simple antigens—a phenomenon now firmly established (Haber, 1967). The capsular polysaccharide of the type II pneumococcus is a highly branched molecule consisting of about 40% rhamnose, 35% glucose, and 16% glucuronic acid (Barker et al., 1965). Glucuronic acid, though present in the smallest proportion, occupies most if not all of the terminal nonreducing positions in the side chains (Butler and Stacey, 1955). Almost all of the antibody in a horse anti-SII serum could be specifically precipitated by a hemocyanin–glucuronide conjugate, demonstrating an almost exclusive specificity for determinants in which glucuronic acid is the main component (Corneil and Wofsy, 1967). A component of an antigenic determinant which plays a major role in defining the specificity of antibodies is referred to as "immunodominant" (Lüderitz et al., 1966). Hence, glucuronic acid is the immunodominant group of the SII polysaccharide.

Nonetheless, a polysaccharide from *Escherichia coli* which also contained terminal nonreducing glucuronyl residues precipitated only 13% of the anti-SII; a different fraction of 12% cross-reacted with dextran (Zolla and Goodman, 1967). Fractional precipitation with the glucuronyl–hemocyanin conjugate preferentially removed the fraction reactive with *E. coli* polysaccharide prior to the portion reactive with dextran. Glucuronic acid proved to be more effective than isomaltose in inhibiting the cross-reaction with *E. coli* polysaccharide, while the reverse held in the cross-reaction with dextran. Thus, glucose was immunodominant in the specificity of a fraction of the antibody which was nonetheless precipitable by a glucuronyl determinant.

In the above, inhibition of the quantitative precipitin reaction between antibody and a cross-reacting antigen proved to be a powerful aid in unraveling the specificities of the antibody fractions. However, a note of caution about the interpretation of inhibition studies of cross-reactions in general is warranted. Reactivity with a hapten is always dictated by the specificity of the antibody and may be unrelated to the structure of the cross-reacting antigen. Thus, the cross-reaction of a horse anti-type II pneumococcus serum with dextran was inhibited more effectively by glucuronic acid than by isomaltose (Goodman and Kabat, 1960), even though dextrans contain only glucose. In this case, glucuronic acid played an immunodominant role even in the fraction of antibody precipitated by the dextran. This example serves to illustrate the important point that inhibition studies cannot be used to draw conclusions about the structure of cross-reacting antigens, as they can for homologous antigens.

2. Antigenic Determinants and Antibody Combining Sites 135

A second approach involves the degradation of complex macromolecular antigens in order to obtain fragments which hopefully represent single, intact antigenic determinants, the structure of which may then be elucidated. The earliest studies of this kind were on silk fibroin (Cebra, 1961) and serum albumin (Lapresle and Webb, 1964, 1965; Press and Porter, 1962), the smallest active fragments of the latter having molecular weights of about 7000. One of these had two partial or complete determinants, while a second possessed only a single site; but when coupled to an insoluble adsorbent the latter peptide removed only 1% of the total antibody (Lapresle and Webb, 1965). A blatant disadvantage of this approach is the rather narrow possibility of obtaining intact determinants unfettered by immunologically irrelevant parts of the antigen molecule. Thus, this peptide may have removed only 1% of the antibody because it represented only part of a determinant. On the other hand, it could have been a complete but very minor, or weakly immunopotent, determinant. There is also a third possibility: namely, that conformation may have played a central part in the specificity of this determinant, and its conformation in the native protein and on the immunoadsorbent surely differed.

Another example germane to this point was the isolation of four peptides from a chymotryptic digest of apomyoglobin (Crumpton and Wilkinson, 1965), a protein whose highly ordered structure has been extensively characterized. The most active of these inhibited precipitation to the extent of only 15% and even the total digest fell far short of complete inhibition. A tetradecapeptide from a helical region of the molecule possessed little or no helix (Crumpton and Small, 1967) and inhibited precipitation to the extent of only 8%. While emphasis was placed on the ability of a nonhelical peptide to combine with antibody specific for a helical region, the marginal binding observed may have been attributable precisely to the conformational deficiencies of the peptide. On the other hand, larger fragments of apomyoglobin, produced by cleavage with cyanogen bromide at the two methionine residues, possessed activities the sum of which equaled that of the native molecule (Atassi and Saplin, 1968).

The degradative approach has also been taken with antigens other than proteins [e.g., polysaccharides, polyamino acids, and nucleoproteins (Maurer, 1964; Kabat, 1966; Goodman, 1969)], and much of this work will be reviewed in later sections of this chapter.

The third and most productive approach to the delineation of antigenic determinants has employed either natural or synthetic homopolymers of a single amino acid or sugar, synthetic polypeptides fabricated in a defined, premeditated way, or synthetic haptens coupled to macromolecular carriers. Haptens may then be synthesized which precisely mimic the primary structure of the antigenic determinant and their binding with antibody can be assessed by inhibition of the quantitative precipitin reaction. Unfortunately, these antigens must ordinarily be of substantial size in order to be immunogenic, and conformational differences between the integral determinant and the synthetic hapten creep in again. If the efficiency of a ligand is expressed as its molar ratio to the antigen or the antibody for a given level of inhibition (Kabat, 1966), the figure has been found to range from several hundred to several thousand for small haptens (Beiser et al., 1960; Cebra, 1961) and polymers with multiple repeating determinants (Kabat, 1966; Sela, 1966). While this has been interpreted to mean that the antigenic determinant is relatively large (Press and Porter, 1962), or attributable to the multiplicity of repeating units in the antigen (Kabat, 1966), the contribution of other parts of the molecule to the configuration of the determinant must be considered.

A profitable circumvention of this obstacle can be achieved by conjugating haptens to the side chains of protein carriers. Thus, the specificity of antibodies to synthetic glycosylated antigens, components of nucleic acids conjugated to proteins or polypeptides, as well as numerous other hapten–protein conjugates has been studied in great detail (Pressman and Grossberg, 1968). The small haptens are not integral parts of the molecular superstructure of the carrier and consequently conformational considerations are minimized. However, in most cases they are also incomplete determinants, which limits their utility. Perhaps the most reliable information about the size of an antigenic determinant was derived from the use of a series of peptides of defined size and structure coupled to protein carriers (B. Schechter et al., 1970), which will be expanded upon later.

Thus, the nature of antigenic determinants has been probed from the vantage point of cross-reactions, degradation of complex antigens, and the application of homopolymers and synthetic antigens. Now we shall proceed to assess the findings of these multifarious labors.

B. Size of the Antigenic Determinant

It has been known since the 1930's that antibody complementarity is directed against limited parts of the antigen molecule, which subsequently became known as antigenic determinants. Landsteiner

2. Antigenic Determinants and Antibody Combining Sites

and van der Scheer (1938) used haptens composed of two moieties linked to the same benzene ring, such as arsanilic and succinanilic acids, or glycine and leucine in aminoisophthalylglycylleucine, which were diazotized to protein carriers. They found that antibodies raised by these antigens were specific for one or the other, but not both groups. These findings led Campbell and Bulman (1952) to calculate the size of an antibody combining site as not exceeding 700 Å. However, other studies with azoproteins and, more recently, dinitrophenylated and penicilloyl proteins (Eisen and Siskind, 1964; Levine, 1963) showed that the hapten linked to the amino acid to which it was joined in the protein was always a better inhibitor than the free hapten, indicating that the antibody combining site was larger than the benzenoid haptens commonly used. These complex antigens did not permit further assessment of the size of an antigenic determinant.

A breakthrough of sorts occurred when it was shown that dextran, a polysaccharide composed of a single sugar, glucose, is immunogenic in man (Kabat and Berg, 1953; Maurer, 1953). Some dextrans are essentially single long chains with very few branch points and provide antigens for which the size of antigenic determinants could be estimated by using an ordered series of oligosaccharides as inhibitors of the dextran–antidextran precipitin reaction (Table II). Thus, using oligosaccharides of the isomaltose series up to the heptaose, it was found with six different sera that the hexasaccharide was the best inhibitor, isomaltoheptaose being no better on a molar basis (Kabat, 1966). In its most extended form, the dimensions of isomaltohexaose

TABLE II

Estimations of the Size of Sequentially Defined Antigenic Determinants Based on Hapten Inhibition Assay

Antigen	Species	Determinant	Reference
Dextran	Man	Isomaltohexaose	Kabat, 1966
Dextran	Rabbit	≦Isomaltohexaose	Mage and Kabat, 1963
Poly-γ-D-glutamic acid (killed *B. anthracis*)	Rabbit	Hexaglutamic acid	Goodman et al., 1968
Polyalanyl-bovine serum albumin	Rabbit	Pentaalanine	Sage et al., 1964
Polylysyl-rabbit serum albumin	Rabbit	Penta- or hexalysine	Arnon et al., 1965
Polylysyl-phosphoryl-bovine serum albumin	Rabbit	Pentalysine	Van Vunakis et al., 1966
α-DNP-(lysine)$_{11}$	Guinea pig	α-DNP-heptalysine	Schlossman et al., 1968
α-DNP-polylysine	Guinea pig	α-DNP-trilysine	Schlossman et al., 1968
(D-Ala)$_n$-Gly-RNase	Rabbit	Tetrapeptide	B. Schechter et al., 1970
Denatured DNA	Man (L.E. sera)	Pentanucleotide	Stollar et al., 1962

are $34 \times 12 \times 7$ Å. This was taken to be the maximum size of the antigenic determinant of dextran and, by extrapolation, the approximate size of the complementary region of the antibody.

The antibodies produced in response to dextran possessed combining sites with different relative binding affinity for oligosaccharides of the isomaltose series. This has been interpreted to mean that the sites vary in the extent of their complementary regions, the upper limit being complementary to the hexasaccharide (Kabat, 1966). This interpretation is open to question, as several lines of evidence raise the possibility that enhanced binding with haptens of increasing size does not necessarily reflect the size of the antigenic determinant, but rather the approach to a conformation for which the antibody site is complementary. This preferred conformation could involve only a portion of the total hapten in direct binding with antibody, the remainder being essential for the assumption of the required configuration.

A specific illustration can be found in results with guinea pig antibody to polymers of α-DNP-lysine (Schlossman *et al.*, 1968). Antibodies to a mixture of peptides with an average chain length of 11 amino acids were maximally inhibited by α-DNP-heptalysine when the trimer to the nonamer were assayed. In contrast, polymers of α-DNP-lysine with 60 or more residues elicited antibody inhibited most efficiently by the tripeptide when the same series of oligomers was tested (Table II). Specificity in both cases was directed against the terminal α-DNP-lysine sequence. It seems unlikely that the size of the antibody combining site would vary so dramatically with the size of the immunogen. The observations are more reasonably explicable on the basis of conformational differences in the determinants of the large and small polymers. In the latter case, peptides up to the nonapeptide were no better than the tripeptide in approximating the correct conformation. Some support for this rests in the observation that the peptides were poorer inhibitors of the anti-α-DNP(Lys)$_{60}$ than of the anti-α-DNP(Lys)$_{11}$ homologous reaction.

A more recent and startling finding from the same laboratory was the detection of a small but perceptible increment in the binding of the homologous DNP-polylysine when two discontinuous series from the dipeptide up to mixtures containing 16–30 residues were assayed with antigen by fluorescence quenching (Levin *et al.*, 1971). One series was substituted at the α amino position while the other had the DNP group on the ϵ amino of the carboxy-terminal lysine. Taken at face value, these findings suggest that a very large, possibly almost infinite, variety of antibodies may be induced to just the polylysine series of immunogens. Since there is no reason to expect that this is restricted to polymers of lysine, it makes one wonder how selection, rather than instruction, could account for such staggering diversity. On the other hand, it may be possible that the observations can be accounted for by different proportions of a relatively small number of antibodies elicited by this family of polypeptides. Still a third possibility is that the increment in binding with the homologous polymer is due to interactions that take place outside the combining site and, consequently, is irrelevant to specificity (see discussion in Section II,C,2). In any event, it seems clear that the observations are explicable in terms of combining site symmetry rather than size.

Numerous other investigations using homopolymers of amino acids (Goodman *et al.*, 1968; Van Vunakis *et al.*, 1966) or multichain-polymer–protein conjugates with average polymer chain lengths of 5 to 8 residues (Sage *et al.*, 1964; Arnon *et al.*, 1965; Schechter *et al.*, 1966) as antigens in hapten inhibition assays have yielded determinant group sizes in reasonable consonance with the dextran model. For example, the size of the region on the capsular polypeptide of *Bacillus anthracis*, poly-γ-D-glutamic acid, was concluded to be equivalent to a hexapeptide, the dimensions of which are $36 \times 10 \times 6$ Å (Goodman *et al.*, 1968), compared to $34 \times 12 \times 7$ Å for isomaltohexaose. It is noteworthy that in the polyglutamic acid system, although penta-Glu and hexa-Glu behaved indistinguishably with several antisera, larger peptides gave additional increments of inhibiting efficiency (Goodman, 1969). These results paralleled the optical rotatory dispersion aspects of a series of γ-linked oligopeptides of glutamic acid and suggested that the specificity of the antibody was directed against a conformation of the randomly coiled polymer reflected by the spectra.

Perhaps the most precise evaluation of determinant group size was obtained using as immunogens proteins to which peptides of defined structure were attached (B. Schechter *et al.*, 1970). Peptides of the form $(D\text{-Ala})_n$-Gly, where n varied from 1 to 4, were coupled to ribonuclease and rabbit serum albumin, which induced peptide-specific antibodies in rabbits. Peptides of the general structure $(D\text{-Ala})_n$ ($n = 1$ to 4), and $(D\text{-Ala})_n$-Gly-ϵ-aminocaproic acid ($n = 1$ to 3) were used as inhibitors of precipitation. From cross-precipitation and inhibition experiments, it was concluded that the antigenic determinant in all instances was a tetrapeptide and that the lysine residue of the protein carrier participated in this determinant only when the conjugated hapten was smaller than a tetrapeptide. The consistency of the results and the improbability of conformational complications with such short peptide chains argue strongly that the antibody combining site is such as to accommodate four amino acid residues. This conclusion is in rather good agreement with studies cited above, and summarized in Table II, involving other antigens in several different species of animals, so we may feel confident that the size of an antigenic determinant has now been defined within very narrow limits. Moreover, IgG and IgM antibodies to poly-D-alanine gave very similar inhibitory patterns with alanyl peptides (Haimovich et al., 1969). In all instances, tetra-D-alanine and penta-D-alanine were equivalent to each other and more efficient than tri-D-alanine. Thus, the combining sites of both classes of antibodies appear to have similar dimensions which can accommodate a tetrapeptide determinant.

As in the example cited earlier of glucuronic acid being a better inhibitor than isomaltose of the cross-reaction between anti-SII antibody and dextran, the structure of the antigenic determinant must be known if misleading interpretations are to be avoided. Thus, it was found that with antibodies to the (D-Ala)$_2$-Gly determinant, peptides of the structure (D-Ala)$_4$ and (D-Ala)$_5$ were better inhibitors than (D-Ala)$_2$-Gly (B. Schechter et al., 1970). Similarly, antibodies to the protein coat of tobacco mosaic virus were bound more effectively by a pentapeptide from the protein to which (Ala)$_5$ was attached than by the specific pentapeptide itself (Benjamini et al., 1968a). Furthermore, although peptides smaller than the pentapeptide showed no detectable binding, the addition of octanoic acid to the amino terminus of a tri- or tetrapeptide produced strong specific binding with antibody (Benjamini et al., 1968b). There have been other findings of a similar nature. Some rabbit antisera to an isomaltotrionic acid derivative of bovine serum albumin gave increasingly efficient binding with oligosaccharides up to isomaltohexaose (Arakatsu et al., 1966). Two chymotryptic peptides of myoglobin which differed in chain length by four amino acids had decidedly different specific inhibitory activities, the larger being more effective (Crumpton and Wilkinson, 1965). This tetrapeptide, Ile-Arg-Leu-Phe, appears to be masked in the intact molecule, although this does not necessarily preclude its forming a part of the antigenic determinant.

A common denominator between these nonspecific appendages is their hydrophobicity. The interpretation that nonspecifically increasing the hydrophobicity of a ligand (Benjamini et al., 1968b) may enhance its binding by antibody is consistent with the view that the active sites of antibody molecules are unusually hydrophobic (Singer and Doolittle, 1966). A further useful test here would be the substitution of a nonspecific hydrophobic group for the masked tetrapeptide of myoglobin, which is itself substantially hydrophobic. The phenomenon does not appear to be universal, since the attachment of octanoyl chains to peptides of glutamic acid did not enhance their binding with antibody to poly-γ-D-glutamic acid (J. W. Goodman, unpublished observations).

C. Factors in Selection of Antigenic Determinants

From the abundant studies of the specificity of antibodies to hapten–carrier conjugates, we may surmise that virtually any structural entity may serve as an antigenic determinant. This does not necessarily imply that the organism is capable of generating an infinite variety of antibodies, but through overlapping cross-reactivities antibodies of sufficient affinity may be produced to any structural determinant. It is assumed that the determinant selects those immunocompetent cells with receptors that bind it with an affinity that exceeds the threshold required for triggering antibody production.

Most antigens of an appreciable size, with molecular weights in excess of several thousand, are multivalent, which means that antibodies are produced to more than one determinant. Even proteins of substantial size, however, seem to possess a limited number of determinants, although the number may be greater than the experimentally determined valency due to steric limitation of the maximum number of antibody molecules which may simultaneously bind to one antigen molecule. A number of rabbit antisera to tobacco mosaic virus protein contained antibodies that had specificities limited to an eicosapeptide region of the molecule (Benjamini et al., 1968a), although the protein consists of 158 amino acids and has a molecular weight of about 17,500. A given antiserum to bovine serum albumin probably has specificity for no more than five or six distinct determinants. Since the specificity of the immune response is capable of such great diversity, there is obviously a selection of determinants in any given situation. Some of the factors involved in selection of antigenic determinants, which is what Sela (1969) has termed "immunopotency," have been identified and will be considered now.

1. Accessibility

Exposure to the aqueous environment is a cardinal factor in the determination of immunopotency. Using multichain synthetic polypeptides with sequences of alanine on the outside and tyrosine

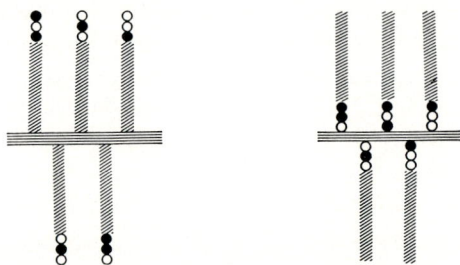

Fig. 2. A multichain copolymer in which L-tyrosine and L-glutamic acid residues are attached to multi-poly-DL-alanyl–poly-L-lysine [poly(Tyr,Glu)-poly(DL-Ala)–poly(Lys)] (left); and one in which tyrosine and glutamic acid are attached directly to the polylysine backbone with alanine peptides on the ends of the side chains (right). Horizontal lines: poly-L-lysine; diagonal hatching: poly-DL-alanine; closed circles: L-tyrosine; open circles: L-glutamic acid. [From Sela (1969). *Science* **166**, 1365. Copyright 1969 by the American Association for the Advancement of Science.]

closer to the backbone, or the reverse (Fig. 2), antibodies to the former proved to be largely alanine-specific while the latter evoked antibodies with a predominant specificity for tyrosine (Fuchs and Sela, 1963). It has also been clearly established that terminal side chains represent the most immunopotent regions of polysaccharides (Kabat, 1966).

The conformation of macromolecules is a primary factor in determining accessibility to the immune apparatus. While it has been conclusively shown that antigenic determinants can reside in the interiors of polysaccharide (Uchida *et al.*, 1963) and polypeptide (Crumpton and Wilkinson, 1965; Gill *et al.*, 1965; Atassi and Saplin, 1968) chains, internal positioning does not preclude exposure to the environment. In the case of myoglobin, the three-dimensional structure of which is known, it was found that peptides from regions that occupy corners of the molecule, and thus were prominently exposed, were important in its immunochemical specificity.

Altering the conformation of synthetic polypeptides by preparing cross-linked derivatives did not perceptibly affect immunogenicity, but produced marked changes in the immunopotency of different antigenic determinants (Gill *et al.*, 1968). In this particular case, the changes could not be formally related to accessibility because the three-dimensional structures of the compounds were obscure, but there is a strong likelihood that this played a pivotal role.

2. CHARGE

Electrical charge has long been considered a dominant factor in specificity (Landsteiner, 1945), although it is evident that completely uncharged molecules can be immunogenic (Kabat, 1961; Sela and

Fuchs, 1965). In a series of investigations of the specificity of antibodies to a number of linear synthetic polypeptides in humans (Maurer et al., 1962), rabbits (Maurer et al., 1963, 1964), and guinea pigs (Maurer and Cashman, 1963), glutamic acid contributed strongly to the specificity of polymers of which it was a part. This was also found to be true of multichain polymers (Fuchs and Sela, 1964).

There is also indirect evidence for the role of electrostatic forces in the specificity of antibodies to synthetic polypeptides containing charged amino acids. It was found that salt concentration and pH strongly influenced the stability of antigen–antibody bonds whereas nonaqueous solvents did not (Gould et al., 1964), prompting the conclusion that the binding between a charged polypeptide and its antibody is primarily electrostatic. However, changes in pH also affected the binding between a completely uncharged polypeptide and its antibody (Sela and Fuchs, 1965), although ionization of the antigen in this case could not be involved. It thus appears likely that varying the pH can alter immunochemical interactions through intramolecular changes in the antibody molecule which do not necessarily directly involve the combining sites. Although nonaqueous solvents strongly influenced the uncharged antigen system, in contrast to the charged one, which suggests that charged groups, when present, contribute to the stabilization of antigen–antibody complexes, this effect may also take place outside the combining site. It has been shown that the net charge of antibody molecules produced against a specific determinant is dictated by the net charge of the antigen and is independent of the specificity of the antibody (Sela and Mozes, 1966). It is assumed that nonspecific interaction between the antigen molecule and the surface of an immunocompetent cell may contribute to the selection of antibody-producing cells by antigen. Consequently, the electrostatic interaction between charged antigens and their homologous antibodies may, at least in part, occur outside the active site.

Despite difficulties in interpretation of some of the experimental data, the conclusion that charged groups play an important role in the selection of antigenic determinants appears justified. However, the interdependence of charge and accessibility should be kept in mind. In general, it might be expected that charged residues, being hydrophilic, would be in closer contact with the environment than nonpolar groups, subject to other conformational restrictions.

3. GENETIC FACTORS

A growing body of evidence has been accumulating which attests to a genetic control of the ability to produce antibodies of different specificity against the same antigen. Some of the earliest evidence for this phenomenon accrued from a comparison of the specificity of anti-insulin antibodies from strain 2 and strain 13 guinea pigs (Arquilla and Finn, 1963, 1965). The ability of antibodies from the two strains to bind to an insoluble insulin–cellulose conjugate which had been saturated with antibodies from a reference rabbit antiserum was assessed by a hemolytic assay. It was found that strain 2 antisera contained antibodies that bound to sites on the insulin molecule that were not covered by the rabbit antibody, whereas strain 13 antisera did not. The results indicate that strain 2 guinea pigs produce antibody to determinants on the insulin molecule to which strain 13 animals do not respond. They are subject to the criticism that, since the assay detected only hemolytic antibody, what appears to be a qualitative difference could, in fact, be a quantitative difference. However, further support for a real genetic difference was obtained through the use of modified insulin derivatives. Removal of the eight C-terminal residues from the β chain of insulin caused a much greater loss of reactivity with strain 13 than with strain 2 antisera to native insulin. Conversely, substitution of the N-terminal α-amino groups of both chains with fluorescein resulted in a preferential loss of reactivity with strain 2 antisera, suggesting that antibodies produced by the two strains are largely specific for opposite ends of the insulin molecule (Arquilla et al., 1967).

More recently, evidence has been obtained which demonstrates genetic control of the specificity of antibodies against the same branched synthetic polypeptide in two genetically different strains of mice (McDevitt and Benacerraf, 1969). Animals immunized with poly(Phe,Glu)-poly(Pro)--poly(Lys) [(Phe,G)-Pro-L] produced antibodies which were assayed for binding with the polypeptides poly(Phe,Glu)-poly(DL-Ala)--poly(Lys) [(Phe,G)-A-L] and poly(Tyr,Glu)-poly(Pro)--poly(Lys) [(T,G)-Pro-L]. Antibodies specific for (T,G) and (Phe,G) sequences do not cross-react to an appreciable extent. Mice of strain SJL produce anti-(Phe,G)-Pro-L antibodies which bind (T,G)-Pro-L much better than do antibodies from strain DBA/1. On the other hand, DBA/1 antisera react much better with (Phe,G)-A-L than do antisera from SJL mice. These results indicate that determinants in the terminal poly(Phe,Glu) side chain were more immunopotent in DBA/1 mice than in SJL mice, while the most immunopotent determinant for SJL animals resided in the internal poly(Pro) chains. Studies of backcrosses between the F1 hybrids and parental strains showed that the ability to produce antibodies which bound (Phe,G)-A-L was linked to the DBA/1 H-2 histocompatibility locus whereas the ability to produce antibodies

2. Antigenic Determinants and Antibody Combining Sites

which bound (T,G)-Pro-L was not linked to the H-2 locus of SJL mice. The nature of this genetic control and the mechanism of its expression are still inadequately understood and are under intensive investigation.

Returning to the observations of Levin *et al.* (1971) that guinea pig antibodies to DNP-polylysines can discriminate between the homologous polymer and polymers which differ slightly in size, guinea pigs can be divided into two classes on the basis of response to poly-L-lysine. Responders develop cellular immunity to polylysine, which is immunogenic in such animals and can serve as a carrier for the DNP hapten. On the other hand, nonresponders never develop cellular immunity to this polypeptide and it acts as a hapten in these guinea pigs. Strain 2 guinea pigs are all responders, strain 13 guinea pigs are all nonresponders, and other strains contain mixtures of the two. Hartley strain animals, for example, are composed of about 75% responders and 25% nonresponders to poly-L-lysine. When responders and nonresponders were immunized with the series of α-DNP-oligolysines used by these investigators incorporated in Freund's adjuvant containing a strain of mycobacteria which induced anti-DNP antibody even in nonresponders (but no cellular immunity to polylysine, so it is likely that the adjuvant itself served as a carrier), it was found that whereas responder antibody could discriminate between the homologous and heterologous polymers, nonresponder antibody could not. Thus, the genetic difference here is expressed at two different levels, antigen recognition, or immunogenicity, and antibody specificity. Genetic differences at these two levels are also being observed with increasing frequency in mice (McDevitt and Benacerraf, 1969).

D. Factors Determining Immunodominance

In the preceding section we have considered the factors that may determine why a particular region of a molecule acts as an antigenic determinant in a given situation while others do not. We have referred to determinants which induce relatively large quantities of antibody as "immunopotent" (Sela, 1969). Immunopotency, then, is a quantitative expression of the strength of an antigenic determinant. Now, given a particular determinant that from earlier considerations may be the size of a tetrapeptide, the components of that determinant will share unequally in determining the affinity of reactivity with antibody. The degree of this influence on reactivity with antibody, and hence specificity of the determinant, alluded to earlier, has been termed "immunodominance" (Lüderitz et al., 1966). Upon reflection, it becomes apparent that factors that play crucial roles in determining immunopotency, such as accessibility and conformation, are also influential in determining immunodominance. The overlap, or twilight zone, between immunopotency and immunodominance is illustrated by the absence of reciprocal serologic cross-reactivity between lysozyme and its reduced and S-carboxymethylated derivative (Thompson et al., 1972). The native and denatured forms have identical amino acid sequences and it is not known whether the same regions of the two forms, which may now have different conformations, are immunopotent, or if previously immunosilent regions of the native protein are expressed in the denatured molecule.

Using antigens that are better defined, it is possible to show that conformation can play a central role in immunodominance. When polymerized, the tripeptide L-tyrosyl-L-alanyl-L-glutamic acid forms an α-helix under physiological conditions. The same tripeptide has also been attached to a branched synthetic polypeptide consisting of a backbone of polylysine and side chains of polyalanine (Fig. 3). The tripeptide itself does not possess an ordered conformation. Using the two polymers to immunize rabbits, antisera were obtained which showed almost no cross-reaction (Sela et al., 1967). The tripeptide proved to be an efficient inhibitor of the precipitin reaction between the branched polymer and its homologous antibody, but was inactive in the helical polymer system. Thus, the immunodominant feature of the helical polymer was its conformation rather than a particular amino acid residue of the determinant. In what follows we will consider other examples of the role of conformation in immunodominance.

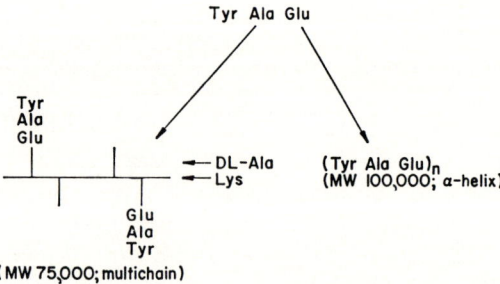

Fig. 3. A synthetic branched polymer in which peptides of sequence Tyr-Ala-Glu are attached to the amino groups of side chains in multi-poly-DL-ananyl--poly-L-lysine (left) and a periodic polymer of the tripeptide Tyr-Ala-Glu (right). [From Sela (1969). Science 166, 1365. Copyright 1969 by the American Association for the Advancement of Science.]

1. Accessibility

Sequential determinants can be defined as those whose specificity is dictated by the sequence of subunits within the determinant, rather than the macromolecular superstructure of the whole antigen. In such cases, components of the determinant (haptens) can bind with antibody, the reaction being demonstrable either directly by such methods as equilibrium dialysis or fluorescence quenching, or indirectly by inhibition of the reaction between antigen and antibody. Sequential determinants may either be composed of terminal or internal sequences of macromolecules, or they may be artificially added to antigens, as in the case of the tripeptide, L-Tyr-L-Ala-L-Glu.

When the antigenic determinant is composed of terminal sequences, the terminal residue of the sequence is almost invariably the immunodominant group. This was recognized quite early when it was shown that the terminal amino acid of a peptide (Landsteiner, 1945) and the terminal monosaccharide of a glycoside (Goebel et al., 1934), when coupled to proteins, played a dominant role in specificity. As already mentioned, in SII polysaccharide, glucuronic acid, which occurs almost exclusively at the terminal, nonreducing ends of the side chains, is the immunodominant sugar in the specificity of most of the antibodies studied. The extensive studies of Heidelberger (1956) with polysaccharide antigens serve to reinforce this principle.

Systems employing synthetic antigens have furnished substantial supportive evidence. The series of $(D-Ala)_n$-Gly peptides coupled to ribonuclease by B. Schechter et al. (1970) elicited antibodies for which the amino-terminal amino acid residue, the most exposed element of the determinant, was immunodominant. In another study of great relevance, chains of L-alanine were coupled to protein either through the terminal α amino group or the C-terminal carboxyl group (I. Schechter et al., 1971). Antibodies elicited by one conjugate did not cross-precipitate with the oppositely coupled conjugate. Furthermore, antibodies against the conjugate with free amino groups did not bind strongly peptides in which the amino terminal end was altered, whereas amides of L-alanyl peptides were very good ligands. Conversely, antibodies elicited by the conjugate with free carboxyl groups did not bind the peptide amides well. Here again, the most exposed, or terminal, portion of the chain appears to constitute the immunodominant group. While both types of antibody reacted with free peptides of L-alanine, it is likely that the peptides were oriented in opposite directions in the respective combining sites.

The contribution to binding with antibody of each amino acid residue in the antigenic determinants of poly-L- and poly-D-alanyl protein conjugates, which contained an average of 4 to 8 alanine residues per chain, was analyzed by comparing the binding of peptides of equal size which differed from one another in a particular feature (I. Schechter, 1971). The antibody combining site was considered to consist of distinct subsites, each of which interacts with a discrete portion of the antigenic determinant. The subsite concept has been used to advantage in mapping the binding sites of proteolytic enzymes. For example, it was found that papain interacts with a sequence of 7 amino acid residues in a substrate peptide, 4 on one side of the catalytic point and 3 on the other (Berger et al., 1971). Hence, the active site of this enzyme is composed of 7 subsites. Since anti-polyalanyl antibodies have combining sites which accommodate 4 alanine residues (Section II,B), the combining site can be divided into 4 subsites.

Antibodies were fractionated by immunoadsorption and subsequent serial elution with di-, tri- and tetraalanine peptides. In each purified antibody fraction, the association constants of series of alanine peptides of increasing size were measured by equilibrium dialysis. The binding energy contributed by the β-methyl side chain of alanine was estimated by using peptides in which a particular alanine residue was replaced by glycine. Stereospecificity and space-filling requirements in each subsite were also assessed. The results showed that the terminal alanine residue contributed the greatest binding energy with a declining gradient along the chain. In addition, each subsite exhibited a marked degree of heterogeneity with respect to interaction with an alanine residue. The same subsite in the three antibody fractions and the various subsites within the same fraction all behaved differently with the series of peptides. The use of paired haptens of equal size which differ from each other in a particular feature can provide detailed information about the fine architecture of antigenic determinants and antibody combining sites which cannot be obtained by studying the effects of elongating a homologous series of haptens.

Even when specificity is directed toward an internal sequence of an antigen, there is a gradient of binding energy for different parts of the determinant. In the classical investigation of the dextran–antidextran system by Kabat (1966), a dextran containing very few branch points presumably elicited antibody directed largely or exclusively against interior sequences of glucose. Taking the hexasaccharide as the determinant, the relative contribution to the total binding energy made by each glucose unit was evaluated by com-

2. Antigenic Determinants and Antibody Combining Sites

paring the inhibitory efficiencies on a molar basis of a series of oligosaccharides. The values obtained indicated that the first glucose contributed 40%, the first two glucoses 60%, and the first three glucoses 90% of the binding energy of the hexasaccharide. Similar decrements in binding energy occurred with other essentially linear polysaccharide antigens such as SIII (Mage and Kabat, 1963). In general, then, it may be concluded that all determinants exhibit a gradient of immunodominance, and that when the determinant is comprised of a terminal sequence, the gradient decreases from the most exposed portion inward.

2. Optical Configuration

Antibodies exhibit a pronounced stereospecificity (Landsteiner, 1945; Pressman and Grossberg, 1968). While polyamino acids of the D optical configuration are very weakly or nonimmunogenic, D-amino acids can serve as partial or complete determinants when either appended to immunogenic carriers or integrally incorporated into synthetic polypeptides. In general, cross-reactivity based on precipitation between antibodies to determinants of L-amino acids and their D counterparts has not been observed (Sage *et al.*, 1964; Arnon *et al.*, 1965; Schechter *et al.*, 1966). While a recent report suggests that enantiomorphic polypeptides can cross-react weakly by precipitation (Gill *et al.*, 1967), the data do not exclude slight racemization of the test polymers as a possible explanation for the observed cross-reactivity. By hapten inhibition of precipitation between poly-γ-D-glutamic acid and its homologous antibody, there was no distinction in inhibiting capacity between D- and L-glutamic acids (Goodman and Nitecki, 1966). However, when the eight possible dipeptides of glutamic acid were assayed, those of the D series were distinctly superior. A number of polypeptides containing L- but no D-glutamic acid were unable to precipitate the antibody, but could significantly inhibit precipitation, albeit very inefficiently. It thus appears that stereospecificity, while strong, may not be absolute.

In at least some situations, D-amino acids may be more immunopotent or immunodominant than their stereoisomeric counterparts. Most of the antibody formed to poly-DL-alanyl proteins, in which the polypeptides were mixtures of the two isomers, was specific for sequences of D- rather than of L-amino acids. This conclusion stemmed from finding that the antisera cross-reacted with poly-D- or poly-DL-alanyl peptides conjugated to heterologous proteins, but reacted poorly with conjugates of the L-isomer (Schechter and Sela,

1965). It is probable that D-amino acids formed the immunodominant groups of determinants comprised of both isomers.

3. Conformation

An example has already been given of the influence conformation may exert in immunodominance, but its role in specificity is so profound that it warrants more detailed consideration. It should be reiterated at this point that the distinction between immunopotency and immunodominance in this context is extremely vague. I have chosen to consider what follows within the framework of immunodominance, but the alternative might be equally valid.

There are examples of determinants that depend for their immunochemical reactivity on the quaternary structure of the antigen. Studies with the hemoglobin molecule revealed that the oxygenated form of human hemoglobin Al showed greater complement fixation with antiserum than the reduced form, and this has been attributed to the difference in quaternary structure between the two forms (Reichlin et al., 1964, 1965a). The isolated α or β chains failed to fix complement with anti-A serum, but regained activity when hybridized with chains of the complementary type from canine hemoglobin, even though the canine chains themselves were inert toward the antiserum (Reichlin et al., 1965b). The heterologous chains were undoubtedly responsible for the assumption of a conformation approximating that of the native molecule. Additional experiments showed that while antisera prepared against isolated α and β chains do not appreciably cross-react, the reactivity of an anti-α chain serum with α chains by themselves or combined in tetramers with β chains from various sources or with γ chains were all different (Reichlin et al., 1966).

There are other examples of specificity which are dependent on quaternary structure, including antigenic determinants of immunoglobulin molecules which require for their expression association between heavy and light polypeptide chains (Seligmann and Mihaesco, 1967).

Examples of the effect of altering tertiary structure on immunodominance are more abundant. The pronounced change in the specificity of lysozyme upon reduction of its disulfide bridges followed by carboxymethylation of the sulfhydryl groups has already been mentioned. Similarly, performic acid-oxidized ribonuclease cross-reacts weakly, if at all, with antiserum prepared against native ribonuclease and *vice versa* (Brown et al., 1967). In general, the more extensively a molecule is denatured, the weaker will be its cross-reactivity with antisera to the native form, which, in turn, discloses that the antigenic determinants of globular proteins are, for the most part, dependent on conformation.

A novel series of experiments which demonstrated conformation-dependent specificity made use of a synthetic conjugate between a peptide encompassing residues 64 to 83 of hen egg lysozyme, designated the "loop" peptide because it contained a disulfide bridge between residues 64 and 80, and a branched polypeptide, multi-poly-DL-alanyl–poly-L-lysine (Arnon and Sela, 1969). This antigen raised antibodies that reacted with native lysozyme, demonstrable by inhibition of the homologous antigen–antibody reaction as well as by removal of antibodies on an immunoadsorbent prepared from lysozyme and bromoacetyl cellulose. Some of the antibodies evoked by immunization with native lysozyme could be isolated with an immunoadsorbent containing the loop peptide. These antibodies could be inhibited from reacting with lysozyme by the loop peptide, but not by its reduced and carboxymethylated derivative. Thus, opening the loop destroyed the antigenic determinant involved.

Another synthetic antigen, this one a polymer of repeating subunits, (Pro-Gly-Pro)$_n$, has the triple-stranded helical character of collagen (Sela et al., 1967). Guinea pig and rabbit antisera to the synthetic polymers cross-reacted with collagen from several sources by passive cutaneous anaphylaxis, and a reciprocal cross-reactivity with anti-collagen antisera also occurred. The basis for this cross-reactivity probably resides in conformational similarities between the synthetic polymer and collagen, but since collagen contains about 30% glycine and 13–15% proline, the data do not exclude cross-reactivity on the basis of sequential determinants.

Antibodies specific for determinants in the same sequential region of the staphylococcal nuclease molecule were prepared both by immunization with polypeptide fragments of nuclease and by immunization with intact nuclease followed by isolation of antibodies on immunoadsorbent columns bearing the corresponding fragments (Sachs et al., 1972). The specificities of the antibodies formed against the native protein and its fragments showed marked differences by quantitative precipitin and enzyme inhibition assays which could be attributed to conformational differences between the immunizing antigens. For one thing, antibodies formed against native nuclease readily inhibited enzyme activity whereas antibodies formed against the appropriate fragment did not. For another, antibody-induced inactivation of the enzyme was inefficiently inhibited by the appropriate fragment, suggesting that only a small fraction of the fragment molecules was bound by antibody combining sites at any given time. If this poor efficiency of binding was due to conformational differences between the antigenic determinant in the fragment and in native nuclease, then increasing the similarity between the two would be expected to increase the inhibitory capacity of the fragment. This was borne out by mixing the fragment with a complementing fragment from another part of the nuclease sequence. The two fragments combine and produce physical characteristics suggestive of the ordered structure of native nuclease. The addition of increasing concentrations of the complementing fragment, which carried no immunologic activity itself, enhanced the inhibition of inactivation by a fixed quantity of the specific fragment.

The results were interpreted as signifying that antinative nuclease antibodies react only with determinants that are in their native ordered conformation. It was plausibly proposed that the fragments of nuclease exist in solution in a variety of disordered or random conformations in equilibrium with the native conformation, which is generated by spontaneous and reversible folding of the polypeptide chain. Only those conformations approximating the native form will be bound with sufficient affinity by the antibody combining site. Once bound, the peptide should be stabilized in the native conformation. Indeed, antibodies to the helical polypeptide $(Tyr-Ala-Glu)_n$ (Fig. 3) have been shown to "induce" increased helicity in the oligopeptide $(Tyr-Ala-Glu)_{13}$, presumably by stabilizing the helical conformation of bound peptide and causing a shift in equilibrium of the conformational forms of remaining free peptide (B. Schechter *et al.*, 1972).

Antibodies to a sequence even as small as a nonapeptide may be heavily conformation-dependent. Rabbits immunized with a branch-chain copolymer of bradykinin and poly-L-lysine responded with antibodies that bound bradykinin. When synthetic analogues of bradykinin were assayed for binding, it was found that alterations in charge or hydrophobicity of amino acid side chains produced little effect, whereas substitutions at positions which had an obligatory influence on conformation (proline or glycine) profoundly altered binding (Spragg *et al.*, 1967).

There is thus abundant evidence for the existence of antibodies with specificity for conformation-dependent features of antigen molecules, as well as antibodies whose specificity is directed against sequential determinants. To reiterate, in the latter situation, antibodies will normally react with small fragments of the antigen, while in the former situation disruption of the original conformation of the antigen will result in very weak or negligible binding. Consequently, the determinants of globular proteins have been difficult to delineate in detail, whereas the deployment of natural or synthetic fibrous (i.e., linear or randomly coiled) molecules and peptidyl–protein conjugates has met with greater success. Such antigens have provided us with the most solid information concerning the size and nature of antigenic determinants.

IV. The Antibody Combining Site

A. *The Concept of Complementarity*

The idea that antigens and antibodies unite because of a structural complementarity analogous to that of a key fitting a lock was first articulated by Paul Ehrlich during the early years of the twentieth century. Emil Fischer proposed much the same mechanism for the binding of substrates by enzymes. Later, instructive theories of antibody formation postulated that the antigen provided a keylike template around which the antibody molecule was folded in locklike fashion.

Actually, structural complementarity in biologic phenomena is probably as ancient as biology itself. The replication of DNA and the synthesis of messenger RNA occur through the copying of partial or complete strands of DNA. The formation and stabilization of the DNA helical duplex depends on the complementarity of the bases. The propensity of cells for their own kind is undoubtedly due to surface complementarity, about which little is known as yet at the molecular level. A fascinating example of this is the mating of compatible strains of yeast through the specific interaction of surface macromolecules. The soluble surface molecules, which have been partially purified and characterized, have been shown to inhibit the mating process (Crandall and Brock, 1968), reminiscent of the inhibition of immune agglutination by soluble antigen. It seems plausible that the immune response, a much later phylogenetic development than the appearance of unicellular organisms, had its origin in primitive recognition systems of this kind.

The principle of complementarity led to predictions about the size of the antibody combining site, based on reactivity with haptens, upon which we have already remarked. These predictions rely on a model of the antibody combining site which is similar to that of the active sites of enzymes for their substrates. The enzyme lysozyme has been crystallized from egg white and its intimate three-dimensional structure has been elucidated by X-ray diffraction (Phillips, 1966). The single polypeptide chain of lysozyme is folded to form a cleft that accommodates its substrate, a polysaccharide constructed of alternating sequences of N-acetyl-D-glucosamine and N-acetylmuramic acid in β-(1 → 4) linkage. The crevice can accommodate six sugar rings, or three of the disaccharide subunits, which occupy very definite positions therein, stabilized by noncovalent interactions with the atoms of amino acids forming the crevice. It appears that the conformation of the enzyme is altered upon contact with the substrate, which results in a greater degree of complementarity.

Much less is known about the active sites of antibody molecules, principally due to their heterogeneity which has retarded crystallization and X-ray diffraction analysis. However, progress is being made in the crystallization of myeloma proteins for which ligands have been found (Inbar et al., 1971), techniques are being perfected for the more-or-less routine induction of relatively homogeneous antibody (Krause, 1970), and even hapten–protein conjugates that ordinarily induce very heterogeneous responses occasionally raise antibodies that are crystallizable (Nisonoff et al., 1967). Very recently, crystals have been obtained from fragments produced by pepsin digestion of mouse myeloma proteins that bind phosphorylcholine. Crystals from one of these diffracted X-rays to a resolution of about 2.7 Å and bound one mole of hapten per mole of fragment (Rudikoff et al., 1972). Therefore, it may be anticipated that we will have a portrait of an antibody combining site as detailed as that of the active site of lysozyme in the not-too-distant future.

However, up to the present time attempts to observe direct effects of ligand-binding on the structure of the antibody molecule have been disappointing. Circular dichroism spectroscopy could not detect conformational changes in the papain-generated univalent fragments of rabbit anti-DNP antibody upon binding with DNP-lysine, although the antibody had a high affinity for the hapten ($K \approx 10^9$ liters/mole) (Cathou et al., 1968). On the other hand, hapten did stabilize the conformation of such antibody, since circular dichroism bands which disappeared rapidly from the spectra of unbound antibody in 4 M guanidine-HCl were lost much more gradually in the presence of hapten (Cathou and Werner, 1970). Such stabilization suggests that the antibody site is not confined to a very limited segment of the macromolecule, but is formed by the folding of polypeptide chains in such a way as to juxtapose regions that are distantly related in the linear sequence. However, in order to proceed beyond

2. Antigenic Determinants and Antibody Combining Sites

this gossamer image, we must draw inferences from what is known about the structure of antibody molecules.

B. The Structure of Immunoglobulin Molecules

Although precise localization of the antibody combining site to a circumscribed part of immunoglobulin molecules has not yet been conclusively established, elucidation of the molecular structure of antibodies has progressed so rapidly in recent years that strong inferences may be confidently drawn. The structure of immunoglobulins is treated in depth elsewhere in this series, so only those aspects bearing directly on the combining site itself will be briefly considered here.

It is now firmly established that all immunoglobulin molecules are composed of heavy (H) and light (L) polypeptide chains. The IgG class of immunoglobulins is comprised of a pair of each type of chain, arranged so that the molecule is bilaterally symmetrical (Fig. 4). The amino-terminal sequence of about 110 residues of both H and L chains is highly variable; these V regions comprise half the L chain and one-quarter of the H chain. Each class of immunoglobulins

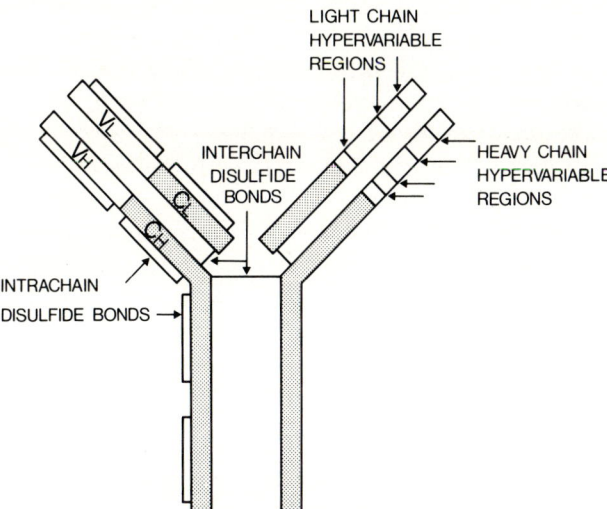

Fig. 4. Schematic model of an IgG immunoglobulin molecule illustrating the polypeptide chain structure and the approximate positions of the hypervariable regions in heavy and light chains. V_L and V_H: variable region of light and heavy chain, respectively; C_L and C_H: constant region of light and heavy chain, respectively.

has a distinctive sequence for the constant region of the H chain, although minor variations in sequence within a class have led to the recognition of subclasses. Some classes of immunoglobulins (IgM and IgA) are larger molecules made up of polymers of the basic four-chain unit. The two classes of L chains, κ and λ, are common to all classes of immunoglobulins and thus can pair with any class of heavy chain. All κ chains have identical sequences in their carboxy-terminal half, which differs markedly from the distinctive sequence of the carboxy-terminal half of all λ chains. The only exception to this constancy is a single position within the constant half of each class which defines either an allotypic or an isotypic variation. Despite their extreme variability, the variable regions of light chains can be placed into subgroups based on patterns of amino acid sequence. Thus far, no κ variable region subgroup has been found associated with a λ constant region, or vice versa. Thus, the variable region, as well as the constant region, is distinctive for each class of light chain.

It is believed that there are a small number of germ-line structural genes for the constant region of each class of polypeptide chain, in all likelihood a single gene for each subclass. Family studies in species for which genetic markers on the different classes of polypeptide chains have been identified have demonstrated that the heavy chain genes fall within one linkage group, while the genes for κ and λ chains segregate independently from heavy chain genes and from each other. There is a large, as yet unidentified, number of V-region genes in separate sets for heavy, κ, and λ chains. The question of a germ-line origin or somatic generation of this diverse assortment of V-region genes is undecided and is the subject of substantial controversy at present. However, there is convincing evidence that the polypeptide chains are coded for by separate genes for the variable and constant regions and that the different classes of H chains, in contrast to L chains, share the same pool of V genes. This evidence emanates from the identity of V-region allotypes of rabbit γ (IgG) and μ (IgM) heavy chains (Koshland et al., 1969), as well as from the apparent identity of the amino acid sequences of the V regions from the γ and μ chains of IgG and IgM myeloma proteins from a single human subject (Wang et al., 1970).

There is general agreement that the antibody combining site is formed by the variable regions of the H and L chains and that the complex heterogeneity of antibodies is, for the most part, a reflection of the degree of variability that occurs at well over 70% of the positions within these sequences of about 110 residues. For one thing, upon enzymatic fragmentation of antibody molecules, activity is found only in fragments that include the variable regions. Indeed, a fragment of a mouse IgA myeloma protein which apparently included only the variable regions possessed antigen-binding activity (Inbar et al., 1972). For another, when small but significant differences in the total amino acid compositions of different antibodies from the same rabbit were initially demonstrated (Koshland and Englberger, 1963), it was found that these differences were confined to the N-terminal portions of H and L chains where variability is known to occur (Koshland, 1966). Further, the antibodies to two highly cross-reacting determinants, arsonic and phosphonic acids, showed no significant compositional differences, while antibodies to other non-cross-reacting anionic determinants did (Koshland et al., 1967). These findings certainly suggest that the observed differences are related to specificity and hence to the combining site, but it is important to appreciate that they represent a minimum value for the magnitude of primary structural differences related to specificity. This becomes apparent when one considers that proteins of identical composition can have entirely different sequences, although such an extreme case would hardly be encountered in nature. Yet another line of evidence for the location of the combining site within the variable regions derives from affinity-labeling studies in which the hapten becomes covalently bound to amino acid residues of the antibody molecule (Singer and Doolittle, 1966). The evidence that coupling takes place while the hapten is within the combining site is compelling, and the hapten has invariably been found on residues from the V regions of H and L chains.

This latter point, namely, the association of the hapten with both types of chains in affinity-labeling experiments, has been used as an argument for the participation of the variable regions of both H and L chains in the antibody combining site. However, when isolated H and L chains have been tested separately for antigen-binding activity, only the H chains have shown this capacity to any substantial degree. In a few instances, isolated L chains have been shown to possess weak intrinsic binding activity, but very sensitive techniques have been required to demonstrate it. In one case, rabbit L chains neutralized bacteriophage provided antibody to the L chain was added. Antibody against H chains had no effect on the neutralization produced by the L chain fraction (Goodman and Donch, 1965). In another approach, enhancement of the fluorescence of the hapten, 4-azonaphthalene-1-sulfonate, was observed when L chains from specific antibody were present. This hapten is one of a group of compounds that show negligible fluorescence in polar solvents but fluoresce strongly in hydrophobic solvents or when bound to proteins. The enhancement curves given by L chains and H chains were qualitatively different, indicating that the activity of L chains was not due to contamination by minute quantities of H chain (Yoo et al., 1967). The highest activity of isolated L chains yet reported has been for a preparation of horse diphtherial antitoxin from which this fraction possessed 5–10% of the activity of the intact antibody (Mangalo et al., 1966).

The difficulties attending substantiation of the intrinsic binding activity of isolated H or L chains stem from incomplete separation of the chains under conditions that permit retention of demonstrable activity. Contamination of the H chain fraction by small amounts of L chain is common, since dissociation is often incomplete in mildly dissociating solvents. More rigorous conditions which effect complete dissociation produce extensive denaturation of the isolated chains. Even small amounts of L chain might be expected to restore appreciable activity to H chain fractions, particularly if the antibodies of highest affinity are the most difficult to dissociate. The isolation of L chains free of H chains is not as subject to this limitation, but it is conceivable that L chains are more easily denatured than H chains, rendering the demonstration of binding activity more difficult. At any rate, the combined evidence appears to favor the specific participation of both chains in the antibody combining site.

C. The Location of the Antibody Combining Site

Given the formidable evidence that the antibody combining site is somehow constructed of the variable regions of heavy and light chains of immunoglobulin molecules, a natural question that arises is whether the entire variable regions are involved or whether the binding site can be further circumscribed within these regions. Upon cursory inspection of sequence data, the variable regions show no gradient of variability across their span; the positions at which variation occurs appear to be randomly distributed. However, when the variable region subgroups of light chains, for which much more sequence data are available than for heavy chains, were initially recognized, it was noted that certain positions showed a remarkably high degree of variability relative to the background (Milstein and Pink, 1970). As sequence data accumulated, two regions of hypervariability could be identified, immediately following each of the two cysteine residues at positions 23 and 88 which form the intrachain disulfide loop of the variable region (Fig. 4). It was particularly noteworthy that these two regions were brought into close proximity by the disulfide bridge and that they were also the locations of insertions or deletions (Milstein and Pink, 1970; Kabat, 1970).

A detailed statistical analysis was made by Wu and Kabat (1970) of the variability at each position from the sequence data available on 77 Bence Jones proteins and immunoglobulin light chains, considering human and mouse κ and human λ chains of various subgroups as a single population aligned for maximum homology. Defining variability as

$$\frac{\text{number of different amino acids at a given position}}{\text{frequency of the most common amino acid at that position}}$$

three hypervariable regions were found which encompassed residues 24 to 34, 50 to 56, and 89 to 97 (Fig. 5). It was suggested that at least the first and third of these regions, since they are brought into juxtaposition by the disulfide bridge, and possibly all three, together with similar hypervariable stretches in the heavy chain, might form the complementarity regions which actually make contact with the antigenic determinant.

It was proposed that the remaining residues of the variable regions would serve a structural function in establishing the three-dimensional folding of the site. According to this model, the combining sites of all antibodies should have essentially the same position and

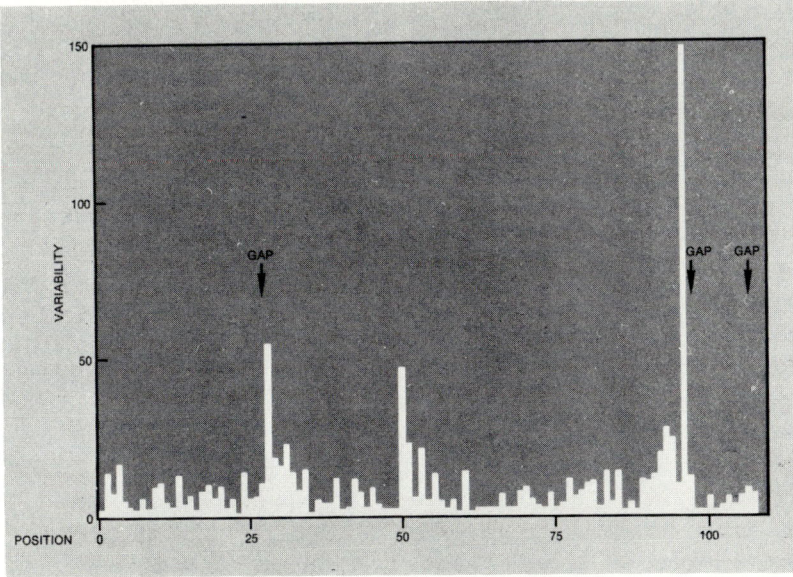

Fig. 5. The variability at different amino acid residue positions for the variable region of human and mouse light chains. (From Wu and Kabat, 1970.)

dimensions, but the intimate topology within the site would vary, depending on the amino acid sequences of the hypervariable regions.

Experimental data from other sources have tended to support this concept and to reinforce the significance of the hypervariable regions. Affinity-labeling techniques using different reagents have labeled residues in each hypervariable region (Goetzl and Metzger, 1970; Franek, 1971; Ray and Cebra, 1972; Haimovich et al., 1972). It is particularly significant that labeled residues have never been found far from the hypervariable regions. In most cases the label in light chains has been located between residues 30 to 40 and/or 80 to 100.

Entirely different support for the significance of the hypervariable regions can be found in the unusually small λ V-gene pool in mice. Of 10 mouse λ chains analyzed by amino acid composition of peptides, 6 had apparently identical sequences in the variable regions while the remaining 4 had substitutions only in one or another of the three hypervariable regions (Weigert et al., 1970). These findings strengthen the view that the hypervariable regions are intimately associated with antibody specificity.

Although amino acid sequence data for the variable regions of heavy chains are more fragmentary than for light chains, there is likewise evidence for three or four hypervariable regions in human and rabbit heavy chains (Press and Hogg, 1969; Capra, 1971; Kehoe and Capra, 1971; Mole et al., 1971). These appear to span residues 31 to 37, 50 to 60, 86 to 91, and 101 to 109 and are indicated in the schematic diagram in Fig. 4.

If the hypervariable regions do indeed represent the contact points of the antibody combining site with the antigenic determinant, then despite their distance from one another in the linear sequence they must be brought within sufficient proximity in the three-dimensional structure of the antibody molecule to be spanned by a tetra- to hexapeptide or -saccharide. It is immediately apparent that the first and third hypervariable regions would be brought into very close proximity by the disulfide bridge between cysteines 23 and 88. A model of the variable region of κ light chains was constructed on the basis of X-ray diffraction data for the orientation in space of each amino acid residue in six nonimmunoglobulin proteins for which such information was available (Kabat and Wu, 1972). The data were assembled in the form of tripeptide tables in which the (ϕ, ψ) angles of amino acid n were related to the neighboring residues $(n-1)$ and $(n+1)$. This rationale is based on the postulate that nearest neighbors profoundly

2. Antigenic Determinants and Antibody Combining Sites 161

influence and largely determine the orientation in space of a given amino acid in a polypeptide chain. On that basis, it was possible to tabulate the coordinates for any amino acid located in the middle of a tripeptide which occurred in at least one of the six reference proteins. It is important to recognize that factors other than nearest neighbors will influence the orientation of a given amino acid. For example, coordinates may be very different for a given triplet, depending on whether it is located within or outside a helical domain. Thus, of the 8000 possible tripeptides (20^3), (ϕ, ψ) angles were available for 1067 from the six reference proteins, and two or more sets of values were obtained for 130 of these which were recurrent. When a given tripeptide had several sets of values, in some instances they were very similar while in others distinctly different. For example, of 111 tripeptide sequences with two sets of values, for only 27 did the two values fall within ±15°. In addition, a number of tripeptide sequences occurred in the κ chains which had no exact counterpart in the reference proteins. This could be anticipated since only 1067 of the possible 8000 tripeptides appeared in the reference proteins. In order to compensate for this inadequacy, a hierarchy of criteria was established, ranging in reliability from highest, for instances in which the κ tripeptide was found in the reference proteins, to lowest, for which only the dipeptide sequences $(n-1)$ $(n)(-)$ and $(-)(n)(n+1)$ occurred in the reference proteins. The set of angles chosen for residue n was the one for which data of highest reliability were available, except in seven instances in which preferred choices produced a structure that would not accommodate the amino acid side chains. In such cases, data from a criterion lower in the hierarchy were used.

Despite the obvious limitations and approximations of this approach, a model of the variable region emerged in which the cysteine residues at positions 23 and 88 were, surprisingly enough, sufficiently close in space for the disulfide bond to form. The first and third hypervariable regions could well form part of a cleft, which in conjunction with analogous regions of the heavy chain might constitute the antibody combining site. Even the second hypervariable region (residues 50 to 56) was only about 30 to 35 Å from some of the residues in the third hypervariable region. This is about the span of the most extended form of a hexasaccharide, so it is not inconceivable that contact amino acids might be provided by all three areas of extreme variability.

However, at this stage it must be emphasized that the above portrait of the antibody combining site, and, indeed, even the relevance of the hypervariable regions to complementarity is inferential and still belongs in the realm of thoughtful speculation. The issue will not be settled until we have a high resolution X-ray diffraction pattern of an antibody embracing its antigenic determinant. That time should not be far off.

V. Immunogenic Determinants

A. *Haptens and Immunogens*

In the first section of this chapter, the structural features of antigens which determine the specificity of humoral antibody have been considered. These antigenic or haptenic determinants can react with antibody formed against the intact antigen molecule, but they are usually unable to induce antibody formation, or, for that matter, an immune response of any kind. This is illustrated by the response pattern of rabbits to poly-γ-D-glutamic acid (Goodman and Nitecki, 1967). The polypeptide, though of molecular weight 35,000, was unable to induce antibody formation by itself, but when it was electrostatically complexed with methylated bovine serum albumin an antigen was formed which readily provoked the formation of antibody precipitable by the pure polypeptide. Animals which were actively producing anti-polypeptide antibody in response to the complex were nonetheless refractory to subsequent challenge with the free polypeptide in the sense that it neither induced additional anti-polypeptide antibody nor served as a carrier for a second hapten, p-amino-p'-dimethylaminoazobenzene, which was linked to the polypeptide using a carbodiimide coupling agent. Immunization with electrostatic complexes of the dihaptenic conjugates and methylated albumin raised antibody against each hapten, demonstrating the functional activity of each component of the conjugate.

Thus, the multivalent polypeptide was not "recognized" as an immunogen, even by animals that had already mounted an antibody response against it, and the addition of a second type of haptenic determinant did not alter this unresponsiveness. While evidence has been presented which indicates that at least two determinants are required for a humoral immune response (Rajewsky *et al.*, 1969), this is a necessary but insufficient condition unless other requirements are satisfied. These findings underscore the now firmly established principle that immunogenicity is a rigid genetically determined property, and an animal cannot be conditioned to recognize a hapten as an antigen. Very similar results have been obtained with polylysine in guinea pigs, where it was additionally shown that induction of tolerance to the carrier abrogated the anti-hapten response to complexes of the two (Green et al., 1968).

An established and significant disparity between haptens and immunogens is that cellular immunity can be induced and elicited only by the latter (Eisen, 1959; Borek et al., 1963), although responses with a distinct anti-hapten component have occasionally been observed (Benacerraf and Gell, 1959; Paul et al., 1968; Phair and Kantor, 1970; Henney, 1970). This type of immunity, in contrast to humoral immunity, can be transferred by lymphoid cells but not by serum from an immune donor. As one of many examples, animals that have produced circulating antibody to polyglutamic acid by virtue of immunization with hapten–carrier complexes do not exhibit delayed cutaneous hypersensitivity *in vivo* or a proliferative response by lymphoid cells in culture upon challenge with the pure polypeptide, whereas these reactions are invariably elicited by the carrier (Roelants et al., 1969; Roelants and Goodman, 1970). Thus, while there are apparently antibody-forming cells for haptenic determinants, haptens as a rule do not induce cellular immunity, cannot serve as carriers for other haptens, and induce antibody formation only when introduced on immunogenic carriers.

Another cardinal characteristic of the anti-hapten response is its strict carrier specificity. A secondary response to the hapten can usually be elicited only when it is administered on the same carrier molecule that served for priming (Ovary and Benacerraf, 1963; Dutton and Bulman, 1964). If the same hapten to which the animal was primed is given on an immunologically unrelated second carrier, the animal shows no immunologic memory for the hapten and makes a typical primary response. Here, too, exceptions have been noted wherein heterologous carriers triggered secondary anti-hapten responses. With most (Steiner and Eisen, 1966; Brownstone et al., 1966; Paul et al., 1967; Klinman, 1971), but not all (Rittenberg and Campbell, 1968) such exceptions, the heterologous carrier provoked a relatively weak secondary response. It is not yet clear how significant carrier cross-reactivity at the level of cellular immunity may be in anamnestic responses to heterologous carriers, since cross-reactivity has usually been assessed only at the level of humoral immunity. Antibody affinity and cross-reactivity increase with time after immunization, and mature anti-hapten memory is less carrier-specific than immature memory (Paul et al., 1967; Kontiainen and Mäkelä,

1971). It is also possible that high-affinity anti-hapten cells are superior to low-affinity cells in capturing antigen without external concentrating mechanisms which involve the carrier and carrier-specific cells.

B. Dichotomy of Humoral and Cellular Immunity

An immunogenic molecule will, in most instances, induce both humoral and cellular immune responses. When hapten–carrier conjugates are used for immunization, it can readily be shown that cellular immunity is confined to the carrier or the intact conjugate, whereas antibodies directed against the conjugated hapten as well as against antigenic determinants native to the carrier molecule are ordinarily formed.

Although little has been done by way of systematically comparing the cross-reactivity of native antigens at cellular and humoral levels, a few examples have recently been cited of proteins which cross-react cellularly but not serologically. Hen egg-white lysozyme and bovine α-lactalbumin have considerable chemical homology but little or no serologic cross-reactivity with antisera from rabbits or guinea pigs. In contrast, they cross-react strongly when assayed by antigen-induced blast transformation in cell culture or by delayed hypersensitivity reactions *in vivo* (Maron *et al.*, 1972). Similarly, humoral cross-reactivity between *Ascaris* and mammalian collagens, which have a triple helix structure but differ radically in molecular organization, was negligible whereas cell-mediated cross-reactivity was substantial (Michaeli *et al.*, 1972).

While there is usually little or no humoral cross-reactivity between a native protein and its extensively denatured derivatives (Section II,D,3), in several such instances significant cellular cross-reactivity has been demonstrated. Gell and Benacerraf (1959) found that native and heat-denatured proteins produced delayed hypersensitivity to either material in guinea pigs under circumstances where immediate skin reactivity was either weak or absent. Moreover, immunization with relatively large quantities of bovine or human serum albumin led to cross-sensitization of the delayed type only, whereas both humoral and cellular reactions could be elicited by the homologous antigen. It was concluded that delayed hypersensitivity is a more sensitive and less specific manifestation of immunity than reactions of antigen with conventional antibody.

Additional evidence for a dichotomy of humoral and cellular specificity has been obtained using chemically modified proteins. Lysozyme and its reduced and S-carboxymethylated derivative, CM-lysozyme, did not cross-react serologically (Gerwing and Thompson, 1968; Young and Leung, 1970), but showed strong cross-reactivity on the basis of delayed hypersensitivity reactions in guinea pigs, and spleen cells obtained from animals immunized with either form of the protein made essentially equivalent proliferative responses to both antigens (Thompson et al., 1972). In addition, cross-tolerance between the native and modified forms of lysozyme was observed.

Parallel findings have been obtained using flagellin from a strain of *Salmonella* and its acetoacetylated derivatives, which did not cross-react serologically but showed a significant degree of cross-reactivity with respect to delayed hypersensitivity (Parish, 1971a,b). Delayed hypersensitivity to polymerized flagellin (POL) of one specificity could be transferred to normal or lethally irradiated syngeneic mice by lymphoid cells activated by POL of another serologic specificity (Cooper, 1972). The transfer was completely abrogated by saturating the cells with POL labeled with ^{125}I to a specific activity sufficient to kill cells which bound substantial numbers of molecules (Cooper and Ada, 1972). This effect has been called "antigen-induced cell suicide." Cells activated by POL of one serologic specificity were completely inactivated by [^{125}I]POL of the same or a serologically non-cross-reacting specificity, but not at all by a completely unrelated protein, [^{125}I]hemocyanin.

On the other hand, Rajewsky and Pohlit (1971) concluded that the specificities of humoral and cellular immunity were qualitatively similar after finding that the capacity of heterologous albumins to serve as carriers for a secondary anti-hapten response correlated with their serologic cross-reactivity with the carrier used for priming. A complication in comparing these findings with the divergent results above is that delayed skin reactivity and carrier activity, while manifestations of cellular immunity, may be mediated by different cell populations.

C. The Specificity of Humoral and Cellular Immunity

The work discussed above was performed with large proteins, the structural similarities and disparities of which are obscure. It has thus not been possible to identify the structural determinants involved in humoral and cellular immunity employing these materials. As a consequence, there are two possible interpretations of the findings: (1) that cellular immunity has a broader, less exquisite specificity than that of conventional antibody (Gell and Benacerraf, 1959; Salvin and Smith, 1960) or (2) that the structural determinants of the antigen involved in humoral and cellular immunity need not be the same. According to the second hypothesis, antigens that do not share haptenic determinants would not cross-react at the humoral level but might do so at the level of cellular immunity, without implying a qualitative or even quantitative difference in the nature of specificity of the two systems.

Investigations using well-defined antigens of characterized structure are clearly needed to distinguish between these alternative possibilities. Efforts in this direction have proved quite productive and tend to support the interpretation that humoral and cellular specificities may be directed against different determinants of the antigen molecule. Bovine glucagon, a polypeptide of 29 amino acids whose structure has been completely delineated, proved to be immunogenic in guinea pigs (Senyk et al., 1971). Using isolated tryptic peptides of the hormone (Fig. 6) to explore its immunologic determinants, it was found that antisera from all of more than two dozen immunized animals were specific for the amino-terminal heptadecapeptide and showed little or no reactivity with the carboxy-terminal undecapeptide.

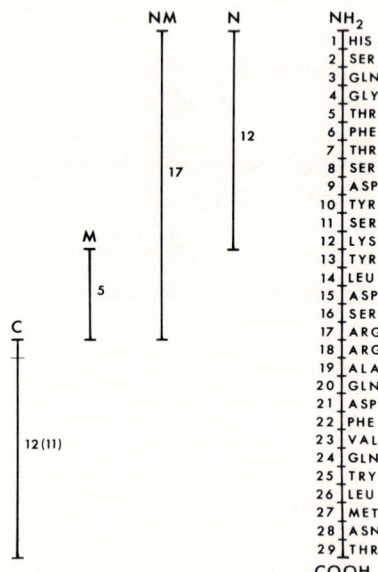

Fig. 6. The structure of bovine glucagon and its fragments produced by digestion with trypsin. (From Senyk et al., 1971.)

TABLE III

Cellular Immune Response of Guinea Pigs to Glucagon[a]

Test antigen	Average delayed skin reaction (mm)	Inhibition of cell migration (%)[b]	Lymphocyte stimulation[c]	
			Range	Mean
Glucagon	14 (20)[d]	65 (8)	2.3–26.0	10.9 (13)
N	3 (6)	21 (3)	—	—
M	0 (6)	0 (3)	—	—
NM	8 (6)	55 (3)	0.7–1.1	0.8 (6)
C	12 (6)	75 (3)	2.7–20.0	8.8 (13)

[a] From Senyk et al. (1971).
[b] The figures were derived from the following equation:

$$\left(1 - \frac{\text{migration of cells in chambers containing antigen}}{\text{migration of cells in chambers without antigen}}\right) \times 100$$

[c] Ratio of [^{14}C]thymidine incorporation in cultures with antigen present relative to cultures without antigen from the same animal.
[d] Parentheses indicate number of animals tested.

Assays for cellular immunity revealed that both fragments elicited delayed cutaneous reactions and inhibited the migration of peritoneal cells from immune animals, although the smaller carboxy-terminal peptide seemed to have a higher specific activity in these semiquantitative assays (Table III). However, only intact glucagon and its carboxy-terminal fragment stimulated lymphoid cells to synthesize DNA (Table III). These findings demonstrated a functional dissection of the antigen into two parts, one of which housed the major antigenic or haptenic determinant while the other carried the major determinant for cellular immunity. Of course, this distinction need not be and, in fact, is not absolute. The anti-glucagon antibodies were heterogeneous in specificity and a minor population in a significant fraction of the antisera bound the carboxy-terminal peptide. Furthermore, guinea pigs immunized with glucagon–protein conjugates in which glucagon was linked via the tyrosine residues at positions 10 and 13 made antibodies specific for one or more determinants in the carboxy-terminal region (Senyk et al., 1972). This can be understood on the basis of the importance of accessibility in immunopotency and the extreme diversity of the antibody response. In conjugated form, glucagon behaves like a conventional hapten and does not induce cellular immunity. Conversely, the amino-terminal fragment elicited delayed hypersensitivity. An apparent dissociation between different manifestations of cellular immunity was observed in that this peptide was unable to provoke a proliferative response by lymphoid cells in culture. Similar observations have been made with other protein (Spitler et al., 1970) as well as with polysaccharide (Chaparas et al., 1970) antigens. It is still unknown whether these different activities are expressed by the same or by different populations of cells.

A series of peptides initiated at the carboxy-terminal position of glucagon was synthesized to determine the smallest peptide with demonstrable transforming activity for cells from animals immunized with the native hormone. Activity declined sharply with peptides smaller than the undecapeptide, but was still significant in one instance with the heptapeptide (Table IV). Of particular interest, the pattern of reactivity varied from animal to animal. With most, the undecapeptide was markedly more active than the dodecapeptide, but cells from one guinea pig did not distinguish between the two. This kind of variation bears a strong resemblance to that seen in the specificities of populations of antibody molecules from different animals.

Guinea pigs responsive to poly-L-lysine develop cellular immunity when immunized with polymers larger than the hexapeptide. An uninterrupted sequence of at least 7 L-lysine residues appears to be required for immunogenicity; substitution of a residue of the D configuration causes loss of activity in a nonapeptide with the sequence L_4DL_4, whereas peptides of sequence L_7DL and LDL_7 are fully active.

TABLE IV

Stimulation of Lymph Node Cell Cultures from Glucagon-Sensitized Guinea Pigs by Natural and Synthetic Peptides

	Maximum stimulation given by[a]									
					Synthetic peptides					
Animal	Glucagon	C	C_1[b]	C_2[c]	Dodeca-	Undeca-	Deca-	Nona-	Octa-	Hepta-
1	15.0	15.7	1.0	16.0	1.1	9.0	1.3	1.0	0.9	1.1
2	15.0	12.7	10.5	10.2	4.3	4.3	1.8	1.1	1.1	1.0
3	23.0	18.5	–	–	11.5	14.1	8.8	4.3	3.3	2.1
4	7.3	11.6	–	–	6.3	11.6	5.2	1.7	1.1	1.3
5	9.0	8.8	–	–	1.2	5.1	0.9	0.9	0.9	0.8
6	16.5	12.8	–	–	2.0	3.4	1.1	1.1	1.0	1.1

[a] Ratio of [^{14}C]thymidine incorporation in cultures with antigen present relative to cultures without antigen from the same animal.
[b] Natural carboxy-terminal dodecapeptide of glucagon.
[c] Natural carboxy-terminal undecapeptide of glucagon.

2. Antigenic Determinants and Antibody Combining Sites

TABLE V

Immunogenicity of Derivatives of L-Tyrosine-Azobenzene

Structure	R	Name	Immunogenicity[a]

H$_2$N—CH—COOH
      |
     CH$_2$
      |
  [phenyl]—N=N—[phenyl]—R
      |
     OH
	—AsO$_3$H$_2$	-p-arsonate	+

	—COOH	-p-carboxylate	−
	—SO$_3$H	-p-sulfonate	+
	—NH—CO—CH$_3$	-p-acetamide	−
	—SO$_2$NH$_2$	-p-sulfonamide	−
	—NO$_2$	-p-nitro	−
	—N(CH$_3$)$_3$Cl	-p-trimethylammonium chloride	+

[a] Induction of delayed cutaneous sensitivity.

A comparison was made of the responses to a series of DNP-nonalysines in which the positions of the DNP group and D-lysine residues varied (Schlossman et al., 1969). Lymph node cells from responder guinea pigs immunized with α-DNP-Lys$_9$ (L$_9$), α-DNP-Lys$_9$ (L$_7$DL), α-DNP-Lys$_9$ (LDL$_7$), 5-ε-DNP-Lys$_9$ (L$_9$), 9-ε-DNP-Lys$_9$ (L$_9$), or Lys$_9$ (L$_9$) could discriminate between these peptides and made maximal proliferative responses to the homologous immunogen.

Another low molecular weight compound, L-tyrosine-p-azobenzenearsonate (ABA-L-Tyr), induces cellular immunity in guinea pigs (Leskowitz et al., 1966). In an investigation of the structural requirements for immunogenicity of this molecule, a series of analogs in which substitutions were made for the arsonate group (Table V) was prepared and used for immunization (Alkan et al., 1972). The results showed that other charged moieties could substitute for arsonate without loss of immunogenicity. However, modification at this position yielded molecules with distinctive specificities. There was little or no cross-reactivity on the basis of elicitation of delayed cutaneous reactions between compounds containing arsonate, sulfonate, carboxylate, acetamide, sulfonamide, nitro-, or trimethylammonium substituents. Moreover, lymph node cultures from guinea pigs immunized with ABA-L-Tyr or one of the p-azobenzenearsonate substituted tetrapeptides ABA-L-Tyr-(L-Tyr)$_3$, ABA-L-Tyr-(L-Ala)$_3$, and (L-Tyr)$_3$-L-Tyr-ABA made maximal proliferative responses to the homologous immunogen (Becker et al., 1973).

Thus, in the rare instances in which cellular immunity has been induced by molecules small enough to permit the elucidation of structure-specificity relationships, the specificities of cellular and humoral immunity appear to be comparably discriminatory.

Why, then, is cross-reactivity at the cellular level often retained after humoral cross-reactivity has disappeared, as with modified or denatured protein antigens? One would anticipate that if specificity for different determinants was entirely responsible, then cellular immunity should disappear first in about half the instances. The answer to this question is not yet at hand, but it may lie in the relative affinities of the antigen-recognition sites. In the case of humoral immunity, the recognition site is the antibody combining site. It has been established that the average affinity of antibody for its antigenic determinant usually increases during the course of the response (Eisen and Siskind, 1964). It has also been frequently observed that the specificity of antisera decreases with progressive immunization (Hooker and Boyd, 1941). Affinity could readily account for the observed changes in specificity since antibodies of high affinity should be capable of displaying a wider range of cross-reactions than those of low affinity. In the case of cellular immunity, the recognition structure is a receptor on the surface of a cell. The affinities of antigen receptors have not yet been determined, principally because the numbers of receptors per cell or per preparation have not been accurately quantitated. If the affinities of antigen receptors on cells that mediate cellular immunity prove to be appreciably greater than observed antibody affinities, it could account for the greater cross-reactivity, without loss of discriminatory power, of cellular immune reactions. Such a finding would also be consistent with observations that cells that mediate cellular immunity are more readily rendered unresponsive by antigen than those which secrete antibody (Weigle, 1973). However, this issue will be resolved only when the affinities of cell receptors have been accurately determined.

D. Cell Cooperation in the Immune Response

The dichotomy between humoral and cellular immunity can be readily understood on the basis of a mechanism involving the expression of these activities by immunocompetent cells of different lineage. Lucid evidence for such a mechanism was initially obtained from studies with avian species, which have a clearly differentiated immune system (Warner et al., 1962). Bursectomy early in life ablated humoral responsiveness without significantly impairing cellular immunity, whereas early thymectomy eradicated cellular immunity. Experiments with mice have substantiated the role of thymic lymphocytes in cellular immunity, although the bursal equivalent in mammals has not yet been positively identified (Miller et al., 1971). About the same time, it was also shown that neonatal thymectomy impaired the antibody response to most, but not all, antigens (Humphrey et al., 1964), and that immunologic responsiveness could be fully restored to neonatally thymectomized or thymectomized and irradiated adult mice by implantation of a thymic graft from a syngeneic donor (Leuchars et al., 1965), although thymic lymphocytes themselves did not produce antibody (Davies et al., 1967). This latter point was hammered home by the work of Miller and his colleagues who reconstituted thymectomized, irradiated mice with bone marrow and either thymocytes or thoracic duct lymphocytes, which could be distinguished on the basis of chromosomal or allotypic markers (Miller et al., 1971). These investigations clearly established that the antibody response resulted from the interaction of a cell derived from the thymus, which specifically recognized antigen but did not secrete antibody, with another cell derived from the bone marrow, the actual precursor of the antibody-producing cell. These two functionally distinct, antigen-specific cells have come to be designated T and B cells, respectively.

Although a detailed review of the cellular work leading to our understanding of cooperation is beyond the province of the subject matter here, this brief sketch serves to illustrate its compatibility with the character of the immune response to haptens and carriers. Thus, T cells recognize structural features of carriers and cooperate with B cells which recognize haptenic determinants, whether they be conjugated to, or integral parts of, the antigen molecule. The "carrier effect" referred to earlier, wherein the hapten must be administered on the homologous carrier in order to obtain a secondary anti-hapten response, is due to the requirement for a primed or expanded population of T "helper" cells (Raff, 1970). If an animal is primed to the hapten and carrier separately by injection with hapten–carrier$_1$ and –carrier$_2$, then a secondary response will follow challenge with hapten–carrier$_2$ (Rajewsky et al., 1969). Similarly, a more intense anti-hapten response can be obtained by pretreatment with the carrier alone (Alkan et al., 1971).

Specific recognition of the antigen appears to take place via receptors at the cell surface. The chemical nature of the T-cell receptor is still at issue, but there is convincing evidence that the B-cell receptor is conventional antibody identical to the secretory product of the cell (Roelants, 1972). The nature of the cooperative and inductive processes is also enshrouded in mystery. It has been proposed

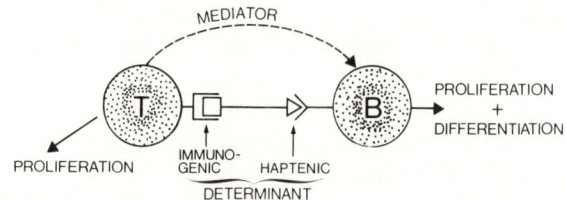

Fig. 7. A minimum model of cooperation between two antigen-specific cells leading to a humoral antibody response. The T cell is induced by a signal from an immunogenic determinant to proliferate and release a non-antigen-specific humoral mediator which exerts a concentration-dependent effect on the B cell. This, in concert with a second signal from a haptenic determinant, triggers the B cell to proliferate and differentiate into an antibody-producing cell.

that the T cell concentrates and focuses haptenic determinants for the B cell (Mitchison, 1969), perhaps in a way which produces allosteric changes in the membrane of the B cell, signaling its differentiation (Bretscher and Cohn, 1970). However, there is strong evidence that the T cell, when acted upon by antigen, releases a nonspecific (and, hence, nonantibody) humoral factor which, in concert with antigen, activates the B cell (Schimpl and Wecker, 1972).

Whatever the mechanism of the cooperative process, it is clear that the two cells must be brought into close proximity, if not into actual contact, since hapten and carrier must be administered on the same molecule in order to obtain an anti-hapten response. The idea has emerged, owing chiefly to Mitchison (1969), that antigen might serve this function by bridging the cells, and a skeletal model based on this concept is depicted in Fig. 7.

E. Carrier Activity of Determinants That Induce Cellular Immunity

Consideration of the character of the immune response and the principles of cell cooperation lead logically to the prediction that any molecule capable of inducing a cellular immune response should be able to serve as a carrier for a hapten. There are several examples of molecules about the size of an antigenic determinant which exhibit this behavior. One of these, ABA-L-Tyr (Section III,B), induces cellular immunity without discernible antibody formation (Leskowitz *et al.*, 1966; Alkan *et al.*, 1971; Nauciel and Raynaud, 1971), even by the extremely sensitive passive neutralization of bacteriophage technique (Becker *et al.*, 1973). This accords with expectations in that a unideterminant antigen, though capable of interacting with T and B lymphocytes, should be unable to mediate cooperation between them. The result also implies that cooperation between T cells is not essential for their activation, but its occurrence cannot be excluded. Indeed, there is evidence of synergy between thymocytes and peripheral blood lymphocytes of thymic origin in the graft-versus-host reaction, although each cell type is capable of some activity in the absence of the other (Asofsky et al., 1971).

Conjugates of ABA-L-Tyr and the multivalent hapten poly-γ-D-glutamic acid raised humoral anti-hapten antibody and cellular immunity directed against the ABA-L-Tyr determinant (Alkan et al., 1971). Lymphoid cells in culture were transformed more efficiently by the homologous conjugate than by free ABA-L-Tyr, but the polyglutamic acid hapten itself had no transforming activity. Similar observations have been made using conventional hapten–protein conjugates (Davie and Paul, 1970). Moreover, prior immunization with ABA-L-Tyr potentiated the anti-hapten response, paralleling the effect obtained with protein carriers (Rajewsky et al., 1969). Thus, in this instance a molecule of molecular weight 409 served as a carrier for a hapten with an average molecular weight of about 35,000, the reverse of the customary relationship.

Better defined, small bifunctional antigen molecules composed of one ABA-L-Tyr immunogenic determinant and one dinitrophenyl haptenic determinant separated by spacers of varying size permitted an exploration of the spatial requirements between hapten and carrier for an anti-hapten response (Alkan et al., 1972). The spacer employed was 6-aminocaproic acid (SAC), a flexible chain of six carbon atoms with an extended span of 8 Å. One or a series of spacers could be linked in stepwise fashion through the amino group of tyrosine, leaving the amino group of the terminal spacer available for reaction with 2,4-dinitrofluorobenzene. Guinea pigs immunized with such conjugates developed cellular immunity directed against the ABA-L-Tyr determinant and antibody specific for the DNP determinant. The magnitude of the anti-DNP response was similar whether the two determinants were separated by one or three SAC spacers, but was significantly weaker when the determinants were joined without a spacer. Thus, cooperation could apparently be mediated by an antigen in which the carrier and haptenic moieties were separated by less than 8 Å.

This result appears paradoxical in light of the size of an antigenic determinant and evidence that the receptor for the cellular immune response exhibits specificity for more than just ABA-L-Tyr, based on the proliferative responses of lymph node cells to a series of ABA-Tyr peptides (Becker *et al.*, 1973). However, the orientation of the ABA group in the various peptides might be sufficiently different to account for the observed specificity. In addition, it is still not known if proliferative responses can be equated with helper activity, so the specificity of the former may not necessarily apply to T cells which cooperate in the antibody response.

In dealing with the immunogenicity of small molecules like ABA-L-Tyr, the specter of artifact looms large and must be given scrupulous consideration. Could the cellular immune response to ABA-L-Tyr be due to adherence to autologous proteins, which might thereby be modified sufficiently to serve as carriers? Could the antihapten response to the bifunctional antigens be an indirect consequence of transconjugation from ABA-L-Tyr to autologous proteins? It is known that the deliberate covalent substitution of autologous serum proteins renders the conjugates immunogenic (Davie and Paul, 1970). While such *in vivo* processes are difficult to conclusively exclude, the character of the response to ABA-L-Tyr speaks against them. The relevant points are the following:

1. ABA-L-Tyr engenders a pure cellular immune response. It would be expected to behave like a hapten if it induced a response consequent to attachment to proteins.

2. ABA conjugates of polypeptides containing D-amino acids did not induce cellular immunity specific for ABA-Tyr (Leskowitz *et al.*, 1966), although peptides comprised of D-amino acids are potent haptenic determinants (Section II,D,2). There appears to be no *a priori* basis for believing that conjugates of L-amino acids would be chemically more reactive in attaching to autologous proteins than conjugates of D-amino acids. While ABA-D-Tyr itself did induce cellular immunity (Leskowitz *et al.*, 1966), this may be tied to the observation that antibody against poly-γ-D-glutamic acid did not discriminate between the enantiomorphic forms of the free amino acid but discriminated very well between the various dipeptides of L- and D-glutamic acid (Section II,D,2) (Goodman and Nitecki, 1966). The thesis that "antigen recognition" may be unable to discriminate between enantiomorphic forms of a single amino acid is supported by the observation that cellular immunity induced by ABA-D-Tyr was elicitable by ABA-L-polypeptide conjugates but not by their D counterparts (Leskowitz *et al.*, 1966).

3. Haptenic conjugates of ABA-L-Tyr are chemically stable in the physiological pH range. The cellular immune response to these con-

jugates manifests specificity for the original immunogen, minimizing the possibility that transconjugation precedes induction.

4. The anti-DNP antibody response to ABA-L-Tyr-SAC-DNP is significantly less heterogeneous by isoelectric focusing than the response to DNP–protein conjugates (Roelants and Goodman, 1974). This is in good agreement with other findings wherein relatively simple antigens often give rise to relatively homogeneous antibody populations (Haber, 1967). If the DNP group of the bifunctional antigen was transconjugated to a variety of autologous proteins, the reverse would be anticipated.

As already noted (Section IV,C), homopolymers of L-lysine containing at least seven residues induce cellular immunity in responder guinea pigs. DNP conjugates of immunogenic oligolysyl peptides induce anti-DNP antibody responses (Schlossman et al., 1965). Smaller peptides that do not induce cellular immunity do not act as carriers for the DNP haptenic determinant. These examples, though few in number, provide persuasive evidence for the carrier activity of determinants that induce cellular immunity.

F. The Libraries of Haptenic and Immunogenic Determinants

What has gone before leads inexorably to the conclusion that the diversity of determinants to which T cells are responsive is more restricted than the universe of B-cell determinants. Otherwise, the compounds that are haptens would be immunogenic and there would be no such entity as a hapten. However, "immunogenicity" is an operational term and only defines a response that is detectable under a given set of conditions. In order to understand why, for example, dinitrophenyl-6-aminocaproyl-L-tyrosine is a potent hapten but an extremely poor immunogen, in contrast to L-tyrosine-p-azobenzenearsonate, which is of comparable molecular size and is both a potent hapten and a strong immunogen (Alkan et al., 1972), one must distinguish between at least two possibilities. First, the libraries of genetic information in T- and B-cell populations may differ, permitting B cells to respond to a much greater variety of antigenic signals. This suggests that the generation of diversity in the two lymphocyte populations is independently regulated, a not altogether comfortable premise. Second, there may be stringent requirements for the presentation of determinants to T cells in order to activate them. In this, the macrophage may play a determining role, since antigens associated with macrophages are more immunogenic than comparable doses of free antigen (Unanue, 1972).

There is a substantial body of literature concerned with "hapten-specific" T-cell activity, a careful review of which would be appropriate at this juncture. Mice immunized with nitroiodophenacetyl chicken globulin (NIP-CG) conjugates and others with DNP–ovalbumin conjugates were used as donors of spleen cells for syngeneic irradiated recipient mice (Mitchison et al., 1971). The secondary response of mice which received a mixture of the donor cells was tested by injecting an unrelated carrier which had been substituted with the same two haptens. Such animals made a stronger anti-hapten response than did control recipients injected with a mixture of the singly substituted conjugates. This was taken to signify carrier activity by the haptenic determinants. However, antibody-forming cells were also transferred, and it has been shown that in some circumstances antibody to one determinant can exert a "carrier-like" effect in the antibody response to other determinants on the same antigen molecule (Janeway, 1972; Pincus et al., 1973). This complication has been given careful consideration by Mitchison, and it has been shown that the level of humoral anti-hapten antibody bears no relationship to helper activity (Mitchison, 1971a). However, small amounts of passively administered antibody were more effective than larger doses in mimicking the carrier effect (Pincus et al., 1973). The effect of antibody is very difficult to adequately control, because under some circumstances antibody may suppress the immune response while under others it apparently enhances. The net result may depend on quantity, affinity, and immunoglobulin class (Henry and Jerne, 1968) of the antibody; simulation of conditions in experimental and control animals under these circumstances would prove difficult, if not impossible.

Underscoring this limitation is the finding that when thymus cells rather than spleen cells from mice immunized with hapten–protein conjugates were transferred to recipients that had been treated with anti-lymphocyte serum, a helper effect could not be detected (Mitchison, 1971b). In these experiments, the donors of helper cells were lethally irradiated mice reconstituted with syngeneic thymus and immunized with DNP–protein conjugates. The recipients were treated with anti-lymphocyte serum to suppress their T-cell activity and, after receiving "helper" cells, were immunized with DNP-heterologous carrier conjugates. Helper activity was based on the anti-carrier antibody response. The inability of thymic cells from animals immunized with hapten–protein conjugates to provide help in this system casts doubt on the existence of hapten-specific T-cell help and supports the alternative interpretation that antibody may have been responsible for the effects observed in the earlier experiments (Mitchison et al., 1971).

On the other hand, skin painting the donors of thymic cells with fluorodinitrobenzene instead of immunizing them with DNP–protein conjugates did provide a helper effect (Mitchison, 1971b). Skin painting with chemically reactive compounds induces an apparent hapten-specific cellular immunity and has been shown to engender carrier activity by the hapten in recipients of spleen cells from sensitized mice (Taylor and Iverson, 1971). The difficulty here is that the compound reacts with an indeterminate number of proteins in the tissues of the painted animal, forming conjugates that are immunogenic by virtue of chemical modification. It has been established that haptenated autologous proteins are immunogenic and that the immunochemical specificity is directed at new determinants of the carrier arising as a consequence of modification, as well as at the hapten itself (Rubin, 1973). Consequently, it is extremely difficult to exclude cross-reactivity at the T-cell level between one or more of the myriad of modified autologous proteins, which may be the inducers of the cellular immune response, and the hapten–protein conjugate used to assess hapten-specific helper activity. The upshot of this is that it is enormously difficult to establish hapten-specific T-cell activity using such an ill-defined system.

Evidence other than helper activity for a T-cell response to the NIP determinant was found by evaluating the contribution of the hapten to the stimulation of DNA synthesis by thymus cells from mice immunized with NIP-mouse γ-globulin conjugates (Moorhead et al., 1973). Activated T cells were secured by injecting syngeneic thymic cells intravenously into irradiated recipients, immunizing the mice, and using the spleens as a source of such cells. The cells responded in vitro to the homologous conjugate, but not to the unmodified autologous protein carrier. This of itself is inconclusive, since cellular recognition may be directed against new carrier determinants resulting from haptenic modification (Rubin, 1973). The telling point in these experiments was that the response to the conjugate could be partially inhibited by NIP coupled to ϵ-aminocaproic acid. Therefore, if the in vitro response was entirely attributable to T cells, the results clearly demonstrate T-cell recognition of the NIP determinant. However, since B cells can apparently participate in the in vitro proliferative response to antigen (Moorhead et al., 1973), this remains a moot point in that it is based on the assumption of null

B-cell activity in the spleens of irradiated mice reconstituted with thymic cells.

Another approach, which suffers from much the same shortcomings as skin painting, but to a lesser degree, involves immunization with hapten-conjugated mycobacteria. Complete Freund's adjuvant, of which mycobacteria comprise the cardinal component, induces strong cellular immunity to antigens with which it is mixed, and immunity to tubercle bacilli is the classical example of delayed hypersensitivity, affording a plausible basis for the hypothesis that a more intimate association between the antigenic determinant and the bacterial cell might enhance the cellular immune response. It was observed some time ago that trinitrophenylated mycobacteria induced strong hapten-specific delayed sensitivity in guinea pigs, precedent to the appearance of circulating antibody (Benacerraf and Gell, 1959). It is of interest that conventional conjugates of the hapten with heterologous or homologous proteins also induced delayed sensitivity, though they were less satisfactory in this regard than mycobacterial conjugates. In the light of present knowledge, these observations suggest T-cell recognition of the TNP group and, further, that the manifest diversity of T-cell specificities may be expanded by appropriate presentation of the antigenic determinant.

The observations pertaining to picrylated mycobacteria have recently been confirmed and extended, using a variety of haptens coupled to *Mycobacterium butyricum* (Trefts et al., 1973). These haptenated mycobacteria regularly induced in guinea pigs hapten-specific skin reactivity of the delayed type, the capacity for lymphoid cells from immune animals to make a hapten-specific proliferative response in culture, and lymphoid cells with a capacity to lyse erythrocytes coated with hapten. Although the possibility that these activities derive from B cells and/or circulating antibody has not been entirely excluded, they are generally attributed to T cells and suggest that this mode of immunization may be an extremely effective way to trigger the response of such cells to determinants which are normally haptenic.

Exploration of hapten binding using [2,4-^{125}I]dinitrophenyl human IgG revealed a surprisingly large fraction of radiolabeled cells in preparations from normal mouse spleen (0.99%) and thymus (0.15%) (Lawrence et al., 1973). The binding of haptenated protein could be inhibited by DNP–lysine and other DNP conjugates, pointing to a specificity for the DNP determinant. Treatment of the thymic cell preparations with anti-θ serum, which is specifically cytotoxic for T cells, reduced the proportion of antigen-binding cells, indicating that the binding by thymic cell preparations was not wholly attributable to immigrant B cells. In addition, antigen binding by thymic cells could be inhibited with anti-mouse μ-chain serum but not with anti-γ-chain serum, whereas spleen cells were inhibited with both antisera. These findings are consistent with the relatively large proportion of myeloma proteins that bind DNP (Potter, 1971), as well as with other investigations that indicate that the antigen receptor on mouse T cells may be identical or similar to IgM immunoglobulin (Marchalonis et al., 1972; Roelants et al., 1973). However, these results should be interpreted very cautiously with respect to hapten recognition by T cells. Antigen binding is not necessarily indicative of immunologic function; it is conceivable that IgM might be passively bound to the surfaces of all or a subpopulation of T cells which have not produced it. Another important consideration evolves from quantitative inhibition experiments which indicated that DNP binding by thymic cells was less avid than by spleen cells (Lawrence et al., 1973). This low avidity binding might possibly result from interaction between the relatively hydrophobic ligand and a conservative hydrophobic patch near the active site of the IgM molecule which may not be directly related to antigen specificity (Singer and Doolittle, 1966). An interpretation along these lines is even more palatable in view of the very high frequency of DNP-binding thymic cells from unimmunized animals. At any rate, a correlation between antigen binding and immunologic activity must be demonstrated before these observations can be granted relevance to antigen recognition.

Thus, in sum, we are left with a collection of observations suggesting but not firmly establishing that the library of T-cell specificities may be larger than heretofore recognized and perhaps comparable to B-cell diversity. However, it is indisputable that T-cell activity in the form of cellular immunity is difficult to switch on under normal circumstances with molecules the size of one or several determinants. The basis for this difficulty is still obscure.

VI. Concluding Remarks

The nature and dimensions of haptenic determinants of antigen molecules is a subject that has received much attention during the past two decades and is now reasonably solved. The use of homopolymers of amino acids or sugars and peptidyl proteins as antigens has established that the determinant is composed of four to six amino acid or sugar residues which contribute unequally to binding with the antibody combining site. The optical configuration and conformation of the determinant figure heavily in its immunochemical specificity.

These properties bear a strong resemblance to those of the contact regions of enzyme substrates. Six sugar residues entirely fill the combining site of lysozyme (Chipman and Sharon, 1969). Here, too, estimates of the contribution of a given residue in the site to the total free energy of association of a saccharide with the enzyme indicate unequal contribution by the various residues, but a continuous gradient has not been observed, in contrast to the situation with haptenic determinants and antibody combining sites. The proteolytic enzyme papain interacts with a sequence of seven amino acids in a polypeptide substrate, and limited data indicate unequal contribution to binding by different subsites in the ligand (Berger et al., 1971). The evidence converges toward a coherent image of the dimensions of ligands involved in binding with active sites of proteins.

Until the mid-1960's, what was known about antibody combining sites was largely inferred on the basis of complementarity with haptenic determinants. Since then, physicochemical studies, amino acid sequence data, and affinity-labeling experiments have combined to establish quite firmly that antibody combining sites are formed from a relatively small number of amino acids located in sequentially distant parts of the variable regions of heavy and light polypeptide chains. These amino acids occur in two hypervariable sequences C-terminal to the half-cystines of the intrachain disulfide bridge in the variable region of each chain. One or two other hypervariable regions may also be involved, and indications are that heavy chains may contain somewhat more hypervariable positions than light chains. The precise location of all hypervariable regions remains somewhat uncertain, particularly for the heavy chain. Based on these findings, it is probable that the amino acid residues lining the combining site are centered around positions 30 and 96 on each of the two polypeptide chains. Additional noteworthy features are the presence of very stable sequences near the two half-cystine residues adjacent to the hypervariable stretches, as well as hydrophobic areas nearby (Porter, 1972). The last feature is consistent with earlier observations that affinity-labeled peptides were unusually hydrophobic (Singer and Doolittle, 1966).

It may again prove instructive to compare this model of the antibody combining site with the known structures of enzymes and their combining sites, all of which appear to be clefts or grooves

2. Antigenic Determinants and Antibody Combining Sites

formed by the folding of polypeptide chains so that sequentially distant regions are brought into close proximity. The clefts are lined with perhaps 10 to 20 residues. Hartley (1970) has made an interesting comparison of the catalytic sites of chymotrypsin, trypsin, and elastase which illustrates how readily the specificity of binding of small molecules by proteins may be altered. These sites differ only in that serine at position 189 in chymotrypsin is replaced by aspartic acid in trypsin and the glycine residue at position 216 is replaced in elastase by valine. The latter substitution effectively blocks the subsite that accepts an aromatic or basic residue in chymotrypsin and trypsin, respectively. These small changes against an otherwise similar background alter the specificity of binding from that of a peptide containing an aromatic or leucine residue by chymotrypsin to that of a peptide containing a basic residue by trypsin, and, finally, to much less specific binding of any peptide by elastase.

From consideration of the structure–specificity relationships of these enzymes, there is no difficulty in envisaging an antibody combining site as a cleft or groove within which an enormous range of specificities might be attained by variation at 20 or so amino acid positions. When the background variability of the variable regions is coupled with the hypervariable stretches which are postulated to actually reside within the site, the possibilities of variation in the topology of the site may easily be as great as the range that antibody heterogeneity demands. Determination of the steric structure of an antibody molecule binding its ligand should complete our understanding of the antibody combining site. This promises to be achieved over the near term as crystallization of immunoglobulins, into which considerable effort is being poured, progresses.

In contrast to haptenic determinants, elucidation of the nature and dimensions of immunogenic determinants is still in its infancy. Only a few small, structurally defined, unideterminant molecules have thus far been shown to be immunogenic. While their intrinsic immunogenicity may still be open to question, the evidence that they function in much the same way as macromolecular, multideterminant antigens is growing and has become rather persuasive. The crux of this issue is that little is known as yet of the pathway of any antigen from the time of administration to the appearance of a detectable host response.

The essential requisite for immunogenicity appears to be recognition by one or more clones of T cells. Unideterminant antigens do not by themselves induce a significant antibody response, but do induce a cellular immune response and serve as carriers for haptens.

The haptenic determinant of bifunctional antigen molecules may either be different from (Alkan *et al.*, 1972) or the same as (Bush *et al.*, 1972) the carrier determinant. These findings are consistent with the two antigen-specific cell model of cooperation in the antibody response which is now almost universally accepted. On the basis of a T-cell response to presumably unideterminant antigens, it is postulated that cooperation between T cells is not required for their activation.

Why do many potent haptenic determinants fail to activate significant T-cell responses? Evidence is emerging which indicates that such activation may take place by special means of antigen presentation—for example, in the form of mycobacterial–hapten conjugates (Section IV,F). However, even if true, this begs the question of a distinction between the diversity of T-cell and B-cell populations with respect to antigen specificity. Such a distinction apparently exists, and its mechanistic origin is a central issue in immunology. If speculation is permissible, then it seems reasonable that molecules which do not interact above a threshold affinity with antigen-receptors on T cells cannot trigger a response and consequently are haptens, regardless of the affinity of their interaction with B-cell receptors. Rigorous methods of presenting the hapten to the T cell may overcome this energy barrier, at least temporarily, but it exists nonetheless. This problem cannot be resolved until the affinity of antigen receptors on cells can be determined in much the same way antibody molecules have been characterized. Then it will be possible to compare the affinities of T-cell receptors for an authentic immunogenic determinant like L-tyrosine-*p*-azobenzenearsonate with one to which T-cell activity has been artificially generated, as in the case of haptenated mycobacteria. If the hypothesis is correct, then the affinity of the former should be significantly higher than that of the latter.

Assuming this to be the case, what might account for the absence of high affinity T cells for haptenic determinants? Either they are never generated or they disappear during development. The former explanation, of necessity, postulates independent generation of diversity in T-cell and B-cell populations. However, it is clear that T cells are more readily rendered unresponsive than B cells (Weigle, 1973). Could the apparent absence of T-cell responsiveness to many determinants which are potent haptens be due to induced tolerance by exposure to cross-reactive determinants which are present at paralyzing dose levels in the environment? These and other intriguing questions await experimental elucidation.

Acknowledgment

Much of this chapter was written during a sabbatical leave at the Basel Institute for Immunology, Basel, Switzerland. I thank the Institute and its personnel for the gracious cooperation I received there.

References

Alkan, S. S., Nitecki, D. E., and Goodman, J. W. (1971). *J. Immunol.* **107**, 353.
Alkan, S. S., Williams, E. B., Nitecki, D. E., and Goodman, J. W. (1972). *J. Exp. Med.* **135**, 1228.
Arakatsu, Y., Ashwell, G., and Kabat, E. A. (1966). *J. Immunol.* **97**, 858.
Arnon, R., and Sela, M. (1969). *Proc. Nat. Acad. Sci. U. S.* **62**, 163.
Arnon, R., Sela, M., Yaron, A., and Sober, H. A. (1965). *Biochemistry* **4**, 948.
Arquilla, E. R., and Finn, J. (1963). *Science* **142**, 400.
Arquilla, E. R., and Finn, J. (1965). *J. Exp. Med.* **122**, 771.
Arquilla, E. R., Miles, P., Knapp, S., Hamlin, J., and Bromer, W. (1967). *Vox Sang.* **13**, 32.
Asofsky, R., Cantor, H., and Tigelaar, R. E. (1971). *In* "Progress in Immunology" (B. Amos, ed.), pp. 369–381. Academic Press, New York.
Atassi, M. Z., and Saplin, B. J. (1968). *Biochemistry* **7**, 688.
Avery, O. T., and Goebel, W. F. (1929). *J. Exp. Med.* **50**, 533.
Barker, S. A., Somers, P. J., Stacey, M., and Hopton, J. W. (1965). *Carbohyd. Res.* **1**, 106.
Becker, M. J., Levin, H., and Sela, M. (1973). *Eur. J. Immunol.* **3**, 131.
Beiser, S. M., Burke, G. C., and Tannenbaum, S. W. (1960). *J. Mol. Biol.* **2**, 125.
Benacerraf, B., and Gell, P. G. H. (1959). *Immunology* **2**, 219.
Benjamini, E., Shimizu, M., Young, J. D., and Leung, C. Y. (1968a). *Biochemistry* **7**, 1253.
Benjamini, E., Shimizu, M., Young, J. D., and Leung, C. Y. (1968b). *Biochemistry* **7**, 1261.
Berger, A., Schechter, I., Benderli, H., and Kurn, N. (1971). *Proc. Eur. Symp. Peptides, 10th, 1969* pp. 290–309.
Borek, F., Silverstein, A. M., and Gell, P. G. H. (1963). *Proc. Soc. Exp. Biol. Med.* **114**, 266.
Bretscher, P., and Cohn, M. (1970). *Science* **169**, 1042.
Brown, R. K., McEwan, M., Nickoryak, C. A., and Polkowski, J. (1967). *J. Biol. Chem.* **242**, 3007.
Brownstone, A., Mitchison, N. A., and Pitt-Rivers, R. (1966). *Immunology* **10**, 481.
Bush, M. E., Alkan, S. S., Nitecki, D. E., and Goodman, J. W. (1972). *J. Exp. Med.* **136**, 1478.
Butler, K., and Stacey, M. (1955). *J. Chem. Soc., London* p. 1537.
Campbell, D. H., and Bulman, N. (1952). *Fortschr. Chem. Org. Naturst.* **9**, 443.
Capra, J. D. (1971). *Nature (London), New Biol.* **230**, 61.
Cathou, R. E., and Werner, T. C. (1970). *Biochemistry* **9**, 3149.
Cathou, R. E., Kulczycki, A., and Haber, E. (1968). *Biochemistry* **7**, 3958.

Cebra, J. J. (1961). *J. Immunol.* **86**, 205.
Chaparas, S. D., Thor, D. E., Godfrey, H. P., Baer, H., and Hedrick, S. R. (1970). *Science* **170**, 637.
Chipman, D. M., and Sharon, N. (1969). *Science* **165**, 454.
Cooper, M. G. (1972). *Scand. J. Immunol.* **1**, 237.
Cooper, M. G., and Ada, G. L. (1972). *Scand. J. Immunol.* **1**, 247.
Corneil, I., and Wofsy, L. (1967). *Immunochemistry* **4**, 183.
Crandall, M. A., and Brock, T. D. (1968). *Science* **161**, 473.
Crumpton, M. J., and Small, P. A., Jr. (1967). *J. Mol. Biol.* **26**, 143.
Crumpton, M. J., and Wilkinson, J. M. (1965). *Biochem. J.* **94**, 545.
Davie, J. M., and Paul, W. E. (1970). *Cell. Immunol.* **1**, 404.
Davies, A. J. S., Leuchars, E., Wallis, V., Marchant, R., and Elliott, E. V. (1967). *Transplantation* **5**, 222.
Dutton, R. W., and Bulman, H. N. (1964). *Immunology* **7**, 54.
Eisen, H. N. (1959). *In* "Cellular and Humoral Aspects of the Hypersensitive State" (K. S. Lawrence, ed.), p. 89. Harper (Hoeber), New York.
Eisen, H. N., and Siskind, G. W. (1964). *Biochemistry* **3**, 996.
Franek, F. (1971). *Eur. J. Biochem.* **19**, 176.
Fuchs, S., and Sela, M. (1963). *Biochem. J.* **87**, 70.
Fuchs, S., and Sela, M. (1964). *Biochem. J.* **93**, 566.
Gell, P. G. H., and Benacerraf, B. (1959). *Immunology* **2**, 64.
Gerwing, J., and Thompson, K. (1968). *Biochemistry* **7**, 3888.
Gill, T. J., III, Kunz, H. W., and Marfey, P. S. (1965). *J. Biol. Chem.* **240**, 3227.
Gill, T. J., III, Kunz, H. W., and Papermaster, D. S. (1967). *J. Biol. Chem.* **242**, 3308.
Gill, T. J., III, Papermaster, D. S., Kunz, H. W., and Marfey, P. S. (1968). *J. Biol. Chem.* **243**, 287.
Goebel, W. F., Avery, O. T., and Babers, F. H. (1934). *J. Exp. Med.* **60**, 599.
Goetzl, E. J., and Metzger, H. (1970). *Biochemistry* **9**, 3862.
Goodman, J. W. (1969). *Immunochemistry* **6**, 139.
Goodman, J. W., and Donch, J. J. (1965). *Immunochemistry* **2**, 351.
Goodman, J. W., and Kabat, E. A. (1960). *J. Immunol.* **84**, 347.
Goodman, J. W., and Nitecki, D. E. (1966). *Biochemistry* **5**, 667.
Goodman, J. W., and Nitecki, D. E. (1967). *Immunology* **13**, 577.
Goodman, J. W., Nitecki, D. E., and Stoltenberg, I. M. (1968). *Biochemistry* **7**, 706.
Gould, H. J., Gill, T. J., III, and Kunz, H. W. (1964). *J. Biol. Chem.* **239**, 3071.
Green, I., Paul, W. E., and Benacerraf, B. (1968). *J. Exp. Med.* **127**, 43.
Haber, E. (1967). *Annu. Rev. Biochem.* **37**, 497.
Haimovich, J., Schechter, I., and Sela, M. (1969). *Eur. J. Biochem.* **7**, 537.
Haimovich, J., Eisen, H. N., Hurwitz, E., and Givol, D. (1972). *Biochemistry* **11**, 2389.
Hartley, B. S. (1970). *Phil. Trans. Roy. Soc. London* **257**, 77.
Heidelberger, M. (1956). "Lectures in Immunochemistry." Academic Press, New York.
Henney, C. S. (1970). *J. Immunol.* **105**, 919.
Henry, C., and Jerne, N. K. (1968). *J. Exp. Med.* **128**, 133.
Hooker, S. B., and Boyd, W. C. (1941). *Proc. Soc. Exp. Biol. Med.* **47**, 187.
Humphrey, J. H., Parrott, D. M. V., and East, J. (1964). *Immunology* **7**, 419.
Inbar, D., Rotman, M., and Givol, D. (1971). *J. Biol. Chem.* **246**, 6272.
Inbar, D., Hochman, J., and Givol, D. (1972). *Proc. Nat. Acad. Sci. U. S.* **69**, 2659.
Janeway, C. A., Jr. (1972). *Fed. Proc., Fed. Amer. Soc. Exp. Biol.* **31**, 746.
Kabat, E. A. (1961). "Experimental Immunochemistry," 2nd ed. Thomas, Springfield, Illinois.

Kabat, E. A. (1966). *J. Immunol.* **97**, 1.
Kabat, E. A. (1970). *Ann. N. Y. Acad. Sci.* **169**, 43.
Kabat, E. A., and Berg, D. (1953). *J. Immunol.* **70**, 514.
Kabat, E. A., and Wu, T. T. (1972). *Proc. Nat. Acad. Sci. U. S.* **69**, 960.
Karush, F. (1956). *J. Amer. Chem. Soc.* **78**, 5519.
Karush, F. (1957). *J. Amer. Chem. Soc.* **79**, 3380.
Kehoe, J. M., and Capra, J. D. (1971). *Proc. Nat. Acad. Sci. U. S.* **68**, 2019.
Klinman, N. R. (1971). *J. Exp. Med.* **133**, 963.
Kontiainen, S., and Mäkelä, O. (1971). *Immunology* **20**, 101.
Koshland, M. E. (1966). *J. Cell. Comp. Physiol.* **67**, Suppl. 1, 33.
Koshland, M. E., and Englberger, F. M. (1963). *Proc. Nat. Acad. Sci. U. S.* **50**, 61.
Koshland, M. E., Ochoa, P., and Katagiri, J. (1967). *Fed. Proc., Fed. Amer. Soc. Exp. Biol.* **26**, 311.
Koshland, M. E., David, J. J., and Fujita, N. J. (1969). *Proc. Nat. Acad. Sci. U. S.* **63**, 1274.
Krause, R. M. (1970). *Fed. Proc., Fed. Amer. Soc. Exp. Biol.* **29**, 59.
Landsteiner, K. (1945). "The Specificity of Serological Reactions," 2nd ed. Harvard Univ. Press, Cambridge, Massachusetts.
Landsteiner, K., and van der Scheer, J. (1931). *J. Exp. Med.* **54**, 295.
Landsteiner, K., and van der Scheer, J. (1934). *J. Exp. Med.* **59**, 751.
Landsteiner, K., and van der Scheer, J. (1938). *J. Exp. Med.* **67**, 709.
Lapresle, C., and Webb, T. (1964). *Bull. Soc. Chim. Biol.* **46**, 1701.
Lapresle, C., and Webb, T. (1965). *Biochem. J.* **95**, 245.
Lawrence, D. A., Spiegelberg, H. L., and Weigle, W. O. (1973). *J. Exp. Med.* **137**, 470.
Leskowitz, S., Jones, V., and Zak, S. (1966). *J. Exp. Med.* **123**, 229.
Leuchars, E., Cross, A. M., and Dukor, P. (1965). *Transplantation* **3**, 28.
Levin, H. A., Levine, H., and Schlossman, S. F. (1971). *J. Exp. Med.* **133**, 1199.
Levine, B. B. (1963). *J. Exp. Med.* **117**, 161.
Little, J. R., and Eisen, H. N. (1965). *Fed. Proc., Fed. Amer. Soc. Exp. Biol.* **24**, 333.
Lüderitz, O., Staub, A. M., and Westphal, O. (1966). *Bacteriol. Rev.* **30**, 192.
McDevitt, H. O., and Benacerraf, B. (1969). *Advan. Immunol.* **11**, 31.
Mage, R. G., and Kabat, E. A. (1963). *J. Immunol.* **91**, 637.
Mangalo, R., Iscaki, S., and Raynaud, M. (1966). *C. R. Acad. Sci.* **263**, 204.
Marchalonis, J. J., Atwell, J. L., and Cone, R. E. (1972). *Nature (London)* **235**, 240.
Maron, E., Webb, C., Teitelbaum, D., and Arnon, R. (1972). *Eur. J. Immunol.* **2**, 294.
Maurer, P. H. (1953). *Proc. Soc. Exp. Biol. Med.* **83**, 879.
Maurer, P. H. (1964). *Progr. Allergy* **8**, 1.
Maurer, P. H., and Cashman, T. (1963). *J. Immunol.* **90**, 393.
Maurer, P. H., Gerulat, B. F., and Pinchuck, P. (1962). *J. Exp. Med.* **116**, 521.
Maurer, P. H., Gerulat, B. F., and Pinchuck, P. (1963). *J. Immunol.* **90**, 388.
Maurer, P. H., Gerulat, B. F., and Pinchuck, P. (1964). *J. Biol. Chem.* **239**, 992.
Michaeli, D., Senyk, G., Maoz, A., and Fuchs, S. (1972). *J. Immunol.* **109**, 103.
Miller, J. F. A. P., Basten, A., Sprent, J., and Cheers, C. (1971). *Cell. Immunol.* **2**, 469.
Milstein, C., and Pink, J. R. L. (1970). *Progr. Biophys. Mol. Biol.* **21**, 209.
Mitchison, N. A. (1969). *In* "Mediators of Cellular Immunity" (H. S. Lawrence and M. Landy, eds.), pp. 71–80. Academic Press, New York.
Mitchison, N. A. (1971a). *Eur. J. Immunol.* **1**, 18.
Mitchison, N. A. (1971b). *Eur. J. Immunol.* **1**, 68.
Mitchison, N. A., Rajewsky, K., and Taylor, R. B. (1971). *In* "Developmental Aspects of Antibody Formation and Structure" (J. Sterzl and I. Riha, eds.), Vol. 2, p. 547. Academic Press, New York.

Mole, L. E., Jackson, S. A., Porter, R. R., and Wilkinson, J. M. (1971). *Biochem. J.* **124**, 301.
Moorhead, J. W., Walters, C. S., and Claman, H. N. (1973). *J. Exp. Med.* **137**, 411.
Nauciel, C., and Raynaud, M. (1971). *Eur. J. Immunol.* **1**, 257.
Nisonoff, A., Zappacosta, S., and Jureziz, R. (1967). *Cold Spring Harbor Symp. Quant. Biol.* **32**, 89.
Ovary, Z., and Benacerraf, B. (1963). *Proc. Soc. Exp. Biol. Med.* **114**, 72.
Parish, C. R. (1971a). *J. Exp. Med.* **134**, 1.
Parish, C. R. (1971b). *J. Exp. Med.* **134**, 21.
Paul, W. E., Siskind, G. W., Benacerraf, B., and Ovary, Z. (1967). *J. Immunol.* **99**, 760.
Paul, W. E., Siskind, G. W., and Benacerraf, B. (1968). *J. Exp. Med.* **127**, 25.
Phair, J. P., and Kantor, F. S. (1970). *J. Immunol.* **105**, 417.
Phillips, D. C. (1966). *Sci. Amer.* **215**, 78.
Pincus, C., Miller, G., and Nussenzweig, V. (1973). *J. Immunol.* **110**, 301.
Porter, R. R. (1972). *Contemp. Top. Immunochem.* **1**, 145.
Potter, M. (1971). *Ann. N. Y. Acad. Sci.* **190**, 306.
Press, E. M., and Hogg, N. M. (1969). *Nature (London)* **223**, 807.
Press, E. M., and Porter, R. R. (1962). *Biochem. J.* **83**, 172.
Pressman, D., and Grossberg, A. L. (1968). "The Structural Basis of Antibody Specificity." Benjamin, New York.
Pressman, D., Siegel, M., and Hall, L. A. R. (1954). *J. Amer. Chem. Soc.* **76**, 6336.
Raff, M. C. (1970). *Nature (London)* **226**, 1257.
Rajewsky, K., and Pohlit, H. (1971). *In* "Progress in Immunology" (B. Amos, ed.), pp. 337–354. Academic Press, New York.
Rajewsky, K., Schirrmacher, V., Nase, S., and Jerne, N. K. (1969). *J. Exp. Med.* **129**, 1131.
Ray, A., and Cebra, J. J. (1972). *Biochemistry* **11**, 3647.
Reichlin, M., Bucci, E., Antonini, E., Wyman, J., and Rossi-Fanelli, A. (1964). *J. Mol. Biol.* **9**, 785.
Reichlin, M., Bucci, E., Wyman, J., Antonini, E., and Rossi-Fanelli, A. (1965a). *J. Mol. Biol.* **11**, 775.
Reichlin, M., Bucci, E., Fronticelli, C., Wyman, J., Antonini, E., and Rossi-Fanelli, A. (1965b). *J. Mol. Biol.* **12**, 774.
Reichlin, M., Bucci, E., Fronticelli, C., Jeffries, W., Antonini, E., Ioppolo, C., and Rossi-Fanelli, A. (1966). *J. Mol. Biol.* **17**, 18.
Rittenberg, M. B., and Campbell, D. H. (1968). *J. Exp. Med.* **127**, 717.
Roelants, G. E. (1972). *Curr. Top. Microbiol. Immunol.* **59**, 135.
Roelants, G. E., and Goodman, J. W. (1970). *Nature (London)* **227**, 175.
Roelants, G. E., and Goodman, J. W. (1974). *J. Immunol.* **112**, 883.
Roelants, G. E., Senyk, G., and Goodman, J. W. (1969). *Isr. J. Med. Sci.* **5**, 196.
Roelants, G. E., Forni, L., and Pernis, B. (1973). *J. Exp. Med.* **137**, 1060.
Rubin, B. (1973). *Eur. J. Immunol.* **3**, 26.
Rudikoff, S., Potter, M., Segal, D. M., Padlan, E. A., and Davies, D. R. (1972). *Proc. Nat. Acad. Sci. U. S.* **69**, 3689.
Sachs, D. H., Schechter, A. N., Eastlake, A., and Anfinsen, C. B. (1972). *Proc. Nat. Acad. Sci. U. S.* **69**, 3790.
Sage, H. J., Deutsch, G. F., Fasman, G., and Levine, L. (1964). *Immunochemistry* **1**, 133.
Salvin, S. B., and Smith, R. F. (1960). *J. Exp. Med.* **111**, 465.
Schechter, B., Schechter, I., and Sela, M. (1970). *J. Biol. Chem.* **245**, 1438.
Schechter, B., Conway-Jacobs, A., and Sela, M. (1972). *Eur. J. Biochem.* **20**, 321.

Schechter, I. (1971). *Ann. N. Y. Acad. Sci.* **190**, 394.
Schechter, I., and Sela, M. (1965). *Biochim. Biophys. Acta* **104**, 301.
Schechter, I., Schechter, B., and Sela, M. (1966). *Biochim. Biophys. Acta* **127**, 438.
Schechter, I., Clerici, E., and Zazepizki, E. (1971). *Eur. J. Biochem.* **18**, 561.
Schimpl, A., and Wecker, E. (1972). *Nature (London), New Biol.* **237**, 15.
Schlossman, S. F., Yaron, A., Ben Efraim, S., and Sober, H. A. (1965). *Biochemistry* **4**, 1638.
Schlossman, S. F., Levine H., and Yaron, A. (1968). *Biochemistry* **7**, 1.
Schlossman, S. F., Herman, J., and Yaron, A. (1969). *J. Exp. Med.* **130**, 1031.
Sela, M. (1966). *Advan. Immunol.* **5**, 29.
Sela, M. (1969). *Science* **166**, 1365.
Sela, M., and Fuchs, S. (1965). *Mol. Cell. Basis Antibody Form., Proc. Symp., 1964* p. 43.
Sela, M., and Mozes, S. (1966). *Proc. Nat. Acad. Sci. U. S.* **55**, 445.
Sela, M., Schechter, B., Schechter, I., and Borek, F. (1967). *Cold Spring Harbor Symp. Quant. Biol.* **32**, 537.
Seligmann, M., and Mihaesco, C. (1967). *Rev. Fr. Etud. Clin. Biol.* **12**, 851.
Senyk, G., Williams, E. B., Nitecki, D. E., and Goodman, J. W. (1971). *J. Exp. Med.* **133**, 1294.
Senyk, G., Nitecki, D. E., Spitler, L., and Goodman, J. W. (1972). *Immunochemistry* **9**, 97.
Singer, S. J., and Doolittle, R. F. (1966). *Science* **153**, 13.
Spitler, L., Benjamini, E., Young, J. D., Kaplan, H., and Fudenberg, H. H. (1970). *J. Exp. Med.* **131**, 133.
Spragg, J., Schroeder, E., Stewart, J. M., Austen, K. F., and Haber, E. (1967). *Biochemistry* **6**, 3933.
Steiner, L. A., and Eisen, H. N. (1966). *Bacteriol. Rev.* **30**, 383.
Stollar, B. D., Levine, L., Lehrer, H. I., and Van Vunakis, H. (1962). *Proc. Nat. Acad. Sci. U. S.* **48**, 874.
Taylor, R. B., and Iverson, G. M. (1971). *Proc. Roy. Soc., Ser. B.* **176**, 393.
Thompson, K., Harris, M., Benjamini, E., Mitchell, G., and Noble, M. (1972). *Nature (London), New Biol.* **238**, 20.
Trefts, P., Alkan, S. S., Koren, H. S., Nitecki, D. E., Goodman, J. W., and Mishell, R. I. (1973). Unpublished observations.
Uchida, T., Robbins, P. W., and Luria, S. E. (1963). *Biochemistry* **2**, 663.
Unanue, E. R. (1972). *Advan. Immunol.* **15**, 95.
Van Vunakis, H., Kaplan, J., Lehrer, H., and Levine, L. (1966). *Immunochemistry* **3**, 393.
Wang, A. C., Wilson, S. K., Hopper, J. E., Fudenberg, H. H., and Nisonoff, A. (1970). *Proc. Nat. Acad. Sci. U. S.* **66**, 337.
Warner, N. L., Szenberg, A., and Burnet, F. M. (1962). *Aust. J. Exp. Biol. Med. Sci.* **40**, 373.
Weigert, M. G., Cesari, I. M., Yonkovich, S. J., and Cohn, M. (1970). *Nature (London)* **228**, 1045.
Weigle, W. O. (1973). *Advan. Immunol.* **16**, 61.
Wells, H. G., and Osborne, T. B. (1913). *J. Infec. Dis.* **12**, 341.
Wu, T. T., and Kabat, E. A. (1970). *J. Exp. Med.* **132**, 211.
Yoo, T. J., Roholt, O. A., and Pressman, D. (1967). *Cold Spring Harbor Symp. Quant. Biol.* **32**, 117.
Young, J. D., and Leung, C. Y. (1970). *Biochemistry* **9**, 2755.
Zolla, S. B., and Goodman, J. W. (1967). *Immunochemistry* **4**, 135.

CHAPTER 3

Lymphocytic Receptors for Antigens

G. L. ADA AND P. L. EY

I. Introduction	190
II. Historical	191
III. Two Classes of Lymphocytes	193
A. Origin	193
B. Membrane Markers of T and B Lymphocytes	194
C. Function	196
D. Stimulation	197
IV. The Lymphocyte Plasma Membrane	197
A. Structure	197
B. Properties	199
V. Relevant Properties of Immunoglobulins	201
A. Shape and Size	202
B. Functional Activity of Immunoglobulins	204
VI. Immunoglobulins on the Lymphocyte Plasma Membrane	206
A. Techniques for Studying Membrane Ig of Lymphocytes	207
B. Ig on B Cells	208
C. On Cells of Thymic Origin	214
VII. The Binding of Antigen to Lymphocytes	217
A. Rosette Formation	217
B. Binding of Radiolabeled and Other Antigens	219
VIII. Specificity and Immunocompetence of ABC	232
A. Depletion and Enrichment of ABC	233
B. Specific Inactivation ("Suicide") of ABC	235
C. Membrane Modulation	240
IX. Receptors on Lymphocytes for Antigens	242
A. Ig as Antigen Receptor	243
B. The Ir Gene Product	247
C. Histocompatibility Antigens	250
X. Antigens, The Antigen–Receptor Complex, and Mitogens	251
A. The Reaction of Antigen with IgMs Receptors	251
B. Conditions for Stimulation of B Cells by Antigen	252
C. Conditions for Induction of Tolerance in B Cells	254

    D. Summary of B Cell Activation and Tolerance 256
    E. T Cell Tolerance and Activation 257
XI. Inside the B Cell 257
    A. Flip-Flop Mechanisms 257
    B. Allosteric Changes in the IgMs Receptor 258
    C. Cooperative versus Allosteric Effects 258
    D. Intracellular Messengers 259
    References 260

Abbreviations

T cell	thymus-derived lymphocyte	NNP	4-hydroxy-3,5-dinitro-phenacetyl
B cell	bone marrow (or bursa)-derived lymphocyte	LPS	lipopolysaccharide
ABC	antigen-binding cell	ATS	anti-thymocyte serum
C_3	third component of complement	GVH	graft versus host
		BSA	bovine serum albumin
C^1	activated complement	HSA	human serum albumin
RBC	red blood cell(s)	GPA	guinea pig albumin
RFC	rosette forming cell(s)	HGG	human γ-globulin
SRBC	sheep RBC	OA	ovalbumin
Con A	concanavalin A	GL	copolymer of L-glutamic acid and L-lysine
Ig	immunoglobulin		
^{3}HTdr	[^{3}H]thymidine	TGAL	poly(Tyr,Glu)-poly(DL-Ala)-poly(Lys)
NP40	Nonidet P-40		
DNP	2,4-dinitrophenol	TIGAL	heavily iodinated TGAL

I. Introduction

The reaction of antigen with lymphocytes is an event of central importance to immunology. It is highly specific and is believed to involve special receptors on the surface of the lymphocyte. This review asks: "What are these receptors for antigen, and how do they function?" To answer this question, we shall consider the following topics:

1. The properties of lymphocytes and of the lymphocytic plasma membrane

2. The identity and properties of candidates for the receptor for antigen

3. The nature of the reaction between antigen and lymphocytes

4. Properties of antigens which are relevant to cell activation or inactivation

5. Possible mechanisms of activation/inactivation

3. Lymphocytic Receptors for Antigens

As in other branches of science, immunology has its prophets who have proposed hypotheses or theories. As far as receptors for antigens are concerned, some of these have and will continue to influence the thinking and experimentation of many other immunologists for some time to come. The ideas of early workers in this field are of particular interest, especially in relation to our present concepts, and we start by discussing these.

II. Historical

In 1900, the German immunologist Paul Ehrlich proposed in the Croonian lecture to the Royal Society that the body contained cells which "are equipped with certain atomic groups, whose function especially consists in fixing to themselves certain foodstuffs." Some of these groups (termed "side-chains") were proposed to unite with toxins which, by chance, possessed haptophore groups corresponding to those of foodstuffs. Thus, it was proposed that "antitoxines are merely certain of the protoplasm 'side chains', which have been produced in excess and pushed off into the blood." This proposal inferred that "side-chains" or, as we now call them, *receptors*, of specific patterns preexisted in the body—the substance did not confer this pattern on a cell. It was in part a selective theory though Ehrlich did not envisage the unique segregation of specific receptors on lymphocytes now known to exist. In view of recent findings, however, Ehrlich's prediction must be regarded as remarkable.

The first serious criticism of Ehrlich's ideas came from work carried out by a number of chemists, notably Landsteiner (1936) who synthesized a variety of components which acted as *haptens* if coupled to a suitable *carrier*. Injection of the complex induced the formation of antibodies some of which had a specificity directed toward the hapten. To these workers it seemed inconceivable that cells in the body contained receptors of the appropriate specificity to correspond with any antigenic determinant which was either already known or perhaps might be synthesized in the future. Their viewpoints resulted in the formation of theories for antibody formation which have been termed Instructive or Directive Theories. In essence, it was proposed that the antigen or part thereof entered the cell and acted as a template upon which "normal" globulin molecules were molded to form a complementary pattern to the antigen. In this way, antibody molecules with specific antigen binding regions were formed. In retrospect, it seems that there would be no need for a potential antibody forming cell to possess specific receptors on its surface and that any cell capable of producing "normal" globulin molecules could, upon instruction, produce specific antibody molecules. This theory, in various forms, was promoted by many distinguished workers, such as Haurowitz, Pauling, Mudd, and Alexander and it remained unchallenged until the mid-1950's.

Three publications (Jerne, 1955; Talmage, 1957; Burnet, 1957) drew attention to other possibilities. Jerne proposed that γ-globulin molecules present in the body fluids possessed reactive sites that could unite with all known and any potential antigenic determinants, save those present on self components in the body. Extrinsic antigen acted as "a selective carrier of spontaneously circulating antibody to a system of cells which reproduce this antibody." Replicas of the "natural" antibody were produced and secreted once the antigen antibody complex was taken into the cell. As Talmage pointed out, Jerne's theory was in many ways similar to Ehrlich's theory—both being selective rather than instructive. Jerne's theory, though initially attractive, had a major disadvantage. It seemed unlikely that antibody on being taken into a cell would spontaneously initiate production of its own kind by that cell. Talmage thought that cell replication, a prominent feature of the immune response, must be linked more closely to antibody production than was suggested by Jerne's proposal; thus the replicating elements would be cellular in character, rather than the antibody molecule per se.

Though his experimental work had for some time been mainly concerned with viruses, Burnet had been intensely interested in the mechanism of antibody production, particularly the manner in which extrinsic material (nonself) was distinguished from the bodies own components (self). He had argued (Burnet and Fenner, 1949) that this was primarily a biologic rather than a chemical phenomenon and at the mid-1950's had been impressed with recent evidence that adaptive enzymes were genetically determined and "not a 'transcript' of patterns introduced by substrate or inducer molecule" (Burnet, 1959).

Jerne's hypothesis and Talmage's comments acted as a catalyst on Burnet. By switching the emphasis from extracellular globulin (natural antibody) to the lymphocyte, Burnet immediately overcame the main disadvantages of Jerne's proposal but in addition proposed new concepts for which there was at that time little precedence. Two of the three main points of Burnet's proposal—subsequently to be called the Clonal Selection Theory—can be stated as follows.

1. Prior to meeting an antigen, the body already possesses cells (lymphocytes) that have, at their surface, receptors (antibody molecules) that recognize determinants on antigen. Individual lymphocytes make antibody of only one or a limited number of antigen binding specificities.

2. Cells with specific receptors, upon reacting with the appropriate antigen, proliferate and become antibody secreting cells.

It is difficult to overestimate the importance of this concept to the development of immunology. It was the subject of controversy, sometimes bitter, for nearly 10 years, until its first general acceptance at the Cold Spring Harbor meeting in 1967 (Jerne, 1967). Evidence forthcoming in the last six years has further substantiated the concept.

III. Two Classes of Lymphocytes

A. Origin

The thymus is the first organ to become lymphoid in the embryo. While still epithelial in nature, the thymus is colonized by large hemocytoblast-like cells which migrate into it and are the ancestors of the lymphocyte. Cells of similar morphology also colonize the *anlagen* of organs such as the fetal liver, spleen, and the avian bursa of Fabricius. Seeding of stem cells into lymphoid organs continues into and throughout adult life. In adults, the major source of stem cells is the bone marrow although the spleen is also a source.

In adults, the only organs that can with certainty be regarded as primary lymphoid organs are the thymus and the avian bursa. There are three features that characterize these organs. (1) They have a large component of epithelial cells, which may have an inductive role throughout life. (2) In these organs, the intensity of lymphopoiesis as measured by mitosis of the primitive lymphoid cells, is largely independent of antigen stimulation. (3) Both lymphoid cells which can respond to antigen and activated cells, such as antibody secretors, are a minor component. There does not appear to be an exact equivalent of the avian bursa in other vertebrates. It is thought that the bone marrow serves this role in these situations.

Cells are seeded from the primary to the secondary lymphoid organs (spleen, lymph nodes, etc.). Cells of thymic origin in the periphery are called T cells or T lymphocytes. Other lymphoid cells are referred to as B lymphocytes or B cells which indicates that in birds they are derived from the bursa or, in other vertebrates, probably from the bone marrow.

B. Membrane Markers of T and B Lymphocytes

Although T and B lymphocytes are morphologically very similar, they can be distinguished either by functional tests or by surface properties, particularly surface antigens. Little is known of the physical or chemical properties of the plasma membrane of either cell, however, for although plasma membranes have been purified from lymph node cells and thymocytes (Allan and Crumpton, 1970; Ferber et al., 1972), their isolation from pure populations of T and B cells has not yet been reported. Structural differences have been shown by freeze-fracture studies (Mandel, 1972) and Santer et al. (1973) have reported that the cell coat or glycocalyx of thymocytes is twice as thick as that of B lymphocytes. T and B cells have also been separated by electrophoresis, which probably depends largely upon the amount of sialic acid present on the cell surface (Zeiller et al., 1971; Nordling et al., 1972; Wioland et al., 1972).

Some of the known differences between the plasma membranes of T and B lymphocytes are based on antigenic properties (Boyse, 1971; Raff, 1971; Takahashi et al., 1971) and are listed in Table I. In the mouse, H-2 alloantigens are present on both types of cell (Boyse, 1971). Thymocytes express a number of surface antigens (TL, Ly-A/B, θ) of which some are masked or repressed either partially (θ) or completely (TL) in mature T lymphocytes. Certain of these antigens have been isolated and characterized after dissolving membrane proteins by citraconylation (Eshhar et al., 1971, 1972; Bustin et al., 1972) or by direct isolation from cells enzymatically labeled with ^{125}I (Vitetta and Uhr, 1973; Atwell et al., 1973). None of the thymocyte antigens (except H-2) can normally be detected on mouse B lymphocytes although Schlesinger (1970) has reported that neuraminidase treatment of mouse spleen or bone marrow cells increases their susceptibility to anti-θ serum and complement. Most B cells can be identified by their possession of (a) large amounts of surface Ig, (b) the heteroantigen "mouse bone marrow lymphocyte antigen" (MBLA) (Raff et al., 1971), and (c) of receptors for Fc (Basten et al., 1972a; Paraskevas et al., 1972) and modified C_3 (Bianco et al., 1970). However, Anderson and Grey (1974) have since reported the presence of Fc receptors on some T lymphocytes.

The presence of these markers on cells can sometimes be utilized

TABLE I

Some Markers That Distinguish Mouse T and B Lymphocytes[a]

Marker	Thymocytes	T lymphocytes	B lymphocytes
Antigenic (detected by antibody binding)			
Thymocyte leukemic antigen (TL)	+	−	−
Theta (θ)	++	+	−
Ly-A, Ly-B	+	+	−
H-2 alloantigens	+	+	+
Ig	±	±	++
Mouse bone marrow lymphocyte antigen (MBLA)	−	−	+
Receptors			
C_3	−	−	+
Fc	−	−	+
In vitro stimulation by:			
PHA	+	+	−
Con A (mon)	+	+	−
(aggregate)	+	+	+
LPS	−	−	+
PWM	±	++	++

[a] Information taken in part from Basten and Howard, 1973; Boyse, 1971; World Health Organization, 1973.

TABLE II

Sources of T and B Lymphocytes

Cell class	Source
B lymphocytes	Congenitally athymic mice (nu/nu)
	ATXBM (adult thymectomized, X-irradiated, bone marrow reconstituted) mouse spleen, lymph nodes, etc.
	Mice treated with ATS (anti-thymoctic serum)[a]
	Spleen, lymph node cells treated with anti-θ serum and complement[a]
T lymphocytes	Hormonally bursectomized chickens
	Normal thymocytes or thymic cells from cortisone treated mice
	Spleens, etc., from X-irradiated mice previously given thymocytes or thymic cells from cortisone treated mice
	Spleen, etc., cells treated with anti-Ig sera and complement[a]
	Removal of cells from spleens, etc., bearing receptors for C_3 or Fc[a]

[a] These treatments in particular may cause severe depletion rather than the complete removal of the cell type.

to prepare either *in vitro* suspensions of lymphocytes enriched for one or the other class of lymphocyte, or *in vivo* situations where one or the other class of lymphocyte is absent or depleted. Commonly used sources of such lymphocyte preparations are outlined in Table II and have been used by many workers whose studies are later discussed.

C. Function

To establish beyond doubt that a given membrane component is a receptor for antigen, it is necessary to devise biologic tests that can be used to analyze the role of the component in question. Table III outlines the main functions of T and B lymphocytes which may be used in such experiments. B cells obviously have one overriding function—antibody production—which can be detected either as humoral antibody levels or by the enumeration of antibody secreting cells (plaque forming cells—PFC).

There are three major biologic activities attributed to T cells. First is the rejection of "foreign" cells which may be grafted cells, tumors, or virus-infected cells. In only one syngeneic system—virus infected target cells in tissue culture—is there clear evidence that T cells are cytotoxic for the target cells and even here the relevance of this finding to the *in vivo* activity of the T cell is not clear. On the other hand, it is established beyond doubt that T cells, when activated, liberate a range of substances which in turn affect the behavior of macrophages

TABLE III

Function of T and B Lymphocytes

Cell type	Function	Examples	Mechanisms
T lymphocytes	Rejection of "foreign" cells	Allografts Tumors Virus-infected cells	Cytotoxicity? Cytotoxicity? Cytotoxicity? (*in vitro*)
	Activation of macrophages	Delayed type hypersensitivity; resistance to infection	Release of pharmacologically active substances.
	Cooperation with B cells	Helper activity; suppressor activity	Secretion of antigen-Ig complexes?
B lymphocytes	Production of "humoral" antibody		

or their precursors. Finally, T cells can cooperate with B cells either to enhance or to suppress antibody formation. T cells can also suppress the activity of other T cells.

In this very brief statement on lymphocyte activity, it is worthwhile to stress two aspects. (1) Unlike B cells, there is as yet no assay available which enumerates active T cells. (2) With one exception—cytotoxicity assays—the measurement of T cell activity is indirect as it is based on the final activity of other cells.

D. Stimulation

Unprimed or memory T and B cells need to go through at least one stage of differentiation and division before they can act either as a helper cell of antibody secretor respectively (see review, Katz and Benacerraf, 1972). An early elegant experiment was that reported by Dutton and Mishell (1967) which showed that uptake of ^{3}HTdr of high specific radioactivity caused radiation damage to the antibody producing cells, preventing their replication.

Recent experiments (Feldmann and Basten, 1972b) have shown that treatment of unprimed and of memory T cells with mitomycin prevented the expression of helper activity in a cell collaboration system. Cells that demonstrate helper activity have been variously reported to be either susceptible or resistant to radiation damage. A possible explanation of the different results is the recent demonstration that helper cells, if exposed to radiation prior to injection into a lethally irradiated host, are radiation-sensitive. If such cells are first injected into the host and the latter lethally irradiated 24 hours later, the helper activity is intact. These authors suggest that such irradiation may have a subtle damaging effect on the helper cell, possibly influencing its ability to home to lymphoid organs.

IV. The Lymphocyte Plasma Membrane

A. Structure

Cell membranes vary considerably in character and composition, but all contain phospholipid and protein. Much of the phospholipid is arranged as a bilayer about 4.5 nm thick, in which hydrophobic fatty acid chains interact at the internal face and ionic or polar moieties face the aqueous milieu on each side (Fig. 1A) (Engelman,

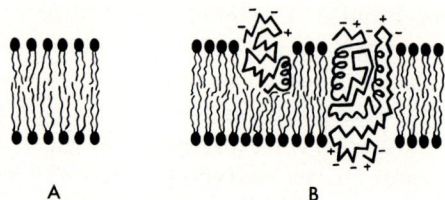

Fig. 1. (A) Schematic cross-sectional view of a phospholipid bilayer. The filled circles represent the ionic and polar hydrophilic head groups of the phospholipid molecules. The wavy lines represent the hydrophobic fatty acid chains. From S. J. Singer and G. L. Nicolson, *Science* (1972) **175**, 720. Copyright 1972 by the American Association for the Advancement of Science. (B) The lipid-globular protein mosaic model of membrane structure: schematic cross-sectional view. The integral proteins (or lipoproteins) of the membrane are largely globular and are intercalated into a matrix consisting of a discontinuous lipid bilayer. The ionic and polar heads of the lipids and the ionic residues of the proteins are all in contact with the aqueous phase. The fatty acid chains of the lipids and the hydrophobic residues of the proteins provide an interior hydrophobic core to the membrane. From S. J. Singer and G. L. Nicolson, *Amer. J. Pathol.* (1971) **65**, 427.

1970; Tourtellotte *et al.*, 1970; Wilkins *et al.*, 1971). Various models have been proposed to explain the interaction of proteins and other membrane components with the lipid matrix in intact membranes. The "fluid mosaic" model (Singer and Nicolson, 1971, 1972) is at present the most acceptable. In this model the bilayer is considered to be a viscous two-dimensional fluid in which proteins and other components are "dissolved" (Fig. 1B). The latter may be of two types: (1) *Peripheral components*, i.e., easily removed intact from the membrane. These are probably not strongly associated with membrane lipid, but held only by weak, noncovalent forces. (2) *Integral components*, i.e., not easily removed from the membrane. These are often insoluble in neutral aqueous buffers and probably interact strongly with membrane lipids.

Both peripheral and integral components should diffuse in the lateral plane of the membrane, at a rate depending on the size and shape of the component and particularly on the viscosity of the lipid matrix. The latter is markedly temperature-dependent in the range 10°–25°C (see Singer and Nicolson, 1972). In this context, cell membranes are dynamic entities whose components interact randomly with one another. The membranes constitute barriers to the passage of polar or ionic molecules as the latter cannot permeate the lipid matrix without the mediation of specific or nonspecific transport proteins which may form hydrophilic channels through the bilayer (Rothschild and Stanley, 1972).

It seems clear that certain membrane proteins span the plasma membrane so that portions of the proteins are exposed on both of its surfaces. The length of these molecules must be at least 8 nm, as most cell membranes are 7.5–9.0 nm thick. Two such proteins occur in human RBC (Marchesi et al., 1972; Bretscher, 1973). The first has a molecular weight of about 100,000, of which 10% is carbohydrate. It is thought that most of this molecule is buried within the membrane. The second, a glycoprotein named glycophorin, consists of a single polypeptide chain of about 200 amino acids to which approximately 130 sugar residues are attached at several sites on its N-terminal half. These residues are exposed extracellularly and account for >80% of the carbohydrate, including >90% of the sialic acid, found on the RBC surface (Kathan and Winzler, 1963; Winzler, 1969). The C-terminal end of the polypeptide is exposed on the intracellular side of the membrane (Bretscher, 1971). Threonine and serine account for >25% of the amino acids in this protein (Kathan and Winzler, 1963) and a hydrophobic sequence 23 amino acids long was recently determined (Segrest et al., 1972). This sequence, in the middle part of the polypeptide, is believed to exist *in situ* in an α-helical conformation. If so, it would be about 35 nm long—sufficient to span most of the lipid bilayer. The possession of a long hydrophobic sequence could possibly be a property common to other integral membrane proteins, particularly those which extend across the lipid bilayer.

One or both of the above-mentioned glycoproteins are believed to account for the surface particles seen on freeze-etched RBC by electron microscopy (Pinto da Silva and Branton, 1970; Pinto da Silva, 1972; Tillack et al., 1972). Similar particles have been observed on thymocytes (Mandel, 1972) and lymphocytes (Scott and Marchesi, 1972; Loor, 1973). These particles could represent a variety of proteins that may or may not span the plasma membrane. Some may be involved in reactions that stimulate the cell, but this has yet to be shown.

B. Properties

1. MEMBRANE MODULATION

Considerable experimental evidence exists to support the concept of a dynamic plasma membrane. This comes mainly from the changes that can occur in the distribution of membrane components if viable cells are incubated with polyvalent macromolecules which adhere to the cell surfaces. Redistribution or modulation of membrane components has been observed in a variety of mammalian cells (e.g., Frye and Edidin, 1970; Leonard, 1973) and it is therefore characteristic of other cells as well as lymphocytes. This does not mean that it is immunologically unimportant. The phenomenon may be a mechanism by which plasma membranes are "cleared" of debris and reutilized, but it might equally be a means of cellular activation common to many types of cells. This aspect is discussed in Section VIII,C.

When lymphocytes are incubated at 37°C with certain labeled antibodies, antigens, or mitogens, the label is initially distributed randomly over the surface of the cells. However, it rapidly aggregates into numerous "patches" before forming a large aggregate, termed a "cap," which may be endocytosed (e.g., Smith and Hollers, 1970; Osunkoya *et al.*, 1970; Taylor *et al.*, 1971; Loor *et al.*, 1972; Unanue *et al.*, 1972a,b; Kourilsky *et al.*, 1972; de Petris and Raff, 1972, 1973; Diener and Paetkau, 1972; Raff *et al.*, 1973; Loor, 1973). The essential findings of these studies are as follows:

Aggregation of membrane components into *patches* occurs via a temperature-sensitive, nonmetabolic process which almost certainly involves cross-linkage of individual components. For instance, divalent antibodies specific for surface antigens induce patch formation whereas their monovalent Fab fragments cannot do so unless they are themselves crosslinked by a divalent anti-Fab antibody. Crosslinkage, at least to the stage of patches, is probably a result of diffusion as it is markedly inhibited at temperatures <15–20°C (due to increased viscosity of the lipid matrix) but not by metabolic poisons.

Capping (which involves aggregation of patches) and endocytosis of the cap are both inhibited at low temperatures or with substances that inhibit oxidative phosphorylation, but not by those that only inhibit macromolecule synthesis. These characteristics, together with reports that caps form over the tail (or uropod) of motile cells, suggest that cell motility is necessary for cap formation (Smith and Hollers, 1970; Greaves *et al.*, 1972; Stobo *et al.*, 1972). There is increasing evidence that different components on the surface of a lymphocyte can cap independently of each other (Taylor *et al.*, 1971; Preud'homme *et al.*, 1972; Neauport-Sautes *et al.*, 1973; Bernoco *et al.*, 1972).

Substances such as Con A or sugars at high concentrations inhibit capping of membrane-bound fluorescent anti-Ig antibodies, possibly by extensively cross-linking membrane glycoproteins and glycolipids and immobilizing the membrane (Loor *et al.*, 1972; Yahara and

3. Lymphocytic Receptors for Antigens

Edelman, 1972). Con A itself can be capped and endocytosed (Smith and Hollers, 1970; Greaves *et al.*, 1972; Karnovsky *et al.*, 1972; Stobo *et al.*, 1972) but it has on another occasion remained uncapped (Yahara and Edelman, 1972). Perhaps capping of Con A and also its effect on the capping of surface Ig are concentration-dependent. It is difficult to see how Con A could immobilize the membrane if it becomes capped itself.

2. TURNOVER AND RELEASE OF MEMBRANE COMPONENTS

A variety of plasma membrane components are lost or released at 37°C into the extracellular medium by lymphocytes whose surface components are labeled with ^{125}I (Cone *et al.*, 1971; Vitetta and Uhr, 1972a,b; Jones, 1973). Similarly, a proportion of the complexes formed by binding anti-Ig antibodies to lymphocytes are released from the cells at 37°C (Wilson, 1972; Wilson *et al.*, 1972; Engers and Unanue, 1973; Ey, 1973b). However, those complexes not released are capped, endocytosed, and degraded intracellularly (Melchers and Andersson, 1973; Engers and Unanue, 1973; Ey, 1973b). Replacement of surface Ig by the cell occurs over a period of 5–20 hours (Loor *et al.*, 1972; Elson *et al.*, 1973; Hütteroth *et al.*, 1973; Melchers and Andersson, 1973; Diener and Paetkau, 1972).

The significance of the loss of membrane components from cells is difficult to establish. The losses may reflect active turnover of the components and/or the release of important soluble factors. They may equally well represent loss from dead or dying cells or, especially in the case of cell-bound antibodies, loss of cytophilically bound antibody or of cytophilic Ig to which antibody is attached.

V. Relevant Properties of Immunoglobulins

Knowing some of the properties of membranes, we might postulate that a membrane receptor should have certain properties. One of these obviously is that the binding site(s) for antigen should protrude from the extracellular surface of the membrane. Another is that the molecule should be large enough and have appropriate chemical properties to be held in the membrane. It may also be desirable for the receptor molecule to span the membrane so that a portion protrudes into the cell. This could have advantages for subsequent signal generation (Section XI).

As will become evident in later sections, IgMs is the likely receptor for antigen on "virgin" B cells. Unfortunately, there is little physical data available on IgMs, particularly concerning shape. As IgG closely approximates to it in size and presumably general structure, we present a summary of our knowledge of the size and shape of IgG molecules in the belief that these findings will be applicable to IgMs.

A. Shape and Size

IgG molecules have been observed by electron microscopy, their structure studied by X-ray crystallography and their shape measured in free solution. Valentine and Green (1967) mixed anti-DNP IgG molecules with a divalent hapten (bis-N-DNP-octamethylenediamine) which could serve as a link between IgG molecules. Electron microscopy showed hapten-linked trimers, each IgG molecule being in the shape of the letter Y. The dimensions are shown in Fig. 2. Depending on the polymeric size of the complexes seen, the angle, α, between the Fab arms varied from 10° to 180°. Green (1969) has since suggested that the length of the Fab fragment is 7 nm (70 Å) and that for antibody molecules in free solution, α is less than 60°. These results confirmed and extended the earlier work of Feinstein and Rowe (1965) who also showed a hinged structure.

The binding sites for antigen are clearly at the tip of each Fab subunit which measures some 3.5 nm across. The binding site for antigen of Fab subunits examined by X-ray crystallography is thought to be about $3 \times 1.5 \times 1.5$ nm (Poljak, 1973). It is of considerable interest that estimates of the binding sites of polysaccharides (Kabat, 1966) or proteins (Maurer, 1964; Sage et al., 1964; Haber et al., 1967)

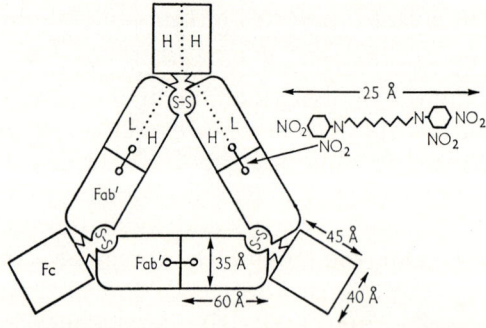

Fig. 2. Scale diagram of a hapten-linked trimer of IgG immunoglobulin molecules. From R. C. Valentine and N. M. Green, *J. Mol. Biol.* (1967) **27**, 615.

TABLE IV

Size and Shape of IgG

Source of IgG	Length of Fab (nm)	Size of α[a]	Physical state	Technique	Reference
Rabbit	6	Variable (10–180°)	Hapten–Ig complex; dried on grid	Electron microscopy	Valentine and Green, 1967
	7	<60°	Freeze-dried on grid	Electron microscopy	Green, 1969
Human myeloma IgG$_1$	9.8	180° invariant	Crystal	Small angle x-ray scatter	Pilz et al., 1970
Human myeloma IgG$_1$	7	180° invariant	Crystal	X-ray crystallography	Sarma et al., 1971
Rabbit	6	130–180°	Free in solution	Electric birefringence	Cathou and O'Konski, 1970
Rabbit hybrid IgG	7 (assumed)	80° (α minimum)	Free in solution	Singlet-singlet energy transfer	Werner et al., 1972

[a] α, Angle between the Fab arms of IgG.

for antibody are within the ranges 3.5 × 1.0–1.5 × 0.6–1.0 nm suggesting that most of the tip of each Fab subunit may be involved in antigen binding. Preliminary interpretation of a 0.6 nm resolution X-ray crystallographic analysis of Fab from the IgG New has shown clearly the presence of two "domains," as forecast on the basis of sequence data. These are believed to correspond to the variable and constant regions of the light and heavy chains in the Fab unit (Poljak, 1973). At the beginning of the variable domain, the two chains jointly define a cavitylike space which has dimensions compatible with the above requirements of an antigen binding site.

The shape and size of IgG molecules have been examined by various techniques and some results are quoted in Table IV. The Fab subunit is probably about 7 nm in length. When in crystalline form, α (the angle between the Fab subunit in IgG) is 180°. In free solution it seems to vary between 80° and 180°. Electron microscopy suggests α may be as low as 10° in antigen:antibody complexes and less than 60° when IgG is examined. It seems likely that these low angles may be in part due to distribution of the Fab arms of the molecule during drying on a grid; that the very low angles observed with the complexes may be caused in part by the binding to antigen cannot be excluded. Assuming α (minimum) = 80°, the distance between binding sites in IgG would be about 9 nm. Because of the difficulty in obtaining suitable heavy atom substitution in the Fc piece of IgG, detailed X-ray crystallographic data have not yet been obtained.

IgM exists mainly in two forms: as a 7 S molecule (IgMs), similar in general size and composition to IgG, and as a 19 S molecule consisting of five IgMs subunits (Miller and Metzger, 1965; Lamm and Small, 1966; review, Metzger, 1970). It was proposed that the subunits formed a circular, thermodynamically stable pentamer (Miller and Metzger, 1966) and electron microscopy (Svehag et al., 1967; Shelton and McIntire, 1970) has confirmed this. Thus the molecule is starlike, with a diameter of 25–40 nm. Frequently one diameter was smaller than another. The length of individual arms varied which suggests that the subunits of the molecule are free to move relative to each other. IgM with anti-RBC activity has been viewed attached to RBC and has the appearance of umbrella spokes (Feinstein and Munn, 1969). Svehag et al. (1967) found the center of the molecule to be ringlike but Shelton and McIntire observed a dense center. As the Fc moieties contribute mainly to this region, Shelton and McIntire speculated that the high content of carbohydrate present on the molecule together with the presence of the J chain contribute to the density of the inner part of the molecule.

The approximate dimensions of the IgMs molecule are shown in Fig. 3. For comparative purposes, we have drawn the molecule as being "buried" within the plasma membrane. If these dimensions are correct, then it is clear that IgMs molecules are sufficiently large to span the membrane so that part of the Fc moiety could extend into the cytoplasm while the Fab binding sites remain exposed extracellularly.

B. Functional Activity of Immunoglobulins

1. Fab Subunits

Immunoglobulins are oligofunctional molecules and a fascinating aspect is that their functions are qualitatively distributed between the different portions of the molecules. The antigen binding property is clearly a function of the Fab subunits. Thus, all studies using affinity labeling techniques (see reviews by Porter, 1972; Givol, 1973) indicate that the binding site is a function of the variable region of the light and heavy chains; this, together with the electron microscopic and X-ray crystallographic data suggest that the antigen binding site is an exclusive function of the N-terminal domain of the Fab subunit.

We know of no evidence that indicates any direct functional activity to the C-terminal domain of the Fab subunit. Similarly the Fc subunit appears to be uninvolved in the antigen binding activity.

3. Lymphocytic Receptors for Antigens

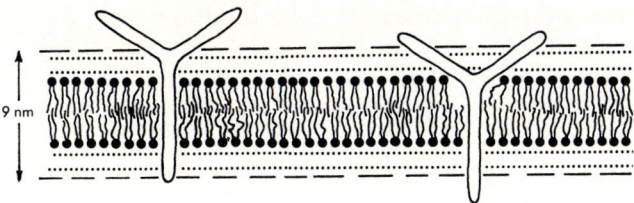

Fig. 3. Schematic cross-sectional view of a plasma membrane containing IgMs molecules. Components have been drawn to scale according to their approximate dimensions: lipid bilayer thickness, 4.5 nm; thickness of whole membrane, 9 nm, maximum. The dimensions of the IgMs molecules are assumed to be similar to those of IgM subunits (see Metzger, 1970). The broken lines represent the outer boundaries of the membrane and are *not* meant to suggest that a continuous layer of material overlies the lipid matrix. Analyses suggest that the IgD molecule would be of a similar size to IgMs.

The Fab subunits have identical properties and each may react with one antigenic determinant. The binding energy of a Fab subunit is defined as its affinity for a determinant. The affinity of an intact antibody molecule is independent of the number of such binding sites. The ability of an antibody molecule to bind antigen is expressed as its avidity and is a function of both affinity and the number of binding sites. Thus, an IgM antibody molecule (5–10 binding sites) with the same affinity as an IgG antibody molecule (2 binding sites) would exhibit greater avidity. The effect would be quite substantial. Thus the avidity of binding of antigen by a divalent antibody would be 10^4 to 10^5 fold higher than by a monovalent antibody (Hornick and Karush, 1972). Presumably the avidity would be still higher in the case of the IgM compared to IgMs molecule. The diameter of the IgM molecule is large (25–40 nm) so that such molecules could display very high avidity.

2. The Fc Subunit

The Fc subunit has several distinct functional activities. The first is cytophilic activity—the ability to bind to cell surfaces. Some but not all IgG preparations (Berken and Benacerraf, 1966) and a 7 S IgM molecule thought to be released from T cells (Cone *et al.*, 1974; Feldmann and Basten, 1972a) adsorb to the plasma membrane of macrophages. The Fc subunit of a guinea pig cytophilic antibody binds stoichiometrically to macrophages (Liew, 1971). B lymphocytes also possess receptors for the Fc portion of Ig molecules, particularly mouse IgG_1 (Basten *et al.*, 1972a). Dukor *et al.*, (1971) have found that a subpopulation of B cells bind antibody-coated RBC in the presence of C^1.

Some, but not all classes, of Ig and particularly IgM bind complement and this is a function solely of the Fc piece. It has been established that the N-terminal domain of the Fc piece is involved. A single molecule of IgM attached to a cell surface is sufficient to fix C^1 whereas "doublets" of IgG on the cell surface are required (Humphrey and Dourmashkin, 1965; Borsos and Rapp, 1965).

Finally, Stevens and Williamson (1974) have recently demonstrated that γ-chain messenger RNA can bind specifically to IgG molecules, thus maintaining a feedback mechanism for controlling the level of H_2L_2 in the cell. The binding is relatively strong and these authors suggest that there is a conserved binding site for any H_2L_2 molecule on the RNA molecule coding for any H chain. A search of the literature on γ-chain sequences showed that the sequence starting at Cys 425, namely, Cys-Ser-Val-Met-His-Glu-Ala-Leu-His-Asn-$\genfrac{}{}{0pt}{}{\text{His}}{\text{Arg}}$, would be consistent with their model. It is particularly interesting that a related sequence starting at residue 536 — Cys-Val-Val-Ala-His-Glu-Ala-Leu-Pro-Asn-Arg — occurs in a μ chain (Putnam et al., 1973). As the length of the μ chain is 576 residues, an IgMs molecule situated in the membrane might well have this sequence exposed in the cytoplasm.

VI. Immunoglobulins on the Lymphocyte Plasma Membrane

The presence of Ig on lymphocytes was clearly demonstrated by Sell and Gell (1965) who induced transformation of rabbit lymphocytes into blast cells following treatment with anti-Ig allotype sera. Van Furth et al. (1966) shortly afterwards found that some small mouse lymphocytes displayed weak immunofluorescence for IgM. Klein et al. (1968) first reported the presence of 7 S IgM (IgMs) on Burkitt lymphoma cells. These findings opened the way for more detailed studies. In this section we will be concerned mainly with those procedures that directly show the presence of Ig on lymphocytes. Others have reviewed earlier findings (Greaves and Hogg, 1971; Pernis et al., 1970) so this section will deal mainly with overall findings, and particularly with those reports that quantitate their findings.

In most, if not all, vertebrates, the lymphocyte population can be divided into two groups on the basis of their binding of anti-Ig reagents: those that bind large amounts, i.e., possess much, readily demonstrable Ig, and those that bind little of these reagents. Until very recently the former were usually identified as B cells and the latter as T cells. As much of the work to be discussed is based on this criterion, we will observe it but wish to acknowledge that recent evidence (e.g., Lamelin et al., 1972; Stobo et al., 1973; Parish and Hayward, 1974a,b) indicates other overlapping populations. Future work should seek to check the identity of these cells by additional criteria.

A. Techniques for Studying Membrane Ig of Lymphocytes

Almost all techniques used to detect Ig on the surface of lymphocytes rely at some stage on the use of specific antibody which may however be used at different stages in the investigation.

The use of antibody may be indirect and measure secondary effects such as lymphocyte transformation (Sell and Gell, 1965; Sell, 1970; Greaves, 1970), complement-mediated cytolysis (Takahashi et al., 1971), altered electrophoretic mobility (Bert et al., 1969), and by suppression of immune responses (Gardner et al., 1974) or reduction in antigen binding (Byrt and Ada, 1969).

Direct procedures involve the reaction of purified anti-Ig chain antibody with live lymphocytes. Techniques used are immunofluorescence (Raff et al., 1970) or rosette formation using RBC coated with antibody (Coombs et al., 1969). Alternatively, intact or disrupted lymphocytes may be used in antibody consumption tests as inhibitors in the reaction between radiolabeled Ig chain and antibody.

Components present in the plasma membrane may be radiolabeled biosynthetically (Vitetta and Uhr, 1972a,b, 1973; Melchers and Andersson, 1973; Lisowska-Bernstein et al., 1973) or, if exposed, labeled with ^{125}I using lactoperoxidase (Baur et al., 1971); Marchalonis et al., 1972). With this approach, the membrane must be solubilized and the labeled membrane components reacted with antibody.

With several of the above approaches, quantitation and details of the nature of the Ig associated with the lymphocyte can be achieved if the membrane is disrupted and the labeled component or complex isolated and identified. For isolating preformed complexes, a solvent should be used which will not cause dissociation. Nonionic detergents, such as Nonidet P-40 and Triton X-100 are frequently used for this purpose. Of these, NP40 is very popular (Melchers and Andersson, 1973; Parkhouse, 1973; Vitetta and Uhr, 1973) but may not be suitable for universal application as some membranes, e.g., nuclear, are resistant (Marchalonis and Cone, 1973). If labeled Ig is to be isolated from the membrane, Marchalonis and Cone (1973) recommend the use of an acetic acid/urea solvent at 37° to dissolve the membrane and then dialysis of the extract against nondissociating buffers before immunoprecipitation is performed. Possible dangers with this solvent are (1) denaturation during extraction, requiring renaturation to occur during dialysis and (2) losses and/or contamination during immune precipitation. Grey et al. (1972b) and Jensenius and Williams (1973b) report that the use of nonionic detergents yields higher recoveries of B and T cell Ig.

Other approaches that should be tried for the isolation of membrane associated Ig are treatment of intact cells with citraconic anhydride (Eshhar et al., 1971, 1972; Bustin et al., 1972) or prior isolation of the plasma membrane before solution in a detergent such as deoxycholate (Allan and Crumpton, 1970, 1971, 1973).

B. Ig on B Cells

1. Synthesis and Secretion of IgM by B Lymphocytes

Recently, the synthesis and secretion of IgM by normal cells has been investigated and is reported here because of the accumulating evidence that, in mice, IgM is the major Ig found associated with the lymphocyte plasma membrane. Recent reviews (Melchers and Andersson, 1973; Parkhouse, 1973) have summarized much of the relevant information.

Melchers and Andersson (1973) found that "capped" membrane bound Ig was insoluble in the detergent NP40 used to disrupt the lymphocyte plasma membrane. The ability to isolate membrane-bound as well as intracellular and secreted IgM enabled a study of the synthesis and secretion of IgM by B lymphocytes. Spleen cells of congenitally athymic (nu/nu) mice were pulse labeled with [^{3}H]leucine, -mannose, -galactose, or -fucose and chased in nonradioactive medium for various periods. The synthesis and secretion of IgM by large and small B cells, separated by velocity sedimentation in albumin gradients, has also been studied (Andersson et al., 1974; Melchers and Andersson, 1974). The chief findings are represented diagrammatically in Fig. 4 and are summarized below.

a. By Unstimulated nu/nu Mouse Spleen Cells. Populations of unstimulated B cells synthesize IgM but not IgG in detectable amounts. *Large B cells*, which constitute approximately 1% of B cells in nu/nu spleens, synthesize on a cell/cell basis 10–100 times more

3. Lymphocytic Receptors for Antigens

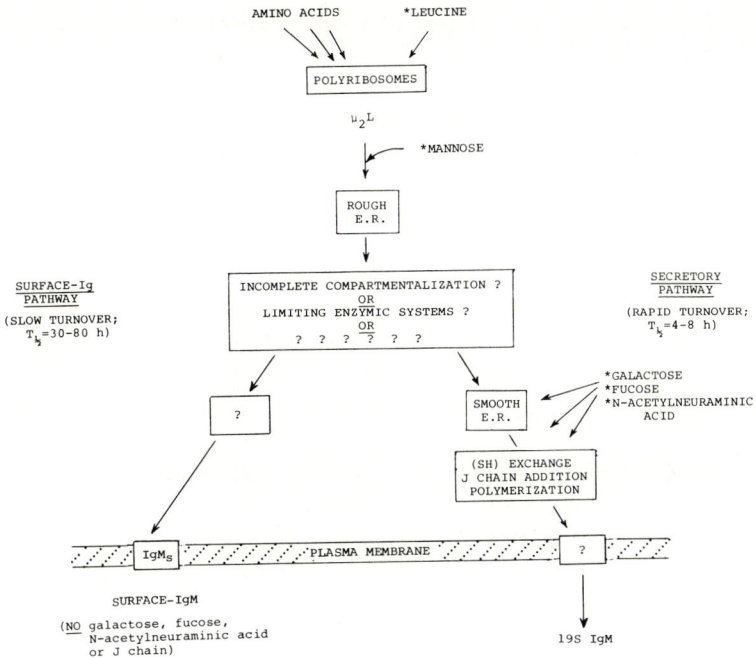

Fig. 4. Proposed pathways of synthesis and secretion of IgM in B lymphocytes. Constructed from data of Melchers and Andersson (1973) and Della Corte and Parkhouse (1973).

IgM than small B cells and secrete this IgM (half-life about 4 hours) in the form of 19 S pentameric molecules containing the complete complement of sugar residues found associated with serum 19 S IgM. These sugar residues are acquired sequentially by newly synthesized intracellular 7–8 S IgM (IgMs) molecules during their passage to the cell surface, where they are polymerized and immediately secreted. *Small B cells* constitute about 99% of B cells in unstimulated nu/nu spleens and contain IgMs molecules that are synthesized at approximately 20 molecules/minutes/cell and shed *without polymerization* with a half-life of 20–80 hours. These 7–8 S molecules, 90% of which are situated in the plasma membrane and accessible to extracellular anti-Ig antibody, contain the "core" sugars galactosamine and mannose attached to the μ chains, but *not* the penultimate galactose and terminal fucose residues common to secreted 19 S IgM.

b. By Lipopolysaccharide-Stimulated nu/nu Mouse Spleen Cells. The action of mitogens such as lipopolysaccharide in transforming B lymphocytes is thought to be analogous to triggering of antigen-specific B cells by antigen, except on a non-antigen-specific basis. *In vitro* incubation of B cells in the presence of mitogenic concentrations of *E. coli* lipopolysaccharide (LPS) causes the surface-IgMs of B cells to aggregate and disappear from the cell surface during the first 30 minutes of culture. This IgM is slowly digested by proteases, presumably after being capped and endocytosed. *De novo* synthesis refurnishes the original number of surface-IgM molecules within 12 hours, after which time more and more molecules appear on the surface. By 40–60 hours there is 35–100 times more IgM on the surface of the cells than was originally present before stimulation. As judged by immunofluorescence, more than half the cells have increased quantities of surface-IgM, most of which is turned over with a half-life of about 4 hours and once secreted, as 19 S IgM, contains the complete carbohydrate content of serum 19 S IgM. Although the rate of total cellular protein as well as IgM synthesis increases with increasing time of exposure to LPS, the ratio of synthesis of IgM/total protein increases steadily with time, as does the incorporation of mannose, galactose, and fucose into all intracellular and secreted proteins. Pokeweed mitogen has also been observed to selectively increase IgM synthesis in mouse B lymphocytes (Parkhouse *et al.*, 1972).

Surface IgM thus differs from secreted 19 S IgM in two important ways. First, it lacks the semiterminal galactose and terminal fucose and *N*-acetylneuraminic acid carbohydrate residues found in all secreted 19 S IgM. Second, surface IgM molecules are 7 S IgM subunits (IgMs).

It has been suggested (Melchers and Andersson, 1973) that the addition of the missing carbohydrate residues to IgMs molecules may alter their conformation and allow polymerization and secretion. However, IgMs molecules lacking a full carbohydrate complement can be polymerized *in vitro* by the covalent addition of a joining (J) chain in the presence of a disulfide-exchange system (Della Corte and Parkhouse, 1973). Nevertheless, the addition of these residues may increase the affinity of the IgMs molecule for the disulfide-exchange system so that the IgM is rapidly and efficiently polymerized. Furthermore, IgMs molecules are probably rather hydrophobic, considering their stability in the plasma membrane. It is possible that the addition of carbohydrate residues may decrease

3. Lymphocytic Receptors for Antigens

the hydrophobic nature of IgMs. Thus, if these residues were added in the proximity of both the cell surface and a disulfide-exchange system, altered IgMs molecules would be rapidly polymerized and secreted. Molecules acquiring only an incomplete carbohydrate complement, perhaps as a result of a rate-limiting enzyme system or because of prior compartmentalization, would not be readily polymerized and would remain as stable entities within the surface membrane.

2. Ig Class on Lymphocyte Membranes

B cells bind antilight chain Ig which in the mouse is mainly anti-κ Ig. It is generally found that B cells bind anti-Fab and anti-μ Ig well (e.g., Raff, 1970; Pernis et al., 1970; Vitetta et al., 1971). Some have found that individual cells may bind antibody with specificities against different heavy chains (e.g., in mice, Greaves, 1970; in sheep, Ey, 1973a).

As B cells possess receptors for Fc, is some membrane associated Ig adsorbed from the medium? This can be examined in several ways.

a. Is the membrane bound Ig synthesized by the cell? This is clearly so for IgMs (Vitetta and Uhr, 1972a; Melchers and Andersson, 1973; Parkhouse, 1973); both these latter groups, however, failed to find membrane bound IgG, although the cells were found to synthesize and secrete IgG. We do not know of any report that clearly demonstrates *synthesis* of membrane bound IgG (or IgA or IgE) in cells from unprimed animals. Recently, it has been reported that some μ negative cells may have α chains in their membrane (Jones et al., 1974) and there are now several well-documented claims that human (Rowe et al., 1973; Kubo et al., 1974) lymphocytes have IgD in their plasma membrane. Some lymphocytes have IgM and IgD. It is unlikely that the IgD is simply adsorbed onto the membrane.

b. Is there replacement of surface Ig after capping? This is observed for IgM. Preud'homme and Seligmann (1972) reported IgG bound to surface IgM of cells from a case of lymphoproliferative disorder; on redistribution and capping, only IgM reappeared. The IgM and IgD that is found on some human lymphocytes cap independently and both reappear on the cell surface after capping.

c. If Ig is adsorbed to B cells, it might be shed during incubation at 37°. Ey (1973a,b) found (presumably) B cells in sheep lymph to possess both IgG and IgM on the cell surface. When the cells were incubated at 37° for up to 20 hours in Ig-free medium, some IgM and larger amounts of IgG appeared in the medium. After 20 hours, there was almost the same amount as initially of membrane bound IgM whereas the amount of surface IgG had decreased by 90–95%, suggesting that the latter had been simply adsorbed to the cell.

d. Some human lymphoma cells have been found to have IgM, IgA, and IgG on their surface when first isolated; after serial passage in nu/nu mice, only IgM is detected (Klein et al., 1968; Povlsen et al., 1973).

These results suggest that in unprimed animals of most species, either B cells will be found to have IgM as the predominant, if not sole, Ig on their surface or that there are relatively few B cells that have Ig other than IgM on their surface. B cells from primed animals have not been examined so far in the above detail but it may be found that other Ig classes are present on their surface. Ey (1973b) found sheep lymph cells to contain small amounts of IgM as well as IgMs. It is not yet established whether IgM may serve as a receptor.

3. Quantitation of Ig

Table V contains data from recent reports where attempts have been made to quantitate Ig on B cells. We have not included values based primarily either on immunofluorescence or radioiosotopic labeling of cell surface components as we consider these techniques are less amenable to quantitation than others mentioned in Table V. The techniques reported in Table V are either the use of cells as inhibitors, or grain counts and/or bulk scintillation counting of cells that have reacted with labeled purified reagents. Apart from again noting that IgM is the major Ig found, the point of interest is the very large spread of values for numbers of molecules of IgM found. This varies over at least a 50-fold range. All methods have inherent difficulties, but such a large range is unexpected. On average, it would seem that the value may be a five number figure, but is it closer to 10^5 or to 10^6? If Ig in the membrane is IgMs and if it behaves as a molecule in free solution, then the Fab arms may spread over an area about 10 nm in diameter. A lymphocyte of diameter 8×10^{-3} mm, if smooth like a ball at 0°, will have a surface area $10 \times 20 \times 10^6$ nm². This could accommodate side by side 2×10^6 Ig molecules. As Ig is only one of many protein molecules at the cell surface and as much of the surface is probably lipid in nature, this would suggest that estimates in Table V above $1-2 \times 10^5$ are probably too high. At present, we cannot get closer than this to "correct" values.

TABLE V
Quantitation of Ig on B Lymphocytes

Cell source	Procedure	Reagent used for quantitation	Ig found	Surface Ig (7 S)	Anti-Ig bound (IgG)	Reference
Mouse spleen	Immunofluorescence[a] Inhibition by cells in radioimmunoassay[b]	Anti-IgG$_2$ Anti-κ Anti-κ	— N.D.[c] Mainly IgM	5–143 11–57[d] 140–392[d]	—	Rabellino et al., 1971 Unanue et al., 1971 Grey et al., 1972a
Mouse spleen	Radioautography[a] Saturation with anti-Ig[b] Bulk scintillation counting[b]	Anti-κ	Mainly IgM	—	about 60	Nossal et al., 1972
Human Burkitt lymphoma	Immunofluorescence[a] Inhibition of IgM-coated RBC hemagglutination[b]	Anti-μ Anti-κ	Mainly IgM	about 80	—	Klein et al., 1970
Sheep lymph cells	Radioautography[a] Inhibition by cells in radioimmunoassay[b]	Anti-μ Anti-γ	IgM IgG	27–130 11–27	—	Ey, 1973a
Rat lymph cells	Saturation with peroxidase coupled anti-Ig[b]	Anti-IgG	—	—	about 220	Avrameas and Guilbert, 1971
Rat TDL	Radioautography[a] Grain counts and bulk scintillation counting[b]	Anti-Fab Anti-μ	Mainly IgM	—	20–150 8–60	Jensenius and Williams, 1974a
Cultured human lymphocytes (cloned)	Inhibition by cells in radioimmunoassay[b]	Anti-γ	IgG[e]	about 100	—	Lerner et al., 1972
Rabbit blood	Radioautography[b] (single dose, i.e., nonsaturated)	Anti-allotype	—	—	7–40	Jones et al., 1970

[a] Technique used to determine proportion of B cells. [b] Technique used to quantitate surface Ig. [c] N.D., not determined. [d] Calculated from N content of precipitates. [e] Have not assayed for IgM.

4. Ig on Precursor B Cells

Ig can be readily detected on the surface of cells present in some primary lymphoid organs, the most clear-cut case being lymphocyte-like cells in the avian bursa, of which almost 100% bind anti-light chain sera (Kincade *et al.*, 1971). Cells in this organ synthesize IgM as early as the eighteenth day of embryonic development and the organ, as a whole, is more active than spleen in this regard until at least day 7 after hatching when Ig synthesis in the spleen becomes apparent (Thorbecke *et al.*, 1968). Following the work of Moore and Owen (1965, 1966) these authors postulated that immigrant cells settled in the bursa and, under the influences of a bursal epithelial hormone, differentiated into Ig bearing cells. Kincade and colleagues (1970) found that administration of anti-μ chain sera to 13-day embryos resulted in an absence of IgM containing cells in the bursa 3–6 days later. The production of this IgM seemed to be independent of the presence of antigen.

In vertebrates other than birds, Ig bearing cells occur in several tissues and can be detected 3 days before birth in liver, spleen, and bone marrow. A rapid influx of Ig bearing cells into lymph nodes occurs shortly after birth (Nossal and Pike, 1973).

C. On Cells of Thymic Origin

" . . . Our data provides evidence that approximately equal amounts of immunoglobulin can be isolated from the surface of T cells and B cells . . . " (Marchalonis and Cone, 1973).

"Thymocytes and T lymphocytes have little or no Ig on their surface and do not synthesize detectable amounts of Ig. We, therefore, suggest that T cells may have an antigen specific receptor other than Ig" (Vitetta and Uhr, 1973).

These two statements describe the state of affairs in this area in 1973. In the work we will discuss, four situations have been examined: thymocytes, T cells, activated T cells, and thymomas.

1. Biosynthesis of Ig by T Cells

To our knowledge, no worker or group has provided evidence for the biosynthesis of Ig by T cells in conditions where it was certain that B cells of their products were missing. Both Anderson and Dresser (1972) and Vitetta *et al.* (1973) have found up to 2% of plasma cells in thymus. Kirov and Ada (1974) have found thymus cells to contain between 0.1 and 1% of cells which bind anti-light

3. Lymphocytic Receptors for Antigens

chain Ig and which were mostly resistant to lysis by anti-θ antibody and complement. Vitetta et al. (1973) and Lisowska-Bernstein et al. (1973) looked for synthesis of Ig by T cells without success. In the former case, their system was sufficiently sensitive to detect readily B cells present to 0.5% in a total population of 10^9 thymocytes.

Various thymomas have been tested for short-term in vitro Ig synthesis. Of 19 radiation-induced Balb/C, NZB, and NZW thymomas examined, twelve showed no light or heavy chain synthesis, six showed traces of light chain synthesis and one made small amounts of IgM (Harris et al., 1973). It would be unwise, however, to extrapolate from thymomas to normal cells of thymic origin. Possibly every cell in the body has the genetic information for the synthesis of Ig molecules yet few do so.

It has been reported by a number of workers that upon incubation of ^{125}I-labeled lymphocytes at 37°, labeled Ig molecules are shed into the supernatant (e.g., Marchalonis and Cone, 1973). There seems no way of determining whether this "shed" Ig comes from all or only a (perhaps minor) fraction of the cells. Vitetta and Uhr (1973) have suggested that shedding could be a characteristic of dying cells.

Thus, at present, there does not seem to be any substantial evidence of synthesis of Ig by normal cells of thymic origin.

2. Detection of Ig on T Cells

We know of no exception to the finding that exposure of T cells from unprimed animals to labeled anti-Ig reagents results in a much lesser extent of binding than is seen with B cells (e.g., Hämmerling and Rajewsky, 1971; Bankhurst and Warner, 1971; Nossal et al., 1972; Unanue et al., 1972b; Kirov and Ada, 1974). Some differences were reported. Bankhurst and Warner (1971) found that up to 17% of thymocytes and 50% of peripheral T cells possessed surface Ig. Nossal et al. (1972) found that, although nearly all mouse T lymphocytes could be labeled with anti-κ and anti-μ reagents, the binding capacity was 100–400 times less than that of B cells. Exposing rat thymocytes to saturating doses of (Fab')$_2$ anti-Ig reagents, Jensenius and Williams (1974a) found that anti-γ chain bound rather better (300 molecules/cell) than did anti-μ chain antibody (60 molecules/cell).

The small amount of Ig found by many workers raises the possibility that this is a type of antibody produced by B cells which is cytophilic for both T cells and macrophages. Recent work by Webb and Cooper (1973) lends credence to this possibility. T cells from bursectomized chickens failed either to bind labeled antigens or to form rosettes (Cooper, 1971), but gained this ability if the chickens were transfused with plasma from immunized normal chickens. The Ig which adsorbed to T cells had light and μ chain determinants.

Using the lactoperoxidase technique of surface labeling and acetic acid/urea to dissolve membranes, Marchalonis and colleagues (see review, Marchalonis and Cone, 1973) have found that T cells apparently contain as much Ig as do B cells. At least three other groups using similar, if not identical, techniques have found very little Ig on T cells (Vitetta and Uhr, 1973; Grey et al., 1972b; Lisowska-Bernstein et al., 1973). It is not possible for us to explain the different results although, in a careful appraisal of the technique, Lisowska-Bernstein et al. (1973) pointed to some possible sources of error, such as contamination of the immune precipitate.

We believe there may be another substantial source of error. If the surface labeling approach is used, we see no way of judging the *proportion* of Ig molecules labeled or the *competition* of other cell surface components for the reagent. For example, if both B and T cells had the same ratio of Ig/other surface proteins but (1) B cells had *more* surface protein available for iodination and (2) the available iodide was limiting (as it is using carrier-free iodide), then the technique could yield similar estimates for the amount of Ig per T or B cell.

To explain the low binding of anti-Ig antibody to T cell surface Ig, Marchalonis et al. (1972) proposed that much of the Ig molecule was "buried" in the glyocalyx of the T cell and unavailable to anti-Ig reagents but accessible still to specific antigen. This notion would agree with the inhibition of T cell rosette formation by anti-Ig reagents directed to different regions of the molecule (Hogg and Greaves, 1972). Marchalonis and Cone (1973) suggest that the buried regions of the T cell Ig would still be accessible to labeling with ^{125}I using lactoperoxidase. This was based on the belief that the latter is achieved by short-lived iodide radicals or molecular iodine. However, at neutral pH, the reaction between lactoperoxidase (MW 77,000) and tyrosine shows stereospecificity, indicating that tyrosine must bind to the enzyme to be iodinated (Morrison and Bayse, 1970; Bayse and Morrison, 1971). Thus, iodination with lactoperoxidase might still be subject to much the same accessibility restrictions as labeling with anti-light chain or anti-Fab reagents.

Marchalonis and Cone (1973) cite two other major pieces of evidence in favor of their claim for large amounts of Ig on T cells. (1) Lethally irradiated mice, given syngeneic thymic cells and allogeneic cells, produce large numbers of T cells activated against histocompatibility antigens. Cells isolated from the thoracic duct are almost entirely (>99%) θ-positive and Cone et al. (1972) found these shed large amounts of IgM with specific anti-H-2 activity. It seems likely that in this case, the specific antibody is cytophilic and is derived from plasma cells resident in lymphoid organs (and not in the lymph) and these cells are the progeny of precursors present in the inoculum of thymic cells (Lisowska-Bernstein et al., 1973). (2) The IgM secreted by T cells is particularly cytophilic for macrophages, more so than would be expected if it came from contaminating B cells. The work of Webb and Cooper (1973), quoted earlier in this section, suggests that this is an unreliable argument.

In conclusion, most workers in the field of T cell Ig have produced evidence that at least a proportion of thymocytes and most if not all T cells have on their surface small amounts of Ig, but much less than that present on B cells. Some or all of this may be cytophilic. One group of workers has stated that thymocytes and T cells have as much surface Ig as do B cells. The lack of confirmation of these results by three other groups suggest that (1) possible deficiencies in technical procedures and/or (2) differences in specificity of sera used by the various groups have contributed to the different findings.

VII. The Binding of Antigen to Lymphocytes

So far in this review we have discussed some general properties of lymphocytes, the nature of the plasma membrane of cells, the size and shape of Ig molecules (particularly IgMs, the subunit of IgM), and those experiments that have shown or attempted to show the presence of Ig in the lymphocyte plasma membrane. These sections have provided us with a picture of the lymphocyte, a cell waiting to express its potential. This it does by coming into contact with an external reagent, the antigen. The first step in responding to the antigen is to bind it and the next two sections discuss the binding of antigens to lymphocytes and the way this reaction has been used to demonstrate the specificity and competence of individual lymphocytes. The consideration of this and earlier data then allows us to nominate the properties that a lymphocyte receptor for antigen should possess and to examine critically proposed candidates.

A. Rosette Formation

Nota et al. (1964) and Zaalberg (1964) observed that when SRBC were mixed with cells from mouse lymphoid tissues, some nucleated cells bound SRBC to form "rosettes." This was initially considered to be simply a more sensitive means of detecting specific antibody secreting cells, but it soon became clear that rosette forming cells were present in small numbers in lymphoid cell populations from unprimed animals. The standard procedure for forming rosettes is to mix the lymphoid cells with about a 10-fold excess of RBC. As the number of RBC that can attach to a lymphocyte is limited, the number of rosettes observed should be largely independent of concentration of RBC, provided an excess is present. In unprimed spleen cell populations, most rosette forming cells were small lymphocytes. After immunization, over 50% of such cells were medium lymphocytes. Macrophages could also form rosettes due to the presence of cytophilic antibody. When prepared at low temperatures to minimise rosette formation by antibody secreting cells, rosettes formed are specific as tested by formation in the presence of two morphologically different types of red cells (Biozzi *et al.*, 1966; Laskov, 1968; Bach *et al.*, 1971; Greaves, 1971). The mean number of RFC in unprimed mouse spleen cells is about 1/1000 and usually increases about 10-fold at the peak of a primary response (see Roelants, 1972a).

Erythrocytes or other particles such as bentonite (Baker *et al.*, 1966) can be coated with antigens and RFC for these antigens studied by particle adhesion. Roelants has listed the incidence of RFC for five antigens and one hapten in unprimed mouse spleen cells. They range from $1-100/10^5$ cells.

There is a complete agreement that B cells of the appropriate specificity may form rosettes. Despite many contributions from several laboratories, there is not complete agreement whether T cells form rosettes. The subject has been reviewed by Roelants (1972b) and Bach (1973). The evidence for and against can be briefly summarized as follows.

It has been shown that following administration of ATS to mice or treatment of normal mouse lymphocyte populations with anti-θ serum and complement, there is a significant drop in the incidence of RFC formed. On this basis, up to 60% of rosette forming cells were claimed to be T cells. Similarly, in primed mice, figures between 25 and 50% were found (e.g., Bach *et al.*, 1971; Möller and Greaves, 1971; Wilson and Miller, 1971).

RFC, formed with RBC coated with *E. coli* lipopolysaccharide which is a thymus independent antigen, were not suppressed by anti-θ and complement (Möller and Sjöberg, 1972).

In immunized, irradiated mouse chimeras, cells identified as being

3. Lymphocytic Receptors for Antigens

of thymic origin by T-cell chromosomal or H-2 markers and which are sensitive to anti-θ form rosettes (Charreire et al., 1973, quoted by Bach, 1973). There are however two other groups of observations that raise difficulties.

Using an anti-θ serum raised in congenic mice, Takahashi et al. (1971) found that they could not inhibit the formation of rosettes by normal mouse spleen cells by pretreating the cells with anti-θ (no complement). These authors considered that if T cells did become RFC, they lost their T cell marker in the change from thymocyte to T cell. Greaves and Raff (1971), however, showed that such anti-θ could inhibit RFC in the presence of thymocyte-absorbed anti-θ serum, indicating the need for additional antibody, perhaps an autoantibody.

Good et al. (1971), Crone et al. (1972), and Hemmingson and Alm (1972) report that neonatally bursectomized chickens immunized with SRBC do not form rosettes. As mentioned earlier, Webb and Cooper (1973) also find T cells in bursectomized chickens do not form rosettes, and describe experiments suggesting that rosette formation by T cells may be due to cytophilic antibody.

Greaves and Hogg (1971) found that the formation of rosettes by T cells from normal mice could be inhibited by anti-κ but not by anti-μ, -γ or -α sera. Rosette formation by T cells from immunized mice could also be inhibited by anti-μ sera and some evidence implicated the hinge region of the μ chain being accessible on primed T cells.

B. Binding of Radiolabeled and Other Antigens

Naor and Sulitzeanu (1967) designed an experiment to test directly the Clonal Selection Theory. It was argued that if individual lymphocytes were monodeterminant, only a very small fraction of a population of lymphocytes would bind a given antigen; if however individual lymphocytes were multideterminant, then a large proportion, if not all cells, would bind some of the antigen. Normal mouse spleen cells were exposed at 0° to a low concentration of [^{125}I]BSA (specific activity about 100 μCi/ug) for 1 hour, and then washed thoroughly, smeared, and examined by radioautography. Of 5×10^3 cells examined, 3 showed more than 20 grains, a larger proportion of cells showed between 5 and 19 grains, but more than 99% showed no more than the background level of grains (<4). When cells were exposed to a mixture of four different labeled albumins, the number of labeled cells was about equal to the sum of labeled cells found for each antigen. Further, the binding of [^{125}I]BSA could be inhibited by 1000-fold excess of BSA but not by the same excess of HSA. These findings were consistent with the notion of monodeterminant lymphocytes.

Byrt and Ada (1969) extended these observations using different antigens, particularly bacterial flagellin (MW 40,000) and hemocyanin from *J. lalandii* which is a pentameric protein of unit MW 90,000. In general (though there are differences), similar binding patterns to those seen by Naor and Sulitzeanu were observed. In addition, the effect of various parameters such as antigen dose, time of exposure, specific activity, and effect of anti-Ig reagents on binding were studied.

Detection of antigen binding cells is now a standard procedure in immunology. Most follow the technique described by Byrt and Ada (1969) which was based on that of Naor and Sulitzeanu (1967). Briefly, lymphoid cells (about 10^8/ml) in neutral buffer containing fetal calf serum and 15 mM sodium azide at 0° are mixed with labeled antigen and kept at 0° for 30 minutes. The cells are then centrifuged through gradients of fetal calf serum to remove unbound antigen. As measured by bulk scintillation counting, the radioactivity in the cell pellet is less than 1% of the total. The cells are then smeared on a coated glass slide. After fixation, the slide is dipped in photographic emulsion, dried, and exposed for periods of days or weeks at 4°. The emulsion is then developed, and the slide is stained and mounted for examination. The number of grains associated with a cell is usually counted or estimated by the observer, although recently a mechanical attachment to a microscope has become available for this purpose (Rogers, 1972).

Results using this technique have been reviewed by Sulitzeanu (1968, 1971), Ada (1970), Paul and Davie (1971), and Roelants (1972b). Because of the increasing use of the technique, it is not feasible to mention individually all findings; rather, an attempt will be made to extract major findings from the mass of literature. Before doing so, however, we wish to make three main points.

First, the reaction of an antigen, preferably of low molecular weight (see Section VII,B,8), with a lymphocyte and the study of factors that influence this reaction is the most direct method of determining the nature of the receptor for antigen on the cell surface. It is most desirable to achieve a positive relationship between this binding and functional activity of the cell. The final analysis will be of the isolated complex between antigen and receptor.

Second, in contrast to rosette formation, there are many variables associated with the antigen binding test. These include conditions of incubation, the specific activity and concentration of the labeled antigen, the type of photographic emulsion, and the time of exposure. Few workers have included all this data in their protocols; it is more usual to make comparisons simply within a laboratory. It is desirable (Roelants, 1972b) to state not only the number of labeled cells but the number of molecules of antigen per cell. This latter figure can be calculated from grain numbers (Ada et al., 1966). Complete exchangeability of data between laboratories would only be obtained if a standard labeled antigen and animal strain were available worldwide. All results with other systems could be expressed relative to the standard. In the absence of this, strict comparisons cannot be made. Differences in values obtained with T cells in several laboratories probably reflect the need for such a standard.

Third, within laboratories, the binding patterns of antigen are frequently found to differ. Factors such as size, the monomeric versus oligomeric versus polymeric nature of the antigen, and the past antigenic history of the host may play a role.

Some of the major findings will now be discussed.

1. Do B and T Cells Bind Labeled Antigens?

The answer is yes, though until recently some have experienced difficulty in demonstrating labeled T cells. It seems certain that, with the reaction conditions used in most laboratories, the labeled cells seen in unprimed animals are mainly, if not exclusively, B cells. Thus, under conditions where antigen binding cells (ABC) to [^{125}I]BSA were detected in the white blood cells of normal patients, none was seen in the WBC of agammaglobulinaemic patients (Naor et al., 1969). Conversely, congenitally athymic (nu/nu) mouse spleens were found to possess large numbers of cells binding four different labeled antigens (Dwyer et al., 1971). It seems that to detect T-ABC, more sensitive methods are necessary. For example, using a labeled antigen (specific activity 20–50 μCi/μg, 100–500 ng/ml) and exposing for 3–6 days will detect many B-ABC and few T-ABC. T-ABC (primed mice) have been most clearly seen using labeled antigens (specific activity 150–300 μCi/μg, 2.5 μg/ml) and exposing for 2–4 days (Roelants et al., 1973). That is, for equally short exposure periods, effective labeling of T cells may require antigen concentrations and specific activities about five-fold higher than for B cells, yielding a differential factor of 25-fold. The best documented examples of T-ABC are those in which polymeric or oligomeric antigens are used, e.g., KLH (Roelants, 1972a; Engers and Unanue,

1973) or TGAL (Hämmerling and McDevitt, 1974). C. De Luca (personal communication) observes T-ABC if the lymphocytes are pretreated with glutaraldehyde before exposure to the antigen. It is thought this might minimize rapid shedding of the antigen–receptor complex from the T lymphocyte.

As most characteristics of the binding reaction have been determined by observing B cells, most subsequent comments will refer in particular to B cells.

2. Temperature of the Binding Reaction

Low temperatures of reaction were initially chosen to minimize metabolic events that might follow the binding of antigen to the cell, and also to minimize uptake of antigen by phagocytic cells, such as macrophages and polymorphs. There are two recent reports where 37°C has also been used. Diener and Paetkau (1972) used polymerized flagellin, biosynthetically labeled with tritium, as an antigen. This has a low specific activity (0.15 $\mu Ci/\mu g$) so high concentrations and long exposure times were used. These workers detected no labeled cells when the cells were exposed to the antigen at 0°C, but only after they had been incubated (with the antigen) at 37°C for periods up to 6 hours. More recently, Hämmerling et al. (1973) found a threefold increase in the incidence of T-binding cells for TGAL if the reaction was carried out at 37°C, rather than at 0°C. These results are not necessarily in conflict with those of other workers, as they might be explained, first, in terms of different sensitivities of ABC detection, and, second, by accumulation at 37°C of labeled antigen within the cells as a result of capping and pinocytosis of bound antigen. The latter possibility seems likely as the increase in T-binding cells observed at 37°C by Hämmerling et al. was inhibited by sodium azide.

3. A Hierarchy of Binding Cells

It has been consistently observed that, when radioautographs of labeled cells are examined, there is a hierarchy of binding cells, some binding more antigen than others. More lightly labeled than heavily labeled cells are usually seen.

4. Concentration of Antigen

The number of ABC observed in a population of lymphocytes from unprimed mice is a function of the concentration of the antigen used. At low concentration (1–10 ng/ml) the incidence may be very small but it increases with increasing concentration of antigen. Using hemocyanin (*J. lalandii*), Ada (1970) judged the limit to be about 1–2% but high backgrounds caused difficulties in interpretation. This level was reached at concentrations of antigen higher that 1 μg/ml. Using an entirely different technique, Edelman *et al.* (1971) found that about 1% of lymphocytes would bind to antigen-coated threads, similar values being found for a number of different antigens. Microscopy showed that the surface area of the threads occupied by bound cells was only a fraction of the total area available, thus simulating conditions of antigen excess. Miller *et al.* (1971) studied the binding patterns of the enzyme β-galactosidase for which a sensitive assay is available. The activity of the enzyme is known to be unaffected by binding to antibody. Using saturating levels, it was found that 1–2% of mouse spleen and bone marrow cells bound this antigen. In contrast to these results, Rolley and Marchalonis (1972) have reported that up to 10% of mouse spleen cells bound homologous hemoglobin substituted with DNP if the cells were exposed to very high amounts (up to 50 μg) of the conjugate. (However, see also Section VII,B,4.)

The antigens quoted above are multideterminant, the number of determinants varying according to the molecular weight. Thus, for *J. lalandii* hemocyanin (90,000 MW for the monomer), the number of determinants might be 10–20 (Crumpton, 1974). Roelants and colleagues (Roelants and Rydén, 1974; Roelants *et al.*, 1974) have examined the relationship between antigen concentration and incidence of labeled cells using the polypeptide TIGAL which can be regarded as a polymer with repeating similar, if not identical, antigenic determinants. The incidence of labeled cells increased with increasing concentration of TIGAL until a maximum number was reached at 1.5–2 μg/ml. In two experiments, the figure was, for B cells, 40 and 7 cell/10^4 cells, i.e., about 10% of the figure for hemocyanin, as expected on the basis of number of determinants. However, the concentration of protein at which the maximum number of binding cells was found was about the *same* for hemocyanin and TIGAL, as expected.

To our knowledge, Diener and Paektau (1972) is the only group which has not found an increase in the incidence of binding cells with increasing antigen concentration. As mentioned earlier (Section VII,B,2), their system may measure uptake rather than binding of antigen.

5. Number of Receptors on B Cells

Few workers using isotopically labeled antigens have attempted to estimate the number of receptors available to the antigens because the specific activity of their antigen preparations is usually too high for use under saturating conditions. For example, using ^{125}I-labeled antigens of specific activity about 20 μCi/μg, it can be calculated that, for 4 days exposure, 1 grain over a cell represents about 150 molecules of the antigen(Hämmerling et al., 1973; Byrt and Ada, 1969). Numbers above 15,000 molecules would result in more than 100 grains over a small lymphocyte. With specific activity of 300 μCi/ug, it is more difficult still. Miller et al. (1971), using β-galactosidase, estimate that up to 10^6 molecules can be bound to an individual cell. In view of the molecular weight of 540,000 and calculations for receptors in Table V, this estimate may be considerably too high. Later work (C. De Luca, personal communication) indicates that cells that bind such large amounts of this antigen are a very small proportion of all cells binding this antigen.

6. The Specificity of the Receptors

This can be considered in various ways. One approach has involved estimating the affinity of cell receptors for the antigen concerned. Davie et al. (1971; Davie and Paul, 1971) measured the inhibition of binding by DNP-lysine of DNP-guinea pig albumin to cells from nonimmune and immune guinea pigs. In nonimmune cells, the 50% inhibition point was achieved at about 5×10^{-4} M. For cells taken from guinea pigs 21 days after priming, the figure was about 5×10^{-7} M and this decreased to $<10^{-10}$ M at 28 days. The incidence of binding cells in the unimmunized guinea pigs was about $2/10^4$ cells. These results indicate a maturation in affinity during immunization. Perhaps cells with receptors of low affinity gave rise to progeny cells, most of which had receptors of high affinity (Cunningham, 1974); or the progeny was derived only from precursor cells with receptors of high affinity so that the great majority (>99%) of cells that, in unimmunized pigs, bound the antigens, were not stimulated to differentiate and proliferate. The concept that ABC in unimmunized hosts are a mixture of cells with receptors of different affinities for the antigen is entirely consistent with the hierarchy of binding cells observed by most workers, e.g., Ada (1970).

It has been found by many workers in this field that the binding of labeled antigens to B cells can be inhibited by prior or simultaneous exposure of the cells to unlabeled antigens of the same but not a different specificity. The amount of specific antigen needed can be very high—between 10^3- and 10^4-fold. Attempts to use such data to es-

3. Lymphocytic Receptors for Antigens

timate the number of receptors on B lymphocytes gave unreasonably high values (Byrt and Ada, 1969).

If exposed to serologically distinct antigens under saturating conditions for each, it might be expected that occasionally cells would be found which bound both antigens. Miller *et al.* (1971) mixed lymphocytes with saturating doses of two enzymes, β-galactosidase and horseradish peroxidase and found a small proportion of cells that bound both enzymes. The fact that the binding of each enzyme by individual cells was in discrete areas on the cell suggested to the authors that these double binding cells possessed receptors of at least two different specificities. It seems equally likely that the separate areas of antigen binding was an aggregation of receptors due to patching and that these cells might have receptors of a single specificity but of low affinity for either or both enzymes.

The question arises whether the high proportion of ABC observed under saturating conditions of antigen is meaningful in terms of a functional role the cells might play for the antigen concerned. In addition, β-galactosidase is an oligomer and the recent demonstration that polymeric antigens may act as nonspecific mitogens raises doubts as to the specificity of binding of large amounts of these antigens. This will be discussed later (Section X).

7. Binding of Antigens by Cells of Thymic Origin

The presence in the thymus of ABC for soluble antigens was described by Byrt and Ada (1969), who found their incidence to be lower than in the spleen. As indicated earlier, the detection of cells of thymic origin which bind labeled antigens requires either higher doses and/or higher specific activity of the antigen concerned than is the case with B cells. There are two reports of the number of binding cells found when saturating conditions of antigens are used. Miller *et al.* (1971) found that in mouse spleen and thymus, respectively, there were (per 10^4 lymphocytes) 230 and 22 cells binding β-galactosidase and 440 and 42 cells binding horseradish peroxidase. The thymic binding cells were recovered in the cortisone resistant fraction. Roelants and Rydén (1974) found, under saturating conditions, between two and three TIGAL binding T cells per 10^4 cells. Below saturating levels of antigen they found that T and B cells from unprimed mice had similar avidities for this antigen. Möller *et al.* (1973) reached similar conclusions using hapten inhibition of rosette formation.

Lawrence *et al.* (1973) have reported that HGG (MW about 15,000) heavily substituted with DNP (DNP_{57}-HGG) binds to a much higher proportion (0.15%) of thymocytes than does the carrier alone (<0.02%) or DNP_{14}-OA(<0.02%). The binding is specific for DNP and could be inhibited by anti-μ chain serum. The reason for the high incidence of ABC is obscure as DNP_{37}-D-GL is reputedly a thymus independent antigen (Katz et al., 1972).

8. Inhibition of Binding of Antigen by Anti-Ig Sera

The binding of labeled antigens to mouse lymphocytes can be inhibited if the lymphocytes are pretreated with a polyvalent anti-Ig sera (Byrt and Ada, 1969). The only antisera found to be effective as inhibitors were those directed against light and μ chains (Warner et al., 1970). In the absence of specific functional tests, the ability to inhibit binding of antigens to cells has come to be regarded as the strictest test for the specificity of the antigen binding reaction, indicating that the receptor for antigen is Ig. This argument becomes less valid as the size of the antigen relative to the receptor Ig molecule increases. With large or polymeric antigens, a possible interpretation is that the "true receptor" for the antigen is adjacent to the Ig present in the cell and the reaction with anti-Ig sterically blocks access of the antigen both to Ig and to the adjacent receptor. This possibility is less likely when the antigen is both monovalent and of low MW and the Fab fraction of anti-Ig is used, but, to our knowledge, this combination has not been used.

As shown in Table V, IgMs has been shown to be the dominant Ig present on rodent B lymphocytes and, to our knowledge, blocking of antigen binding to such lymphocytes is achieved only with anti-light and/or anti-μ chain Ig. Surprisingly the situation differs in guinea pigs where anti-IgG_2 was most effective in inhibiting the binding of DNP-GPA to spleen cells (Davie and Paul, 1971).

9. Antigen Binding Cells in Immune Animals

Naor and Sulitzeanu (1969a) reported an increase in the number of antigen binding cells during immunization. Using BSA as the antigen, they found that the incidence of binding cells in spleens for labeled BSA rose from 0.05% in unimmunized to 0.45% early in the immune response and to 4% in a hyperimmune response. About a tenfold rise early in the immune response is commonly (Ada et al., 1971) but not always seen (e.g., Cooper et al., 1972). Naor and Sulitzeanu showed that an increase in the number of binding cells did not occur if normal cells from mice passively immunized with antiserum were exposed to labeled BSA. In view of the more recent finding by Basten and colleagues of a receptor for Fc on B lymphocytes and the passive binding of antigen–antibody complexes to such cells, the possibility of cytophilic binding of Ig cells from mice undergoing an immune response is difficult to eliminate, as much of the antibody being produced may be cytophilic and not recovered in the serum used for passive immunization.

Using inhibition of antigen binding by antisera to different heavy claims as an index, Hämmerling *et al.* (1973) have looked at the changes in classes of IgG present on B cells during an immune response. They counted the number of ABC to TGAL in high (CWB) and low (C_3H) responder mice to this antigen. Some of the results are summarized in Table VI. Unprimed mice of both strains had similar numbers of ABC to the antigen and anti-μ serum was a more effective inhibitor of binding than antisera to other heavy chains. After a single injection of antigen in FCA, there was in both strains a fourfold increase in the incidence of ABC. Both strains only produced IgM, but with cells taken at 21 days, anti-μ serum was less effective, and anti-γ_1 and -γ_2 sera more effective in inhibiting antigen binding. At 21 days, TGAL was again injected. The responder but *not* the nonresponder mice showed a two- to threefold increase in ABC and production of humoral IgG. The inhibition of binding (by antibody) characteristics of both populations of ABC was relatively unchanged compared to those seen following the primary response. The point made by the authors is that, although the nonresponder mice did not make IgG, the relative amounts of different IgG classes on their B cells changed during immunization as though the cells in the low responder mice *intrinsically* had the ability to switch to IgG production, this switch being triggered by antigens. On the other hand, the sensitivity of the method for detection of antibody was not great so that both strains of mice may have made sufficient cytophilic IgG to apparently alter the characteristics of the cells.

The nature of the binding of antigen to primed T cells has been investigated by Roelants (1972a). Spleen cells from either normal or primed mice were reacted with ^{125}I-labeled *M. squinado* hemocyanin or TGAL after having been exposed to either anti-θ or normal AKR serum and complement. The specific activities of the antigens varied from 130–400 μCi/μg. In unprimed mice, few if any of the heavy binding cells (<50 molecules antigen/cell) but about 40% of light binders (10–50 molecules per cell) were suppressed by anti-θ treatment. In primed (6 months) mice, all the lightly labeled and up to 45% of the heavily labeled cells were deleted by anti-θ treatment.

TABLE VI
Inhibition by Anti-Ig of Binding of TGAL to Spleen Cells from Responder (CWB) and Nonresponder (C_3H) Mice[a]

Mouse strains	Nonimmune			Primed (day 21)			Boosted (day 21, tested day 31)		
	Incidence ABC/10^{-4} cells	Antiserum	Inhibition (%)	Incidence ABC/10^{-4} cells	Antiserum	Inhibition (%)	Incidence ABC/10^{-4} cells	Antiserum	Inhibition (%)
CWB	12	Polyvalent	75	47	Polyvalent	100	93	Polyvalent	96
	12	IgM[b]	58	47	IgM	42	93	IgM	33
	12	IgG_1[b]	16	47	IgG_1	32	93	IgG_1	44
	12	IgG_2[b]	−16	47	IgG_2	38	93	IgG_2	39
C_3H	11	Polyvalent	91	46	Polyvalent	100	54	Polyvalent	92
	11	IgM	55	46	IgM	28	54	IgM	22
	11	IgG_1	0	46	IgG_1	30	54	IgG_1	28
	11	IgG_2	−36	46	IgG_2	15	54	IgG_2	31

[a] Data taken from Hämmerling et al. (1973).
[b] The antisera were stated to be heavy chain class specific.

3. Lymphocytic Receptors for Antigens

The results suggested that, in unprimed mice, T cells bound up to 50 molecules of antigen whereas B cells bound up to 5000 molecules (under their conditions of assay); T lymphocytes in primed mice bound up to 750 molecules of antigen. This suggests a "maturation" process for T cells or accretion of cytophilic antibody by T cell during immunization, although the possibility of rare T cells in unprimed mice which bind more antigen was not eliminated.

10. Differentiation of Ig Bearing Lymphocytes

Kincade and Cooper (1971) studied the appearance in chick organs of cells that could bind anti-light chain, anti-μ or anti-γ chain Ig labeled with a fluorochrome. Cells binding anti-μ and anti-L chain Ig appeared in the bursa of 14-day-old embryos whereas cells binding anti-γ Ig did not appear until 21 days, i.e., at hatching. This sequence also occurred in the spleen, but on the third and eighth day after hatching. The authors noted that many bursal cells contained both IgG and IgM on the surface whereas this was the exception for spleen cells. It should be remembered that immunofluorescence is a rather less sensitive method than radioautography for this purpose.

Stutman (1973) and Nossal and Pike (1973) have made similar studies in mice. Stutman used the ability of anti-Ig sera to transform Ig bearing cells and scanned for blasts, whereas Nossal and Pike enumerated anti-Ig binding cells. Similar results were obtained and in summary suggested that Ig bearing cells could first be detected in the fetus some 3–5 days before birth at all major sites of erythromyelopoiesis, i.e., in liver, spleen, and bone marrow. A rapid influx of such cells into lymph nodes occurred shortly after birth and at no time were many seen in the thymus. Osmond and Nossal (1974a,b) have since examined lymphocyte differentiation in bone marrow in more detail. They found, in essence, two populations of lymphocytes in bone marrow: one that bound anti-Ig reagents and one that did not. Neither was sensitive to anti-θ serum and complement. The two populations were present in about equal numbers in bone marrow but the Ig-negative cells were seen in only small numbers in spleen or lymph node of adult animals.

The possible relationship between the two classes of bone marrow lymphocytes was investigated by a double-labeling procedure. All were exposed to ^{3}HTdr and ^{131}I-labeled anti-Ig and examined by radioautography. The anti-Ig binding cells were almost exclusively nondividing small lymphocytes. After injections of ^{3}HTdr, 90% of small lymphocytes became labeled by 48 hours. The earliest cells to label were the Ig-negative cells while Ig bearing cells howed a lag of 1½ days, and heavy binders nearly 2 days. The results suggest Ig molecules are not detectable on the surface of newly formed lymphocytes but they appear in increasing numbers during a subsequent maturation process.

It remains a matter of some concern that some of these results were not confirmed using the Fab fragment of anti-Ig as it is well known that B cells bind Ig through a receptor for Fc.

11. The Appearance during Fetal Life of ABC

Dwyer et al. (1972) studied the incidence of binding cells for ^{125}I-labeled flagellin and *J. lalandii* hemocyanin in human and mouse thymic cells, taken at different ages of fetal and natal life. Cells from fetal human thymus, taken as early as 12 weeks after gestation, reacted with flagellin to the extent that nearly 2% were classed as specific binding cells. The figure for hemocyanin was 0.1%. Cells from fetal mouse thymus showed the contrary pattern, 0.03% for flagellin and 0.03% for hemocyanin. In each situation, the binding of these antigens to the cell could be inhibited by pretreatment of the cells with anti-μ chain sera (up to 100%) or anti-κ sera (up to 60%) but not with anti-γ sera. The incidence of binding cells in the thymus decreased during natal life. Experiments were carried out *in vivo* and *in vitro* to exclude a role for cytophilic antibody in these results.

Decker et al. (1973) have looked at the binding of β-galactosidase and horseradish peroxidase binding cells in chicken, rabbit, and mouse tissues in early and late fetuses and in adults. These findings suggested that, from the very earliest time that the macroscopic organ can be dissected out, a nearly adult proportion of cells that could bind these antigens was found. Antigen binding by mouse fetal thymus cells was inhibited to 70% by anti-mouse κ chain sera, a similar degree of inhibition to that found with adult thymocytes. In late fetal life, the proportion of binders in thymus compared to spleen could be higher or lower, depending on the species. Similar levels of antigen binding cells were found in tissues of germ-free and immunoglobulin-free piglets. Again in the organs studied, binding could be inhibited by anti-pig Ig serum. The results suggest that ABC appear in large numbers in the absence of both antigenic stimulation and circulating immunoglobulin. In bursectomized chickens, the incidence of cells binding β-galactosidase increased in the thymus and bone marrow but decreased 60% in spleen.

The results of these two groups have some puzzling features.

3. Lymphocytic Receptors for Antigens

Despite the failure of every worker in the field to demonstrate the binding of significant amounts of anti-Ig sera to more than a very small proportion of thymic cells, high proportions of binding cells for some antigens are found and the binding can be inhibited by anti-κ and particularly anti-μ antibody. For example, Nossal and Pike (1973) failed to find anti-Ig binding cells in mouse thymus at any stage of development yet Dwyer et al. (1972) found up to 2% in 12-week-old human thymus cells and 0.34% of mouse fetal thymus cells binding hemocyanin. Both binding patterns could be inhibited by anti-Ig sera. The results of Decker et al. (1973), particularly in bursectomized chickens, are clearly inconsistent with those of three other groups (Good et al., 1971; Crone et al., 1972; Hemmingson and Alm, 1972) who fail to find rosette formation with thymus cells from such chickens.

It is difficult to assess the significance of these findings, particularly those relating to the binding of antigen to fetal thymocytes. One of the greatest needs is a test directly relating antigen binding to the function of the cells.

12. ANTIGEN BINDING CELLS IN TOLERANCE

As findings in the field have been recently discussed in some detail elsewhere (Ada and Cooper, 1974), they will be only summarized here. It is clear that tolerance to an antigen may be a property of either or both T and B lymphocytes. In view of our comments earlier on the relative ease of binding of antigens to these two cell classes, it might be expected, using conditions frequently chosen in this procedure, that one of two results might be found. If tolerance is a B cell lesion, there might be a deletion of specific cells so that antigen binding cells are significantly decreased. This has been observed in two cases, to our knowledge.

Guinea pigs (or mice) may be rendered tolerant to DNP if DNP-D-GL is administered. This reagent does not react with T cells and the evidence suggests strongly that this is B cell tolerance (Katz et al., 1971, 1972; Nossal et al., 1973). At least in guinea pigs, there is a significant depression in the number of binding cells for DNP. There are several important features about these findings. (1) Tolerance is induced by remarkably small amounts of the antigen. (2) The tolerance is stable in transfer of cells to lethally irradiated recipients and is not reversible if the cells are treated with trypsin. (3) Tolerance can be rapidly induced even using primed B cells. (4) Calculations indicate that, on the average, the spacing interval between DNP residues on DNP-D-GL is about 1.0 nm.

The second example (Louis et al., 1973) is tolerance to HGG in mice. In this model, the function of both B and T cells may be affected. Under conditions where it is known that B cells are affected, there is a progressive decrease in the number of tolerogen binding cells as tolerance in the B cell population develops.

Studies of high zone tolerance to BSA have yielded different results. G. L. Ada and N. A. Mitchison (unpublished) found a slight decrease (35%) in binding cells to BSA present in such mice, whereas Humphrey *et al.* (1971) did not. Naor and Sulitzeanu (1969b) found that adult mice given a total of 60 mg of BSA from birth lacked BSA binding cells but they thought this might be due to masking of the cell receptors by the BSA. In view of more recent knowledge of cell capping by antigen (Diener and Paetkau, 1972), it seems likely that simple masking of cells is not a sufficient explanation for these findings, so that these cells might have been deleted.

There is one situation where a deficiency of θ-sensitive rosette forming cells has been observed. This is in mice tolerant of NNP_{12}-BSA (Möller and Sjöberg, 1972). It will be of interest to see if this observation is extended to other models.

Several groups have reported states of tolerance in mice where there is no indication of a significant decrease in antigen binding cells or rosettes. Ada *et al.* (1971) and Cooper *et al.* (1972) have reported that rats tolerant of flagellin and mice high zone tolerant of hemocyanin *(J. lalandii)* have normal levels of specific antigen binding cells. In both cases there is substantial evidence that the lesion is in T cells but it has yet to be shown that B cells are unaffected.

There is a category of tolerant states in which clearly the lesion is in B cells but, unlike the cases quoted above, transfer of cells results in a rapid breakage of tolerance. In both cases—pneumococcal polysaccharide (Howard, 1972) and lipopolysaccharide (Sjöberg, 1972)—there is not a significant decrease in the number of rosette forming cells (using antigen-coated RBC). The numbers in fact may be increased. The mechanism involved here is unknown, although it has been suggested (J. Howard, personal communication) that formation of antigen–antibody (receptor) complexes at the cell surface is unstable so that the cells are "held in check" and not deleted.

VIII. Specificity and Immunocompetence of ABC

Although the data on ABC presented in the previous section are entirely consistent with the notion that cells specifically binding antigens were relevant in the immune response, direct evidence was needed for this. Several approaches have been successful. One was to selectively enrich or deplete populations of lymphocytes for cells binding to particular antigens, using column or batch separation techniques. Another was to show specific inactivation of cells by radiolabeled antigen.

A. Depletion and Enrichment of ABC

1. COLUMN CHROMATOGRAPHY

The first experiments (e.g., Wigzell and Andersson, 1969) involved passing a suspension of unprimed lymphoid cells through columns packed with glass or plastic beads coated with one of a number of antigens. It was a general finding that cells in the column effluent were less able, upon transfer into inactivated recipients, to respond to the homologous antigen compared to the original population. The loss was selective and was prevented if soluble homologous antigen was present. Similarly, cells from immunized animals could be depleted both of memory cells and of PFC, but not of helper activity, a T cell function (Wigzell, 1971). Thus, B cells seemed to be preferentially bound. It was difficult to recover cells from the column and the only reasonably effective way was agitation of the column contents in a flask. The yield of cells was poor and the damage rate high.

The most successful approach has been the use of polyacrylamide beads to which the hapten phenyl-β-lactoside (lac) was attached via a spacer molecule (Truffa-Bachi and Wofsy, 1970; Wofsy et al., 1971; Henry et al., 1972). When spleen cells from immune mice were passed through the column, 99% of the cells were recovered in the effluent which contained all anti-SRBC PFC and anti-β-glucoside PFC but only 20% of anti-lac PFC. About 50% of the latter was recovered when the column was eluted with 15 μM lac, yielding an enrichment of 500-fold. Lac-specific B cells could also be removed from normal spleen cells in this way. The effluent from such columns was active in transfer experiments, provided there was helper activity.

A modification of this technique has been described by De Luca et al. (1972). Lymphoid cells were incubated with the enzyme β-galactosidase, the excess enzyme removed, and the cell preparation passed through a column containing polyacrylamide beads coated with the substrate, phenyl-β-thiogalactoside. ABC that had bound the enzyme were retarded rather than retained on the column, and after several passages an enrichment of up to 150-fold could be obtained, although the losses were considerable.

An interesting variant that offers more hope is the use of Sephadex G-200 beads to which anti-Ig antibody had been coupled (Schlossman and Hudson, 1973). Ig-positive cells (B) were retained on passage through this column and could be completely recovered by digesting the column contents with dextranase.

The results obtained with these techniques suggest that the receptors on B cells are readily available for coupling to antigen attached to insoluble supports, in contrast to those on T cells. The results, particularly of Wofsy and colleagues, support strongly the concept of restricted specificity of receptors on individual B lymphocytes.

2. Batch Procedures

Batching procedures have been used to deplete cell suspensions of particular specificities as an alternative procedure to column chromatography. Davie and Paul (1970, 1971) and Davie *et al.* (1971) mixed spleen cell suspensions from guinea pigs immune to DNP with agarose beads coated with various DNP-substituted proteins. After 1 hour, the beads were allowed to settle and the cells in the supernatant assayed. Anti-DNP producing cells and cells binding labeled guinea pig albumin substituted with DNP (DNP-GPA) were depleted. Cells which could be stimulated by DNP-GPA to incorporate ^{3}HTdr were depleted only if beads coated with GPA were used.

Nylon fibers have also been used to separate ABC from other cells (Edelman *et al.*, 1971; Rutishauser *et. al.*, 1972). The fibers were coated with antigen and moved backward and forward in a suspension of lymphoid cells. For different antigens, up to 1% of cells bound to the fibers but up to 50% of these bound nonspecifically. There was a rise of 2- to 3-fold in the number of binding cells when immunized donors were used compared with an increase of 15- to 600-fold in the number of RFC and indirect PFC. Mechanical plucking of the fibers in a medium of low ionic strength was the best way of recovering binding cells.

Rosette formation was early considered to be a very suitable procedure for enrichment and depletion of cells of the appropriate specificity, due to the ease of separation and recovery of rosettes. Three groups (Brody, 1970; Gorczynski *et al.*, 1971; Osoba, 1970) were able to obtain useful enrichment and depletion of B cells in this way and it is surprising that the technique has not been more widely used. Parish and Hayward (1974a,b) have very successfully adapted the technique for separation of cells bearing different surface antigens.

3. Lymphocytic Receptors for Antigens

In summary, all these approaches have strengthened the concept of specificity at the level of individual B and/or T cells.

B. Specific Inactivation ("Suicide") of ABC

A population of T and/or B cells can be depleted selectively for immunocompetence to a given antigen by inactivation of cells which specifically bind that antigen.

The initial experiments were described independently by two groups in 1969. Byrt and Ada (1969) wished to devise a test to demonstrate that ABC were functionally important. It had been shown by Dutton and Mishell (1967) that the formation of antibody producing cells during an immune response could be prevented by exposing the responding cells to ^{3}HTdr of high specific activity. By analogy with this work, Ada and Byrt (1969) reckoned that cells that bound sufficient radiolabeled antigen, if exposed to the radiation for a suitable period, would be damaged and be unable to replicate, a process that characterizes the immune response. To demonstrate selective inactivation, two serologically unrelated preparations of polymerized flagellin were chosen and labeled with ^{125}I. Separate mouse spleen cell preparations, treated with one or the other (30 minutes, 4°; removal of non-cell-associated antigen; storage for 16 hours at 4°), were transferred to lethally irradiated mice and challenged with nonradioactive antigen of both serologic specificities. The antibody response to the labeled antigen used was abolished or significantly reduced without affecting the response to the other. It was claimed, therefore, that at least some of the lymphocytes that bind radioactive antigens are cells that take part in an antibody response; that at any one time most or all of the cells in the mouse spleen that can be stimulated to produce antibody within eight days are able to bind antigen *in vitro;* that the specificity of inactivation is difficult to reconcile with any theory other than one requiring cell populations with a very restricted potential for antigenic stimulation; and that the ability to inactivate selectively particular cells in mixed populations should prove useful for assessing the contribution of such cells in the immune response.

In contrast, Humphrey wished to extend earlier observations (McDevitt *et al.*, 1966; Nossal *et al.*, 1965) that, in draining lymph nodes of animals injected with radioactive antigen, antibody containing and/or secreting cells contained very few molecules of labeled antigen (from <15 to <4 molecules in specific cells). Using TIGAL in which iodine atoms form part of the antigenic determinant and iodinating to very high specific activities (>2.5 mCi/μg, some 100-fold greater than is usually achieved with naturally occurring proteins), Humphrey and Keller (1971) found that injection of their labeled antigen failed to elicit either a primary or a secondary response to TIGAL. The effect was specific, and on subsequent injection (by an alternative route) of nonradioactive TIGAL the mice gave a normal primary response. This suggested that the radioactive antigen killed a proportion but not all cells that possessed sufficiently avid receptors to bind immunologically significant amounts of antigen. Subsequent work (Humphrey et al., 1971) established the correctness of the interpretation.

The mechanism of cell inactivation by this procedure is not known. Possibilities are chromosomal damage, interphase death, or even more subtle changes such as failure of the cells to "home" to appropriate lymphoid organs (see Section II,D). We cannot choose between these possibilities at present. The properties to be desired of an isotope for this purpose cannot at present be defined too clearly except that the extent of radiation penetration should not extend beyond one cell diameter, approximately 8 μm. Clearly ^{125}I is suitable in this respect (Myers and Vanderleeden, 1960; Ada et al., 1966; Humphrey et al., 1971) as the maximum path length of the β electrons is about 10 μm. This also accounts for the reasonably good resolution attained in radioautography with this isotope. If the cells are in a pellet, then cells in the layer immediately surrounding the antigen coated cell may also be damaged. It follows, therefore, that this technique should only be used where the cells to be inactivated occur rarely and possibly less than 1% of the cell population.

It is possible to estimate the dose of radiation delivered to a cell following the binding of ^{125}I-labeled antigen (Humphrey et al., 1971). In a suicide experiment, therefore, it should be possible to estimate the number of cells inactivated by the ^{125}I and, hence, the incidence of immunocompetent cells. Our lack of knowledge of the mechanism of inactivation by ^{125}I or even by X-irradiation makes this task impracticable at present.

Workers using the "suicide" technique have followed mainly the procedure described by Ada and Byrt (1969). Table VII describes some of the published findings, which are discussed under two headings.

1. B Cells

Several groups have inactivated B cells in spleen cell preparations from normal or primed mice and the "suicide" technique is now a

TABLE VII

Summary of Experiments Demonstrating Inactivation ("Suicide") of Mouse Lymphocyte Function by Radiolabeled Antigen

Source and/or type of lymphocyte	Response measured	Function involved	Labeled antigen	Control antigen	Reference
Spleen (B) (unprimed)	Antibody production	Differentiation, replication	POL 1338 POL 870	POL 870 POL 1338	Ada and Byrt, 1969
Activated T lymphocytes	Antibody production	Helper activity	Hemocyanin	Ovalbumin	Roelants and Askonas, 1971
Thymocytes	Antibody production	Helper activity	Fowl IgG	TBC	Basten et al., 1971
B lymphocytes	Antibody production	Differentiation, replication	Fowl IgG	RBC	Basten et al., 1971
Thymocytes	Delayed-type hypersensitivity	Replication	POL 870	POL 1338 Hemocyanin	Cooper and Ada, 1972
Activated T lymphocytes	Delayed-type hypersensitivity	Secretion of active factors	POL 1338 Hemocyanin	POL 870 Hemocyanin POL 870 POL 1338	Cooper and Ada, 1972
Spleen (B) unprimed	Antibody production	Differentiation, replication	KLH	—	Unanue, 1971a
Spleen (B) primed	Antibody production	Differentiation, replication	HGG	KLH	Unanue, 1971a
Spleen (B) primed	Antibody production	Differentiation, replication	TIGAL KLH	KLH TIGAL	Humphrey et al., 1971
Bone marrow	Antibody production	Differentiation, replication	KLH	SRBC	Unanue, 1971b

standard procedure in some laboratories, including the authors'. Initially Ada and Byrt (1969) showed a difference in antibody levels at days 7 or 8 after antigenic challenge. Basten et al. (1971) measured PFC on day 15 after two injections of antigen. Unanue (1971a) and Humphrey et al. (1971) have shown that, even at day 22, the response of animals receiving inactivated cells is diminished, which indicates that both IgM and IgG are affected.

The finding by Unanue (1971b) that immunocompetent cells in bone marrow can be inactivated by this technique is in agreement with the work of Weigle and colleagues showing that *in vivo* bone marrow cells can be rendered tolerant of HGG. Nevertheless, it is somewhat surprising in view of findings (e.g., Osmond and Nossal, 1974a,b) that suggest the presence of a large pool of probable precursor cells which do not bind anti-Ig antibody. Even 10 weeks after reconstitution of the irradiated recipients with the treated bone marrow and three injections of antigen, Unanue found that antibody levels were considerably lower than those of controls. Basten et al. (1971) failed to inactivate bone marrow cells under conditions where spleen B cells were inactivated. Obviously, more work is needed in this area.

2. T Cells

The inactivation of T cell populations for two functional activities has been reported. These are helper activity and delayed type hypersensitivity (DTH).

Humphrey et al. (1971) were unable to show inactivation of the helper activity of T cells primed to KLH. Roelants and Askonas (1971) were successful but only under conditions where limiting numbers of T cells were employed. The effect was clear-cut and specific. Basten et al. (1971) were also able to inactivate thymus cells which took part in helper activity in transfer experiments. The inactivation could be prevented if the cells were preexposed to an antimouse Ig $F(ab')^2$ preparation.

Parish (1971) using rats and Cooper (1972) using mice showed that flagellar H antigens from *Salmonella* could induce DTH reactions. In contrast to B cells which clearly seemed to distinguish between H antigens from different strains of *Salmonella* (as measured by the immobilization technique—Ada et al., 1964), the DTH reaction in rats or mice sensitized with antigen of one specificity could be elicited equally well with H antigens of the same or a different specificity. Subsequent work (Langman, 1972) showed that these proteins contained two classes of antigenic determinants, one which was unique to a given strain—Hv determinants—and one which was common to all strains—Hc determinants. With the two strains commonly used, SL 870 (*S. typhimurium*) and SW 1338 (*S. adelaide*), B cells seemed to preferentially recognize Hv compared to Hc so that antibody titers were always higher to Hv than to Hc. This accorded with the results obtained by Ada and Byrt (1969) showing specificity at the B cell level. The cross-reactivity observed by Parish (1971) and of Cooper (1972) suggested T cells might only recognize Hc determinants. This interpretation was strengthened when Cooper and Ada (1972) found that T cells from mice sensitized to H antigen of one strain could be inactivated by exposure to ^{125}I-labeled antigen of SL 870 or SW 1338 strains, suggesting that the sensitized cells bound either antigen equally well. Inactivation could be prevented if the sensitized cells were preexposed to a concentrated preparation of anti-mouse light chain Ig. Sensitization of thymic cells in X-irradiated mice was prevented if the thymus cells were first exposed, under inactivating conditions, to ^{125}I-labeled H antigen.

3. General Comments

The inactivation of cells using radiolabeled antigens is "not wholly unpredictable" (Humphrey *et al.*, 1971). Clearly some B cells can bind large numbers of antigen molecules, possibly up to 10^5, and yet about 99% of other cells in the same preparation bind very few molecules. The results obtained indicate a restriction in specificity but not necessarily unispecificity at the level of individual cells. One of the future uses of the technique may well be to examine the conditions under which cells with a given specificity reappear after inactivation. The early work of Unanue (1971a) suggests if *very high* specific activities are used (>1 mCi/μg protein), the response to a given antigen may be completely abolished.

The results with T cells are more controversial. It is generally conceded that T cells bind less antigen than B cells, and yet they can be inactivated by this technique. It is possible that T cells that bind large amounts of antigen occur even less frequently than B cells so that they are rarely, if ever, observed in radioautographs. Another possibility is that a majority of labeled antigen attached to T cells in the presence of excess labeled antigen is shed during the washing procedure, preparatory to smearing on a slide for radioautography.

The results as such might be taken to indicate that T cells are more susceptible to radiation damage than are B cells. Much of the evidence in the literature would suggest that at least primed T cells are resistant to X-irradiation (e.g., Katz *et al.*, 1973b). However, thymus cells must replicate at least once before they can act as helpers (Feldmann and Basten, 1972b). An extra difficulty in interpretation is the extent to which cytophilic activity may contribute to the binding of antigen.

A strict comparison of the properties of B and T cells in this regard may have to await the availability of a method of enumerating functionally active T cells, i.e., comparable to the assay of B cells as PFC.

C. Membrane Modulation

Modulation (patching and/or capping) of membrane components, while not directly measuring the immunocompetence of lymphocytes, may indicate certain properties, such as homogeneity of particular components, especially as different components on the cell surface cap independently of each other (Section IV). Using this approach, several groups have carried out ingenious experiments to examine B cell tolerance and the relationship between bound antigen and cell-associated Ig.

Diener and Paetkau (1972) reported that, following exposure of B cells to immunogenic doses (250 ng/ml) of polymerized flagellin labeled with tritium, the bound antigen could be capped and endocytosed. If tolerogenic doses (20 ug/ml) were used, capping did not occur. Under the latter conditions, these authors calculated that about 2×10^6 monomer equivalents bound. Bearing in mind that (1) the polymer consists of 6–8 strands of monomer units; (2) not all monomer units immediately adjacent to the membrane would bind to specific receptors; and (3) B cells may contain only $1-2 \times 10^5$ Ig molecules at their surface (Table V), it seems that exposure to the high concentrations of the polymer probably caused saturation of the receptors so that for steric reasons, modulation could not occur (see also Section IV,B,1).

Ashman (1973) has shown that the appearance of B cell rosettes could be altered by exposure to anti-Ig sera. Capping of the Ig and red cells occurred simultaneously. As the binding of antigens to the cell can also be almost entirely prevented by pretreatment with anti-Ig sera, the question arose whether the antigen could cause the capping of *all* Ig on the cell surface; if so, this would suggest that the cell-associated Ig was entirely of one antigen-binding specificity. Using labeled polymerized flagellin and fluorescent anti-POL and anti-Ig reagents, Raff et al. (1973) exposed spleen cells from normal or immunized mice to high concentrations of antigen at 20° and 37°C

3. Lymphocytic Receptors for Antigens   241

to allow capping to occur. The cells were then exposed at 4° first to rhodamine labeled anti-POL Ig and then fluorescein labeled anti-Ig. More than 95% of POL binders could also be labeled with anti-Ig reagents but not with anti-θ reagent. The anti-Ig label was seen as a cap on the POL binding cells. The incidence of positive B cells was 4–7 cells/10^5 cells in spleens from normal mice and 3–10 cells/10^4 cells in spleens from mice 4–7 days after injection with the antigen.

Although immunofluorescence is not a very sensitive technique for the detection of antigens, the results indicate that, on those cells that bound large amounts of POL, over 90% of the cell associated Ig capped. This suggests that most if not all Ig on the cell surface was of a single antigen binding specificity. There is another, probably less likely explanation. It has recently been demonstrated that polymerized flagellin in high concentration can be mitogenic for B lymphocytes and induce polyclonal antibody production (Coutinho and Möller, 1973). It is not known whether this is a result of the binding to Ig or to other sites on the cell surface. If the former, it could be argued that this antigen, as a polymer, can react with Ig molecules with a variety of antigen binding specificities (i.e., low affinity for POL but overall high avidity), and therefore that the cells observed by Raff and colleagues may have contained Ig of different binding specificities.

A similar approach has been used for T cells. Thus, Ashman and Raff (1973) showed that rosette formation could be inhibited by anti-Ig sera and treatment of formed rosettes with anti-Ig caused capping of the red cells. Direct visualization of Ig on the red cells was not seen.

Roelants and colleagues (Roelants et al., 1973, 1974; Roelants and Rydén, 1974) have also carried out experiments with T cells (regarded as such on the basis of reactivity with anti-θ sera or failure to bind anti-Ig antibody) from unprimed and primed animals. The antigens used were TIGAL and *Maia squinado* hemocyanin, both being iodinated to high specific activity so that in radioautographs one grain corresponded approximately to one molecule of antigen. T cells from normal mice were estimated in one experiment to bind >1200 molecules of antigen and in another to bind up to 50,000 molecules. The degree of labeling of B and T cells from spleens of primed mice "was identical." In both cases, capping of antigen on T cells was observed following exposure to anti-Ig sera. With cells from unprimed mice, the capping procedure was repeated twice.

As Roelants et al. (1973) admit, there are some puzzling features of their work, e.g., the failure to detect binding of anti-Ig to T cells, although this may simply be a reflection of the low sensitivity of immunofluorescence. It is also unclear from their findings the extent to which antigen per se induces capping (e.g., Raff et al., 1973); it seems that this occurs to some extent. In addition, both antigens sued are substantially larger than IgMs or IgG molecules and it might be wondered how, following binding of antigen, anti-Ig molecules gained access to the antigen–Ig complexes. One can also ask if all B cells are Ig-positive; there is increasing evidence this is not so.

Can the results with T cells be explained by cytophilic antibody? In the case of T cells from primed hosts, this seems possible, if not likely as shown in the following experiments. Almost pure populations of T cells, primed to alloantigens, can be collected from thoracic duct lymph (T. TDL) of irradiated F_1 mice injected 4 days earlier with parental thymus cells (Sprent and Miller, 1972a,b,c). A high proportion of these cells stain positively with rabbit anti-mouse Ig reagents as detected by indirect immunofluorescence (Pernis et al., 1974). If these cells are cultured in vitro at 37° for 18 hours, with or without prior treatment with chymotrypsin, surface Ig can no longer be detected on the cells. This behavior is, of course, in contrast to the reappearance of IgM on the surface of B cells after capping and endocytosis or its continual presence during incubation at 37°. It was suggested that this Ig on the T. TDL is cytophilic and derived from B cells contaminating the suspension of donor thymus cells. Thus, T. TDL generated from thymus cells depleted of B cells showed less surface Ig (Hudson et al., quoted by Pernis et al., 1974).

A similar explanation for the results obtained with cells from unprimed mice is less likely, and Roelants and colleagues confidently conclude that the receptor on T cells for antigen is Ig.

IX. Receptors on Lymphocytes for Antigens

We nominate three requirements for a component of the lymphocyte plasma membrane to be identified as a receptor for antigens.

1. It should show specificity.
2. It should be a product of the cell itself.
3. Binding of antigen to the component should be a necessary, but not necessarily sufficient, step in the pathway of events leading to differentiation and proliferation of the cell.

These are strict criteria and we can now examine the credentials of possible candidates for acceptance as the antigen receptor.

A. Ig as Antigen Receptor

1. SPECIFICITY

The results of studies on antigen binding cells, on enrichment, depletion and inactivation procedures, and on antigen-mediated membrane modulation all point to the specificity of individual B cells. It has not formally been shown that individual B cells make V regions for light and heavy chains of a single amino acid sequence but this at least must be considered very likely.

T cell reactions also show considerable specificity, notably those involved in cell mediated immunity (Benacerraf and Levine, 1962; Paul, 1970; Schlossman, 1972). If examined at the level of single cells, there is not as much evidence as exists for B cells. In general terms however, T cell populations show specificity but there are some apparent differences between B and T cells.

a. The recognition of different antigenic determinants on flagellar antigens by T and B cells, as mentioned earlier.

b. Thompson *et al.* (1972) demonstrated that whereas B cells can clearly distinguish between egg-white lysozyme and its reduced and carboxymethlated derivation, CM-lysozyme, T cells apparently did not. Several activities usually considered to be T cell functions, namely, DTH and migration inhibitory factor production, showed cross-reactivity.

c. Cross-tolerance to flagellar antigens (Austin and Nossal, 1966) and to lysozyme and CM-lysozyme (Scibienski *et al.*, 1972) has been shown. Some evidence suggests that the effect observed by Austin and Nossal is at the level of T cells (Ada and Cooper, 1974) and Scibienski, Fong, Davis, and Benjamini (quoted by Scibienski *et al.*, 1972) showed that, in animals tolerant of lysozyme, helper (T) cell activity was absent.

d. Goodman and colleagues (Alkan *et al.*, 1972) have carried out experiments in which they have made use of two haptenic groups which seem to differ in their reactivity for T and B cells.

L-Tyrosine azobenzene-p-arsonate (RAT) induces cellular immunity without antibody production. Guinea pigs injected with RAT conjugated to poly-γ-D-glutamic acid (PGA) produced antibody to PGA, showing that RAT could act as a carrier. On the other hand, DNP functions poorly as a carrier but well as a hapten reacting with B cells. RAT joined by a spacer to DNP is a good immunogen, cellular immunity against RAT and anti-DNP antibody being produced. RAT-RAT compounds failed to induce a humoral response.

The authors considered that RAT molecules separated by a rigid spacer might be more active or there might be a biologic block to self help. The latter does not occur with polymeric antigens such as TGAL.

These exceptions may be more apparent than real in that they may reflect the past antigenic history of the host. For example, the finding that T cells recognize the Hc determinants of flagellar antigens, sometimes in preference to the Hv determinants, may be due to memory T cells accumulating following infections by flagella-bearing organisms.

Despite such findings, we would be reluctant to support the notion that the specificity of antigen recognition by T cells is of quite a different order from that displayed by B cells were it not for recent results from an entirely different type of experiment.

Except in the case of lymphocytes reacting to alloantigen, results from these different experimental systems indicate that the interaction between sensitized T lymphocytes and other somatic cells occurs only in syngeneic or semiallogeneic systems. Thus, histoincompatible T cells do not function as helpers for B cells (Kindred and Shreffler, 1972; Katz *et al.*, 1973b). In addition, maximal proliferation of lymphocytes (T cells?) following exposure *in vitro* of sensitized lymphocytes to antigen-pulsed macrophages occurs only if the two cell types share major histocompatibility antigens (Rosenthal and Shevach, 1973). Finally, T cell-mediated lysis of target cells infected with the specific virus (lymphocyte choriomeningitis (LCM) virus or ectromelia (mousepox) virus) only occurs when the *specifically* activated T cell and the target cell share at least one set of H-2 antigenic specificities (Zinkernagel and Doherty, 1974a; Gardner *et al.*, 1975).

Zinkernagel and Doherty (1974b) have now further analyzed the nature of this interaction. They surmised that this restriction could reflect one of two distinct mechanisms:

1. Two recognition steps between T cell and target cell were necessary, one involving recognition of H-2 antigens and the other of specific viral antigens.

2. The T cell recognized "altered self," that is, H-2 and viral antigen.

Lymphocytes from F_1 infected (immune) mice were found to efficiently lyse virus infected targets of either parent H-2 type. If model 1 were correct, F_1 mice need possess only one clone of sensitized T cells which recognized viral antigen by a specific receptor and like H-2 antigen of either type in a nonimmunologic way. If model 2 were correct, F_1 mice would possess at least two specific clones of T cells, reactive to modified H-2 of one or the other parent type. The models were distinguished by injecting F_1 LCM immune T cells into immunosuppressed LCM-infected mice of either H-2 type and examining the properties of progeny cells.

Proliferation of, for example, F_1 ($H-2^{k/b}$) immune spleen cells with the ability to lyse $H-2^k$ LCM-infected target cells occurred *only* in recipient mice of $H-2^k$ antigenic specificity, thus favoring model 2 hypothesis (if model 1 were correct, the cells should have replicated in hosts of either antigenic specificity). Later work (R. V. Blanden, P. C. Doherty, M. B. C. Dunlop, I. D. Gardner, R. M. Zinkernagel, and C. S. David, personal communication) using H-2 recombinant mouse strains rules out the possibility that allelic exclusion could explain these data. Most importantly, these results also indicate that further replication of the immune T cells in the immunosuppressed mice is dependent upon exposure to virus infected target cells in these hosts and is *not* triggered by free virus.

Shearer (1974) has also found that if spleen cells from congenic mouse strains are cultured *in vitro* with TNP-modified syngeneic spleen cells, cytotoxic T cells are generated which have a specificity directed in part against TNP but primarily against modified syngeneic cell surface components.

Though one should be cautious in extrapolating from these results to the properties of helper T cells and DTH T cells, all of these results do suggest that recognition by T cells may be rather more complicated than recognition by B cells and raises the possibility that the findings from antigen binding studies involving T cells *in vitro* may not be relevant to antigen recognition *in vivo*.

These findings do not tell us the nature of the receptor on cytotoxic T cells. They emphasize, however, that recognition of foreign structures by T cells is a complex process.

2. SYNTHESIS

"Virgin" B cells synthesize the IgMs found at the cell surface (e.g., Melchers and Andersson, 1973). Lymph node cells from normal mice synthesize both IgG and IgM but only IgMs seems to be expressed at the B cell surface (Parkhouse, 1973). Most results suggest that, with unprimed cells, classes of Ig other than IgMs and IgD found associated with the plasma membrane are cytophilic. However, the finding that the target cells for T cell dependent allotypic suppression in mice are B cells suggests strongly that the cell must express some γ chain at the cell surface (Herzenberg et al., 1973; Jacobson et al., 1972). The nature of the Ig present on the surface of primed B cells has yet to be examined in detail.

Two groups (Vitetta et al., 1973; Lisowska-Bernstein et al., 1973) have failed to show synthesis of Ig by T cells under conditions where a contribution by contaminating B cells was excluded. In contrast, Moroz and Hahn (1974) report that 30% of all protein synthesized by human thymocytes *in vitro* is Ig and that this is found (even on the surface of these cells) as noncovalently linked L and μ chains. Because of the lack of interchain disulfide bonds, these authors consider it unlikely that they are measuring IgMs synthesized by contaminating B cells. These results are potentially very interesting but we feel that separate more direct evidence for the total lack of B or plasma cells should be sought.

Roelants et al. (1974) also argue in favor of Ig synthesis by T cells. They found that a small proportion of cells (Ig-negative or θ-positive) from unimmunized mice could bind TIGAL following a prior treatment in which a similar proportion of cells in the population had bound this antigen and had been capped, using anti-Ig sera. If, as the authors claim in this paper, T cells bind as much TIGAL as B cells, it seems difficult to explain the results on the basis of cytophilic antibody. The evidence does not constitute formal proof of Ig synthesis, however, and the argument is weakened if it were to be shown that T cells bind much less antigen than do B cells.

In summary, formal evidence for the synthesis of Ig by T cells is lacking and the circumstantial evidence is not totally convincing.

3. BIOLOGIC FUNCTION OF IG

This is discussed in two parts. First, does anti-Ig antibody interfere with the activity of lymphocytes, as tested by both passive tests and inhibition of active functions? Table VIII is a collection of a variety of assays using both T and B cells. The list is not exhaustive but two points stand out. Inhibition of B cells by anti-Ig sera, with one exception, are all positive. The story with T cells is a collection of assertions and contradictions and we have no means at present of coming to a firm decision.

The most positive evidence will come with a critical analysis of the complex formed when antigen binds to the cell surface, and the relationship between the formation of this complex and stimulation of the cell. Experiments along these lines have yet to be done. Rolley and Marchalonis (1972) have reported the formation of antigen—Ig complexes when mouse spleen cells were exposed to very high concentrations of conjugates of DNP–homologous hemoglobin. Under these conditions up to 10% of cells bound the reagent. This figure is so much higher than the upper limit found by other workers that a high proportion of nonspecific binding may have occurred.

To our knowledge, there are now several experiments that suggest the nature of an antigen–receptor complex released from helper T cells. Feldmann and Basten (1972a) and Feldmann (1973) demonstrated the passage of an antigen–IgMs complex from a compartment containing activated T cells to one containing primed B cells. Two observations have cast doubt on the interpretation put on this work.

1. Some experiments suggest that the complex may come from B cells (Pernis et al., 1974).
2. Experiments of Katz et al. (1973b) showed that T-B cell cooperation did not occur if histoincompatible cells were used. This failure would not be expected if cell cooperation occurred via a soluble complex.

On the other hand, Taussig (1974) has described the preparation of an antigen specific T cell factor capable of totally replacing T cells *in vitro* in the induction of an antibody response to TGAL. Later work (Taussig and Munro, 1974) has shown that the factor could not be removed by an anti-mouse Ig adsorbent but was removed completely by congenically raised anti-H-2 antibodies, suggesting that the cooperative T cell factor is associated with the alloantigens of the strain in which it is produced.

4. SUMMARY

Almost all the evidence supports the concept that Ig acts as the receptor for antigen on B lymphocytes. The final demonstration of this has yet to be done. We believe that most evidence argues against the belief that T cells have as much Ig as B cells but does not exclude the possibility that they contain much less Ig than B cells and that this Ig is the T cell receptor. We can be dogmatic on one point: the nature of the receptor for antigen on T cells can still be regarded as one of the most challenging problems in immunology.

It is clear that other candidates for the T cell receptor should be seriously considered. The first of these is the Ir gene product.

B. The Ir Gene Product

The ability to form immune responses to a variety of antigens is genetically controlled (Benacerraf and McDevitt, 1972; Grumet and

TABLE VIII

Findings for and against Functional Ig on T Lymphocytes

	Assay procedure	B cells	T cells	Activated T cells	References[a]
Detection	Anti-Ig sera				
	^{125}I-labeled	+++	±	±	1–5
	Fluorescent	+++	–	–	6–8
		+++	–	+	9
	Surface ^{125}I-labeling				
		+++	+++	+++	10
		+++	–	–	11–13
	Column enrichment	+++	–	–	14–16
Lysis	Anti-Ig + C^1	+++	–	–	17,18
		–	–	+	19
Inhibition of activity by anti-Ig	Killer T cells			–	20–23
	GVH and/or DTH			+	24–26
				–	15
	MLC			+	27
				–	15,28,29
	Antibody formation	+++			20
Inhibition of antigen binding	By anti-Ig	+++			30–32
		+++	+++	+++	33
		+++	+++		33–36
Inhibition of suicide	By anti-Ig	+++	+++		37
				+++	38
Cytophilic Ig on T cells	Bursectomized chickens		+++		39
	Activated TDL			+++	9
Capping of antigen		+++			40
	By anti-Ig sera		+++	+++	33,35,41

[a] Key to references:
1. Raff *et al.* (1970).
2. Bankhurst and Warner (1971).
3. Nossal *et al.* (1972).
4. Ey (1973a).
5. Jensenius and Williams (1974a).
6. Pernis *et al.* (1970).
7. Raff (1970).
8. Rabellino *et al.* (1971).
9. Pernis *et al.* (1974).
10. Marchalonis and Cone (1973).
11. Vitetta and Uhr (1973).
12. Grey *et al.* (1972b).
13. Lisowska-Bernstein *et al.* (1973).
14. Abdou (1971).

McDevitt, 1974). The antigens that have been used to demonstrate this now number about 25; they are synthetic polypeptides with restricted heterogeneity, weak native antigens or some "strong" protein antigens, such as BSA, used at low concentration. Usually, the immune response (Ir) genes are closely linked to the major histocompatibility system of the species concerned. For example, the response to the polypeptide poly-L-lysine is linked to the strain 2 guinea pig H gene; and the gene controlling the response to TGAL maps between the K end of H-2 and the S_s locus of the mouse H-2 system.

The Ir genes are autosomal dominant so that the hybrid offspring of a high and low responder strain will respond well. High responders show an IgM and an IgG response while low responders exhibit the IgM response only. If the antigen is attached to a carrier, low responders will produce an IgG response but not a specific DTH reaction. Procedures such as neonatal thymectomy which affect T cell functions convert a high responder to a low responder so that they now do not show an IgG response. Conversely, procedures which bypass the need for T cells, such as a GVH reaction, trigger the switch from IgM to IgG production in a low responder strain.

Thus Ir gene products seem to be expressed on T cells. Some experiments suggest that the Ir gene product is not expressed on B cells (Freed et al., 1973) although the evidence is not clear-cut. There is one series of reports, however, which implicate B cells. Shearer and colleagues (e.g., Mozes et al., 1970; Shearer et al., 1971, 1972; Mozes and Shearer, 1971) have demonstrated that the antibody response to a number of synthetic polypeptides by high and low responder mice strains may be a function of the number of B or T precursor cells, and that the structure of the entire immunogenic

---

15. Crone et al. (1972).
16. Wigzell (1971).
17. Miller et al. (1972).
18. Takahashi et al. (1971).
19. Lesley et al. (1971).
20. Cerottini et al. (1971).
21. Chapuis and Brunner (1971).
22. Canty and Wunderlich (1970).
23. Henny et al. (1972a).
24. Mason and Warner (1970).
25. Riethmüller and Rieber (1971).
26. Theis and Thorbecke (1973).
27. Greaves et al. (1971).
28. Roitt (quoted by Crone et al., (1972).
29. Frohland and Natvig (1971).
30. Warner et al. (1970).
31. Dwyer et al. (1971).
32. Dwyer and Mackay (1972).
33. Roelants et al. (1973).
34. Hogg and Greaves (1972).
35. Ashman and Raff (1973).
36. Dwyer et al. (1972).
37. Basten et al. (1971).
38. Cooper and Ada (1972).
39. Webb and Cooper (1973).
40. Raff et al. (1973).
41. Roelants et al. (1974).

macromolecule is important in the expression of the different genetic defects.

Is the Ir gene product an immunoglobulin? This is unlikely because there is no linkage between the genes controlling the constant and variable regions of the heavy chain and either H-2 (mouse) or HL-A (human). Conceivably, there is a new class of H chains, production of which is linked to the H-2 system; or a complex involving Ig light chains and an Ir gene product.

The possibility of determining the nature of the Ir gene product has been enhanced by the recent availability of antisera prepared by reciprocal immunization of two congenic mouse lines which differed in the middle of the H-2 complex (Hauptfeld et al., 1973). In contrast to H-2 antigens which are present in all lymphocytes, the antigens detected by immunofluorescence using these antisera were present only on a subpopulation of lymphocytes present in lymph nodes and spleen, on a small proportion of thymocytes, but not at all on bone marrow cells. The positive cells were thus thought most likely to be T cells. Other and more recent work (e.g., David et al., 1973; Hammerling et al., 1973; Unanue et al., 1974) indicates that these products occur predominantly on B cells, macrophages, and to varying extents on T cells. The interrelationship between these products and the T cell receptor is now the subject of much speculation (e.g., Katz and Benacenaf, 1975) and cannot be reproduced here.

C. Histocompatibility Antigens

Histocompatibility antigens have been suggested as candidates for receptors because specific antisera has been found to interfere with a GVH reaction (e.g., Crone et al., 1972). As these antigens are not found exclusively on lymphocytes, this proposition does not seem per se to be very attractive. One possibility in many minds is the concept of an association between these antigens and an Ig fragment, e.g., light chains, or a common precursor, a molecule of about 11,000 MW. Recent findings of Cresswell et al. (1973) and Tanayaki et al. (1973) are of particular interest as it was found that HL-A2 and HL-A7 antigens solubilized from cultured human lymphocytes by papain possessed two chains, one a glycopeptide of MW 30,000–31,000, the other peptide of 11,000–12,000 MW. These authors consider that these two chains may represent most if not all the HL-A molecule but this cannot be decided with certainty at present. Peterson et al. (1973) have found that the large subunit carries the antigenic specificity of HL-A whereas the small polypeptide chain is very similar if not identical to β_2 microglobulin which occurs in serum and urine. The interesting point is that β_2 microglobulin is a structural and probably an evolutionary analogue to the immunoglobulin domain (Peterson et al., 1972). The temptation to assign a recognition function to these molecules has now become somewhat stronger and has received further impetus from the work of Taussig (1974) and Taussig and Munro (1974).

X. Antigens, The Antigen–Receptor Complex, and Mitogens

In this chapter, we discuss very briefly some properties of antigens that may be of special importance in their reaction with lymphocyte receptors and result in stimulation of the cell or induction of tolerance. Some antigens have the ability to act as nonspecific mitogens and the relationship between this activity and other methods of generating mitogenic effects is discussed.

A. The Reaction of Antigen with IgMs Receptors

As shown by their reaction with soluble antibodies, antigens can have two kinds of regions. One kind, the antigenic determinants or epitopes, includes those regions of the molecule (e.g., amino acid or sugar sequences) with which the binding sites of antibody molecules combine. Most antigens possess other regions which, for steric or other reasons, are not epitopes. Both regions may be involved in determining and maintaining the overall conformation of the molecule (Sela, 1969). We work with two types of antigens: naturally occurring and synthetic. As monomers, naturally occurring antigens usually contain a number of epitopes each of which is different from the others. These differences contribute to the immunogenicity of naturally occurring antigens as they tend to cancel out the ability or inability of an animal to respond to individual epitopes. Increasingly, much of our recent knowledge about immune responses has come from the use of synthetic antigens as there is usually little variation between epitopes. Thus, a polypeptide like TGAL can be regarded as having repeating but similar epitopes. A situation somewhat in between synthetic polypeptides and naturally occurring antigens can be obtained by adding substituents such as DNP to naturally occurring proteins.

As individual B lymphocytes probably possess receptors of only one specificity, each cell should recognize multideterminant monomeric antigens as unideterminant. Thus, to any cell, flagellin contains one epitope but polymeric flagellin contains repeating epitopes, 5 nm apart. If substituted with a hapten such as DNP, the distance between the hapten can be varied. Four situations are thus obtained: monomer and polymer with constant or variable epitope density or frequency per unit distance. Presumably, each epitope can bind to IgMs at the cell surface as easily as it can with soluble antibody. The important point is that the different forms of antigen can have very different effects on the B cell—from nondetectable effects to induction of antibody production or tolerance—which are not to be explained simply on the binding of individual epitopes with individual IgMs molecules. Obviously, other factors are very important in determining the immunogenicity of the molecule.

In discussing the role of other factors, it is useful to start with a model. The most interesting is that put forward by Cohn (1973) and Bretscher (1972) in a series of papers. Briefly, this concept proposes that, to be stimulated, an immunocompetent cell must receive two signals—one from the binding of antigen by (Ig) receptors and the other from a product, associative antibody, of collaborating T cells. Cohn and Bretscher have extensively documented their case and we will discuss the induction of antibody production and tolerance in these terms.

B. Conditions for Stimulation of B Cells by Antigen

Monomeric proteins at least *in vitro* are very poor at stimulating B cells to produce specific antibody. The defect, which is partly in the production of IgG, can be overcome by the addition of specific T cells as predicted by Cohn and Bretscher. On the other hand, polymeric antigens in the apparent absence of T cells can induce antibody production if presented in low concentration. This applies to polymeric antigens that are known to react with T cells (polymerized flagellin; Cooper, 1972) as well as to those believed not to react with T cells pneumococcal polysaccharide; Howard, 1972). In this case, Cohn and Bretscher argue that the need for a second signal is much reduced but still necessary. Two questions arise. What is the nature of the second signal provided by T cells? In what way do polymeric antigens act so that the need for signal 2 is eliminated or at least greatly reduced?

In answer to the first question, work from several laboratories has provided some clues. A subpopulation of B cells carries membrane receptors that bind antigen–antibody–C_3 complexes (Bianco et al., 1970; Dukor et al., 1973). Dukor and Hartmann (quoted Dukor et al., 1973) have proposed that the second signal to B lymphocytes is generated by the interaction of activated C_3 (C_3^1) with the complement receptor. A number of T-independent antigens and B cell mitogens are capable of activating C_3 via a bypass mechanism (Bitter-Suermann et al. quoted Dukor et al., 1973). It was thought then that other bypass activators might be effective B cell mitogens and substitute for the T cell requirements of unrelated antigens. Cobra venom factor has such an activity and was found to substitute for T cells in tissue cultures in restoring a response to SRBC. Furthermore, venom factor coupled to Sepharose interfered with the ability of B cells to form rosettes with complexes of antibody and complement bound to red cells, suggesting that the factor could bind to B cell membranes. On this basis, it would be proposed that T cell factors might include an enzyme capable of activating C_3 and so cause a mitogenic effect.

Pepys (1972) has found that injection of the C_3 cleaving factor from cobra venom into mice caused depletion of C_3 and a depression in the antibody response to two T-dependent antigens but no difference to the response to two T-independent antigens. Possibly, active products produced from C_3 were removed from the circulation and unable to stimulate localized B cells. Lipopolysaccharide is now known to be a B cell mitogen and it has recently been shown (Chiller and Weigle, 1973a,b) that, in mice tolerant of HGG where the lesion is solely in the T cell, tolerance can be broken by administration of lipopolysaccharide with HGG. It is considered that the lipopolysaccharide bypasses the need for T cells in the antibody response to HGG. Lipopolysaccharide and HGG were ineffective at a time when it was known that B cells were tolerant. The mitogenic activity of lipopolysaccharide has been shown to be a function of the lipid A moiety of the molecules (Andersson et al., 1973; Chiller et al., 1973). Lipopolysaccharide is known to integrate into plasma membranes (Rothfield and Romeo, 1971), and possibly lipid A acts by perturbing the conformation of the lipid bilayer or by combining with protein components of the membranes.

Schrader (1973) has also found that polymerized flagellin can act as a B cell stimulator by causing antibody production to another antigen (aggregate-free fowl IgG) which by itself was nonimmunogenic. The fowl IgG had to be present in the incubation medium; otherwise anti-fowl IgG antibody was not produced, a finding in agreement with the observations of Chiller and Weigle, reported above.

Somewhat in contrast with these two sets of results, however, are the recent findings of Coutinho and Möller (1973), who have shown that *in vitro* six different polymeric antigens ("thymus independent" antigens) can act as nonspecific mitogens and induce polyclonal antibody synthesis, as tested using SRBC, HRBC, and SRBC substituted with three different haptens. In each case, there was a significant increase in PFC to the antigen and this occurred in the *absence* of the specific antigens. Large amounts of polymers were added, sufficient at least in the case of polymerized flagellin to cause tolerance of specific B cells. A. J. Cunningham and L. M. Pilarski (personal communication) have found that injections of polymerized flagellin into mice induces the formation of PFC to a variety of RBC.

Though polymeric antigens may conceivably induce a mitogenic signal by binding to receptors other than IgMs, it is simplest to postulate that a mitogenic signal is induced following the binding to IgMs. At very high concentrations, sufficient antigen might bind to a spectrum of B cells with receptors of low affinity for individual epitopes but sufficiently high avidity for the polymer. Some of the polymeric antigens activate C_3. As receptors for activated C_3 characterize a subpopulation of B cells only, it would be of interest to know whether polymeric antigens are mitogenic for all or only a subpopulation of B cells.

In attempting to integrate these results, the main impression gained is that B cell stimulation can occur following a linking together of a proportion of IgMs receptors on the cell surface, thus causing a degree of receptor aggregation which acts as a mitogenic signal. The proportion of receptors involved is not known, but as B cells are stimulated by 1.0–0.1% of the concentration of polymerized flagellin which causes tolerance, it seems that the proportion need only be minor. Whether such a receptor aggregation suffices to stimulate the cell or whether a T cell signal is also needed in not certain.

C. Conditions for Induction of Tolerance in B Cells

There are a number of examples in the literature in which B cell tolerance occurs. The examples are diverse and have been discussed in some detail elsewhere (Ada and Cooper, 1974). If more attention is paid to *in vitro* experiments because of the greater difficulties of interpreting many *in vivo* experiments, there seems to be at least four distinct situations where B cell tolerance occurs.

1. OVERLOADING

An example is the exposure of B cells to polymerized flagellin—low doses stimulate whereas high doses tolerize. The most

3. Lymphocytic Receptors for Antigens

likely explanation (Section VIII,C) is that most, if not all of the IgMs receptors are binding the polymer so that effective membrane modulation is prevented—the cell membrane is *paralyzed*. (It is noteworthy that exposure of the cells *in vitro* to high concentrations of monomeric proteins does *not* result in tolerance.) It is not known whether cells held in this state persist or die. It seems that the antigen is not capped and endocytosed (Diener and Paetkau, 1972) so it would be of interest to see if the cell could be reactivated by signal 2.

2. HAPTEN ON NONIMMUNOGENIC CARRIERS

Schechter *et al.* (1964) first showed that tolerance could be induced to a molecule which by itself is a nonimmunogenic (poly-DL-alanine) and this has been followed up in recent years by the demonstrations (Havas, 1969; Borel, 1971) that tolerance to haptenic determinants may be induced if the injected complex is composed of haptens conjugated to a nonimmunogenic carrier. Carriers used have been poorly immunogenic proteins, e.g., HGG, self proteins (e.g., NIP-mouse RBC; Hamilton and Miller, 1973), or polymers that react poorly if at all with T cells, e.g., pneumococcal polysaccharide and the polypeptide, D-GL. In some of these cases it could be argued that T cells are completely uninvolved so that signal 2 is absent and tolerance is induced. Similarly, injection of large quantities of antigen into mice lacking T cells should result in tolerance and this has been found (Mitchell *et al.*, 1974). In general, these findings support the Cohn–Bretscher hypothesis.

3. EPITOPE DENSITY

Two findings in particular suggest that epitope density may be important. Polymerized flagellin was substituted with DNP to different extents and B cells exposed to different concentrations of the complexes. At high concentrations (>10 ug/ml) antibody production or tolerance could be induced. When the average epitope (DNP) spacing was 5 nm, anti-DNP antibody was produced; tolerance occurred when this spacing was reduced to 1.5–2 nm.

DNP-D-GL in which the epitope spacing is very small, possibly 1 group per nanometer, is a very effective tolerogen, low concentrations (μg) *in vitro* and small amounts (ng) *in vivo* inducing tolerance. Injection of DNP-D-GL results in fewer DNP-binding cells and the compound is effective both in primed and unprimed hosts (e.g., Katz *et al.*, 1972). An allogeneic reaction (provision of signal 2?) prevents tolerance induction.

With the first example, it seems likely that a majority if not all IgMs receptors on the affected cells are occupied as high concentrations of the tolerogen were needed. This may not be the case when DNP-D-GL was used and it seems likely that only a small proportion of receptors were occupied. In the latter case, it seems possible that the very high density of epitopes creates a microzone of paralysis, by extensive cross-linkage of receptors so that both binding sites of individual IgMs molecules are occupied. It seems doubtful that both binding sites of individual IgMs molecules are linked to adjacent DNP groups on the GL backbone as the value of the angle α might be impossibly small.

4. Tolerance with Antigen–Antibody Complexes

Antigen–antibody complexes composed of monomeric proteins and antibody in well-defined ratios may induce tolerance in B cells *in vitro* at both high and very low (2-200 pg/ml) concentrations (Diener and Feldmann, 1972). The epitope spacing in such complexes is almost certainly low (>5 nm) but complexes of this nature may be rigid structures and could possibly impose restraints upon the fluidity of the membrane.

D. Summary of B Cell Activation and Tolerance

Table IX summarizes the results of this Section. It seems reasonable to propose that too much polymer results in macroparalysis. Below this level, induction of antibody production occurs: monomeric proteins require additional factors to induce signal 2 whereas

TABLE IX

Summary of Some Conditions That Lead to Induction of Antibody Production or Tolerance

Immunogen	Dose	Signal 2	Result	Comment
Monomeric protein		—	Nil	
		+++	Antibody	Signal 2 by mitogens or T cells
Polymeric protein	Low	— or ±	Antibody	Overloading
	High	— or ±	Tolerance	*Macro*paralysis
Hapten–nonimmunogenic protein		—	Tolerance	
Immunogen with very high epitope density	Low	— or ±	Tolerance	*Micro*paralysis?
Antigen–antibody complex	Low or high	— or ±	Tolerance	

polymers largely bypass this signal, perhaps inducing it themselves. There is a third situation which, if only for convenience, we term microparalysis because probably only a minor proportion of a cell's receptors bind the tolerogen. At least in the case of DNP-D-GL, the cell apparently disappears so the effect may be toxic. Finally, haptens attached to nonimmunogenic proteins, where the contribution by T cells is possibly absent, are tolerogenic.

The results in this section were discussed in terms of the Cohn–Bretscher hypothesis. While unproved, this hypothesis serves as a most useful framework on which to base further experiments.

E. T Cell Tolerance and Activation

In this section we have attempted to interpret biologic responses (antibody formation, tolerance) in terms of antigen reacting with cell receptors of known identity. Although something is known about the activation of and induction of tolerance in T cells, we think it premature to discuss mechanisms while the nature and disposition of the receptor for antigen on these cells is so uncertain.

XI. Inside the B Cell

In the last section, immunity and tolerance were discussed in terms of events initiated on the extracellular side of the plasma membrane. We wish now to comment briefly on possible events inside the cell. A number of mechanisms has been proposed for the transfer of information from outside to inside the cell. We discuss briefly a few of them in terms of B lymphocytes.

A. Flip-Flop Mechanisms

A neat method for the transfer of extracellular molecules through a membrane is the concept of the receptor–molecule complex turning 180° through the plane of the membrane so that the molecule is delivered to the inside of the cell. There are reasons to believe that such a mechanism does not need to happen in order for lymphocytes to be stimulated by antigens. Thus, it has been shown that mitogens attached covalently to large rigid surfaces such as Sepharose beads (Greaves and Bauminger, 1972; Andersson and Melchers, 1973) or plastic dishes (Andersson et al., 1972) were able to stimulate B lymphocytes. The phytohemagglutinin from *Ricinus communis* which inhibits DNA and protein synthesis in rat ascites tumor cells is active whether free or attached to Sepharose (Onozaki et al., 1972).

To our knowledge, there is no definitive evidence demonstrating transfer of molecules in this manner. In the case of antigen bound to IgMs receptors, it can be argued that the role of antigen is to select certain cells simply by binding to them and that intracellular processes involved in the activation of those cells involve mechanisms shared by many other systems.

B. Allosteric Changes in the IgMs Receptor

It is often suggested that antigen may act by inducing a conformational change in the receptor molecule, i.e., binding of antigen to IgMs may cause a change in the Fc fragment of the molecule. This change might liberate a molecule previously bound to the Fc piece which could then initiate some activation process; or it might cause an inhibitor molecule to bind to the receptor, thus effectively activating the cell.

The reaction between haptens and IgG molecules has been widely studied and to our knowledge there is no data to suggest a conformational change in the Fc fragment. Admittedly, the situation may differ in the case of the IgMs molecule but there is no a priori reason to believe this. If such a change did occur, one possibility, suggested by the work of Stevens and Williamson (Section V,B,2) on mRNA for the γ chain, is that the mRNA for μ chain might be released from the Fc fragment of the IgMs molecule.

Apropos of both this and the next subsection, it should be pointed out that the IgMs molecule might be favored as a receptor because of the length of the μ chain. The Fc fragment of IgG may be only two-thirds as long as the Fc piece of IgMs so that IgG might be quite unsuited to be a receptor.

C. Cooperative versus Allosteric Effects

Cell activation might be initiated by a degree of membrane modulation, brought about by cross-linking of the IgMs molecules (Section X,B). Furthermore, the μ chain is sufficiently long so that the C terminal end of the Fc fragment could extend into the cytoplasm (Fig. 3). If each Fc fragment possessed one binding site for a cytoplasmic molecule, then the juxtaposition of two or more Fc pieces might allow multipoint binding of the cytoplasmic molecules if they had two or more determinants of similar specificity. In view of the strong possibility that IgD may also act as a receptor on B cells, it is of particular interest that the molecular weight of the heavy chain of IgD has been estimated to be 69,000 and 63,000 (Dorrington and Tanford, 1970). This most likely means that it also is sufficiently long to span the membrane.

Alternatively, one could envisage a molecule (e.g., inactive enzyme or enzymatic subunit) attached to the C-terminal end of the Fc moiety of each IgMs receptor. Aggregation of these following extracellular cross-linkage of the receptors might initiate cooperative/allosteric changes within the molecule which might activate it (e.g., Monod et al., 1965; Koshland, 1966).

The following arguments could be used to support such a notion. (1) Lymphocyte DNA synthesis can be stimulated in vitro by incubating cells with divalent but not with monovalent (Fab') anti-Ig (Fanger et al., 1970; Greaves, 1970). This suggests that the bringing together of at least two Fc fragments might be a critical event. (2) Binding and activation of the complement system seems to occur if two or three Fc pieces are brought together. (3) The avidity would increase with the number of binding sites.

Evidence for such mechanisms might be obtained by analyzing the antigen–receptor complexes isolated following the use of a monomeric versus oligomeric antigen. Such a mechanism also requires receptors to span the membrane and would be favored if this could be shown to apply to IgMs.

D. Intracellular Messengers

Many workers have considered that, in analogy with hormonal activation of cells, extracellular signals may activate membrane associated adenyl cyclase which converts intracellular ATP into cyclic AMP (cAMP). The latter compound may activate kinases which in turn influence the transcription of DNA.

Recent experimental work investigating the nature of intracellular messengers has almost exclusively been concerned with the activity of T cells where our knowledge about the nature of and disposition of antigen receptors is the subject of controversy. It is becoming increasingly clear that these mechanisms are important. Thus, Winchurch et al. (1971) found that poly(AU) stimulates the appearance of

AFC in a tissue culture system and attributed the effect to cAMP mediated events. Smith *et al.* (1971) and Cross (quoted by Smith *et al.*, 1971) found that small amounts of cAMP or particularly dibutyryl cAMP increased the uptake of ^{3}HTdr by lymphocytes from peripheral blood. Hadden *et al.* (1972) found that exposure of human peripheral blood lymphocytes to either PHA or concanavalin A induced a 10- to 50-fold increase in the level of cGMP within the first 20 minutes exposure to the mitogens. No change in the level of cAMP was seen in these cells. As binding of PHA to lymphocytes is complete within about 30 minutes, the rise in cGMP seems to be an immediate result of this event. Based on work of Otten *et al.* (1971) and Sheppard (1972), Hadden and colleagues suggest that cAMP may have a regulatory influence that limits or perhaps inhibits mitogenic effects. It has also been concluded that the capacity of allosensitized T cells to destroy target cells bearing donor alloantigens is modulated by the relative levels of cyclic AMP and cyclic GMP in these T cells. Increases in cyclic AMP inhibit whereas depletion enhances cytotoxicity. In contrast, cholinergic agents that elevate cyclic GMP enhance cytotoxicity. It seems that the levels of these cyclic nucleotides at the time of contact between T cell and target cell determine the extent of cytotoxicity (Henny and Lichtenstein, 1971; Henny *et al.*, 1972b; Strom *et al.*, 1972, 1973).

It may be dangerous to extrapolate these findings to B cells and even more foolhardy to suggest the relationship between cGMP and cAMP to that of activation and tolerance induction by antigen in B cells. But if we exclude overloading of the cell as a mechanism for tolerance induction, it is not unlikely that the activation and inactivation of B cells may involve two different intracellular pathways which are common to all lymphocytes. The *specificity* of the immune system would seem to be entirely at the level of the receptor, and as such is a purely extracellular phenomenon.

Acknowledgments

We would like to acknowledge helpful discussions with our colleagues, particularly M. J. Crumpton and A. J. Cunningham, and the generosity of many scientists who have sent preprints of their work.

References

Abdou, N. I. (1971). *J. Immunol.* **107**, 1637.
Ada, G. L. (1970). *Transplant. Rev.* **5**, 105.
Ada, G. L., and Byrt, P. (1969). *Nature (London)* **222**, 1291.

Ada, G. L., and Cooper, M. G. (1974). *Res. Immunochem. Immunobiol.* **5** (in press).
Ada, G. L., Nossal, G. J. V., Pye, J., and Abbot, A. (1964). *Aust. J. Exp. Biol. Med. Sci.* **42**, 267.
Ada, G. L., Humphrey, J. H., Askonas, B. A., McDevitt, H. O., and Nossal, G. V. J. (1966). *Exp. Cell Res.* **41**, 557.
Ada, G. L., Byrt, P., Mandel, T., and Warner, N. (1971). *In* "Developmental Aspects of Antibody Formation and Structure" (J. Sterzl and I. Riha, eds.), Vol. 2, p. 503. Academic Press, New York.
Alkan, S. S., Bush, M. E., Nitecki, D. E., and Goodman, J. W. (1972). *J. Exp. Med.* **136**, 387.
Allan, D., and Crumpton, M. J. (1970). *Biochem. J.* **120**, 133.
Allan, D., and Crumpton, M. J. (1971). *Biochem. J.* **123**, 967.
Allan, D., and Crumpton, M. J. (1973). *Exp. Cell Res.* **78**, 271.
Anderson, C. L., and Grey, H. M. (1974). *J. Exp. Med.* **139**, 1175.
Anderson, H. R., and Dresser, D. W. (1972). *Eur. J. Immunol.* **2**, 410.
Andersson, J., and Melchers, F. (1973). *Proc. Nat. Acad. Sci. U. S.* **70**, 416.
Andersson, J., Edelman, G. M., Möller, G., and Sjöberg, O. (1972). *Eur. J. Immunol.* **2**, 233.
Andersson, J., Melchers, F., Gelanos, C., and Lüderitz, O. (1973). *J. Exp. Med.* **137**, 943.
Andersson, J., Lafleur, L., and Melchers, F. (1974). *Eur. J. Immunol.* **4**, 170.
Ashman, R. F. (1973) *J. Immunol.* **111**, 212.
Ashman, R. F., and Raff, M. C. (1973). *J. Exp. Med.* **137**, 69.
Atwell, J. L., Cone, R. E., and Marchalonis, J. J. (1973). *Nature (London)* (in press).
Austin, C. M., and Nossal, G. J. V. (1966). *Aust. J. Exp. Biol. Med. Sci.* **44**, 341.
Avrameas, S., and Guilbert, B. (1971). *Eur. J. Immunol.* **1**, 394.
Bach, J. F. (1973). *Contemp. Top. Immunobiol.* **2**, 189.
Bach, J. F., Reyes, F., Dardenne, M., Fournier, C., and Muller, J. Y. (1971). *In* "Cell Interactions and Receptor Antibodies in Immune Responses" (O. Mäkelä, A. Cross, and T. U. Kosunen, eds.), p. 111. Academic Press, New York.
Baker, P. J., Bernstein, M., Pasanen, V., and Landy, M. (1966). *J. Immunol.* **97**, 767.
Bankhurst, A. D., and Warner, N. L. (1971). *J. Immunol.* **107**, 368.
Basten, A., and Howard, J. G. (1973). *Contemp. Top. Immunobiol.* **2**, 265.
Basten, A., Miller, J. F. A. P., Warner, N. L., and Pye, J. (1971). *Nature (London), New Biol.* **231**, 104.
Basten, A., Miller, J. F. A. P., Sprent, J., and Pye, J. (1972a). *J. Exp. Med.* **135**, 610.
Basten, A., Warner, N., and Mandel, T. (1972b). *J. Exp. Med.* **135**, 627.
Baur, S., Vitetta, E., Sherr, C. J., Schenkein, I., and Uhr, J. W. (1971). *J. Immunol.* **106**, 1133.
Bayse, G. S., and Morrison, M. (1971). *Arch. Biochem. Biophys.* **145**, 143.
Benacerraf, B., and Levine, B. B. (1962). *J. Exp. Med.* **115**, 1023.
Benacerraf, B., and McDevitt, H. O. (1972). *Science* **175**, 273.
Berken, A., and Benacerraf, B. (1966). *J. Exp. Med.* **123**, 119.
Bernoco, D., Cullen, S., Scudeller, G., Trinchieri, G., and Ceppellini, C. (1972). *In* "Histocompatibility Testing" (Dausset, ed.), p. 527. *Proc. 5th Int. Workshop Conf.* Munksgaard, Copenhagen.
Bert, G., Massaro, A. L., DiCossano, D. L., and Maja, M. (1969). *Immunology* **17**, 1.
Bianco, C., Patrick, R., and Nussenzweig, V. (1970). *J. Exp. Med.* **132**, 702.
Biozzi, G., Stiffel, C., Mouton, D., Liacopoulos-Briot, M., Decreusefond, C., and Bouthiller, Y. (1966). *Ann. Inst. Pasteur, Paris* **110**, 7.
Borel, Y. (1971). *Nature (London), New Biol.* **230**, 180.

Borsos, T., and Rapp, H. J. (1965). *J. Immunol.* **95**, 559.
Boyse, E. A. (1971). *In* "Immune Surveillance" (R. T. Smith and M. Landy, eds.), p. 1. Academic Press, New York.
Bretscher, M. S. (1971). *Nature (London), New Biol.* **231**, 229.
Bretscher, M. S. (1973). *Science* **181**, 622.
Bretscher, P. (1972). *Transplant. Rev.* **11**, 218.
Brody, T. (1970). *J. Immunol.* **105**, 126.
Burnet, F. M. (1957). *Aust. J. Sci.* **20**, 67.
Burnet, F. M. (1959). "The Clonal Selection Theory of Acquired Immunity," Cambridge Univ. Press, London and New York.
Burnet, F. M., and Fenner, F. (1949). "The Production of Antibodies." Macmillan, New York.
Bustin, M. Eshhar, Z., and Sela, M. (1972). *Eur. J. Biochem.* **31**, 541.
Byrt, P., and Ada, G. L. (1969). *Immunology* **17**, 503.
Canty, T. G., and Wunderlich, J. R. (1970). *J. Nat. Cancer Inst.* **45**, 761.
Cathou, R. E., and O'Konski, C. T. (1970). *J. Mol. Biol.* **11**, 125.
Cerottini, J. C., Nordin, A. A., and Brunner, K. T. (1971). *J. Exp. Med.* **134**, 553.
Chapuis, B., and Brunner, K. T. (1971). *Int. Arch. Allergy Appl. Immunol.* **40**, 322.
Chiller, J. M., and Weigle, W. O. (1973a). *J. Immunol.* **110**, 1051.
Chiller, J. M., and Weigle, W. O. (1973b). *J. Exp. Med.* **137**, 740.
Chiller, J. M., Skidmore, B. J., Morrison, D. C., and Weigle, W. O. (1973). *Proc. Nat. Acad. Sci. U. S.* **70**, 2129.
Cohn, M. (1973). *In* "Genetic Control of Immune Responsiveness" (H. O. McDevitt and M. Landy, eds.), p. 367. Academic Press, New York.
Cone, R. E., Marchalonis, J. J., and Rolley, R. T. (1971). *J. Exp. Med.* **134**, 1373.
Cone, R. E., Sprent, J., and Marchalonis, J. J. (1972). *Proc. Nat. Acad. Sci. U. S.* **69**, 2556.
Cone, R. E., Feldmann, M., Marchalonis, J. J., and Nossal, G. J. V. (1974). *Immunology* **26**, 49.
Coombs, R. R. A., Feinstein, A., and Wilson, A. B. (1969). *Lancet* **2**, 1157.
Cooper, M. D. (1971). *In* "Morphological and Functional Aspects of Immunity" (K. Lindhahl-Kiessling, G. Alm, and M. Hanna, Jr., eds.), p. 531. Plenum, New York.
Cooper, M. G. (1972). *Scand. J. Immunol.* **1**, 167.
Cooper, M. G., and Ada, G. L. (1972). *Scand. J. Immunol.* **1**, 247.
Cooper, M. G., Ada, G. L., and Langman, R. E. (1972). *Cell. Immunol.* **4**, 289.
Coutinho, A., and Möller, G. (1973). *Nature (London)* (in press).
Cresswell, P., Turner, M. J., and Strominger, J. L. (1973). *Proc. Nat. Acad. Sci. U. S.* **70**, 1603.
Crone, M., Koch, C., and Simonsen, M. (1972). *Transplant. Rev.* **10**, 36.
Crumpton, M. (1974). *In* "The Antigens" (M. Sela, ed.), Vol. 2, p. 1. Academic Press, New York.
Cunningham, A. J. (1974). *Contemp. Top. Mol. Immunol.* **3**, 1.
David, C. S., Shreffler, D. C., and Frelinger, J. A. (1973). *Proc. Nat. Acad. Sci. U.S.* **70**, 2509.
Davie, J. M., and Paul, W. E. (1970). *Cell. Immunol.* **1**, 404.
Davie, J. M., and Paul, W. E. (1971). *J. Exp. Med.* **134**, 495.
Davie, J. M., Rosenthal, A. S., and Paul, W. E. (1971). *J. Exp. Med.* **134**, 517.
Decker, J., Clarke, J., MacPherson, L., Weinstein, R., and Sercarz, E. (1973). *In* "Microenvironmental Aspects of Immunity" (B. D. Jankovic and K. Isakovic, eds.). Plenum, New York.

Della Corte, E., and Parkhouse, R. M. E. (1973). *Biochem. J.* **136**, 597.
De Luca, C., Yowell, R. L., and Miller, A. (1972). *In* "Proceedings of the Fourth International Conference on Lymphatic Tissue and Germinal Centers in Immune Reactions." Plenum, New York (in press).
de Petris, S., and Raff, M. C. (1972). *Eur. J. Immunol.* **2**, 523.
de Petris, S., and Raff, M. C. (1973). *Nature (London), New Biol.* **241**, 257.
Diener, E., and Feldmann, M. (1972). *Transplant. Rev.* **8**, 76.
Diener, E., and Paetkau, V. H. (1972). *Proc. Nat. Acad. Sci. U. S.* **69**, 2364.
Dorrington, K. J., and Tanford, C. (1970). *Adv. Immunol.* **12**, 333.
Dukor, P., Bianco, C., and Nussenzweig, V. (1971). *Eur. J. Immunol.* **1**, 491.
Dukor, P., Probst, H., and Bitter-Saermann, D. (1973). *J. Exp. Med.* (in press).
Dutton, R. W., and Mishell, R. I. (1967). *J. Exp. Med.* **126**, 443.
Dwyer, J. M., and Mackay, I. R. (1972). *Clin. Exp. Immunol.* **10**, 581.
Dwyer, J. M., Mason, S., Warner, N. L., and Mackay, I. R. (1971). *Nature (London)* **234**, 252.
Dwyer, J. M., Warner, N. L., and Mackay, I. R. (1972). *J. Immunol.* **108**, 1439.
Edelman, G. M., Rutishauser, U., and Millette, C. F. (1971). *Proc. Nat. Acad. Sci. U. S.* **68**, 2153.
Ehrlich, P. (1900). *Proc. Roy. Soc., Ser. B* **66**, 424.
Elson, C. J., Singh, J., and Taylor, R. B. (1973). *Scand. J. Immunol.* **2**, 143.
Engelman, D. M. (1970). *J. Mol. Biol.* **47**, 115.
Engers, H. D., and Unanue, E. R. (1973). *J. Immunol.* **110**, 465.
Eshhar, Z., Gafni, M., Givol, D., and Sela, M. (1971). *Eur. J. Immunol.* **1**, 323.
Eshhar, Z., Waks, T., Bustin, M., and Sela, M. (1972). *Isr. J. Med. Sci.* **8**, 643.
Ey, P. L. (1973a). *Eur. J. Immunol.* **3**, 37.
Ey, P. L. (1973b). *Eur. J. Immunol.* **3**, 402.
Fanger, M. W., Hart, D. A., Wells, J. V., and Nisonoff, A. (1970). *J. Immunol.* **105**, 1484.
Feinstein, A., and Munn, E. (1969). *Nature (London)* **224**, 1307.
Feinstein, A., and Rowe, A. J. (1965). *Nature (London)* **205**, 147.
Feldmann, M. (1973). *Nature (London), New Biol.* **242**, 82.
Feldmann, M., and Basten, A. (1972a). *J. Exp. Med.* **136**, 739.
Feldmann, M., and Basten, A. (1972b). *Eur. J. Immunol.* **2**, 213.
Ferber, E., Resch, K., Wallach, D. F. H., and Imm, W. (1972). *Biochim. Biophys. Acta* **266**, 494.
Freed, J. H., Bechtol, K. B., Hertzenberg, L. A., and McDevitt, H. O. (1973). *Transplant. Proc.* (in press).
Fröhland, S., and Natvig, J. B. (1971). *Int. Arch. Allergy Appl. Immunol.* **41**, 248.
Frye, L. D., and Edidin, M. (1970). *J. Cell Sci.* **7**, 319.
Gardner, I., Bowern, N., and Blanden, R. V. (1974). *Eur. J. Immunol.* **4**, 68.
Gardner, I. D., Bowern, N. A., and Blanden, R. V. (1975). *Eur. J. Immunol.* **5** (in press).
Givol, D. (1973). *Contemp. Top. Mol. Immunol.* **2**, 27.
Good, R. A., Smith, R. T., and Landy, M. (1971). *In* "Immune Surveillance" (R. T. Smith and M. Landy, eds.), p. 123. Academic Press, New York.
Gorczynski, R. M., Miller, R. G., and Phillips, R. A. (1971). *Immunology* **20**, 693.
Greaves, M. F. (1970). *Transplant. Rev.* **5**, 45.
Greaves, M. F. (1971). *Eur. J. Immunol.* **1**, 186.
Greaves, M. F., and Bauminger, S. (1972). *Nature (London), New Biol.* **235**, 67.
Greaves, M. F., and Hogg, N. M. (1971). *Progr. Immunol.* **1**, 111.
Greaves, M. F., and Raff, M. (1971). *Nature (London)* **233**, 239.
Greaves, M. F., Torrigiani, G., and Roitt, I. M. (1971). *Clin. Exp. Immunol.* **9**, 313.

Greaves, M. F., Bauminger, S., and Janossy, G. (1972). *Clin. Exp. Immunol.* **10**, 537.
Green, N. M. (1969). *Advan. Immunol.* **11**, 1.
Grey, H. M., Colon, S., Campbell, P., and Rabellino, E. (1972a). *J. Immunol.* **109**, 776.
Grey, H. M., Kubo, R. T., and Cerottini, J. C. (1972b). *J. Exp. Med.* **136**, 1323.
Grumet, F. C., and McDevitt, H. O. (1974). *Contemp. Top. Immunobiol.* **3** (in press).
Haber, E., Richards, F. F., Spragg, J., Austen, K. F., Vallotton, M., and Page, L. B. (1967). *Cold Spring Harbor Symp. Quant. Biol.* **32**, 299.
Hadden, J. W., Hadden, E. M., Haddox, M. K., and Goldberg, N. D. (1972). *Proc. Nat. Acad. Sci. U. S.* **69**, 3024.
Hamilton, J. A., and Miller, J. F. A. P. (1973). *Eur. J. Immunol.* **3**, 457.
Hämmerling, G., and McDevitt, H. O. (1974). *J. Immunol.* **112**, 1734.
Hämmerling, G. J., Masuda, T., and McDevitt, H. O. (1973). *J. Exp. Med.* **137**, 1180.
Hämmerling, U., and Rajewsky, K. (1971). *Eur. J. Immunol.* **1**, 447.
Harris, A. W., Bankhurst, A. D., Mason, S., and Warner, N. L. (1973). *J. Immunol.* **110**, 431.
Hauptfeld, V., Klein, D., and Klein, J. (1973). *Science* **181**, 167.
Havas, H. F. (1969). *Immunology* **17**, 819.
Hemmingson, E. J., and Alm, G. V. (1972). *Eur. J. Immunol.* **2**, 379.
Henny, C. S., and Lichtenstein, L. M. (1971). *J. Immunol.* **107**, 610.
Henny, C. S., Clayburgh, J., Cole, G. A., and Prendergast, R. A. (1972a). *Immunol. Commun.* **1**, 93.
Henny, C. S., Bourne, H. R., and Lichtenstein, L. M. (1972b). *J. Immunol.* **108**, 1526.
Henry, C., Kimura, J., and Wofsy, L. (1972). *Proc. Nat. Acad. U. S.* **69**, 34.
Herzenberg, L. A., Chan, E. L., Ravitch, M. M., Riblet, R. J., and Herzenberg, L. A. (1973). *J. Exp. Med.* **137**, 1311.
Hogg, N. M., and Greaves, M. F. (1972). *Immunology* **22**, 967.
Hornick, C. L., and Karush, F. (1972). *Immunochemistry* **9**, 325.
Howard, J. (1972). *Transplant. Rev.* **8**, 50.
Humphrey, J. H., and Dourmashkin, R. R. (1965). *Complement, Ciba Found. Symp., 1964* (G. E. W. Wolstenholme and J. Knight, eds.), p. 175 Churchill, London.
Humphrey, J. H., and Keller, H. U. (1971). In "Developmental Aspects of Antibody Formation and Structure" (J. Sterzl and I. Riha, eds.), Vol. 2, p. 485. Academic Press, New York.
Humphrey, J. H., Roelants, G., and Willcox, N. (1971). In "Cell Interactions and Receptor Antibodies in Immune Responses" (O. Mäkelä, A. Cross, and T. U. Kosunen, eds.), p. 123. Academic Press, New York.
Hütteroth, T. H., Cleve, H., and Litwin, S. D. (1973). *J. Immunol.* **110**, 1325.
Jacobson, E. B., Herzenberg, L. A., Riblet, R., and Herzenberg, L. A. (1972). *J. Exp. Med.* **135**, 1163.
Jensenius, J. C., and Williams, A. F. (1974a). *Eur. J. Immunol.* **4**, 91.
Jensenius, J. C., and Williams, A. F. (1974b). *Eur. J. Immunol.* **4**, 98.
Jerne, N. (1955). *Proc. Nat. Acad. Sci. U. S.* **41**, 849.
Jerne, N. (1967). *Cold Spring Harbor Symp. Quant. Biol.* **32**, 591.
Jones, G. (1973). *J. Immunol.* **110**, 1526.
Jones, G., Marcuson, E. C., and Roitt, I. M. (1970). *Nature (London)* **227**, 1051.
Jones, P. P., Craig, S. W., Cebra, J. J., and Herzenberg, L. A. (1974). *J. Exp. Med.* **140**, 452.
Kabat, E. A. (1966). *J. Immunol.* **97**, 1.
Karnovsky, M. J., Unanue, E. R., and Leventhal, M. (1972). *J. Exp. Med.* **136**, 907.
Kathan, R. H., and Winzler, R. J. (1963). *J. Biol. Chem.* **238**, 21.
Katz, D. H., and Benacerraf, B. (1972). *Advan. Immunol.* **15**, 2.
Katz, D. H., and Benacerraf, B. (1975). *Transplant. Rev.* **22** (in press).

3. Lymphocytic Receptors for Antigens

Katz, D. H., Davie, J. M., Paul, W. E., and Benacerraf, B. (1971). *J. Exp. Med.* **134**, 201.
Katz, D. H., Hamaoka, T., and Benacerraf, B. (1972). *J. Exp. Med.* **136**, 1404.
Katz, D. H., Hamaoka, T., Dorf, M. E., and Benacerraf, B. (1973a). *Proc. Nat. Acad. Sci. U. S.* **70**, 2624.
Katz, D. H., Hamaoka, T., and Benacerraf, B. (1973b). *J. Exp. Med.* **137**, 1405.
Kincade, P. W., and Cooper, M. D. (1971). *J. Immunol.* **106**, 371.
Kincade, P. W., Lawton, A. R., Bockman, D. E., and Cooper, M. D. (1970). *Proc. Nat. Acad. Sci. U. S.* **67**, 1918.
Kincade, P. W., Lawton, A. R., and Cooper, M. D. (1971). *J. Immunol.* **106**, 1421.
Kindred, B., and Shreffler, D. C. (1972). *J. Immunol.* **109**, 940.
Kirov, S. M., and Ada, G. L. (1974). Submitted for publication.
Klein, E., Klein, G., Nadkarni, J. W., Nadkarni, J. J., Wigzell, H., and Clifford, P. (1968). *Cancer Res.* **28**, 1300.
Klein, E., Eskeland, T., Inuoe, M., Strom, R., and Johansson, B. (1970). *Exp. Cell Res.* **62**, 133.
Koshland, D. (1966). *Biochemistry* **5**, 365.
Kourilsky, F. M., Silvestre, D., Neauport-Sautes, C., Loosfelt, Y., and Dausset, J. (1972). *Eur. J. Immunol.* **2**, 249.
Kubo, R. T., Grey, H. M., and Pirofsky, B. (1974). *J. Immunol.* **112**, 1952.
Lamelin, J.-P., Lisowska-Bernstein, B., Matter, A., Rysen, J. E., and Vassalli, P. (1972). *J. Exp. Med.* **136**, 984.
Lamm, M., and Small, P. A., Jr. (1966). *Biochemistry* **5**, 267.
Landsteiner, K. (1936). "The Specificity of Serological Reactions," 2nd ed. Harvard Univ. Press, Cambridge, Massachusetts.
Langman, R. E. (1972). *Eur. J. Immunol.* **2**, 582.
Laskov, R. (1968). *Nature (London)* **219**, 973.
Lawrence, D. A., Spiegelberg, H. L., and Weigle, W. O. (1973). *J. Exp. Med.* **137**, 470.
Leonard, E. J. (1973). *J. Immunol.* **110**, 1167.
Lerner, R., McConahey, P. J., Jansen, I., and Dixon, F. J. (1972). *J. Exp. Med.* **135**, 136.
Lesley, J. F., Kettman, J. R., and Dutton, R. W. (1971). *J. Exp. Med.* **134**, 618.
Liew, F. Y. (1971). *Immunology* **20**, 817.
Lisowska-Bernstein, B., Rinny, A., and Vassalli, P. (1973). *Proc. Nat. Acad. Sci. U. S.* **70**, 2879.
Loor, F. (1973). *Eur. J. Immunol.* **3**, 112.
Loor, F., Forni, L., and Pernis, B. (1972). *Eur. J. Immunol.* **2**, 203.
Louis, J., Chiller, J. M., and Weigle, W. O. (1973). *J. Exp. Med.* **137**, 461.
McDevitt, H. O., Askonas, B. A., Humphrey, J. H., Schechter, I., and Sela, M. (1966). *Immunology* **11**, 337.
Mandel, T. E. (1972). *Nature (London), New Biol.* **239**, 112.
Marchalonis, J. J., and Cone, R. E. (1973). *Transplant. Rev.* **14**, 3.
Marchalonis, J. J., Cone, R. E., and Atwell, J. L. (1972). *J. Exp. Med.* **135**, 956.
Marchesi, V. T., Segrest, J. P., and Kahane, I. (1972). *In* "Membrane Research" (C. F. Fox, ed.), p. 41. Academic Press, New York.
Mason, S., and Warner, N. L. (1970). *J. Immunol.* **104**, 762.
Maurer, P. H. (1964). *Progr. Allergy* **8**, 1.
Melchers, F., and Andersson, J. (1973). *Transplant. Rev.* **14**, 76.
Melchers, F., and Andersson, J. (1974) *Eur. J. Immunol.* **4**, 181.
Metzger, H. (1970). *Advan. Immunol.* **12**, 57.
Miller, A., Deluca, D., Decker, J., Ezzell, R., and Sercarz, E. E. (1971). *Amer. J. Pathol.* **65**, 415.
Miller, F., and Metzger, H. (1965). *J. Biol. Chem.* **240**, 3325.
Miller, F., and Metzger, H. (1966). *J. Biol. Chem.* **241**, 1732.

Miller, J. F. A. P., Sprent, J., Basten, A., and Warner, N. L. (1972). *Nature (London), New Biol.* **237**, 18.
Mitchell, G. F., Lafleur, L. A., and Andersson, K. (1974). *Scand. J. Immunol.* **3**, 39.
Möller, E., and Greaves, M. F. (1971). *In* "Cell Interactions and Receptor Antibodies in Immune Responses" (O. Mäkelä, A. Cross, and T. U. Kosunen, eds.), p. 101.
Möller, E., and Sjöberg, O. (1972). *Transplant. Rev.* **8**, 26.
Möller, E., Bullock, W. W., and Mäkelä, O. (1973). *Eur. J. Immunol.* **3**, 172.
Monod, J., Wyman, J., and Changeux, J.-P. (1965). *J. Mol. Biol.* **12**, 88.
Moore, M. A. S., and Owen, J. J. T. (1965). *Nature (London)* **208**, 956.
Moore, M. A. S., and Owen, J. J. T. (1966). *Develop. Biol.* **14**, 40.
Moroz, C., and Hahn, Y. (1974). *Proc. Nat. Acad. Sci. U. S.* **70**, 3716.
Morrison, M., and Bayse, G. S. (1970). *Biochemistry* **9**, 2995.
Mozes, E., and Shearer, G. M. (1971). *J. Exp. Med.* **134**, 141.
Mozes, E., Shearer, G. M., and Sela, M. (1970). *J. Exp. Med.* **132**, 613.
Myers, W. G., and Vanderleeden, J. C. (1960). *J. Nucl. Med.* **1**, 149.
Naor, D., and Sulitzeanu, D. (1967). *Nature (London)* **214**, 687.
Naor, D., and Sulitzeanu, D. (1969a). *Isr. J. Med. Sci.* **5**, 217.
Naor, D., and Sulitzeanu, D. (1969b). *Int. Arch. Allergy Appl. Immunol.* **36**, 112.
Naor, D., Bentwich, Z., and Cividalli, G. (1969). *Aust. J. Exp. Biol. Med. Sci.* **47**, 759.
Neauport-Sautes, C. E., Lilly, F., Silvestre, D., and Kourilsky, F. M. (1973). *J. Exp. Med.* **137**, 511.
Nordling, S., Andersson, L. G., and Häyry, P. (1972). *Eur. J. Immunol.* **2**, 405.
Nossal, G. J. V., and Pike, B. (1973). *Immunology* **25**, 33.
Nossal, G. J. V., Ada, G. L., and Austin, C. M. (1965). *J. Exp. Med.* **121**, 945.
Nossal, G. J. V., Warner, N. L., Lewis, H., and Sprent, J. (1972). *J. Exp. Med.* **135**, 405.
Nossal, G. J. V., Pike, B. L., and Katz, D. H. (1973). *J. Exp. Med.* **138**, 312.
Nota, N. R., Liacapoulos-Briot, M., Stiffel, C., and Biozzi, G. (1964). *C. R. Acad. Sci.* **259**, 1277.
Onozaki, K., Tomita, M., Sakurai, Y., and Ukita, T. (1972). *Biochem. Biophys. Res. Commun.* **48**, 783.
Osmond, D., and Nossal, G. J. V. (1974a). *Cell. Immunol.* **13**, 117.
Osmond, D., and Nossal, G. J. V. (1974b). *Cell. Immunol.* **13**, 132.
Osoba, D. (1970). *J. Exp. Med.* **132**, 368.
Osunkoya, B. O., Williams, A. I. O., Adler, W. H., and Smith, R. T. (1970). *West Afr. J. Med. Sci.* **1**, 3.
Otten, J., Johnson, G. S., and Pasten, I. (1971). *Biochem. Biophys. Res. Commun.* **44**, 1192.
Paraskevas, F., Lee, S.-T., Orr, K. B., and Israels, L. G. (1972). *J. Immunol.* **108**, 1319.
Parish, C. R. (1971). *Ann. N. Y. Acad. Sci.* **181**, 108.
Parish, C. R., and Hayward, J. A. (1974a). *Proc. Roy. Soc. Ser. B* **187**, 47.
Parish, C. R., and Hayward, J. A. (1974b). *Proc. Roy. Soc., Ser. B* **187**, 65.
Parkhouse, R. M. E. (1973). *Transplant. Rev.* **14**, 131.
Parkhouse, R. M. E., Janossy, G., and Greaves, M. F. (1972). *Nature (London), New Biol.* **235**, 21.
Paul, W. E. (1970). *Transplant. Rev.* **5**, 130.
Paul, W. E., and Davie, J. M. (1971). *Progr. Immunol.* **1**, 637.
Pepys, M. B. (1972). *Nature (London), New Biol.* **237**, 157.
Pernis, B., Forni, L., and Amante, L. (1970). *J. Exp. Med.* **132**, 1001.
Pernis, B., Miller, J. F. A. P., Forni, L., and Sprent, J. (1974). *Cell. Immunol.* (in press).
Peterson, P. A., Cunningham, B. A., Berggård, I., and Edelman, G. M. (1972). *Proc. Nat. Acad. Sci. U. S.* **69**, 1697.
Peterson, P. A., Rack, L., and Lindblom, J. B. (1973). *Proc. Nat. Acad. Sci. U. S.* **71**, 351.

3. Lymphocytic Receptors for Antigens

Pilz, I., Puchwein, G., Kratky, O., Herbst, M., Haager, O., Gall, W. E., and Edelman, G. M. (1970). *Biochemistry* **9**, 211.
Pinto da Silva, P. (1972). *J. Cell Biol.* **53**, 777.
Pinto da Silva, P., and Branton, D. (1970). *J. Cell Biol.* **45**, 598.
Poljak, R. J. (1973). *Contemp. Top. Mol. Immunol.* **2**, 1.
Porter, R. R. (1972). *Contemp. Top. Immunochem.* **1**, 145.
Povlsen, C. O. Fialkow, P. J., Klein, E., Klein, G., Rygaard, J., and Wiener, F. (1973). *Int. J. Cancer* **11**, 30.
Preud'homme, J. L., and Seligmann, M. (1972). *Proc. Nat. Acad. Sci. U. S.* **69**, 2132.
Preud'homme, J. L., Neauport-Sautes, C., Piat, S., Silvestre, D., and Kourilsky, F. M. (1972). *Eur. J. Immunol.* **2**, 297
Putnam, F. W., Florent, G., Paul, C., Shinoda, T., and Shimizu, A. (1973). *Science* **182**, 287.
Rabellino, E., Colon, S., Grey, H. M., and Unanue, E. R. (1971). *J. Exp. Med.* **133**, 156.
Raff, M. C. (1970). *Immunology* **19**, 637.
Raff, M. C. (1971). *Transplant. Rev.* **6**, 52.
Raff, M. C., Sternberg, M., and Taylor, R. B. (1970). *Nature (London)* **225**, 553.
Raff, M. C., Nase, S., and Mitchison, N. A. (1971). *Nature (London)* **230**, 50.
Raff, M. C., Feldmann, M., and de Petris, S. (1973). *J. Exp. Med.* **137**, 1024.
Riethmüller, G., and Rieber, E.-P. (1971). *Progr. Immunol.* **1**, 127.
Roelants, G. E. (1972a). *Nature (London)* **237**, 252.
Roelants, G. E. (1972b). *Curr. Top. Microbiol. Immunol.* **59**, 135.
Roelants, G. E., and Askonas, B. A. (1971). *Eur. J. Immunol.* **1**, 151.
Roelants, G. E., and Rydén, A. (1974). *Nature (London)* **247**, 104.
Roelants, G. E., Forni, L., and Pernis, B. (1973). *J. Eur. Med.* **137**, 1060.
Roelants, G. E., Rydén, A., Hägg, L.-B., and Loor, F. (1974). *Nature (London)* **247**, 106.
Rogers, A. W. (1972). *J. Microsc. (Paris)* **96**, 141.
Rolley, R. T., and Marchalonis, J. J. (1972). *Transplantation* **14**, 734.
Rosenthal, A. S., and Shevach, E. M. (1973). *J. Exp. Med.* **138**, 1194.
Rothfield, L., and Romeo, D. (1971). *Bacteriol. Rev.* **35**, 14.
Rothschild, K. J., and Stanley, H. E. (1972). In "Membranes and Viruses in Immunopathology" (S. B. Day and R. A. Good, eds.), p. 49. Academic Press, New York.
Rowe, D. S., Hug, K., Forni, L., and Pernis, B. (1973). *J. Exp. Med.* **138**, 965.
Rutishauser, U., Millette, C. F., and Edelman, G. M. (1972). *Proc. Nat. Acad. Sci. U. S.* **69**, 1596.
Sage, H. J., Deutsch, H. F., Fasman, G., and Levine, L. (1964). *Immunochemistry* **1**, 133.
Santer, V., Cone, R. E., and Marchalonis, J. J. (1973). *Exp. Cell Res.* **79**, 404.
Sarma, V. R., Silverton, E. W., Davies, D. R., and Terry, W. D. (1971). *J. Biol. Chem.* **246**, 3753.
Schechter, I., Bauminger, S., and Sela, M. (1964). *Biochim. Biophys. Acta* **93**, 686.
Schlesinger, M. (1970). *Proc. Int. Congr. Trans. Soc.* **3**, 895.
Schlossman, S. F. (1972). *Transplant. Rev.* **10**, 97.
Schlossman, S. F., and Hudson, L. (1973). *J. Immunol.* **110**, 313.
Schrader, J. W. (1973). *J. Exp. Med.* **137**, 844.
Scibienski, R., Fong, S., and Benjamini, E. (1972). *J. Exp. Med.* **136**, 1308.
Scott, R. E., and Marchesi, V. T. (1972). *Cell. Immunol.* **3**, 301.
Segrest, J. P., Jackson, R. L., Marchesi, V. T., Guyer, R. B., and Terry, W. (1972). *Biochem. Biophys. Res. Commun.* **49**, 964.
Sela, M. (1969). *Science* **166**, 1365.

Sell, S. (1970). *Transplant. Rev.* **5**, 19.
Sell, S., and Gell, P. G. H. (1965). *J. Exp. Med.* **122**, 423.
Shearer, G. M. (1974). *Eur. J. Immunol.* **4**, 527.
Shearer, G. M., Mozes, E., and Sela, M. (1971). *J. Exp. Med.* **133**, 126.
Shearer, G. M., Mozes, E., and Sela, M. (1972). *J. Exp. Med.* **135**, 1009.
Shelton, E., and McIntire, K. R. (1970). *J. Mol. Biol.* **47**, 595.
Sheppard, J. R. (1972). *Nature (London), New Biol.* **236**, 14.
Singer, S. J., and Nicolson, G. L. (1971). *Amer. J. Pathol.* **65**, 427.
Singer, S. J., and Nicolson, G. L. (1972). *Science* **175**, 720.
Sjöberg, O. (1972). *J. Exp. Med.* **135**, 850.
Smith, C. W., and Hollers, J. C. (1970). *J. Reticuloendothel. Soc.* **8**, 458.
Smith, J. W., Steiner, A. L., Newberry, W. M., and Parker, C. W. (1971). *J. Clin. Invest.* **50**, 432.
Sprent, J., and Miller, J. F. A. P. (1972a). *Cell. Immunol.* **3**, 213.
Sprent, J., and Miller, J. F. A. P. (1972b). *Cell. Immunol.* **3**, 361.
Sprent, J., and Miller, J. F. A. P. (1972c). *Cell. Immunol.* **3**, 385.
Stevens, R. H., and Williamson, A. R. (1974). *Contemp. Top. Mol. Immunol.* **3**, 85.
Stobo, J. D., Rosenthal, A. S., and Paul, W. E. (1972). *J. Immunol.* **108**, 1.
Stobo, J. D., Rosenthal, A. S., and Paul, W. E. (1973). *J. Exp. Med.* **138**, 71.
Strom, T. B., Deisseroth, A., Morganroth, J., Carpenter, C. B., and Merrill, J. P. (1972). *Proc. Nat. Acad. Sci. U. S.* **69**, 2995.
Strom, T. B., Carpenter, C. B., Garovoy, M. R., Austen, K. F., Merrill, J. P., and Kaliner, M. (1973). *J. Exp. Med.* **138**, 381.
Stutman, O. (1973). *In* "Fourth International Conference on Lymphatic Tissue and Germinal Centers in Immune Reactions." Plenum, New York.
Sulitzeanu, D. (1968). *Bacteriol. Rev.* **32**, 404.
Sulitzeanu, D. (1971). *Curr. Top. Microbiol. Immunol.* **54**, 1.
Svehag, S. E., Chesebro, B., and Bloth, B. (1967). *Science* **158**, 933.
Takahashi, T., Old, L. J., McIntire, K. R., and Boyse, E. A. (1971). *J. Exp. Med.* **134**, 815.
Talmage, D. W. (1957). *Annu. Rev. Med.* **8**, 239.
Tanayaki, N., Katagiri, M., Nakamuro, K., Kreiter, V. P., and Pressman, D. (1973). *Fed. Proc., Fed. Amer. Soc. Exp. Biol.* **32**, 1017.
Taussig, M. J. (1974). *Nature (London)* **248**, 234.
Taussig, M. J., and Munro, A. J. (1974). *Nature (London)* **251**, 63.
Taylor, R. B., Duffus, P. H., Raff, M. C., and de Petris, S. (1971). *Nature (London), New Biol.* **233**, 225.
Theis, G. A., and Thorbecke, G. J. (1973). *J. Immunol.* **110**, 91.
Thompson, K., Harris, M., Benjamini, E., Mitchell, G. F., and Noble, M. (1972). *Nature (London), New Biol.* **238**, 20.
Thorbecke, G. J., Warner, N. L., Hochwald, G. M., and Ohanian, S. H. (1968). *Immunology* **15**, 123.
Tillack, T. W., Scott, R. E., and Marchesi, V. T. (1972). *J. Exp. Med.* **135**, 1209.
Tourtellotte, M. E., Branton, D., and Keith, A. (1970). *Proc. Nat. Acad. Sci. U. S.* **66**, 909.
Truffa-Bachi, P., and Wofsy, L. (1970). *Proc. Nat. Acad. Sci. U. S.* **66**, 685.
Unanue, E. R. (1971a). *J. Immunol.* **107**, 1168.
Unanue, E. R. (1971b). *J. Immunol.* **107**, 1663.
Unanue, E. R., Grey, H. M., Rabellino, E., Campbell, P., and Schmidtke, J. (1971). *J. Exp. Med.* **133**, 1188.

Unanue, E. R., Perkins, W. D., and Karnovsky, M. J. (1972a). *J. Immunol.* **108**, 569.
Unanue, E. R., Perkins, W. D., and Karnovsky, M. J. (1972b). *J. Exp. Med.* **136**, 885.
Unanue, E. R., Dorf, M. E., David, C. S., and Benacerraf, B. (1974). *Proc. Nat. Acad. Sci. U. S.* (in press).
Valentine, R. C., and Green, N. M. (1967). *J. Mol. Biol.* **27**, 615.
Van Furth, R., Schuit, H. R. E., and Hijmans, W. (1966). *Immunology* **11**, 29.
Vitetta, E. S., Baur, S., and Uhr, J. W. (1971). *J. Exp. Med.* **134**, 242.
Vitetta, E. S., and Uhr, J. W. (1972a). *J. Immunol.* **108**, 577.
Vitetta, E. S., and Uhr, J. W. (1972b). *J. Exp. Med.* **136**, 676.
Vitetta, E. S., and Uhr, J. W. (1973). *Transplant. Rev.* **14**, 15.
Vitetta, E. S., Boyse, E. A., and Uhr, J. W. (1973). *Proc. Nat. Acad. Sci. U. S.* **70**, 834.
Warner, N. L., Byrt, P., and Ada, G. L. (1970). *Nature (London)* **226**, 942.
Webb, S. R., and Cooper, M. D. (1973). *J. Immunol.* **111**, 275.
Werner, T. C., Bunting, J. R., and Cathou, R. E. (1972). *Proc. Nat. Acad. Sci. U. S.* **69**, 795.
Wigzell, H. (1971). *In* "Progress in Immunology" (B. Amos, ed.), p. 1105. Academic Press, New York.
Wigzell, H., and Andersson, B. (1969). *J. Exp. Med.* **129**, 23.
Wilkins, M. H. F., Blaurock, A. E., and Engelman, D. M. (1971). *Nature (London)* **230**, 72.
Wilson, J. D. (1972). *Aust. J. Exp. Biol. Med. Sci.* **50**, 199.
Wilson, J. D., and Miller, J. F. A. P. (1971). *Eur. J. Immunol.* **1**, 501.
Wilson, J. D. Nossal, G. J. V., and Lewis, H. (1972). *Eur. J. Immunol.* **2**, 225.
Winchurch, R., Ishizuka, M., Webb, D., and Braun, W. (1971). *J. Immunol.* **106**, 1399.
Winzler, R. J. (1969). *In* "Red Cell Membrane" (G. A. Jamieson and T. J. Greenwalt, eds.), p. 157. Lippincott, Philadelphia, Pennsylvania.
Wioland, M., Sablovic, D., and Burg, C. (1972). *Nature (London)* **237**, 274.
Wofsy, L., Kimura, J., and Truffa-Bachi, P. (1971). *J. Immunol.* **107**, 725.
World Health Organization. (1973). *World Health Organ., Tech. Rep. Ser.* **519**.
Yahara, I., and Edelman, G. M. (1972). *Proc. Nat. Acad. Sci. U.S.* **69**, 608.
Zaalberg, O. B. (1964). *Nature (London)* **202**, 1231.
Zeiller, K., Liebich, H. G., and Hannig, K. (1971). *Eur. J. Immunol.* **1**, 315.
Zinkernagel, R. M., and Doherty, P. C. (1974a). *Nature (London)* **248**, 701.
Zinkernagel, R. M., and Doherty, P. C. (1974b). *Nature (London)* **251**, 547.

CHAPTER 4

Allergens and the Genetics of Allergy

DAVID G. MARSH

I.	Introduction	271
	A. Scope	271
	B. Areas Related to Allergen Research	273
II.	Historical Development (1872–about 1960)	274
	A. General	274
	B. Types of Allergens	275
III.	Nomenclature	280
IV.	Modern Allergen Research	282
	A. Methodology	282
	B. Types of Allergens	290
	C. Theories of Allergenicity	311
	D. Allergenic Valence and Haptens	315
	E. Allergoids	317
V.	Nature of Allergenic Sensitization and Stimulation	320
	A. Exposure, Dosage, and Route of Entry	320
	B. Rates of Release of Allergens from Pollens	324
	C. Artificial Induction of IgE-Mediated Sensitivity	328
VI.	Genetics of Allergy	329
	A. Historical	329
	B. Modern Approaches	332
VII.	Practical Considerations	345
VIII.	Concluding Remarks	347
	References	350

I. Introduction

A. Scope

Recent important developments in immediate hypersensitivity have established this scientific subspecialty as one of the most rapidly advancing branches of immunologic research. Immediate hypersensitivity naturally falls into four main areas of study: (1) characteristics of allergens, the agents which stimulate the production of, and which react with, reaginic antibodies associated with the hypersensitive state; (2) the immunochemical nature and function of reaginic antibodies, including their affinity for basophilic cells; (3) factors controlling the induction and continuation of reaginic antibody biosynthesis; and (4) reaction of allergen with cell-bound reagin and its immunopharmacologic and pathological consequences. While many recent advances have taken place in areas (2), (3), and (4), this review will serve to emphasize the present knowledge and important potential for research into the characteristics of those antigenic substances—known as *atopic allergens* or, simply, *allergens*—which induce the biosynthesis of reaginic antibody in man.

Allergens are generally high molecular weight substances such as proteins, glycoproteins, or carbohydrates of foreign animal or vegetable origin, although they may also be complexes formed by chemical modification of the host's own proteins by "allergenic haptens." Since, from the chemical standpoint, there seems little to differentiate allergens from other antigens, it seems reasonable to ask whether all antigens might have a similar potential to be allergenic. In this review, I will attempt to show that, other than a tendency for allergens to be at the lower end of the molecular weight spectrum of antigens (<40,000 daltons), there is no apparent general chemical feature that characterizes allergens as a subpopulation of antigens.

It is now well established that only certain members of the general population are allergically predisposed and that allergies tend to segregate among the members of particular families. Thus, within the human population it seems reasonable to assume that genetic factors are of great importance in determining an individual's general susceptibility toward allergy. Further important characteristics of allergic sensitization are the *route of entry* of the allergen, which occurs primarily by inhalation or ingestion, and the *allergen dosage*, which is often extremely low (especially for inhaled allergens such as pollens).

The isolation of highly purified allergens and a thorough knowledge of allergen immunochemistry are essential prerequisites for determining the basis for allergic sensitization in man. Furthermore, such research has practical application in improving the testing and treatment of allergic individuals. As a primary orientation, the historical development of allergen immunochemistry will be discussed and a detailed review of physicochemical and immunologic research into the nature of allergens will be made. Recent research and con-

4. Allergens and the Genetics of Allergy

cepts in allergen research will be discussed in the context of their significance to current immunologic thinking. In particular, recent studies of the genetic basis of man's sensitivity to specific highly purified allergens will be evaluated, since this research serves as a prototype for genetic studies of human immune responsiveness under immunogenically limiting situations. This work may well improve our understanding of man's susceptibility and resistance to infections and immunologic diseases.

B. Areas Related to Allergen Research

In order that immunochemical research of allergens can be placed into proper perspective, it is necessary to include a brief summary of important developments in other areas of immediate hypersensitivity.*

The discovery of immunoglobulin E as the principal carrier of reaginic antibody activity in man (Ishizaka et al., 1966; Ishizaka and Ishizaka, 1968) was of primary importance. Subsequently, analogous IgE classes were identified in many other mammalian species (Bloch, 1967). Human allergy research was furthered by the discovery of myeloma IgE (Johansson and Bennich, 1967) which made possible structural studies of IgE (Bennich and Johansson, 1971)† and the rapid development of radioimmunoassay procedures for measuring total IgE concentrations and levels of specific IgE antibodies (Johansson et al., 1968; Gleich et al., 1971; Ishizaka et al., 1970; Wide et al., 1967). Very recently, it has been clearly established that in man, as in many animal species, molecules of the IgG class may also carry reaginic antibody activity, although their possible role in allergic disease is presently not established (Parish, 1973).

The state of immediate hypersensitivity, which results from the biosynthesis of IgE antibody, is characterized by the binding of specific IgE molecules, by their Fc portions, to mast cells and basophils (Ishizaka, 1973). Following subsequent allergenic exposure of the host, the allergen combines with its specific cell-bound IgE antibody, initiating a series of biochemical reactions which lead to the release of chemical mediators (principally histamine) possessing vasodilating and smooth muscle constricting activity. Providing suf-

---

* Research into immunoglobulin E (areas 2 and 3) is reviewed in Vol. I of this treatise (Ishizaka, 1973) and recent reviews of allergen–reagin interaction (area 4) include Osler et al. (1968), Lichtenstein (1972), and Orange and Austen (1969).

† Complete amino acid sequencing of two different IgE myelomas will soon be available from the work of Capra and associates, Mount Sinai School of Medicine, New York, and Bennich and associates, Institute of Biochemistry, Uppsala, Sweden.

ficient allergen and high-affinity antibody is present, this immunologic reaction will normally lead to symptoms characteristic of allergic disease (e.g., rhinitis, asthma, eczema and, occasionally, urticaria or systemic anaphylaxis). This reaction has been classified as Type I hypersensitivity (Gell and Coombs, 1968).

Clearer understanding of the immunopharmacologic processes involved in the release of chemical mediators of allergic reaction came with the development of practical quantitative techniques to study allergic reactions *in vitro* using isolated human leukocytes (Lichtenstein and Osler, 1964; Levy and Osler, 1966) and human or monkey lung fragments passively sensitized with human IgE antibody (Orange and Austen, 1969). A semimicromodification (May *et al.*, 1970) of the basic leukocyte histamine release technique of Lichtenstein and Osler (1964) has also proved to be an invaluable tool in allergen research.

II. Historical Development (1872–about 1960)

A. General

The term "allergy"* (von Pirquet, 1906) was conceived as describing all states of changed immunologic reactivity in animals, including hypersensitivity and immunity. The agents causing such changes, the "allergens," were then considered to encompass a broader spectrum of substances than "antigens," since "allergens comprise, besides the antigens proper, the many protein substances which lead to no production of antibodies but to supersensitivity."† The recognition that immediate hypersensitivity was brought about by the production of reaginic *antibody,* which could be detected in the serum of allergic individuals (Prausnitz and Küstner, 1921), led to an increasingly restrictive usage of the term allergen to this area of research. In an attempt to differentiate the agents provoking immediate and delayed hypersensitivities, Coca and Cooke (1923) introduced the term "atopic allergen" or "atopen"‡ to denote a substance that causes immediate hypersensitivity. Only the former of these terms has achieved any general acceptance.

The common routes by which allergens enter the body are by

---

* Derived from the Greek "allos," meaning a deviation from the original state.

† Translation of part of von Pirquet's (1906) article by Carl Prausnitz, in Gell and Coombs (1968).

‡ The agent causing atopy (Greek "atopia," meaning a strange disease).

4. Allergens and the Genetics of Allergy

inhalation, injection, or ingestion, of which inhalation appears to be the most important in the induction of IgE-mediated allergies. The historical part of this review will deal with only some of the more important early immunochemical research into the nature of these three classes of allergens, and will place particular emphasis on studies of pollen allergens where most of the work was done. Early genetic studies of allergy are reviewed in Section VI.

B. Types of Allergens

1. POLLENS

The term "hay fever" was first used by Bostock (1828) to describe a disease of then unknown etiology. Pollens from certain wind-pollinating plants, which shed prolific amounts of pollen (e.g., grasses and various weeds), were independently shown to be causative agents in hay fever allergies by Wyman (1872) and Blackley (1873).* Serious research in the isolation of allergenic components from pollens began with Kammann's (1904, 1912) pioneering studies of the chemistry of rye grass "Pollentoxin." He extracted the pollen with water or 5% NaCl solution, precipitated a protein fraction from the extract with alcohol, and further fractionated this material by differential salt precipitation. The bulk of the skin reactivity was found to reside in the albumin fraction precipitated between 50 and 100% saturated ammonium sulfate. He further investigated the allergenic stability of the extract toward heating, extreme acid or alkaline pH, and enzymatic degradation (using various proteases and carbohydrases). He found that the principal activity was associated with a relatively stable protein-containing fraction.

Subsequent workers investigated principally the allergenic components extracted from pollens of grasses (Gramineae) and ragweeds (Ambrosieae). Both of these types of pollen have been shown to be the main agents causing hay fever in North America (Koessler, 1914), while grass pollens have been found to be the major causative agents in Europe and many other countries (Blackley, 1873; Wodehouse, 1971). Early work (1904–1960) on the immunochemical properties of pollen allergens has been extensively reviewed by Newell (1941), Bernton (1949), Augustin (1952), and Sherman (1959). Here, I will deal briefly with four of the more interesting controversies that surrounded the early research into the nature of pollen allergens; these

---

* The principal allergy-causing pollens in North America, Europe, and certain other countries have since been reviewed in detail by Wodehouse (1971).

have been resolved to a large extent by recent work. The main controversies centered around whether the allergens were: (1) soluble in anhydrous diethylether (the solvent commonly used to defat pollens in order to facilitate subsequent extraction and fractionation in aqueous solvents); (2) labile toward heat denaturation in neutral aqueous solution; (3) stable or resistant to proteolytic enzyme degradation; (4) dialyzable or nondialyzable.

While the great bulk of grass and ragweed pollen allergens were found to be virtually insoluble in ether and other fat solvents (Coca, 1922; Stull *et al.*, 1930), Milford (1930) and Moore *et al.* (1930) reported that ether extracts of ragweed pollen were skin reactive in *some* ragweed-sensitive individuals. This point was almost completely overlooked until the recent work on ragweed allergen Ra5 (Section IV,C,1,b).

Noon (1911), the originator of desensitization treatment (immunotherapy) of allergies, routinely sterilized the aqueous *grass* pollen extracts he used in treatment by heating them for 10 minutes at 100°. He reported that use of such extracts in the immunotherapy of grass hay fever produced good clinical results. Augustin (1959b) confirmed that many grass pollen allergens are indeed relatively stable toward such drastic heat treatment, whereas other components ("A antigens"), highly antigenic in rabbits, were destroyed by heating. On this basis, she concluded that not all grass pollen antigens are allergenic in man. Most workers investigating *ragweed* pollen extracts observed that the major proportion of skin reactive material was rapidly destroyed on boiling the extracts (Gay, 1926; Stull *et al.*, 1931). The divergence between the observed stabilities of grass and ragweed extracts toward heat treatment suggests that the major allergens in the two types of extract differ widely in their susceptibility to physical denaturation, a point that has subsequently been confirmed (Section IV,B,2).

The principal allergenic activity of both grass and ragweed pollens was generally believed to reside in protein-containing fractions, although the presence of some reactive carbohydrate moieties could not be ruled out (Newell, 1941; Augustin, 1959b). However, the ease with which various proteolytic enzymes destroyed the activity of ragweed and grass pollen extracts remained a matter of considerable dispute (Newell, 1941; Augustin, 1959b).

A further problem which early researchers had great difficulty in resolving, and which led to much controversy, was whether the allergenic constituents of ragweed and grass pollens were dialyzable or nondialyzable (Grove and Coca, 1925; Unger *et al.*, 1932; Goldfarb et al., 1954; Johnson and Padley, 1959). Published physicochemical analyses of impure pollen fractions (Abramson et al., 1942; Johnson and Thorne, 1958) did not serve to clarify the problem.

To some extent, the early controversies arose from researchers equating results from immunochemically quite different extracts of grass and ragweed pollens and from using reagents and research materials (enzymes, dialysis membranes, etc.) of variable, and sometimes questionable, quality. A major problem, however, was that many workers did not fully appreciate that each of the complex pollen extracts contained a great many *different* allergenic components, which not only differed in their physicochemical properties but also, qualitatively and quantitatively, in their allergenic activity in different allergic individuals. The case for multiple allergenic components in pollens had been presented as early as 1925 when Caulfield showed that different ragweed-sensitive people reacted to different degrees to different ragweed fractions, observations that were supported in subsequent studies of various pollen extracts (e.g., Coca and Grove, 1925; Rackemann and Wagner, 1936; Britton et al., 1958). Since relatively little attention was paid to quantitative assay of allergenic reactivity (e.g., by simple skin test titration), it is often impossible to evaluate whether the activity of a particular fraction resided in the main components or minor contaminants.

The antigenic complexity and cross-reactivity of a large number of extracts of pollens important in hay fever were investigated by immunodiffusion analysis using hyperimmune rabbit antisera prepared against individual crude pollen extracts (Wodehouse, 1954, 1955, 1957; Augustin, 1959a; Feinberg, 1960). Although one might have some reservations about equating antigenicity in rabbits with allergenicity in man (cf. Augustin, 1959b), the great antigenic (and potentially, allergenic) complexity of pollen extracts was clearly revealed in these studies. In addition, they showed that pollens from plants of different botanical families [e.g., Gramineae (grass) and Ambrosieae (ragweed)] were antigenically unrelated, whereas pollens from closely related species within a family contained several cross-reacting antigens, in accordance with clinical and experimental observations concerning the allergenic relatedness of such pollens.

2. OTHER INHALANTS

Some early biochemical investigations of inhaled allergens other than pollens were made notably by Spies and associates, who investigated components from cottonseed (*Gossypium herbaceum*) (Spies *et al.*, 1940; Spies and Umberger, 1942) and from the castor bean (*Ricinus communis*) (Spies and Coulson, 1943; Spies *et al.*, 1944), both of which are important allergens in the agricultural industry. Fractionation of cottonseed and castor bean, using primarily salt and solvent precipitation techniques, yielded essentially carbohydrate-free, highly allergenic proteins which were remarkably stable to heat treatment and under conditions of extreme pH (reviewed by Spies, 1973).

Attempts were also made to fractionate the grossly heterogeneous mixture of allergens present in house dust (for reviews, see Walzer, 1939; Sutherland, 1945; Berrens, 1971); not surprisingly, relatively little improvement in allergen purity was achieved by the early salt and solvent precipitation techniques. Preliminary antigenic analysis of an extract of the mold alternaria by Sternberger *et al.* (1956) revealed the antigenic (and, potentially, allergenic) complexity of just one of the common allergenic components of house dust.

3. Inhaled or Injected Allergens

A further important area studied by the early workers was insect allergy, where the allergens may be injected or inhaled. Insects were first recognized as agents causing allergies by Waterhouse (1914), who studied generalized allergic (anaphylactic) reactions to bee stings. Subsequently, insect emanations, and also bites, were found to stimulate allergic reactions in man (Perlman, 1958; Fox *et al.*, 1963). While relatively uncommon, allergic sensitivity to stings of the *Hymenoptera* (includes bees, wasps, and hornets) is an important problem, since it frequently leads to life-threatening generalized reactions. However, relatively few immunochemical studies of insect allergens were performed before 1960 (reviewed by Perlman, 1958; Shulman, 1968). The biochemical work was performed mainly by researchers interested in insect toxicology or physiology rather than allergy (Neumann and Habermann, 1954; Hackman and Goldberg, 1958).

Until relatively recently, horse antiserum to the toxins of common human pathogens (e.g., diphtheria and tetanus) was routinely injected, in large doses, for prophylaxis of disease. This treatment often led to the development of reagin-mediated generalized reactions and other immunologic problems, particularly "serum sickness" (Wright and Hopkins, 1941; Kojis, 1942). Another biologic product, dextran (a polymer of D-glucose produced by the bacterium *Leuconostoc mesenteroides*), used as a plasma volume expander, was

4. Allergens and the Genetics of Allergy

found to cause generalized allergic reactions in some people on first injection. Dextrans from different strains of this bacterium were found to vary considerably in the frequency with which allergic reactions were induced (Pulaski et al., 1951). Subsequently, Kabat et al. (1957) clearly demonstrated that the least allergenic strain contained the highest proportions of $1 \rightarrow 6$ (straight chain) linkages and lowest proportion of very high molecular weight components ($>100,000$ daltons). Dextrans possessing many $1 \rightarrow 3$ and $1 \rightarrow 4$ linkages (branched chains) and a relatively large percentage of high molecular weight material were assumed to be more allergenic due to their greater structural complexity. Preexistent reaginic sensitivity was considered to have possibly developed due to previous exposure to dextran contaminants in commercial sucrose, or to pneumococcal polysaccharides which cross-react with dextran (Kabat et al., 1957). Of particular interest in regard to subsequent genetic studies (Section VI) was the finding that individuals with (IgE-mediated) skin sensitivity to dextran generally had measurable serum (IgG) antidextran antibodies. Not surprisingly, individuals possessing high antibody levels tended to have systemic reactions following infusion with the highly branched-chain dextran.

4. INGESTED ALLERGENS

Adverse immunologic reactions to foods, including the development of reaginic allergies, have been known for a long time (reviewed by Kaufman, 1958; Fries and Lightstone, 1962). Passive transfer of reaginic antibody in serum was first demonstrated using the serum of a fish-allergic individual (Prausnitz and Küstner, 1921). Mainly due to the absence of good immunochemical studies, much is still unknown about the nature of food allergens, and why some food allergies appear to be carried into adulthood more than others. Furthermore, a lack of potent, nontoxic food allergens has led to considerable confusion regarding the significance of skin testing in detecting reaginic sensitivity to food allergens.

Another important class of ingested allergens are the parasitic helminths such as *Ascaris lumbricoides*. Individuals with such parasitic infestations were found to have positive intradermal skin reactions and circulating reaginic antibody to extracts of the respective parasite (Rackemann and Stevens, 1927; Soulsby, 1963). Brunner (1934) and Walzer and associates (Davidson et al., 1947; Kailin et al., 1950) showed that reaginic sensitivity to crude ascaris extract could be induced in 90% of the human population (including the majority of nonallergics) by repeated intradermal administration of the extract.

Largely as a result of this work, ascaris (and other helminthic antigens) achieved the distinction of being regarded as a "universal allergen." This conclusion is critically reevaluated in Section IV,D.

III. Nomenclature

In the context of this chapter, the term "allergen" will denote an agent that commonly causes the induction of reaginic IgE antibody biosynthesis and concomitant allergic sensitivity in man or other animals, under normal conditions of exposure. As previously stated, allergens form part of the family of substances, termed "antigens," which are capable of inducing cellular and humoral antibody responses in animals.* Thus, the induction of IgE biosynthesis is only part of the immune response resulting from stimulation by an allergen. The term "allergenic" will denote only properties associated with IgE, whereas "antigenic" will be used, somewhat restrictively, to denote all other immunologic properties of an antigen/allergen. For some purposes, particularly when dealing with "allergoids" (Section IV,F) it will be necessary to subdivide both allergenic and antigenic properties into their two aspects, namely, "immunogenic"—the capacity of an antigen to stimulate specific antibody biosynthesis, and "reactogenic"—the ability of an antigen to combine with presynthesized antibody (Marsh et al., 1970b).

In the past, the terms "major" and "minor" have been used to describe the relative allergenic importance of different components isolated from crude allergen-containing extracts. Such terminology would seem to imply that a major allergen is more immunogenic and reactogenic than a minor allergen in all subjects displaying sensitivity to the crude extract, and/or that a greater percentage of the allergic subjects are appreciably more sensitive to the major than to the minor allergen. However, recent research has clearly shown that certain pollen components, generally of molecular weight 5000–12,000, are more reactive in some allergic subjects than the so-called major allergens (Marsh et al., 1966, 1973a; Lichtenstein et al., 1969, 1973a). A further complication arises from the observation that different allergenic components (of pollens) are extracted at radically

---

* This does not preclude that probably all antigens induce IgE biosynthesis under appropriate conditions of stimulation (route, dosage, use of certain adjuvants). See Sections V and VI for a discussion of this point.

different rates. Thus, an apparent major allergen (e.g., antigen E of crude ragweed pollen) may not be the major causative agent in specific allergic disease if it is eluted relatively slowly before the allergen particle is swallowed (Marsh *et al.*, 1975a; Section V,B).

In order to clarify the problem of nomenclature, I propose that the term "major allergen" be used only to denote an identified highly purified component to which over 90% of clinically specifically allergic individuals react appreciably in high allergen dilution (e.g., produce a "two-plus" skin reaction following intradermal skin testing with the allergen at a concentration of 10^{-3} μg/ml or lower). This definition includes the possibility that a major allergen, defined on the basis of studies with complex crude allergenic extracts, may not be the principal agent actually provoking allergic symptoms *in vivo*, due to factors such as slow extraction from the allergenic matrix or rapid catabolism of the allergen.

The term "isoallergen" will be used to denote a member of a group of allergens isolated from a specific source, and which possesses experimentally indistinguishable immunologic properties and a closely related physicochemical structure to other isoallergens in the same group (Johnson and Marsh, 1965b). Isoallergens usually differ slightly from one another in isoelectric point (pI) due to minor structural differences such as the nature of their carbohydrate moieties (cf. Morris *et al.*, 1965), or differences in the degree of protein amidation (Johnson and Marsh, 1965a). Other differences may represent genetic variants (e.g., Ra5, Section IV,B,2b). The same terminology will be used for all cases.

The need for a unified nomenclature for purified allergens is becoming increasingly apparent with the proliferation of a confusing variety of trivial names, as greater numbers of articles dealing with allergen purification appear in the literature. Currently, a subcommittee of the WHO Committee on Antigen Standardization is developing a nomenclature system based on the abbreviated Latinized taxonomic name of the allergen source and an arabic numeral indicating the allergenic component in the sequence of its published isolation. For example, under a proposal that is under consideration, a major allergen from short ragweed pollen, known as antigen E (King and Norman, 1962), would become Amb.e.1 (*Ambrosia elatior*, first isolated allergen). It is anticipated that there will be rigid requirements for physical, chemical, and immunologic purity for all allergens included under this system. (Partially purified allergens would be temporarily assigned capital letters rather than arabic numerals.) Unfortunately, at the time of writing this article, it would be premature for the author unilaterally to assign new names to previously isolated allergens. However, the full taxonomic names of all allergen sources will be given.

IV. Modern Allergen Research

A. Methodology

1. FRACTIONATION TECHNIQUES

All the early studies had suggested that most extracts of allergen-containing biologic materials, such as pollens, were highly complex mixtures of allergenic proteins and glycoproteins, together with nonallergenic (or weakly allergenic) pigments, carbohydrates, and low molecular weight (dialyzable) substances (Newell, 1941; Johnson and Thorne, 1958). It is, therefore, not surprising that definitive research into the physical, chemical, and immunologic properties of the diverse allergenic components only became feasible with the development, in the late 1950's, of greatly improved protein fractionation procedures. Particular landmarks were the preparation of ion-exchange celluloses (Peterson and Sober, 1956) and cross-linked dextrans (Porath and Flodin, 1959) — media that could be used for the chromatographic fractionation of proteins with minimal denaturation and nonspecific adsorption effects. Fractionation of mixtures of polyionic macromolecules, such as protein allergens, could be achieved by successive column chromatography on the ion exchangers, diethylaminoethyl- (DEAE-) or carboxymethyl- (CM-) celluloses, followed by molecular size fractionation (gel filtration) on appropriate cross-linked dextran xerogels (Sephadexes).

When beginning the isolation of allergens from a complex biologic extract, a useful approach has been to investigate thoroughly the dialyzability and heat and pH stabilities of the allergically active material before proceeding with fractionation. Preliminary semipreparative electrophoretic fractionation of the crude extract on starch, acrylamide, or agarose gels (Marsh et al., 1970a; Ceska et al., 1972; Belin, 1972b) and small scale gel filtration experiments are followed by qualitative and quantitative assay of the allergenicity of all fractions in a panel of at least ten subjects. This approach enables the investigator to identify the approximate isoelectric point and molecular size of the principal allergenic components. The most effective column chromatographic media may then be selected for subsequent larger scale purification of the allergens. In this manner, a procedure was developed for isolating allergens from the pollen of perennial rye grass (*Lolium perenne*), adapted from the method of Johnson and Marsh (1965a) (Fig. 1). Similar procedures have been devised by other authors (King and Norman, 1962; King *et al.*, 1964; Underdown and Goodfriend, 1969; Goodfriend and Lapkoff, 1972) for isolating allergens from short ragweed pollen (*Ambrosia elatior*). Since the methodology used in the case of rye pollen extract is typical of many of the conventional chromatographic procedures that have been developed for allergen fractionation, it will be described in detail.

Dried pollen from perennial rye grass (*Lolium perenne*) is purchased from a reliable pollen supplier soon after pollination and stored at $-20°$ in a sealed bottle containing dessicant until used. Since the ether-soluble fatty components of grass pollens have been found to be allergenically inactive in most allergic subjects (Britton *et al.*, 1958; Augustin, 1959a) and tend to hinder subsequent purification steps, they are usually removed by extracting the pollen several times with peroxide-free dry diethylether. After removal of excess solvent, water-soluble pollen solids are extracted as thoroughly as possible by gently rocking the pollen with slightly alkaline buffered solution (e.g., 0.125 M NH_4HCO_3,* at $4°$. The extract is dialyzed extensively against 0.002 M ammonium bicarbonate and finally against distilled water in a cellulose casing possessing a small average pore size, such as Visking No. 18 (Craig and King, 1962). The dialyzed extract is concentrated by lyophilization or ultrafiltration.

The low molecular weight grass pollen fraction appears to be nonallergenic in *most* allergic individuals (Johnson and Padley, 1959); but, in the light of recent experience with the low molecular weight ragweed allergen, Ra5 (Marsh *et al.*, 1973b), the dialyzable fraction may well be found to contain some minor allergens to which a small percentage of grass-sensitive people react. If low molecular weight, potentially ether soluble, components are to be conserved, a modified procedure such as that used by Roebber *et al.* (1975) for the isolation of Ra5 should be used (see below).

The extract is routinely examined at all stages in the purification by starch, acrylamide, or agarose gel electrophoresis and by immunodiffusion and immunoelectrophoresis against antisera previously prepared to crude and highly purified grass allergens. The yield of the major Group I allergen (relative to that obtained after

---

* For all fractionation procedures, slightly alkaline, volatile nonultraviolet absorbing buffers, such as ammonium bicarbonate, are preferred. All buffers used must be nontoxic and not cause protein denaturation.

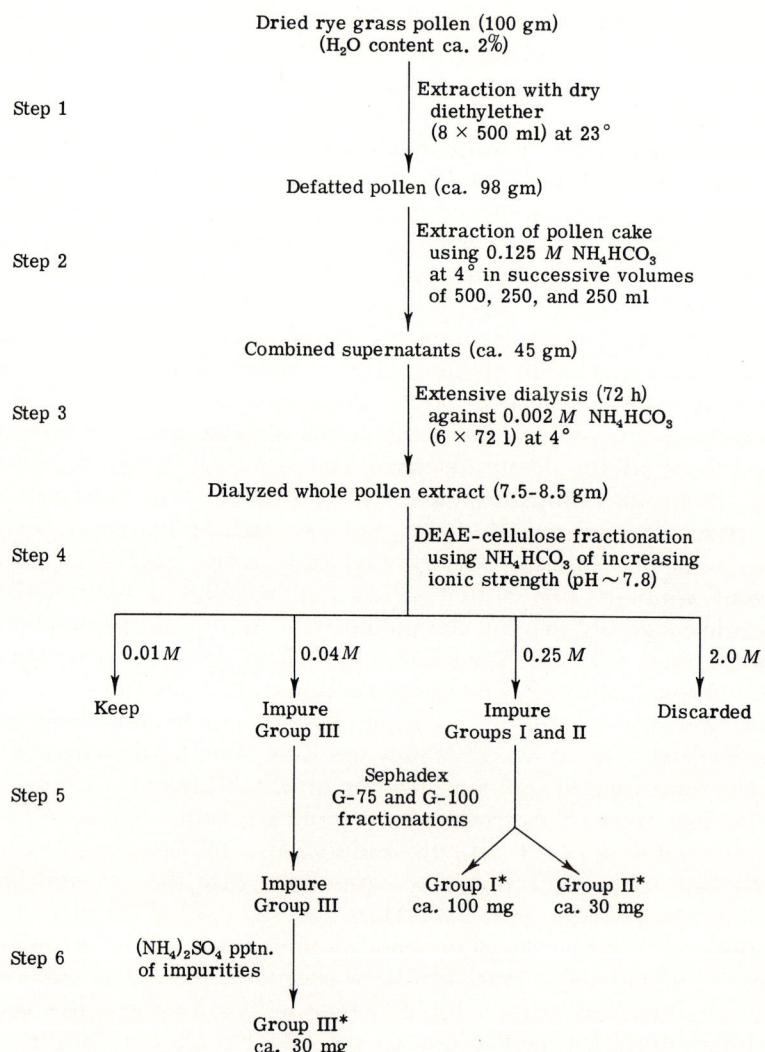

Fig. 1. Schematic outline of methods used to purify rye grass pollen allergens of Groups I, II and III based on modifications of procedures reported by Johnson and Marsh (1965a) and Marsh et al. (1966, 1970a).

* In order to obtain more highly purified materials and to separate component isoallergens, these fractions may be subject to further DEAE-cellulose chromatography or preparative gel electrophoresis or isoelectricfocusing. (From Marsh, 1974, by permission of copyright owners.)

† Use of different types of DEAE-cellulose and different pollen: DEAE ratios may result in the Group III allergen being eluted in the 0.01M buffer.

Step 2) is monitored by radial immunodiffusion analysis (Mancini *et al.*, 1964), using a rye Group I—anti-rye Group I system (Baer *et al.*, 1974).

Subsequent anion exchange chromatography of the dialyzed extract on DEAE-cellulose, Whatman DE52 (Fig. 1, Step 4), is performed as rapidly as possible at 4° on a wide Büchner column to prevent loss of pollen components by irreversible adsorption to the column. The allergen-containing fractions are dialyzed briefly (3–4 hours) against distilled water and lyophilized. They are successively fractionated on Sephadex G-75 and G-100 columns and finally by further DEAE-cellulose, gel electrophoresis, electrofocusing, or salt fractionation steps (Johnson and Marsh, 1965a; Marsh *et al.*, 1970a; Marsh, 1974) to achieve a high degree of allergenic purity and to isolate isoallergenic subcomponents (Section IV,B,2). Three immunochemically distinct groups of allergens, Groups I, II, and III, have so far been isolated from rye grass pollen in this manner.

Various alternative procedures have been used in isolating other allergens; for example, ammonium sulfate precipitation (0.9–1.0 saturation) followed by Sephadex G-25 column fractionation may be used as an alternative to the dialysis Step 3 (Fig. 1), according to King and Norman's (1962) method for fractionating ragweed pollen extract. A minor ragweed allergen, Ra5, was found to possess a relatively low molecular weight (5000) and to be partially soluble in ether, which led to a reevaluation of the original extraction procedure of Lapkoff and Goodfriend (1974). In the new procedure (Roebber *et al.*, 1975), the ether-defatting procedure is omitted. Pollen extraction is carried out for only 30 minutes at room temperature, since the Ra5 component is eluted extremely rapidly from the pollen (Section V,B). No dialysis steps are used in subsequent purification of the allergen.

The great variety of ion-exchange and xerogel chromatographic media, which are now commercially available, permits the allergen chemist to select critically those products that are most appropriate for subsequent chromatographic purification of specific allergens. A further type of chromatographic technique, employing differential solubilization of proteins in an ammonium sulfate gradient, has been employed by King (1972) for the purification of ragweed allergens.

For studies of allergenic specificity, and particularly for genetic studies (Section VI), the isolation of ultra-pure allergens ($\geq 99.9\%$ homogeneity) will be necessary to prevent possible errors arising from the presence of highly allergenic trace impurities. Fortunately, a number of highly discriminating separation procedures, suitable for use in this final stage of purification, are now available. These include acrylamide gel and agarose gel electrophoresis (Ornstein, 1964; Johansson, 1972) and isoelectricfocusing (Vesterberg, 1972, 1973). The latter technique involves separation of components in a pH gradient generated in an ampholyte mixture, and is capable of resolving proteins differing in isoelectic point by only 0.02 pH unit. Most workers have used acrylamide gel as the ampholyte-supporting medium, but the method of Radola (1973), using cooled slabs of Sephadex G-75 paste, appears to offer a highly practical method with regard to the ease with which relatively large samples can be separated and recovered. A further technique that has great potential usefulness in allergen purification is immunoadsorption chromatography (Campbell *et al.*, 1951; Cuatrecasas, 1970).

2. ANALYSIS

The analysis of allergen preparations falls into three categories: physical, chemical, and biologic. In estimating the overall purity of an allergen preparation, at least two or three different assays should be selected from each category. Particular emphasis should be placed on assessing biologic purity and potency. The methodology commonly used is summarized in Table I which, although not an exhaustive list, presents most of the more discriminating techniques presently employed by immunochemists. Many of the methods are widely used and have been described in detail elsewhere (e.g., Williams and Chase, 1967, 1970, 1973). Assays for allergenicity, using leukocyte histamine release, skin testing, and the radioallergosorbent test (RAST), have also been reviewed (e.g., Osler *et al.*, 1968; Stanworth, 1973). I will, therefore, stress only a few of the more important points here. Even the most advanced physicochemical methodology (such as isoelectric focusing) is not sufficiently discriminating to detect minor highly allergenic contaminants, which may be contributing the bulk of the allergenic activity of a purified allergen preparation. On the other hand, assay of allergenic potency alone fails to detect isoallergenic variants (Section III) of an allergen which have experimentally indistinguishable activities. Thus, physical, chemical, and allergenic analysis complement one another. A necessary additional criterion for purity is antigenic analysis employing sera from several different animals hyperimmunized with the crude extract or purified allergen. The most critical analysis of this type is provided by a combination of immunodiffusion and electrophoresis, particularly the recently developed Laurell crossed im-

TABLE I
Analysis of Allergens

Property	Method[a]	General references
Physical		
Molecular size	°a. Sedimentation equilibrium ultracentrifugal analysis	Van Holde and Baldwin (1958)
	°b. Sedimentation-diffusion analysis	Schachman (1959)
	°c. Gel filtration	Porath and Flodin (1959); Andrews (1964)
	°d. SDS gel electrophoresis	Shapiro *et al.* (1967)
Electrical charge	°e. Electrofocusing (on acrylamide/Sephadex)	Vesterberg (1972, 1973); Radola (1973)
	°f. Acrylamide disc electrophoresis	Ornstein (1964); Davis (1964)
	°g. Starch gel electrophoresis	Smithies (1959)
	°h. Agarose gel electrophoresis	Johansson (1972)
Chemical		
N-terminal amino acid	°i. "Dansyl" method	Hirs and Timasheff (1972)
	°j. FDNB method	Hirs and Timasheff (1972)
	°k. Edman degradation	Hirs and Timasheff (1972)
Composition	l. Total amino acid analysis	Hirs and Timasheff (1972)
	°m. Amino acid sequence	Hirs and Timasheff (1972)
	n. Carbohydrate analysis	Dische (1955); Gottschalk (1966)
	o. Other (lipid, prosthetic groupings, etc.)	
Biologic		
Antigenic	°p. Electroimmunoassay and crossed immunoelectrophoresis	Laurell (1972); Minchin Clarke and Freeman (1966)
	°q. Immunoelectrophoresis	Grabar and Burtin (1960)
	°r. Immunodiffusion	Feinberg (1960)
Allergenic	†s. Leukocyte histamine release	Osler *et al.* (1968)
	†t. Radioallergosorbent test (RAST)	Wide *et al.* (1967)
	†u. Quantitative intradermal skin testing	Marsh *et al.* (1972, 1973a)
	v. Semiquantitative prick or scratch skin testing	Squire (1950); Belin (1972a); Marsh *et al.* (1970a); Sherman (1968)
	°w. Allergenic profile of chromatographic fractions[b]	L. Goodfriend (personal communication, 1972)
Other biologic activity	x. Assay for enzymatic activity	

[a] Key: °, used in assessing the purity of allergen samples; †, useful for determining the degree of allergenic contamination in specimens of minor allergens, to which only some of the allergic population is sensitive (cf. Lichtenstein *et al.*, 1969).

[b] See text for details.

munoelectrophoresis technique (Minchin Clarke and Freeman, 1966).

It is advisable to assay the allergenic activity of all fractions, relative to the original crude allergenic extract, at each stage of purification in order that all allergenic components might be recognized and the recovery of biologic activity followed at each step. Semiquantitative prick or scratch testing (Belin, 1972a; Marsh *et al.*, 1970a) in several allergic subjects is particularly useful for this rapid screening procedure. More quantitative assays of highly purified and partially purified fractions are best performed using the leukocyte histamine release technique (Lichtenstein and Osler, 1964; May *et al.*, 1970). In most allergic subjects, there is a good quantitative correlation between prick and intradermal skin testing and between intradermal skin testing and leukocyte histamine release (Belin and Norman, 1974; Norman *et al.*, 1973).

The relative allergenicity of different allergen preparations may be determined from the ratio of the respective concentrations which release 50% of the histamine from allergic human leukocytes in the absence of (toxic) cell lysis (Lichtenstein *et al.*, 1969) or, less precisely, from the ratio of allergen concentrations that produce identical wheal sizes in the central (linear) part of the dose response curve (approximately 0.7–1.3 cm wheal diameter) obtained by quantitative intradermal skin testing with serial dilutions of the allergens (Marsh *et al.*, 1973a). Due to genetic differences between different allergic subjects (Section VI), different individuals exhibit unique response patterns to different allergens (cf. Figs. 2 and 3). Therefore, in order to investigate thoroughly the relative activities of different allergenic fractions, it is necessary to test a number of subjects—preferably at least 6 to 10 when investigating major allergens and 100 or more for some minor allergens (cf. Marsh *et al.*, 1973a).

The recently developed RAST (Wide *et al.*, 1967) employs allergen immunoadsorbents and radiolabeled anti-IgE in the measurement of specific serum IgE antibody. Results from this test correlate surprisingly well with biologic activity measured by leukocyte histamine release or skin test (Lichtenstein *et al.*, 1973b; Norman *et al.*, 1973). The RAST may be used to compare different allergic people's IgE antibody levels to a particular allergen; but, due to current problems of relating the radioimmunoassay units measured in the RAST to absolute amounts of IgE antibody, it cannot, as yet, be used for quantitative comparison of an individual's sensitivity to two different allergens.

Leukocyte histamine release or quantitative skin test assays are

4. Allergens and the Genetics of Allergy

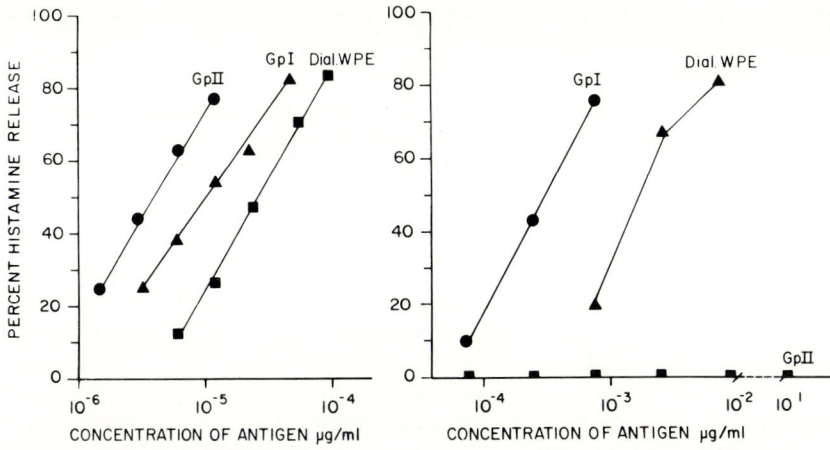

Fig. 2. *In vitro* histamine release assay of the allergenic activity of dialyzed rye whole pollen extract (WPE) and rye Groups I and II using the leukocytes of two highly grass sensitive individuals. The cells of the person on the left are similarly sensitive to both allergens; those of the person on the right are over 100,000 times more sensitive to Group I than Group II. (From Lichtenstein *et al.*, 1969, by permission of copyright owners.)

particularly useful for determining levels of possible trace contamination of a major allergen in a specimen of a minor allergen. Individuals who are highly sensitive to the major but completely insensitive to the minor allergen are selected, and quantitative tests performed with samples of the two preparations. Using this approach, Lichten-

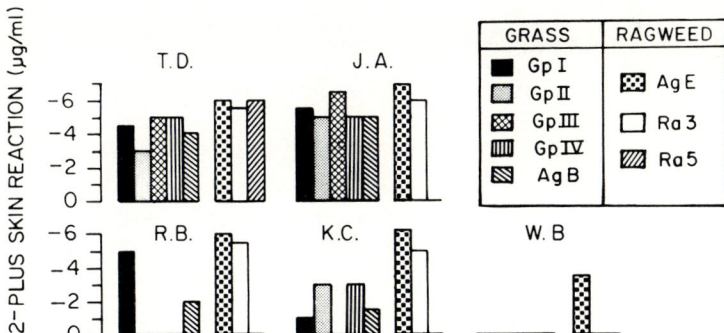

Fig. 3. Comparison of the specific reaginic skin sensitivities of five highly pollen allergic individuals to highly purified grass and ragweed pollen allergens. The vertical bars represent the $\log_{10}$ concentration (μg/ml) of each allergen which elicits a two-plus skin reaction following intradermal skin test (0.05 ml injected). Note the widely different sensitivity patterns for each of the allergic individuals. (From Marsh, 1974, by permission of copyright owners.)

stein *et al.* (1969) demonstrated, by leukocyte histamine release assay, that more than 100,000-fold greater weight proportion of a specimen of rye grass Group II was needed to release the same percent histamine as rye Group I. The specimen of the Group II allergen must, therefore, have contained less than 1 part in 100,000 of the immunochemically distinct major rye Group I allergen. An alternative approach for this type of analysis would be to adapt the radioinhibition method of Yunginger and Gleich (1972). The Group II sample (in high concentration) would be quantitatively compared relative to Group I with respect to its capacity to inhibit the reaction of ^{125}I-labeled Group I with monospecific rabbit anti-Group I.

A particularly critical test for allergenic purity, which looks at the possibility of an allergen preparation being contaminated with other allergen(s) of similar physicochemical properties, has been suggested by L. Goodfriend (personal communication, 1972). The highly purified allergen sample is fractionated separately by ion-exchange and by gel-filtration chromatography, and the peaks of ultraviolet-absorbing material from each chromatographic run are divided into subfractions. The specific allergenic activities of each subfraction (on a weight basis) are tested in several allergic subjects of widely differing sensitivities to the allergen. In any one individual, the specific activities of the subfractions should be indistinguishable if the allergen is pure.

B. Types of Allergens

1. INTRODUCTION

The chemistry of atopic allergens has recently been reviewed in great detail by Berrens (1971); other general reviews have been made by Stanworth (1973) and Spies (1974). Hypersensitivity diseases of the lungs, including IgE-mediated and non-IgE-mediated diseases have recently been discussed in detail by Pepys (1969) and in a New York Academy of Sciences Symposium (Kilburn, 1974). Further more specialized reviews and research publications are cited in Table II. No attempt will be made to review completely the voluminous literature on allergen chemistry and reactivity; it is, however, worthwhile discussing a few of the more interesting research areas and presenting a detailed review of pollen allergens, since this important area is the most advanced in studies of allergen structure and reactivity, allergen–antibody interactions, and the immunogenetics of allergy. The isolation, analysis, and physicochemical properties of most of the allergens which have so far been isolated in a highly purified state are cited in Table III. Most of these allergens are discussed in this and the succeeding sections; others are described in the references cited in Table II.

2. POLLEN ALLERGENS

a. Grass. Due to the abundant and widespread distribution of wind-pollinated species of the family Gramineae (grasses), it seems reasonable to assume that the grasses contribute the most important group of pollens causing allergy. Out of a total of several thousand species, only about 20 abundant grasses produce small wind-distributed pollen particles in sufficient quantity to be important in allergy (Wodehouse, 1971). The grasses have been divided into two main botanical subfamilies, the Festucoideae and the Panicoideae (Hitchcock, 1950), although some botanists make further subdivisions. According to Hitchcock, the two families are comprised of 10 and 4 tribes, respectively. Most tribes consist of several genera, with each genus containing from one to over 100 species. In general, the closer the botanical similarity between species the closer is the antigenic and allergenic cross-reactivity. These observations have been extensively documented by the early researchers (Section II,B,1) and, more recently, by Wright and Clifford (1965) and Marsh *et al.* (1970a).

There are at least 14 distinct antigenic components in extracts of most common grass pollens (Augustin, 1959a; Feinberg, 1960), all of which may be regarded as potential allergens. The first immunochemical studies of grass pollen allergens, employing modern techniques, were reported by Augustin and Hayward (1962). Extracts of the pollens *Phleum pratense* (timothy) and *Dactylis glomerata* (known as either orchard or cocksfoot) were fractionated by a combination of dialysis, acid-NaCl precipitation, and DEAE-cellulose chromatography. Two highly allergenic, immunologically unrelated timothy pollen fractions, T21A-I and T21A-VI, each contained at least two antigenic components when tested against rabbit antiwhole extract serum. Both fractions T21A-I and an analogously prepared, partially related, orchard fraction were highly skin reactive in all patients tested. Conversely, timothy fraction T21A-VI and a similar orchard pollen fraction were extremely reactive in some patients, but unreactive in others. These results demonstrated that there were at least two allergens in each pollen toward which different allergic subjects were differentially sensitive.

None of the preparations contained the heat labile "A antigens"

TABLE II

Selected References[a] for Recent Research in Allergen Structure and Reactivity

Allergen source	Reviews	Research publications[b]
Microbial		
Bacteria	1–3	4–7
Fungi	2, 8, 9	10–13
Algae	9	14
Vegetable		
Pollens (grass, weed, tree)	9, 15, 16	See text
Inhaled dusts		
Castor bean/cotton seed	9, 17	18–20[c]
Other (inc. flour, kapok, ipecac)	2, 9, 21	—
Ingestants (inc. nuts, tomatoes)	9, 17	—
Animal		
Invertebrates		
Parasites (inc. *Ascaris*)	—	22–24
Arachnids (inc. mites)	9	25–28
Insects		
Stings/bites	29, 30	See text
Emanations	9, 29	
Other	—	31
Vertebrates		
Fish	9, 32	33, 34
Birds		
Feces	2	—
Feathers	9	—
Egg proteins	9, 15	—
Mammals		
Danders	9, 15, 35	36, 37
Milk	9, 17, 38	39
Semen	—	40
Chemical		
Penicillin	15, 41–43	—
Aspirin	—	44
Industrial chemicals	45	—
Complex		
House dust	9	14, 26–29, 46

[a] Key:
1. Sherman (1968)
2. Pepys (1969)
3. Norman (1973)
4. Seabury et al. (1973)
5. Pepys et al. (1969)
6. Belin et al. (1970)
7. Belin and Norman (1974)
8. Feinberg (1946)
9. Berrens (1971)
10. Palmstierna et al. (1962)
11. Bonilla-Soto (1969)
12. Axelson (1971)
13. Barker et al. (1967)
14. Bernstein and Safferman (1966)
15. Stanworth (1973)
16. Goldfarb (1964; 1972)
17. Spies (1974)
18. Freedman et al. (1961)
19. Layton et al. (1965)
20. Layton et al. (1966)
21. Schwartz (1952)
22. Ambler and Orr (1972)
23. Hussain et al. (1973)
24. Hogarth-Scott et al. (1973)

4. Allergens and the Genetics of Allergy

which Augustin (1959b) had found to be highly immunogenic in rabbits, but which she believed to be nonallergenic in man (Section II,B,1). Subsequently, O'Sullivan (1968), in Augustin's laboratory, isolated a highly purified preparation of the A antigen from orchard pollen (Table III). This allergenic preparation was pure by immunodiffusion against anti-whole orchard extract, but trace impurities could be detected when the whole orchard extract was allowed to diffuse against anti-A serum. O'Sullivan was not able to obtain a discrete band for the A-antigen by acrylamide gel electrophoresis at pH 8.6, probably because this basic protein did not migrate into the acrylamide gel at this pH. He reported a molecular weight of around 88,000 using a rather imprecise gel diffusion assay; a value of 56,000, which one may calculate from his gel filtration data, is probably nearer the correct value.

Skin tests on four allergic subjects and histamine release assay using human lung passively sensitized with serum from two patients showed that, in different subjects, the purified A antigen was between 10 and $\geq 10,000$ times less active than a crude orchard extract containing the same amount of A antigen. These data suggest that the A antigen is probably a minor allergen, to which only a proportion of the allergic population is sensitive, rather than a "nonallergen," as Augustin (1959b) had suggested. Similar results have been obtained in the author's laboratory using rye Group IV (MW ca. 50,000), a partially purified fraction that has similar physical and immunochemical properties to the orchard A antigen (Marsh, 1974). The reason why such strong antigens (in rabbits) appear to be relatively unimportant allergenically in man may be due to their rather high molecular weight which hinders mucosal membrane permeability (Section V,A).

---

25. Voorhorst et al. (1967)
26. Kawai et al. (1972)
27. Miyamoto (1974)
28. Ricci (1974)
29. Shulman (1968)
30. Habermann (1972)
31. Jyo et al. (1973)
32. Aas (1974)
33. Elsayed and Aas (1971a)
34. Elsayed et al. (1971)
35. Voorhorst (1958)

36. Ohman et al. (1973)
37. Brandt et al. (1973)
38. Spies (1973)
39. Spies et al. (1974)
40. Siraganian et al. (1973)
41. Levine (1966)
42. Batchelor and Dewdney (1968)
43. de Weck (1974)
44. de Weck (1971)
45. Pepys (1973)
46. Vannier and Campbell (1959)

[b] Publications cited are mainly those that add significant additional information to that discussed in the review articles.

[c] References discussing the allergenicity of chlorogenic acid.

TABLE III

Source	Name of fraction	Methods used in purification[a]	Analytical techniques[b]	Pure by criteria[b]	Percent proportion of allergen in source (dry)	
					Theoretical[c]	[Exp. yield]
Pollens						
Gramineae (grasses)						
Lolium perenne (perennial rye)	Group I[e]	Dialysis; DEAE-C; G-75; G-100	b, c, e–j, l, n, p–v	b, c, f–j, q, r	0.63	[0.10]
	Group II	Dialysis; DEAE-C; G-75; G-100	b, c, g–j, l, p–s, u, v	b, c, g, h, q, r, s, u	—	[0.03]
	Group III	Dialysis; DEAE-C; G-75; G-100	c, g–j, q, r, u, v	c, q, r, u	—	[0.03]
Phleum pratense (timothy)	AgB	Salt pptn; EtOH pptn; dialysis; DEAE-C	b, c, f, n, q, r, u	b, c, f, q, r	—	[6% of extractable protein]
Dactylis glomerata (orchard)	A antigen	Salt pptn; G-25; DEAE-C; G-100	c, f, q, r, s, v	c, (q, r)[g]	—	[2% of total][h]
Ambrosieae (ragweeds)						
Ambrosia elatior (short ragweed)	AgE[e]	Salt pptn; G-25; DEAE-C; G-100; TEAE-C	a–c, e–g, j–n, r, s–u	a–c, e, f, g, r	0.48[f] (0.26)	[0.078]
	AgK[e]	Salt pptn; G-25; DEAE-C; G-100; TEAE-C	a, c, e, f, l, n, r, s, u	a, c, e, f, g, r	(0.12)	[0.011]
	Ra3[e]	Salt pptn; G-25; DEAE-C; CM-C; G-50	a–c, f, k–n, q–s, u–w	a, b, c, f, k, m, q–s, u–w	0.081[f]	[0.010]
	Ra5	Salt pptn; DEAE-C CM-S; G-50; P-10	a–c, f, k–n, r, s, u	a, b, c, f, k, m, r, s, u (crystallizes)	0.032[f]	[0.0015][i]
	BPA-R	Salt pptn; G-25; DEAE-C; G-100; CM-S	a, b, c, f, n, q, r, u	a, b, c, f, q, r	(ca. 0.1)	[0.012]
Other						
Ricinus communis (castor bean)	(CB-1A)E	EtOH & PbAc$_2$ pptn; dialysis; EtOH pptn	b, f, l, n, q, r, u	2 ags; 4–5 related elec. cpts.	—	[1.3]
Ascaris suum	Asc-1	Dialysis; G-200; PVC-elec.	a–f, l, n, p–r	a–f, p–r	—	[—]
Gadus callarias (cod: muscle)	M	Dialysis; DEAE-C; G-75; crystn; isoelec. focusing	b, c, e, f, l, n, q, r, t–v	b, c, f, (q, r)[g] (crystallizes)	ca. 0.05–0.1	[0.025]
Ovomucoid (hen: egg white)	VE54B	TCA and EtOH pptn; P-C	b, g, h, l–n, q, r, v	b, g, h, q, r	10–12	[1.8–3.4]
Equus caballus (horse: dander)	b$_2$	Salt pptn; crystn; starch elec.	b, n, q, r, t, v	(q, r)[g]	—	[ca. 7]
Apis mellifica (honey bee venom)	Phospholipase A	Dialysis; G-50; SE-S (3x)	b, c, e–g, i, k–n, r, s, x	b, c, e–g, i, k–m, i (crystallizes)	ca. 15	[2.0]

[a] Abbreviations: DEAE-C, diethylaminoethyl-cellulose; TEAE-C, triethylaminoethyl-cellulose; CM-C, carboxymethyl-cellulose; P-C, phosphate-cellulose; CM-S, carboxymethyl Sephadex; G-25–G-200, Sephadex xerogels; P-10, Biogel xerogel; TCA, trichloroacetic acid; PVC, polyvinyl chloride; NAMA, N-acetylneuraminic acid. [b] For explanation of letter designations, see Table 1. [c] Values determined by less precise methodology cited in parentheses. [d] pI's of isoallergens cited where available. [e] Main isoallergenic variants isolated in a highly purified state. [f] Determined by radial immunodiffusion analy-

Purification and Properties of Some Highly Purified Naturally Occurring Allergens

Percent nitrogen	Percent carbohydrate (principal constituents)	s_{20}^{0} (Svedbergs)	MW^{b,c} (daltons)	pI^d	$E_{1\,cm}^{1\%}$	Principal references
13.3	5.4 (Gal, Man.)	2.89	27,000(1) (32,000(b))	B: 5.25 C: 5.15	15.1	Johnson and Marsh (1965a,b, 1966a,b); Marsh et al. (1966, 1970a); D. G. Marsh (unpublished)
—	—	1.36	11,000(b)	Acidic	10.3	
—	—	—	11,000(c)	Basic	10.6	
14	12.7	1.4	10,500(b) 16,000(c))	Acidic	—	Malley and Dobson (1966); Malley and Harris (1967)
—	—	—	ca. 56,000(c) (88,000)^i	Basic	—	O'Sullivan (1968)
17.1	0.2^j (Ara)	3.05	37,800(a)	B: 5.1 C: 5.0	11.3	King and Norman (1962); King et al. (1964, 1967a)
16.6	<0.6^j (Ara)	—	38,200(a)	A: 5.9	14.8	King (1972)
17.7	7.2 (Ara)	1.72	11,000(a)	8.5	13.1	Underdown and Goodfriend (1969); M. Roebber and L. Goodfriend (personal communication, 1973)
15.8	0.0	—	5,000(a)	9.6	26.3	Lapkoff and Goodfriend (1974); Marsh et al. (1973a)
—	—	—	30,000(a) (28,000(c))	Basic	—	Griffiths and Brunet (1971); M. Roebber and L. Goodfriend (personal communication, 1973)
16.6	5.7	1.98	—	Basic	—	Spies and Coulson (1943, 1964); Morris et al. (1965)
—	8.6	1.86	17,000(a) 18,200(1)	4.8–5.0	—	Hussain et al. (1973)
14.5–14.9	1.46 (Rib, Gal, Man, Glc)	2.11	16,200(b)	4.75	6.0	Aas (1967); Elsayed and Aas (1970, 1971a,b); Elsayed et al. (1971)
13.2	22.9 (Gal, Man, NAc-Glc, NAMA)	2.62	31,500(b)	4.1–4.4	4.1	Bleumink and Young (1969, 1971); Deutsch and Morton (1961)
10.2	9.2 (Gal, Man, NAc, Glc, Fuc)	3.4	34,000^k	4.1	—	Stanworth (1957, 1963)
—	Variable	2.79	19,500(c, k) 14,629(m)	10.5 ± 1.0	—	Shipolini et al. (1971a,b)

sis or radioimmunoassay (in the case of Ra5) on whole (nondefatted) extracts, using appropriate monospecific antisera and antigen standards (Marsh, 1975a). ^{g} Evidence for possible trace impurities with one or more antisera. ^{h} Approximate yield relative to total A antigen content was determined by immunodiffusion analysis. ^{i} Determined by an immunodiffusion method. ^{j} Considered to be contaminants by the authors. ^{k} Osmotic pressure method. ^{l} Using a modified technique yields were increased to 0.01% (Roebber et al., 1975).

Malley and associates (Malley et al., 1962, 1964a,b; Malley and Dobson, 1966; Malley and Harris, 1967) reported the isolation of two further timothy pollen allergens, AgA* and AgB. They also obtained a low molecular weight fraction, AgD, which they believe possesses hapten-like properties (discussed in Section IV,D). The isolation of these fractions was achieved by conventional means, with the exception of their using a phosphate buffer of surprisingly high pH (10.4) for extraction and subsequent fractionation steps.

Immunodiffusion analysis revealed that antigens A and B were partially related; AgA was somewhat impure but AgB was homogeneous by this criterion (see Table III for further analytical details). Antigen B of similar purity, and antigenically identical, to Malley's preparation has also been prepared (by conventional extraction and chromatographic procedures) in the author's laboratory and by B. L. Overell and associates at Bencard Laboratories in England (unpublished observations). A. Malley (personal communication, 1973) reported that AgB consists of three isoallergenic variants; similar results were obtained in the author's laboratory (Marsh, 1974). Malley's antigens A and B had sedimentation coefficients, s_{20}^0, of 2.7 S and 1.4 S, respectively. A molecular weight for AgB of 10,500 was reported by Malley and Harris (1967) using sedimentation-diffusion analysis; a somewhat higher value of 16,000 was obtained by D. G. Marsh (unpublished) by gel filtration on a calibrated Sephadex G-75 column. Although predominantly protein in nature, certain preparations of antigens A and B have been reported to contain carbohydrate and flavanoid pigment.

By intradermal skin test, antigens A and B were found to give positive reactions down to 10^{-7} µg/ml in grass-allergic subjects. Skin reactivity was maintained after exposing the allergens to buffers of pH 4–10.5 (Malley et al., 1962). A quantitative comparison of the skin sensitivities of highly grass-allergic people to AgB and rye Group I (see below) made in the author's laboratory revealed that only 6/13 (42%) of highly Group I-sensitive people were also highly sensitive to AgB (examples cited in Table III). However, a few weakly grass-sensitive people had low sensitivity to AgB in the absence of sensitivity to Group I.†

Three highly purified allergens, Groups I, II, and III, have been isolated from the pollen of *Lolium perenne* (perennial rye grass) by

---

* The A antigen of orchard should not be confused with timothy Antigen A (AgA).

† A two-plus skin reaction at an allergen concentration of 10^{-3} µg/ml or less for a 0.05 ml intradermal injection was taken to indicate high sensitivity and a reaction at 10^{-2} or 10^{-1} µg/ml as low sensitivity.

4. Allergens and the Genetics of Allergy

Marsh and associates (Johnson and Marsh, 1965a,b, 1966a,b; Marsh et al., 1966, 1970a; Marsh and Haddad, 1968; Marsh, 1974: Fig. 1, Table III). A further partially purified fraction, Group IV, which is probably similar to the A antigen of orchard grass pollen, has also been isolated. All of these fractions are antigenically and allergenically distinct from one another and from timothy AgB (Figs. 2–4).

The Group I rye grass allergen consists of four isoallergenic variants (Section III), denoted as I-A, I-B, I-C, and I-D, in the order of decreasing pI value (Johnson and Marsh, 1965b). Highly purified specimens of the principal subcomponents I-B and I-C (pI = 5.25 and 5.15, P. L. Black and D. G. Marsh, unpublished) differ only

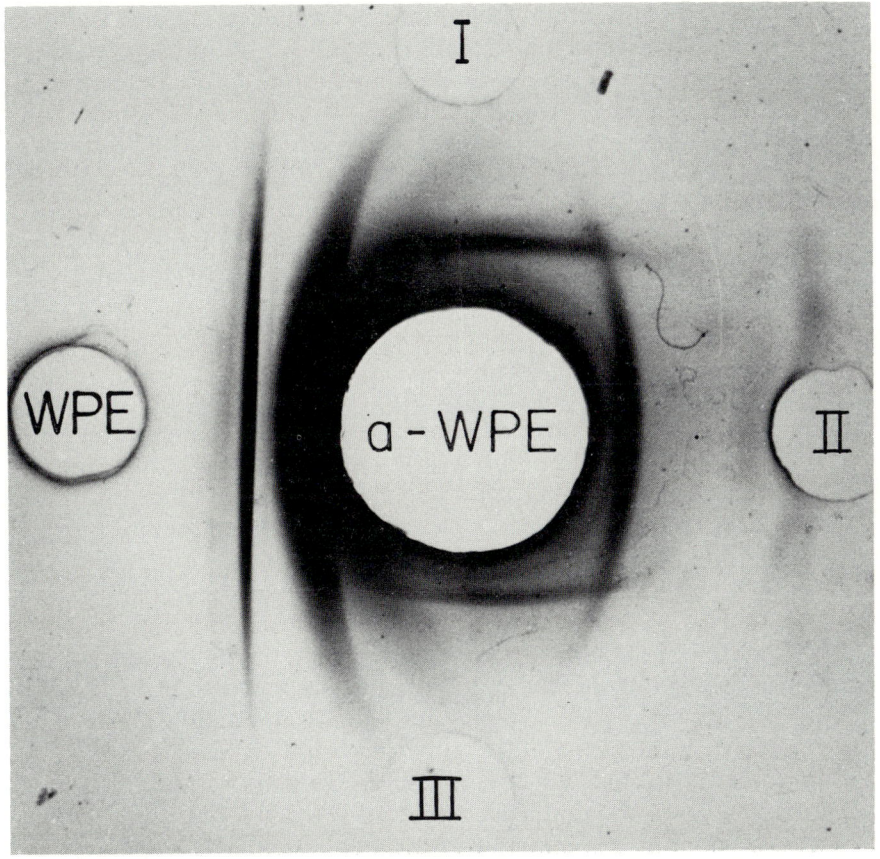

Fig. 4. Immunodiffusion analysis of highly purified rye Groups I, II and III and dialyzed whole rye pollen extract (WPE) against a pooled anti-whole pollen extract (a-WPE). Note the single lines of nonidentity between the three purified antigens.

slightly in their amino acid analyses (Table IV) and tryptic and chymotryptic "fingerprints." The analysis is not yet sufficiently precise to discern whether these minor differences are allotypic or result from deamidation. Both Group II and Group III allergens exist in at least two isoallergenic A and B forms.

Highly purified specimens of rye I-B and I-C (in an early publication termed α and β) are known to be proteins (MW 27,000), containing about 5% carbohydrate which consist mainly of mannose and galactose. Confirmed digestion of I-B with cellulase or β-galactosidase does not reduce the allergenic activity of the molecule which, together with other evidence discussed by Marsh et al. (1966), tends to rule out the possibility that the carbohydrate moiety constitutes an *important* allergenic determinant. On the other hand, complete proteolytic digestion of I-B or I-C completely destroys allergenicity, antigenicity, and hapten-like inhibitory activity. This shows that the protein structure is involved in important immunologic determinants and suggests that portions of the three-dimensional protein structure probably constitute the principal determinants. This conclusion is also supported by preliminary chemical modification studies (Johnson and Marsh, 1966b). In other studies it was found that proteolytic degradation of rye Group II-B (MW 11,000) also destroys allergenicity. The stabilities of rye Group III (MW 11,000) and Group IV (MW ca. 50,000) toward enzymatic degradation have not yet been studied.

Although Group I is remarkably susceptible to proteolytic digestion, it retains its antigenic and allergenic properties after boiling for 30 minutes in neutral solution. Crude rye pollen extract also seems to be quite stable allergenically to heating, as well as to exposure to buffers of pH 3 and 10 (Marsh et al., 1966), suggesting that physically labile allergens such as Group IV do not contribute substantially to the overall biologic activity of the pollen (cf. Augustin, 1959b).

The skin and leukocyte sensitivities of over 250 highly grass pollen allergic individuals to rye Group I have been studied by the author and by Lichtenstein and Norman in the course of studies of pollen allergy; over 95% of these individuals are highly sensitive to rye Group I. In a study of 60 highly grass-sensitive patients, only 2 were much more sensitive to a mixed crude grass extract* than rye Group I. A highly significant association ($p < 0.001$) was found between patients' leukocyte sensitivities to mixed grass and to

* A dialyzed extract of the pollens *Phleum pratense* (timothy), *Dactylis glomerata* (orchard), *Anthoxanthum odoratum* (sweet vernal), *Agrostis alba* (red top), and *Poa pratensis* (june) in the ratios of 3:3:2:1:1.

4. Allergens and the Genetics of Allergy

TABLE IV
Amino Acid Analyses of Some Highly Purified Allergens[a,b]

Amino acid	Lolium perenne (rye)			Ambrosia elatior (short ragweed)					Ascaris suum	Gadus callarias (cod)	Apis mellifica (honey bee) Phospholipase A[c]
	I-B	I-C	AgE-B	AgE-C	AgK-A	Ra3	Ra5[c,d]		Asc-1	M	
Lys	26 11.2	26 11.2	18 5.3	18 5.2	16 4.8	7 6.9	4 8.9		17 12.0	12 10.5	11 8.5
His	3 1.3	3 1.3	6 1.8	6 1.7	11 3.3	3 3.0	0 0.0		6 4.2	1 0.9	6 4.7
Arg	6 2.6	6 2.6	16 4.7	16 4.7	15 4.5	4 4.0	2 4.4		3 2.1	1 0.9	6 4.7
Asx	26 11.2	26 11.2	48 14.2	49 14.3	44 13.3	7 6.9	2 4.4		16 11.3	13 11.4	16 12.4
Thr	17 7.3	16 6.9	17 5.0	18 5.2	22 6.6	8 7.9	0 0.0		7 4.9	1 0.9	10 7.8
Ser	12 5.2	11 4.7	25 7.4	26 7.6	17 5.1	5 5.0	4 8.9		7 4.9	6 5.3	10 7.8
Glx	20 8.9	20 8.9	25 7.4	25 7.3	29 8.8	8 7.9	4 8.9		18 12.8	10 8.8	6 4.7
Pro	13 5.6	14 6.0	15 4.5	15 4.4	16 4.8	10 9.9	3 6.7		6 4.2	10 8.8	5 3.9
Gly	28 12.0	27 11.6	37 10.8	38 11.1	32 9.7	8[c] 7.9	4 8.9		11 7.7	10 8.8	11 8.5
Ala	18 7.7	18 7.7	30 8.9	31 9.0	21 6.3	6 5.9	3 6.7		15 10.7	20 17.5	4 3.1
Half-Cys	6 2.6	6 2.6	7 2.1	7 2.0	9 2.7	3 3.0	8 17.8		0 0.0	1 0.9	8 6.2
Val	14 6.0	14 6.0	23 6.8	24 7.0	23 6.9	6 5.9	4 8.9		9 6.3	7 6.1	5 3.9
Met	2 0.8	2 0.8	7 2.1	7 2.0	9 2.7	1 1.0	0 0.0		0 0.0	1 0.9	3 2.3
Ile	10[e] 4.3	10[e] 4.3	20 5.9	20 5.8	22 6.6	4 4.0	1[e] 2.2		6 4.2	5 4.4	4[e] 3.1
Leu	9 3.9	11 4.7	21 6.2	21 6.1	17 5.1	8 7.9	1 2.2		14 9.6	4 3.5	9 7.0
Tyr	9 3.9	9 3.9	4 1.2	4 1.2	6 1.8	2 2.0	3 6.7		3 2.1	1 0.9	8 6.2
Phe	8 3.4	8 3.4	12 3.6	12 3.5	13 3.9	7 6.9	0 0.0		4 2.8	10 8.8	5 3.9
Trp	6 2.6	6 2.6	6 1.8	6 1.7	9 2.7	4 4.0	2 4.4		0 0.0	1 0.9	2 1.6
Amide	4[f] —	— —	— —	— —	— —	— —	2[f] —		— —	— —	8[f] —
Totals:	233 100.5	233 99.5	337 99.7	343 99.8	331 99.6	101 100.0	45 100.0		142 99.8	114 100.2	129 100.3

[a] Data from Johnson and Marsh (1966a), King et al. (1964, 1967a), Underdown and Goodfriend (1969), Mole et al. (1974), Hussain et al. (1973), Elsayed et al. (1971), and Shipolini et al. (1971b).
[b] The values in regular type are the numbers of each amino acid residue per molecule to the nearest integer, and the values in heavy type are the proportion of each residue per 100 amino acid residues in the protein.
[c] Data derived from amino acid sequence.
[d] A different isoallergenic form of Ra5 contains a substitution of Leu for Val.
[e] N-terminal amino acid where known. No N-terminal could be detected in the case of AgE.
[f] Amide content omitted from total.

Group I (Norman and Lichtenstein, 1973). Group I allergen is rapidly released on extracting native rye and other grass pollens (Section V,C). Also, Group I components that strongly cross-react antigenically and allergenically with rye Group I are found in many grass pollens important in hay fever in temperate regions of the world (Marsh *et al.*, 1970a; Baer *et al.*, 1974). There is, therefore, good reason to believe that Group I components are the major allergens in many grass pollens. Notable exceptions to this rule include members of the subfamily Panicoideae and the tribes Chlorideae (includes *Cynodon dactylon*, bermuda) and Andropogoneae, which are most abundantly found in warmer climates.

A study of 75 unrelated highly grass allergic individuals (D. G. Marsh, unpublished) revealed that 45 (60%) were either more sensitive or similarly sensitive to rye Group II relative to rye Group I. This percentage is similar to preliminary estimates made by Marsh *et al.* (1966, 1970a). Of 61 such subjects studied, 43 (70%) were similarly or more sensitive to Group III than Group I. A much smaller proportion of Group I-sensitive subjects (10/50; 20%) were found to be sensitive to rye Group IV.

There was no evidence for cross-allergenicity or cross-antigenicity between any of the four rye groups or timothy AgB (Marsh *et al.*, 1966, 1970a; Lichtenstein *et al.*, 1969; Marsh, 1974; D. G. Marsh, unpublished; Figs. 2–4). Detailed study of the cross-allergenicity and cross-antigenicity between rye and six other grasses clearly showed that groups of allergens, which strongly cross-react to differing degrees with rye Groups I, II and III, exist in several other temperate grasses. This finding was confirmed in a preliminary physicochemical comparison of the Groups I, II, and III components of rye, fescue, and timothy grass pollens (Marsh and Haddad, 1968).

b. Weed. Almost all abundantly found, wind-pollinated weeds have been implicated in pollen allergy (cf. Sherman, 1968; Wodehouse, 1971). Particularly common families of weeds causing hay fever in the United States and/or Western Europe are Compositae (includes: Ambrosieae, ragweeds, cockleburs, marshelders; Anthemideae, artemisias), Amaranthaceae (pigweeds, water-hemps), Chenopodiaceae (chenopods, salt bushes, Russian thistle), Plantaginaceae (plantains), and Urticaceae (nettles). The most extensively studied allergenic complex is the pollen of *Ambrosia elatior* (short ragweed) which will be considered here in detail. Pollen of the closely related species *Ambrosia trifida* (giant ragweed) has also been studied to some extent (Goldfarb, 1964). Pollen of *Parietaria officinalis* (great nettle), known to be a common allergy-causing agent in the Mediterranean area, has been studied in a preliminary manner by Crifó and Iannetti (1969).

Extracts of various pollens from the botanically related families Amaranthaceae and Chenopodiaceae have been found to be partially related antigenically (Wodehouse, 1957). Using a double antibody radioimmunoassay, Yunginger and Gleich (1972) found components partially related antigenically to antigen E (an important allergen of short ragweed) in commercial pollen extracts of several members of the Compositae family, particularly *Ambrosia trifida* (giant ragweed) and *Ambrosia psilostachya* (western ragweed). These workers also found components in *Franseria acanthicarpa* (false ragweed), *Ambrosia bidentata* (southern ragweed), and *Xanthium commune* (cocklebur) which cross-reacted slightly with AgE.

There are at least 14 antigens in short ragweed pollen extract (Gussoni, 1966). Twenty or more protein bands have been detected by isoelectric focusing (King, 1972; Fig. 5). An important protein allergen, antigen E (AgE), was first isolated by King and Norman (1962); other workers (Callaghan and Goldfarb, 1962; Robbins *et al.*, 1966) isolated fractions which were antigenically identical and physicochemically similar to AgE, although slightly less pure. In subsequent work King *et al.* (1964) found that AgE consisted of two major (IV-B and IV-C) and two minor (IV-A and IV-D) closely related isoallergenic variants (Fig. 4; cf. rye Group I). King and associates reported molecular weights of 37,800 for each of the highly purified IV-B and IV-C variants. The two isoallergens also had very similar amino acid analyses (Table IV). Further physicochemical data is presented in Table III.

King *et al.* (1964) reported that removal of AgE from whole ragweed pollen extract by precipitation with specific rabbit anti-AgE serum removed at least 90% of the allergenic activity of the whole extract. This study and later work suggest that AgE is the major allergen of ragweed pollen, but this conclusion now needs to be reevaluated in the light of recent studies on the release of allergenic components from ragweed pollen grains (Section V,B).

Unlike most grass pollen allergens, AgE is very unstable toward physical denaturation, including lyophilization, heating, 8 M urea treatment, and exposure to buffers outside the range of pH 6–8.5 (King *et al.*, 1964). This instability arises since the AgE molecule is comprised of two fragments, α (MW 21,800) and β (MW 15,700), held together by physical interaction (Griffiths, 1972; King *et al.*, 1974; King, 1974). Under appropriate denaturing conditions the molecule

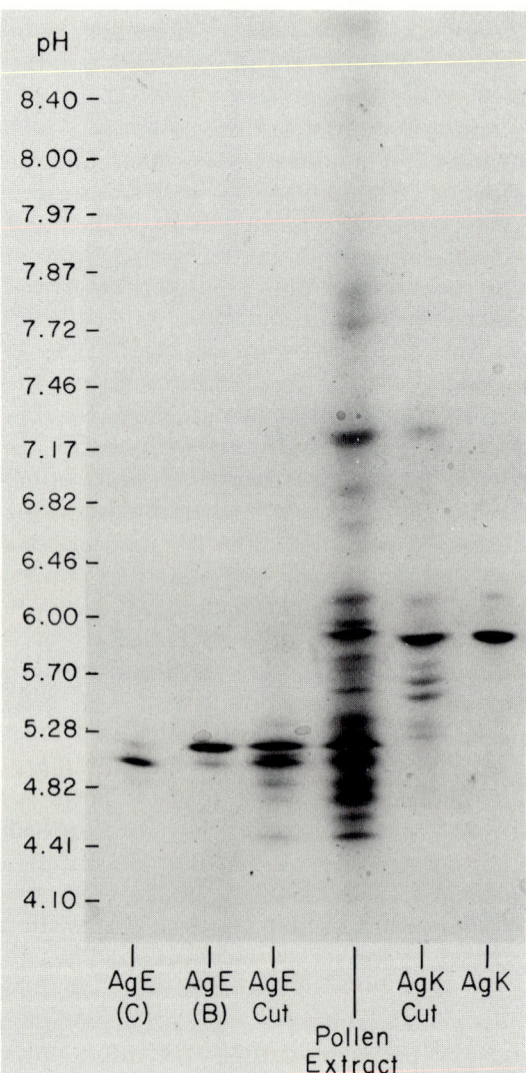

Fig. 5. Isoelectric focusing of ragweed antigens on polyacrylamide gel containing 31% glycerin. The amounts of the combined isoallergenic forms of antigens E and K and of whole ragweed pollen extract (WPE) (shown in the center of the gel) were equivalent to 100 mg of pollen. (From King, 1972, by permission of author and copyright owners.)

breaks apart and subsequently polymerizes, resulting in almost complete loss of biologic activity. The AgE molecule is, however, unusually resistant toward digestion by trypsin, chymotrypsin, or papain at neutral pH, although it is inactivated by pepsin at pH 2 and by the bacterial protease, Nagarse (King et al., 1967b).

Acetylation or succinylation of AgE yields single major derivatives in which two-thirds of the lysine residues are modified (King et al., 1967b). Although the electric charge of the molecule is dramatically altered by this treatment, surprisingly only a 10- to 100-fold loss in allergenicity occurs. Similarly, only a 5- to 20-fold loss in allergenicity occurs if about 50% of the carboxyl groups are discharged by modification with glycinamide or taurine (King et al., 1974). An even more surprising finding is that butyrimidation of 16/18 lysine amino groups of AgE (which produces minimal alteration in electric charge) causes no detectable loss in the allergenic or antigenic properties of the molecule, despite introduction of the bulky butyrimidinyl residues. More extensive substitution of the amino or carboxyl groups or complete reduction and carboxylmethylation of the disulfide bonds of AgE result in almost complete loss of allergenicity and antigenicity. These studies suggest that readily accessible amino and carboxyl groups are not directly involved in the principal immunologic determinants of AgE. However, ionized groups are necessary to retain the native conformation and full biologic activity of the molecule.

King and associates (1967a,b) have also reported the isolation from ragweed of a further highly purified allergen, AgK (MW 38,200), a protein that is partially related antigenically and allergenically to AgE. Like AgE, AgK possesses several isoallergenic forms, the main one being V-A. Analytical details are presented in Tables III and IV and Fig. 5. Based on a quantitative comparison of antigens E and K by leukocyte and intradermal skin test assays, King and associates concluded that AgK was, on average, one-half as potent allergenically as AgE. However, the presence of some unique allergenic determinants on both molecules was evident from the finding that a few patients were either much more, or somewhat less, sensitive to AgE than AgK. These workers concluded that AgK was the second most potent allergen in ragweed pollen.

Goodfriend and collaborators (Underdown and Goodfriend, 1969; M. Roebber and L. Goodfriend, 1970, personal communication, 1973; Lapkoff and Goodfriend, 1974) have studied three basic allergens from ragweed pollen. Allergens Ra3 and Ra5 were isolated in their laboratory; a further fraction, BPA-R, was originally isolated by

Griffiths and Brunet (1971). All three allergens have been obtained in a highly purified state (Tables III and IV). Beside having much more basic isoelectric points than AgE and AgK, these allergens have considerably lower molecular weights (Table III). Component Ra3 is the only purified ragweed component that possesses a substantial carbohydrate moiety (7.2%); other isoallergenic variants of Ra3 possess different proportions of carbohydrate (M. Roebber and L. Goodfriend, 1970, personal communication, 1973).

Allergen Ra5 is of particular importance in genetic studies of allergy (Section VI,B) because of its very simple molecular structure (MW 5000; 45 amino acids). The complete amino acid sequence of Ra5 is now available (Mole et al., 1974; Fig. 6) which will greatly facilitate studies of the chemical nature of its allergenic/antigenic determinants. The molecule possesses an unusually large proportion of half-cystine residues which constitute four disulfide bonds. The cross-linking probably results in a rather rigid three-dimensional structure which may well enhance the immunogenicity of the molecule. The relatively high proportion of the aromatic amino acids tyrosine and tryptophan may also contribute significantly to the immunogenicity of Ra5 (cf. Sela, 1969; Gill, 1972). Of further interest is the finding that Ra5 exists in two different isoallergenic forms; about 30% of the sample of Ra5 sequenced has a substitution of leucine for valine at position 2. Not surprisingly, it has been impossible to distinguish the two forms immunochemically or to separate them by physical techniques such as isoelectric focusing.

Allergens Ra3 and Ra5 are not related immunologically, either to each other or to other isolated ragweed allergens (Lichtenstein et al., 1973a; Marsh et al., 1973a; M. Roebber and L. Goodfriend, personal communication, 1973; Lapkoff and Goodfriend, 1974). Allergen BPA-R, on the other hand, is partially related to AgE (Griffiths and Brunet, 1971; M. Roebber and L. Goodfriend, personal communication, 1973).

```
          1   2   3   4   5   6   7   8   9  10  11  12  13  14
    H2N-Leu Val Pro Cys Ala Trp Ala Gly Asn Val Cys Gly Glu Lys
            Leu

         15  16  17  18  19  20  21  22  23  24  25  26  27  28  29
        Arg Ala Tyr Cys Cys Ser Asp Pro Gly Arg Tyr Cys Pro Trp Gln

         30  31  32  33  34  35  36  37  38  39  40  41  42  43  44  45
        Val Val Cys Tyr Glu Ser Ser Glu Ile Cys Ser Lys Lys Cys Gly Lys-COOH
```

Fig. 6. Amino acid sequence of allergen Ra5 isolated from the pollen of *Ambrosia elatior* (short ragweed). (From Mole et al., 1974.) All half-cystines are known to be involved in disulfide bonds, the position of which is currently being determined.

When sensitivities to minor allergens Ra3 and Ra5 were investigated in populations of highly ragweed-allergic individuals who were also sensitive to AgE (two-plus intradermal skin test at 10^{-2} μg/ml or lower, or 50% histamine release at 10^{-2} μg/ml or lower), the following data were obtained: 65/127 (51%) individuals possessed Ra3/AgE sensitivity weight ratios of 10 or less (molar ratios of ≤35) and 18/105 (17%) individuals possessed Ra5/AgE sensitivity weight ratios of 10 or less (molar ratios of ≤76) (Marsh et al., 1973a, 1975b). Such individuals would generally be regarded as being relatively highly sensitive to the minor allergens Ra3 and Ra5. Despite the structural simplicity of these allergens relative to AgE, in the aforementioned populations 9% were more sensitive to Ra3 than AgE, and 8% (half of the Ra5 sensitive group) were more sensitive to Ra5 than AgE, based on *molar* sensitivity ratios. These ratios are probably low estimates since the populations were selected for high sensitivity to AgE. It is of special interest to note that reactivity to Ra5 tends to occur in an "all-or-none" fashion, suggesting that responsiveness to Ra5 may be under a relatively simple genetic control (Section VI,B). The allergenicity of BPA-R has not yet been thoroughly studied. Comparative data on the skin sensitivities of six unselected allergic individuals to purified ragweed and grass pollen allergens are presented in Fig. 3.

The aforementioned components by no means represent the total allergenic picture for short ragweed. King and Norman (1962) obtained a partially purified acidic fraction, VI_2A (MW ca. 10,000), which was antigenically unrelated to AgE (and probably to the aforementioned basic allergens). Only 16% (4/26) of AgE-sensitive subjects were as sensitive to VI_2A as to AgE. Goldfarb (1968) isolated 16 partially purified, poorly characterized skin reactive fractions by brief (1½ hours at 4°) extraction of nondefatted ragweed pollen. Analysis revealed that three fractions, B4a, B4b, and B1c, which contained little if any AgE, were much more allergenic than other fractions that were rich in AgE. On this basis, Goldfarb questioned the significance of AgE as the only major allergen. Fraction Blc, which contains three basic antigens, is of particular interest since Marsh *et al.* (1975a) have recently observed that certain highly allergenic ragweed components, which are most rapidly eluted from ragweed pollen, are predominantly basic in nature and contain relatively little AgE (see Section V,B for further discussion).

c. *Tree.* Many trees are wind-pollinated and shed prolific amounts of pollen. However, due to shorter pollination seasons and less widespread abundance of individual species, allergy to tree pollens is not as important clinically as allergy to grass or weed pollens, except in certain areas (e.g., birch pollen allergy in Scandinavia). Some antigenic and allergenic cross-reactivity has been found between pollens from members of the same tree family (Rackemann and Wagner, 1936; Segal et al., 1970; Belin, 1972a).

Relatively few attempts have been made to isolate highly purified tree pollen allergens. Herbertson et al. (1958) obtained a partially purified, highly allergenic "B fraction" from the pollen of *Alnus glutenosa* (alder) by chromatography on TEAE- and SE-celluloses. The allergen contained only peptide and pigment and was highly resistant to heat treatment. Belin and Rowley (1971) and Belin (1972 a,b) have more recently studied the allergens of *Betula verrucosa* (birch) pollen. Partially purified preparations of the major allergen were obtained either by Sephadex G-100 or DEAE-cellulose chromatography. By gel-filtration analysis, the molecular weight of the allergen was estimated to be about 20,000. Like the (related?) alder fraction of Herbertson, the birch allergen was thermostable; after heating in neutral solution at 100° for 15–30 minutes, the principal antigen that remained was found to be the major allergen. Of further interest is the observation that this component is extracted from the pollen much more rapidly than other less important allergens (Belin and Rowley, 1971; Belin, 1972a; cf. Section V,B).

3. OTHER ALLERGENS

a. Codfish. First, special mention should be made of the work of Aas and associates (reviewed by Aas, 1974) into the structure and reactivity of the major allergenic fraction, DS 22, from the white muscle of *Gadus callarias* (codfish), an important food allergen in Scandinavia. Using a combination of DEAE-cellulose chromatography, gel filtration, and isoelectricfocusing, these workers were able to isolate several DS 22 subfractions which possessed very similar antigenic and allergenic properties (Elsayed and Aas, 1971a). Their most highly purified subfraction (allergen M), an acidic glycoprotein of MW 16,200, has been studied in great detail (Tables III and IV) and is currently being amino acid sequenced (Aas, 1974). Although physicochemically homogeneous, allergen M gave one major and two minor precipitin bands on immunodiffusion analysis, which is believed to be an artifact (Elsayed and Aas, 1971a).

The different DS 22 components contain amounts of carbohydrate varying from 0.0–1.5%; they also differ in amino acid composition and have significantly different molecular weights (Elsayed et al., 1971). It is of interest that a DS 22 fraction, having an isoelectric point of 4.85 and possessing 28 amino acids, is completely free of carbohydrate, from which the authors deduce that this moiety has "no direct influence" on the allergenic potency of the DS 22 proteins. Allergen and related components are highly biologically active in codfish allergic patients by direct skin and inhalation tests, as well as by passive transfer (P–K) of the serum from fish allergic individuals to nonallergic donors (Aas and Elsayed, 1969; Elsayed and Aas, 1970). Enzymatic removal of the N-terminal (Arg) and/or the C-terminal (Asp, Glu, and Arg) amino acids causes no detectable loss in allergenic or antigenic activity of fraction DS 22; partial loss in immunologic potency occurs following partial proteolytic degradation and complete loss of activity occurs after extensive digestion with most proteolytic enzymes (Aas and Elsayed, 1969). These results are compatible with the major allergenic determinants of the DS 22 fraction comprising portions of the tertiary and quaternary structure of the protein moieties. Further physicochemical and immunologic studies with allergen M and other related DS 22 fractions will undoubtedly prove valuable in elucidating the mechanism of IgE-mediated sensitivity to food allergens.

b. Ascaris. The work of Strejan and associates (Strejan *et al.*, 1973; Hussain *et al.*, 1973) into allergenic components from *Ascaris suum*, a helminthic intestinal parasite that infests swine, also deserve special mention. Strejan's research is important in that he is attempting to work out an animal (rat) model for studying a member of a large group of parasitic allergens which are known to be potent inducers of IgE antibody formation in animals and man (Ambler and Orr, 1972; Phills *et al.*, 1972; Strejan *et al.*, 1973; Hogarth-Scott *et al.*, 1973; Bradbury *et al.*, 1974). Parasitic infestations characteristically give rise to extremely high total IgE levels which can reach as high as 100 μg/ml in the rat (H. Metzger, personal communication) and over 10 μg/ml in man (Johansson *et al.*, 1968); total IgE levels, in nonallergic man are typically 50–250 ng/ml).

Strejan and associates found one component, Asc-1, to be a particularly potent inducer of IgE antibody formation in Sprague-Dawley rats; it was also highly reactogenic in rats sensitized by previous injection of ascaris extract (plus *B. pertussis* adjuvant) or infestation with ascaris. Strejan and associates were particularly thorough in establishing the high degree of homogeneity of Asc-1. They used a wide variety of techniques including the Laurell crossed immunoelectrophoresis method (Minchin Clarke and Freeman, 1966). The molecular weight of Asc-1 was found to be 17,000–19,000 using a variety of different techniques (cf. Table III). A closely related fraction, G50-D2 (MW ca. 10,000), which gives a reaction of antigenic identity with Asc-1 is thought not to be immunogenic in Sprague-Dawley rats, but is highly potent reactogenically in ascaris-sensitized rats (Strejan *et al.*, 1973). It is believed that component G50-D2 might be the monomeric form of Asc-1 (Hussain *et al.*, 1973). This is supported by the finding that Asc-1 dissociates into subunits of MW ca. 8400 in sodium dodecyl sulfate (SDS). It is also interesting to note that Asc-1 appears to be present at all stages of the life cycle of the parasite (Bradbury *et al.*, 1974).

In other work, Strejan *et al.* (1973) have extensively studied the kinetics of induction of IgE and IgG antibody in rats and, more recently, Patrucco and Marsh (1974) have studied the genetics of antibody production to Asc-1 $(DNP)_4$ in inbred mice (Section IV,D). A low molecular weight trypsin inhibitor has also been isolated from ascaris (Fraefel and Acher, 1968). This component is completely sequenced and contains only 66 amino acid residues (MW 7180). It may well turn out to be an interesting allergen.

c. Hymenoptera Venoms. Recent work on allergy to Hymenoptera (bee, wasp, etc.) venoms has established that the anaphylactic reactions following stings are indeed IgE-mediated (Sobotka *et al.*, 1974a; Kern *et al.*, 1974). The major allergen in honey bee venom has been identified by Sobotka *et al.* (1974b) and Elliott *et al.* (1974) as phospholipase A, a highly basic glycoprotein of variable carbohydrate composition which possesses a molecular weight of 19,500 in the monomeric form (Shipolini *et al.*, 1971a). Phospholipase A has been extensively studied in view of its other interesting biologic properties (Habermann, 1972). Recently, detailed physicochemical and amino acid sequence data have been published (Shipolini *et al.*, 1971a,b; Table III). This well-characterized allergen should prove to be a model for studies of injected allergens and improving the immunotherapy of venom allergies. A further bee venom component, mellitin (MW 2840), has been sequenced and synthesized (Habermann, 1972). Mellitin has so far proved to be nonallergenic in several bee-allergic people tested (L. M. Lichtenstein and A. K. Sobotka, personal communication), but it will be of great importance to see whether mellitin-sensitive subjects can be found in the future.

d. Chlorogenic Acid. In 1961, Freedman *et al.* made the surprising announcement that a low molecular weight phenolic constituent of green coffee beans, chlorogenic acid (3-caffeoylquinic acid; MW 354), may be the principal allergen causing sensitivity to green coffee, a common allergy in workers in the coffee industry. This report initiated a heated controversy between the laboratories of Freedman, Sehon, and associates, and those of Layton and associates. Layton *et al.* (1965), having noted the wide occurrence of chlorogenic acid throughout the plant kingdom and in roasted coffee, felt that it was improbable that this compound was an important allergen since allergy toward many natural foodstuffs should be much more widespread than observed clinically. The whole question appears to have been resolved by Layton *et al.* (1966) who showed that commercial chlorogenic acid is contaminated with a small amount of a highly allergenic protein-containing material, and that synthetic or highly purified natural chlorogenic acid is completely nonallergenic in individuals who are highly sensitive to coffee bean extracts. Finally, the nonallergenicity of Layton's samples of chlorogenic acids was also confirmed in an unpublished study by Freedman and associates. The general conclusions were that chlorogenic acid per se was not allergenic; however, the possibility that this compound might act as an allergenic hapten in a small percentage of coffee bean-sensitive individuals could not be completely ruled out.

Important conclusions to be derived from the resolution of this controversy are, first, that ultra-high purity is required to ascertain definitively the allergenic properties of a substance and, second, that many natural allergens are extremely stable—during the isolation of chlorogenic acid, protein-containing allergenic components of coffee beans are carried through several solvent extraction steps without completely losing their activity.

e. Mite and House Dust Allergens. A second controversy has revolved around whether allergen(s) derived from mites of the genus *Dermatophagoides* (particularly *D. pteronyssinus* and *D. farinae*) contribute the major allergens in house dust throughout the world. This question is important since allergy to house dust is probably the most important cause of atopic asthma. Recently, immunotherapy with extracts of *Dermatophagoides* has become fashionable for general treatment of house dust allergy in Europe and Japan. Leading proponents for the overriding role of mite allergens in all house dust allergy include Voorhorst, Spieksma, and associates (Voorhorst *et al.*, 1967; Spieksma and Voorhorst, 1969; Maunsell *et al.*, 1968; Miyamoto *et al.*, 1968). This interpretation has been challenged by Kawai *et al.* (1972) and Marsh and Norman (1974) who found clear evidence that many (although not all) residents of Baltimore, Maryland are principally sensitive to substances in house dust *other* than those derived from *Dermatophagoides*.

The significance of mite allergens in house dust allergy has probably been confused by early reporters finding associations, but failing to present hard evidence of a *causal* relationship, in *large* numbers of dust-allergic people, between allergy to mites and to house dust. In several reports (e.g., Voorhorst et al., 1967; Maunsell et al., 1968) individuals having positive skin tests to house dust were shown to give positive skin tests to mites, without thorough evaluation of the quantitative aspects of each assay and/or of the concentrations of house dust which provoke toxic reactions (see Kawai et al., 1972; Marsh and Norman, 1974). The Baltimore group was unable to find evidence for an important causal association between dust and mite sensitivities (by neutralization of dust-induced histamine release using rabbit anti-mite antibody) except in 1 of 20 dust-sensitive people tested. Furthermore, there was no correlation between sensitivity to mite and to dust allergens as measured either by quantitative histamine release or skin test assays in over 40 dust-allergic individuals. On the other hand, Miyamoto (1974) and Ricci (1974) have recently presented convincing evidence (using RAST inhibition and P-K neutralization assays) for causal association between mite and dust allergy in many Japanese and Italian subjects. Miyamoto, in particular, has presented extensive data showing a close association between the two sensitivities.

The general conclusion to be drawn from this and other data is that the expression of hypersensitivity to house dust is highly complex and multifactorial. Different allergically predisposed individuals develop IgE-mediated sensitivities to widely different degrees to the many possible allergens in house dust depending on (1) the composition of the house dust to which they are exposed (variable from country to country and home to home); (2) the degree and frequency of exposure to dust (i.e., the intensity of the immunization; Section V,A); and (3) the genetic capacity of each individual's IgE-producing system to recognize different house dust components as foreign (Section VI,B). It is, therefore, not surprising to find that allergy to *Dermatophagoides* mites appears to be a significant part of the general house dust allergy picture in areas such as Japan and Italy which have home environments particularly suitable for mite growth (moist, warm climates and little home air conditioning). Conversely, other agents are more important in drier home environments (e.g., U. S. A.). Genetic differences between different populations (e.g., American versus Japanese) and a wide diversity of environmental factors no doubt contribute to the different findings.

C. Theories of Allergenicity

Before the discovery of the role of IgE in atopic allergy, many immunochemists tended to regard allergens and allergenic determinants as a special class apart from antigens and antigenic determinants. This idea can be traced back to the historical view that allergens are a unique subset of antigens (von Pirquet, 1906) and the subsequent findings of Prausnitz and Küstner (1921) and Coca and Cooke (1923) suggesting that these "unique antigens" induce the formation of a unique substance (reagin) which is "no ordinary antibody." These views have, unfortunately, persisted in some quarters up to the present day and have led to the formulation of a number of theories to explain "the unique property of allergens" (Stanworth, 1963, 1973; Berrens, 1971, 1974).

Berrens (1971) has strongly argued that the allergenic activity of a molecule is dependent primarily upon the proportion of N-glycosidically linked sugar residues attached to the ϵ-amino lysines of protein allergens, "optimal specific activity of allergens apparently [being] associated with molecules carrying an optimal proportion of lysine–sugar sites in the reactive Amadori configuration." His view is based mainly on extensive studies of complex allergens isolated from a wide variety of dust, decomposed vegetable and animal components, and other sources, as well as synthetic protein–sugar conjugates containing different proportions of N-glycosidically bound saccharides. Berrens (1974) subsequently went on to elaborate further that such allergens are biologically active through their unusual ability to activate the complement system via a mechanism unlikely to involve IgE.

Berrens' theory seems to fit surprisingly well with impure materials isolated from the various complex allergens and with the synthetic conjugates. The theory fails, however, to explain the exquisite potency of many allergenic substances obtained from pollen, fish, etc., which have no carbohydrate moiety or for which the carbohydrate appears to be unimportant allergenically (Sections IV,B and C); nor does it account for the marked allergenic potency of the highly purified ovomucoid fraction, VE54B [isolated in Berrens' laboratory by his collaborators, Bleumink and Young (1969, 1971; Table III)], which contains carbohydrate but no N-glycosidic linkages. Furthermore, certain protein-free carbohydrates, such as pneumococcal polysaccharides and highly cross-linked dextran, have been shown to be highly allergenic in man (Francis, 1934; Kabat et al., 1957; Section II,B,3). A further major failing is that Berrens' theory does not explain the selectivity of responsiveness of different allergic individuals to different immunochemically distinct allergens isolated from the same allergenic complex. This selectivity is primarily genetic in origin (Section VI).

These objections do not rule out the possibility that N-glycosidic side chains constitute important allergenic determinants in some allergens; but this is clearly not the case for most highly purified allergens so far studied. In his recent publication, Berrens (1974) conceded that the data on pollen and certain other allergens do not fit his original theory. This led him to divide allergens into those that cause perennial symptoms (e.g., dusts), for which he retained his old theory not involving IgE, and those that cause seasonal IgE-mediated allergies (e.g., pollen allergens).

King et al. (1967a,b), Berrens (1971), and Stanworth (1973) have noted that most important allergens are acidic (glyco)proteins with sedimentation coefficients, s_{20}^0, of about 2–4 S. Stanworth (1973) went on to suggest that the notable exceptions of lower molecular weight allergens may well represent "monomeric subunits . . . which re-associate under physiological conditions obtaining in the elicitation of immediate sensitivity reactions." Furthermore, Stanworth speculated that "a dimeric structure is an essential requirement for allergenicity." He argued that duplicate allergenic determinants might be appropriately sighted for the bridging of adjacent cell-bound antibody molecules having the same specificity. Some of Stanworth's proposals contradict experimental data. For example, there have been several reports of acidic *and* basic allergens of MW well below 20,000, which show no tendency to aggregate (e.g., grass Groups II and III, timothy AgB, ragweed Ra3 and Ra5, and codfish allergen M). Furthermore, ragweed AgE tends to disaggregate into fragments of *different* sizes (Griffiths, 1972; King, 1974).

The finding that many allergens are acidic proteins or glycoproteins of MW 20,000–40,000 is not surprising in view of the wide distribution of these compounds in nature and the fact that components of relatively high molecular weight tend to be more immunogenic than compounds of lower molecular weight. The apparent upper molecular weight limit of about 40,000–60,000 for inhaled and ingested allergens might well result from mucosal membranes having a restricted permeability toward higher molecular weight substances (Section V,A). The detailed experimental evidence, particularly for pollen allergens, points to the overriding influence of the genetic capability of the individual's IgE-producing system to recognize the allergen in limiting low dosage (Sections V,A and VI,B). In this regard, the importance of structural features that enhance the immunogenicity of an allergen molecule should not be overlooked. The results of experiments with simple synthetic polypeptide and protein antigens (reviewed by Sela, 1969; Gill, 1972; Borek, 1972) have shown that properties which enhance immunogenicity include (1) high structural complexity, (2) controlled susceptibility toward enzymatic degradation, and (3) the presence of an optimal proportion of immunogenic side chains, particularly aromatic amino acids.

As is the case with most protein antigens, the structurally more complex allergens (e.g., ragweed AgE and grass Group I) are more immunogenic than the less complex allergens (e.g., ragweed Ra5 and grass Group II). This is reflected in the finding that more people are highly sensitive to the more complex than the less complex components. The destruction of the three-dimensional configuration of a protein allergen by proteolytic digestion usually destroys all detectable allergenic properties, due to a loss of immunodominant determinants comprising portions of the exposed secondary and tertiary structure of the molecule (Sections II,B,1 and IV,C; cf. Sela, 1969). Further, recent experiments in inbred mice (Chang and Marsh, 1974) suggest that ragweed AgE, which is not readily degraded by enzymes (Section IV,B,2), is substantially more immunogenic (allergenically and antigenically) than the readily degradable rye Group I allergenic molecule. Despite these observations, the possibility that certain allergenic determinants consist of portions of the primary structure should not be overlooked. In a review of antigen structure, Benjamini *et al.* (1972) report that several antigens are known to possess important sequential (primary structural) determinants.

It seems reasonable to conclude that factors which enhance immunogenicity—in regard to both IgE and IgG antibody production—basically do so by making the conditions of immunization *less limiting*. Thus, as the overall immunogenicity increases, the requirement for an allergic individual to possess a specific immunogenetic constitution becomes less strict and more people develop sensitivity to the allergen (see also Section VI,B).

The above conclusions fit in well with experimental data, and there seems little reason to believe that structural features that are responsible for enhancing the overall immunogenic potency of macromolecules should in any respect differ in regard to whether they stimulate the IgE system or the IgG system. Furthermore, current immunogenetic concepts suggest that the same determinants should be capable of being recognized by both the IgE- and IgG-producing systems of a given allergic individual. Whether this actually happens in practice will depend on the genetic capability of the two systems to respond to the antigenic/allergenic stimulation (Section VI,B,5 and 6), as well as the antigen dosage and frequency and route of immunization (Section V,A).

In any discussion of allergenicity, the apparently unique allergenic potency of components of helminthic parasites (e.g., ascaris) should be raised (cf. Sections II,B,4 and IV,B,3). First, parasitic infestation almost certainly leads to high dosage immunization, which is known to minimize genetic differences in IgE and IgG antibody responsiveness of different mouse strains to complex protein antigens (Levine and Vaz, 1970a; Vaz and Levine, 1970). Second, parasites produce a complex mixture of antigens which should also minimize genetic differences in overall responsiveness. Third, infestation often occurs in the intestines, where IgE-producing plasma cells are located (Tada and Ishizaka, 1970). With these considerations in mind, it is not surprising that most animals and man generally produce high IgE responses to helminthic infestations. High dose immunization of animals and man with crude ascaris, particularly with IgE-stimulating adjuvants, would similarly be expected to produce good IgE antibody responses, especially where animals are selected for this purpose.

Recently, Patrucco and Marsh (1974) investigated the IgE and IgG antibody responses of seven inbred strains of mice, representing six H-2 types, to 1 μg doses (plus alumina) of the potent Asc-1 allergen of Strejan (Section IV,B,3). They found that it behaved no differently from other antigens in that certain strains responded and others did not, and IgE antibody was produced in a manner typical of the established IgE-producing characteristics of each strain. Although further experiments are necessary to compare crude ascaris with other crude antigens, these results suggest that ascaris has no especially unique allergenic properties. The high allergenic potency of Asc-1 (and, perhaps crude ascaris) is most probably accounted for by the general high immunogenic potency of this molecule.

A further interesting point is that most allergens so far discovered have been isolated in at least two or more isoallergenic variants–subcomponents that are structurally similar and allergenically indistinguishable from one another. Examples include grass Groups I, II, and III, timothy grass AgB, ragweed AgE, AgK, Ra3, and Ra5, and castor bean allergen CB-1A. There is probably no specific significance to this finding in terms of *allergenicity;* differences between the variants are probably genetic, or result from deamidation or differences in carbohydrate content (Section III).

Finally, the isolation of two low molecular weight allergens, having molecular weights around 5000—ragweed Ra5 (Lapkoff and Goodfriend, 1974), and a partially purified caddis fly allergen (Shulman, 1968)—demonstrates the existence of natural allergens which pass through most dialysis membranes. The fact that only a small percentage (ca. 17%) of the ragweed-allergic population are sensitive to Ra5 may well account for some of the earlier conflicting reports concerning the dialyzability of ragweed allergens (Section II,B,1). The finding that such low molecular weight allergens exist is not unexpected since polypeptides of even lower molecular weight, e.g., angiotensin (MW 1031), have been reported to be antigenic in animals (Dietrich, 1966). In view of the importance of allergens having a simple molecular structure in elucidating the genetics of immune response in man, it is probable that further low molecular weight allergens will be isolated in the near future.

D. Allergenic Valence and Haptens

An observation by Ovary and Taranta (1963), showing that antigens need to be at least divalent in order to elicit anaphylactic reactions in guinea pigs, led to the general adoption of the "bridging theory" to explain all types of anaphylactic reactions, including allergen–IgE antibody interaction on human basophils and mast cells. This concept has been strongly supported by Levine (1966) and de Weck (1974) who showed at least two penicilloyl groups were generally required to elicit the production of anaphylactic reactions in the guinea pig and man following previous sensitization with penicillin. This concept was supported by Ishizaka and Ishizaka (1969) who demonstrated that *divalent* anti-IgE [whole antibody molecules or (Fab)$_2$ dimer], but not *monovalent* anti-IgE (Fab monomer), was capable of eliciting "reversed" IgE-mediated anaphylactic reactions. On the other hand, certain monovalent haptens, including Levine's penicillin "minor determinant mixture" were found to elicit anaphylactic reactions in some sensitized people and guinea pigs (Levine, 1966; Raffel, 1973; de Weck, 1974); these conflicting reports have generally been attributed to aggregation of the hapten.

Before bridging can be fully accepted as playing an essential role in allergen-mediated reactions in man, further experimental data are required. Experiments using low molecular weight allergens, such as

Ra5, should be particularly useful in testing the hypothesis for highly limiting situations. In order to bridge the Ra5 molecule, two cell-bound IgE antibodies having specificity for *different* determinants on Ra5 must become correctly aligned on the surface of the cell. Monovalent fragments or derivatives of Ra5 should be capable of competitively inhibiting allergic reaction if the bridging concept is valid.

Acceptance of the bridging concept, and early observations that the presence of free hapten in hapten–protein antigen conjugates inhibit formation of anti-hapten antibody, led to the idea that nonreactogenic haptens (or hapten-like substances) might be useful in achieving true desensitization of allergic individuals (Malley *et al.*, 1964b; de Weck, 1974).

Malley and associates (1964a,b; Malley and Harris, 1967) isolated a partially purified glycoprotein–pigment complex, known as antigen D, from the dialyzable fraction of timothy pollen. In high concentration AgD appeared to possess hapten-like properties in that it (1) inhibited precipitin reaction between high molecular weight timothy allergens (notably antigen B) and rabbit anti-timothy sera, (2) prevented timothy anti-timothy PCA reactions in guinea pigs, and (3) inhibited timothy allergen-mediated histamine release from sensitized monkey lung fragments (Malley and Harris, 1967; Malley *et al.*, 1973). It also failed to stimulate the transformation of allergic human lymphocytes *in vitro*. On the other hand, AgD was found to be moderately potent allergenically in some people, which suggests that it may contain a low molecular weight allergen(s) to which only some people are sensitive (cf. data on Ra5, Section IV,B,2). The most dramatic findings were summarized by Malley *et al.* (1973), who reported that most patients treated with AgD exhibit a marked reduction in circulating anti-timothy reaginic antibody, and a dramatic decrease in the responsiveness of their peripheral blood lymphocytes toward challenge with crude timothy antigen *in vitro*. As a group, such patients also showed a marked reduction in symptoms, but attempts to correlate symptom scores with reduction in reaginic titer or decrease in lymphocyte responsiveness were not successful. Other researchers (Feigen *et al.*, 1967; Attallah and Sehon, 1969) have reported hapten-like activity in ragweed pollen dialysates.

Lichtenstein *et al.* (1969) and L. M. Lichtenstein and D. G. Marsh (unpublished) were unable to demonstrate hapten-like activity in dialysates from rye or timothy grass pollens, or in antigen D supplied by Malley. All such low molecular weight compounds were weakly allergenic and, like allergens, had the capability of desensitizing cells under conditions that do not lead to histamine release (Lichtenstein and Osler, 1964); this finding may reconcile some of the apparent anomalies between the results of different laboratories. Previous allergen research clearly shows that the three-dimensional protein structure is involved in allergenic (as well as antigenic) determinants (Section IV,D). Also, each of the many pollen allergens undoubtedly possesses many different determinants (cf. allergoid results, Section IV,E). Thus, it seems unlikely that low molecular weight, especially *purified* low molecular weight, pollen dialysates could contribute any sizable proportion of the determinants to which allergic people are sensitive. On this basis, it is rather difficult to explain the results of Malley and others. Further confirmation and explanation of their findings would, therefore, be desirable.

The most convincing demonstration of the potential usefulness of hapten immunotherapy was presented by de Weck (1974), who showed that high doses of a low molecular weight derivative of penicillin, N^α-formyl-N^ϵ-(α-benzylpenicilloyl)-L-lysine (BPO-FLYS) could be used to prevent anaphylaxis in penicillin-sensitive patients undergoing treatment with prophylactic doses of penicillin. One of de Weck's patients, undergoing successful penicillin plus hapten therapy, manifested urticaria as the dose of *hapten* was reduced. The urticaria faded upon readministration of higher doses of hapten. The BPO-FLYS treatment also led to a loss of skin reactivity to BPO-polylysine and penicillin in almost all patients. These results provide strong practical confirmation for the theoretical basis of hapten immunotherapy in the model system of penicillin sensitivity, where only one major type of chemical determinant (BPO) is involved. However, its practicality as a method for treating allergies toward much more complex multideterminant structures, such as proteins, remains controversial.

E. Allergoids

Studies by Norman, Lichtenstein, and associates and several other groups (reviewed by Norman, 1969; Lichtenstein, 1972) show that immunotherapy of allergic individuals with pollen extracts provides only partial amelioration of symptomatology. Despite extensive research, the immunologic basis for symptomatic relief remains obscure. Whatever the mechanism, most studies have shown that adequately high doses of effective immunogenic material are essential in order that symptoms may be significantly reduced, and this relief is generally accompanied by high levels of serum IgG "blocking antibody." This was the primary consideration that led to the development of "allergoids" as a potential new tool for improving the immunotherapy of human allergic disease. An allergoid has been defined (1) as having greatly reduced allergenic reactivity relative to the native allergen from which it was derived, and (2) as retaining to a high degree other desirable antigenic properties characteristic of the native allergen, including the immunogenic capacity to induce synthesis of allergen-neutralizing blocking antibody in animals and man (Marsh et al., 1970b; Marsh, 1971). Thus, the rationale for developing allergoids as new immunotherapeutic agents has been that relatively high doses could be administered to allergic man without the risk of generalized allergic reaction, and without compromising substantially the desirable immunizing properties characteristic of the native allergen.

Previous attempts to prepare such desirable materials (Stull et al., 1940; Naterman, 1957, 1965) were not very successful; however, Marsh and associates (1970b; Marsh, 1971) were able to establish the practicality of the allergoid concept using the rye Group I allergen as a model. By mild formalin treatment, similar to that used in preparing bacterial toxoids, they were able to reduce the allergenic reactivity of the Group I molecule by 200- to 100,000-fold (variable in different allergic individuals). The most immunogenic product, prepared by treating the allergen with formalin and lysine, retained 60% of the capacity of the native allergen to stimulate the production of blocking antibody in guinea pigs, as measured by the capacity of individual or pooled antisera to neutralize allergen-mediated histamine release in the human leukocyte system. Its capacity to induce IgG blocking antibody formation in nonallergic man was found to be of a similar order of magnitude (Marsh, 1971).

Subsequently, Marsh and co-workers (Haddad et al., 1972; Norman et al., 1972, 1975; Marsh and Lichtenstein, 1975) prepared allergoids from dialyzed crude extracts of grass and short ragweed pollens using modifications of the formalinization procedures used to prepare the Group I allergoids. Initial experiments showed that the crude ragweed and grass allergoids were between 100 and 10,000 times less allergenic than the native allergens from which they were derived. The most immunogenic allergoids were only about 4 times less effective than the respective native allergens with regard to inducing IgG antibody formation in guinea pigs, as measured by a variety of techniques including double antibody radioimmunoassay using appropriate radiolabeled antigens (AgE and crude ragweed or Group I and mixed grass, Marsh and Lichtenstein, 1975).

In a double blind controlled clinical study, comparing the relative efficacies of ragweed allergoid and ragweed allergen in allergic man, the allergoid was somewhat more effective clinically than the allergen, although complete symptomatic relief had still not been achieved (Norman et al., 1975). The allergoid could be administered in substantially greater amounts (averaging 40 times higher) than the allergen without provoking systemic anaphylactic reactions. Preliminary analysis showed that the high dose allergoid treatment was more effective in inducing IgG antibody against native ragweed allergens than was possible with the necessarily more limited dosages of native ragweed allergen (Norman et al., 1975).

Recently, Patterson and associates (1973a,b) have treated ragweed antigen E with glutaraldehyde in an attempt to produce products having comparable properties to those of the formaldehyde-treated allergoids of Marsh and associates. Their most promising preparation was found to be a fraction having a molecular weight range of 0.2–4 million. Experiments in the author's laboratory (Marsh and Lichtenstein, 1975) have also suggested that glutaraldehyde might be used as an alternative to formaldehyde in the preparation of allergoids.

The finding that different allergic people possess widely varying allergoid/allergen sensitivity ratios for derivatives of pure (and crude) allergens strongly suggests that the IgE-producing systems of different individuals recognize different allergenic determinants on the allergen molecules (Marsh et al., 1970b). The importance of exposed surface secondary and tertiary structure in comprising immunodominant allergenic determinants has already been discussed (Section IV,D). It may be assumed that mild formalin treatment modifies surface determinants to different degrees making them less reactive with IgE antibody. Conversely, parenteral administration of much higher doses of allergoid (having greater immunogenicity than the native allergen due to cross-linking) might be expected to stimulate IgG antibody against other determinants, including less extensively modified, partially "buried" determinants; this IgG antibody would be expected to cross-react more extensively with the native allergen than the IgE antibody induced by natural (immunogenically limiting) stimulation, as observed experimentally.

Future development of allergoid immunotherapy promises to improve our theoretical understanding and practical achievement in the therapy of allergic individuals.

V. Nature of Allergenic Sensitization and Stimulation

A. Exposure, Dosage, and Route of Entry

1. CONDITIONS OF IMMUNIZATION

An adequate degree of exposure to an allergen is clearly an essential prerequisite for the development of IgE-mediated sensitivity in predisposed individuals. As discussed in Sections IV,B and VI,B, the overall immunogenicity of the allergen and the individual's genetic constitution determine whether a particular allergen is capable of being recognized under normal (usually immunogenically limiting) exposure and dosage conditions. Phillips (1939) found that two seasons' exposure (each of 1–2 months' duration) was adequate to induce significant reaginic sensitivity to allergens in the pollen of *Beta vulgaris* (sugar beet); severe symptoms were noted soon after pollen exposure in the third year. Similar findings have been reported for allergies to other pollens (Sherman, 1968). The importance of dosage and frequency of allergenic exposure in the development of allergies is evident from a report that 10–20% of bakers and millers are sensitive to wheat flour (Schwartz, 1952), and the finding that workers in the castor bean industry can develop sensitivity to castor bean allergens within 6 months after first exposure (Sherman, 1968). The development of IgE-mediated sensitivity to parasitic allergens (e.g., ascaris) can take place within 10–14 days (Phills *et al.*, 1972), presumably due to the localization of high concentrations of allergen in the vicinity of IgE-producing cells (see below).

Beside the obvious requirement for exposure to allergen, the route of entry and dosage of the allergen are also important parameters in determining the development of IgE antibody response. It now seems clear, particularly from the work of Tada and Ishizaka (1970), that the routes of entry that are most likely to induce IgE antibody formation are via the respiratory or gastrointestinal tracts, since the IgE-producing plasma cells are found predominantly in these locations. The mucosal membranes normally act as barriers against penetration by very high molecular weight allergens. It appears that the molecular weight cut-off above which nasal and alveolar (lung) membranes are impermeable lies somewhere between 40,000 and 60,000 daltons (e.g., Schneeberger, 1974). As expected, no naturally inhaled allergen having a molecular weight of over 60,000 has been discovered. Immunoglobulin E-mediated sensitivity can be found toward injected allergens, such as bee venom, following relatively high dose immunization; approximately 7.5 μg of phospholipase A, out of a total of 50 μg solids, are injected per bee sting [derived from data of L. M. Lichtenstein, A. K. Sobotka, and M. D. Valentine (personal communication) and Shipolini et al. (1971a)].

In the case of inhaled pollen allergens, the mean adult annual dosages of individual allergenic components are probably in the highly limiting nanogram range (Marsh et al., 1973c; Marsh, 1975a). Allergen doses were calculated from rotoslide pollen counts taken in the Baltimore area, physical data on the size and density of pollen grains, and quantitation of the content of individual allergens in grass and ragweed pollen grains. The calculated dosages (Table V) overestimate the actual dosages, by perhaps 10- to 100-fold, since they are based on an improbable 24-hour-a-day outdoor exposure and complete extraction of the allergens in the upper respiratory tract.

It is a well-established fact that exquisite sensitivity to pollen allergens may persist for many years without further allergen contact (Sherman, 1968). The recent experience of L. M. Lichtenstein and associates (personal communication) demonstrates that marked leukocyte sensitivity to phospholipase A (from bee venom) may sometimes persist for 20 years or more without the individual's IgE antibody level being boosted by a further bee sting. While prolonged

TABLE V

Mean Adult Doses of Inhaled Pollen Allergens in the Baltimore Area[a]

Allergen	Total inhaled allergen dosages (μg)[b]		
	Mean annual[c]	Mean hourly[c]	Max. hourly[d]
Ragweed			
AgE	0.9	8×10^{-4}	4×10^{-3}
Ra3	0.15	1×10^{-4}	6×10^{-4}
Ra5	0.06	5×10^{-5}	2×10^{-4}
Grass			
Group I	0.6	6×10^{-4}	2×10^{-3}
Group II	0.3	3×10^{-4}	8×10^{-4}

[a] From Marsh (1975a).
[b] Assumes 24-hour-a-day outdoor exposure and complete extraction of allergens from the pollens.
[c] Based on mean pollen concentrations of 165 grains/m³ for ragweed and 23.0 grains/m³ for grass (derived from rotoslide pollen counts).
[d] Based on maximum pollen concentrations of 736 grains/m³ for ragweed and 58.5 grains/m³ for grass (derived from max. daily rotoslide readings).

persistence of *natural* sensitivity to inhaled or injected allergens is characteristically observed in most allergic people, some appear to lose their sensitivity "spontaneously" by unknown immunologic or immunopharmacologic mechanisms. Conversely, IgE-mediated sensitivity that is artificially induced in nonallergic subjects by high dosages of antigen (Section V,C) is generally short-lived.

The exposure and dosage requirements for the development of IgE-mediated sensitivities to ingested allergens are not clearly understood. Allergic reactions to food, particularly milk and eggs, are more common in children than adults, most children having lost their food allergies by the age of five. This observation has been attributed to a reduced tendency to absorb undigested protein and/or a development of "immunologic tolerance" with age (Kaufman, 1958; Fries and Lightstone, 1962). The recent investigations by Spies (1974) of "new antigens" created by brief peptic digestion of β-lactoglobulin from cow's milk may well prove to be highly relevant to our future understanding of these phenomena.

2. Conditions for Allergic Reaction

We have so far been mainly considering the conditions necessary for the induction of an IgE antibody response. We now turn to factors involved in the presentation of allergens that actually result in IgE-mediated allergic reactions in presensitized individuals.

During the height of the pollination seasons, the mean hourly dosages of individual grass and ragweed pollen allergens provoking allergic reactions (Table V) are similar to those causing positive wheal and flare skin reactions in highly allergic individuals (King *et al.*, 1964; Norman *et al.*, 1973; Marsh *et al.*, 1973a). The size of the allergen-containing particle is also of great importance in determining the primary site of allergic reaction to inhaled allergens. Only about 40–50% of particles of 1 μ diameter are inhaled directly into the lungs and *all* particles of 15 μ or larger are deposited in the nose (mainly on the anterior nares), or in the oropharynx in the case of mouth breathing (Proctor *et al.*, 1969; Bridger and Proctor, 1971). Thus, the smaller sized particles can directly provoke IgE-mediated or other immunologic reactions directly in the lungs, but the larger particles cannot. Bridger and Proctor (1971) demonstrated that nasally inhaled, ^{99}Te-labeled albumin spheres (15–25 μ diameter), similar in size to pollen grains (ragweed, ca. 18 μ diameter; grass, usually 20–40 μ diameter), are cleared from the nasal mucosa within a few minutes; they are carried to the larynx by mucociliary flow and virtually all are swallowed within 30 minutes after being inhaled. Wilson et al. (1973) obtained similar data using high doses (17–79 μg, equivalent to about 2000–8000 grains) of ^{99}Te-labeled grass pollen grains. Following mouth inhalation, radiolabeled pollen was found in the oropharynx, esophagus, and stomach, but *not* in the lung.

The lack of direct contact between the pollen particle and the lung makes it difficult to explain pollen-induced asthma. Involvement of the parasympathetic (vagal) nervous system (Gold, 1973; Nadel, 1973) has been proposed as a possible mechanism (e.g., Marsh, 1973), although Busse et al. (1972) have suggested that fragmented pollen particles of 1–5 μ diameter may be causative agents. The proposed involvement of the vagal reflex system is attractive since this process has a built-in amplification system; local triggering of vagal afferent receptors would be expected to cause widespread bronchoconstriction as a result of signals being transmitted by multiple vagal efferent pathways to different parts of the lungs. In very recent work, G. L. Rosenberg and P. S. Norman (personal communication) challenged ragweed asthmatic patients with several thousand intact ragweed pollen grains under controlled laboratory conditions. Oral challenge produced no asthma and nasal challenge produced hay fever but no asthma. These results tend to rule out the idea that allergen–IgE antibody reactions on mast cells of the upper respiratory tract lead to asthma. A possible solution to the dilemma of explaining natural pollen asthma may be that small allergen-laden "dust" particles are inhaled into the lower respiratory tract, and ensuing allergen-induced release of pharmacologically active mediators such as histamine leads to stimulation of the vagal reflex system.

The doses of allergen which are clinically relevant in provoking allergic reactions can be quite different for different routes of entry of allergen. We have seen that the levels of inhaled allergens which are sufficient to provoke allergic rhinitis and asthma in sensitive subjects are 1 pg/hour or lower (Table V). The quantities of aerosolized pollen extracts which provoke minimal asthmatic reaction in bronchial challenge experiments often used to study "asthma" usually contain microgram quantities of allergens. Thus, such experiments do not reproduce the natural course of an asthmatic attack to pollen from the standpoint of allergen dosage as well as the nonparticulate nature of the allergen. Further relevant findings are described by Bruce et al. (1974).

An observation by Connell (1969) which has relevance to the dosage of allergen needed to provoke allergic rhinitis is known as the "priming effect." Previous intensive exposure to either the same or completely non-cross-reacting pollen allergens leads to a reduction in the dosage of allergen required to induce allergic symptoms.

In the case of injected allergens, allergic symptoms are induced by much higher doses [e.g., microgram quantities in the case of venom allergens (Section V,A) and gram quantities of injected dextran] than is the case for inhaled allergens. Thus, a relatively low level of sensitivity is required in order that some symptoms may be observed following exposure to an injected allergen, and systemic anaphylaxis is common in people who are exquisitely sensitive to such allergens.

B. Rates of Release of Allergens from Pollens

As discussed in the previous section, pollens remain in the upper respiratory tract following inhalation for only about 30 minutes. During this period, the components responsible for provoking allergic reaction must be extracted. Thus, investigation of extraction rates of different allergenic components is of relevance in determining the specificity and intensity of the allergic reaction. Depending on the specificity of IgE antibody responses to the components of an allergenic complex, and the differential amounts of each component extracted in the upper respiratory tract, different individuals having the same sensitivity to a crude ragweed extract (prepared by prolonged extraction *in vitro*) may, in fact, be subjected to quite different *total allergenic loads in vivo*.

Belin (1972a) and Belin and Rowley (1971) were the first workers to study systematically the kinetics of release of allergens from pollen. They clearly showed, by a variety of immunologic and immunofluorescent techniques, that the major birch tree pollen allergen is released very rapidly from the pollen grains. Using a modified radial immunodiffusion allergen technique, release was found to occur through the pores of the pollen grains. In a study of the kinetics of release of different allergens and high molecular weight nondialyzable materials from ragweed pollen, Marsh (1975b) showed that the ragweed component widely considered to be the major allergen, antigen E, is released extremely slowly. Using different batches of pollen, only 1.5–1.7% of the total amount of AgE had been released after 16 minutes vigorous extraction at 23° under physiological conditions *in vitro* (Fig. 7). On the other hand, allergen Ra5 was completely released within the first few minutes of extraction; allergen Ra3 was released at an intermediate rate. If one may presume

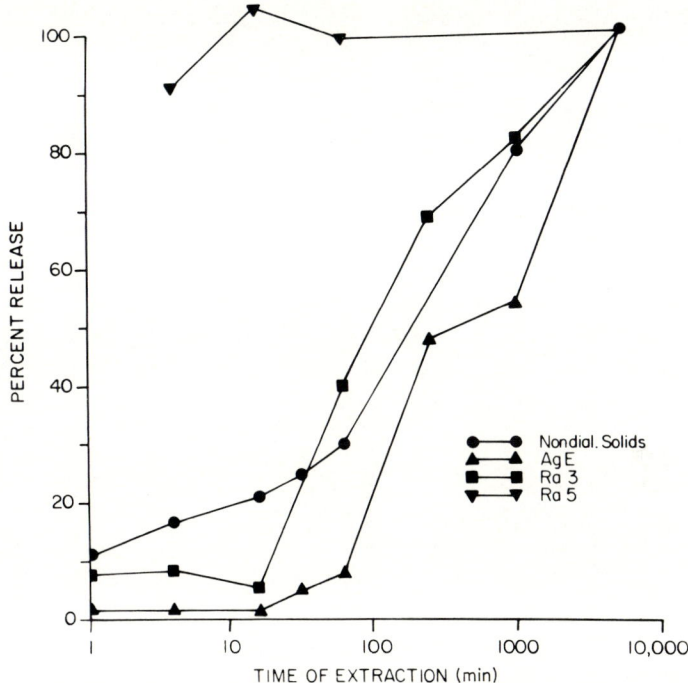

Fig. 7. Kinetics of release of allergens and nondialyzable solids from the pollen of *Ambrosia elatior* (short ragweed). *In vitro* extractions were performed with physiological saline at 23°, except for the longest (4 day) extraction which was performed at 4°. Data for nondialyzable solids was not corrected for possible slight loss of high molecular weight substances through the dialysis tubing. (From Marsh, 1975b.)

that these *in vitro* rates of release resemble the rates *in vivo*, they must have an important bearing on the relative intensities of allergenic stimulation by the different allergens.

To investigate the allergenic significance of ragweed components released at different rates, the biologic activities of extracts prepared by 4-minute, 16-minute, 64-minute, and 4-day extractions were compared (Marsh *et al.*, 1975a). The release of biologically active material, measured by leukocyte histamine release and quantitative intradermal skin testing of 23 ragweed hay fever and 15 ragweed asthmatic patients, did not parallel the release of AgE, as might be expected if AgE were indeed the major ragweed pollen allergen. In most (21/38; 55%) individuals with ragweed hay fever or asthma, the AgE component in the 16-minute extract contributed a negligible proportion ($<1\%$) of the biologic activity of the extract, as can be seen from a comparison of leukocyte sensitivity to AgE versus sensitivity to the 16-minute extract (Fig. 8). In order to facilitate this comparison, the concentration of the 16-minute extract is expressed in terms of its AgE content. People represented by points above the 100-fold difference line are over 100 times more sensitive to combinations of components in the 16-minute extract other than AgE. In another part of the study, it was shown that the 16-minute extract possessed at least 10% of the biologic activity of the 4-day extract in 82% of the patients, and at least 50% of the activity in 47% of the patients. The 16-minute extract used for this study contained only 1.5% of the AgE present in the 4-day extract.

These results strongly suggest that certain rapidly eluted ragweed components contribute a major portion of total biologic activity of ragweed pollen, and lead one to question whether AgE is the princi-

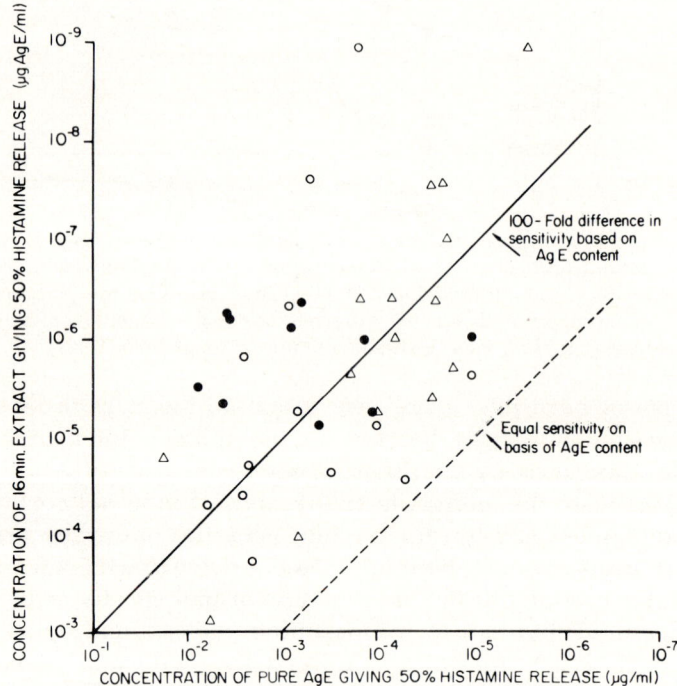

Fig. 8. Analysis of the contribution of Antigen E to the biologic activity of a 16 minute extract of short ragweed pollen. Leukocyte histamine release assays were performed in 23 hay fever (○, untreated; ●, on immunotherapy) and 15 untreated asthmatic (△) patients. The concentration of the 16 minute extract is expressed solely on the basis of its AgE content. Patients represented by symbols above the solid line are over 100-fold more sensitive to components in the 16 minute extract other than AgE. (From Marsh *et al.*, 1975a.)

ple allergen responsible for ragweed allergy (cf. Goldfarb, 1968). In a preliminary analysis of the 16-minute extract, Marsh *et al.* (1975a) showed that a mixture of highly allergenic basic proteins was responsible for the bulk of its allergenic activity.

It may be argued that *in vitro* rates of allergen release do not necessarily correspond to those pertaining *in vivo*, but these studies certainly point to the biologic importance of allergenic components other than AgE in ragweed allergy. On the other hand, these results contradict numerous reports (King *et al.*, 1964; Norman, 1969; Baer *et al.*, 1970; Norman and Lichtenstein, 1973; Norman *et al.*, 1973) suggesting that AgE is by far the most important ragweed allergen. Some of these discrepancies cannot be readily explained, but possible explanations for others have been discussed in detail by Marsh *et al.* (1975a). Among the most important is that several previous studies showed highly significant *associations* between sensitivity to AgE and to the complex mixture of allergens present in crude ragweed extracts without demonstrating quantitative *causal* relationship. Since AgE is such a potent immunogen (Section IV,D), it is quite possible to find virtually all ragweed-allergic people having IgE-mediated sensitivity to this component without it necessarily comprising the bulk of the substances responsible for the allergenic reactivity (reactogenicity) of the crude extract or being the most important component causing allergic disease. Nevertheless, AgE is clearly a useful *indicator* of ragweed allergy and can be used as an index of potency for ragweed extracts (Section VII), since most ragweed allergic subjects' sensitivities to AgE and crude ragweed components are proportional to one another.

In other experiments, Marsh (1975b) showed that the rye grass allergens, Group I, Group II, and timothy AgB, are rapidly eluted from rye grass pollen. It is clear that further experiments along these lines, as well as other attempts to determine the kinetics of allergen release *in vivo*, will lead to a greater understanding of the role of different allergenic constituents in actually provoking allergic disease.

Beside being of great importance allergenically, the rapidly released pollen components probably play a significant role in species recognition during plant fertilization (Knox and Heslop-Harrison, 1971; Knox *et al.*, 1972). "Recognition substances" released from pollens allow pollen tube growth and fertilization *only* of ova from the same species. If this recognition process could be prevented, it is possible that widely different species might be induced to crossfertilize. Thus, pollen allergen research will provide materials and valuable information for future molecular botanical studies.

C. Artificial Induction of IgE-Mediated Sensitivity

In the past, a number of researchers have investigated whether nonallergic individuals can be induced to synthesize IgE antibody and develop IgE-mediated sensitivity following artificial parenteral or intranasal administration of antigen. This work has been reviewed in Marsh *et al.* (1972). The induction of specific IgE response in nonallergic man by parenteral administration of antigen has been studied in detail by Marsh and associates (Marsh, 1971; Marsh *et al.*, 1972; and also by Greenert *et al.* (1971). In experiments designed to compare the immunogenic potencies of native allergen and two allergoids of rye grass Group I, it was found that all nine completely nonatopic individuals studied synthesized IgE antibody which reacted with each of the antigens.

Following four 100-μg doses of antigen with alumina gel and subsequent aqueous booster injections, unexpectedly marked IgE-mediated sensitivity was observed in most subjects, in addition to the anticipated IgG response. The induced reaginic antibody was clearly shown to be IgE. All P–K transfer activity was completely removed either by heating the serum at 56° for 4 hours or adsorbing it with anti-IgE immunoadsorbent, and specific IgE could readily be measured by the RAST assay. The kinetics of IgE-mediated sensitivity following repeated immunizations was studied by leukocyte histamine release assay and skin testing. In addition, total IgE levels and specific anti-rye Group I IgE antibodies were measured. The rise and fall of leukocyte sensitivity to the Group I allergen or allergoid correlated extremely well with the kinetics of the specific serum IgE antibody response as well as with the rise and fall of the total serum IgE level.

Several important differences between naturally and artificially induced IgE-mediated hypersensitivity were found. The artificially induced responses were generally short-lived compared to natural sensitivity, and showed much less specificity for the immunizing allergen—that is to say, using the high doses of antigen and alumina needed to induce response in nonallergic man, the cross-reaction between allergen and allergoid was much greater than in atopic people who are naturally sensitized by limiting low dose exposure. The people who were immunized with the allergoids tended to produce IgE antibody preferentially against the native Group I allergen rather than the allergoid used for immunization. This result suggests that the IgE-producing systems of nonallergic individuals may have been subliminally immunized against the native allergen by natural exposure.

Greenert *et al.* (1971) showed that 37 out of 42 nonatopic individuals immunized with repeated high doses of aqueous crude ragweed extract are capable of synthesizing specific IgE, as well as IgG, antibody. Like Marsh and associates, these workers found no clinical allergy in the artificially sensitized individuals. They suggested that one possible difference between allergic and nonallergic individuals may lie in the relative responsiveness of their tissues and shock organs to allergic stimulation. This interpretation merits further study.

It is worth noting that both the kinetics and specificity of artificially induced IgE antibody response following immunization with high doses of antigen are similar to the high dosage response of inbred mice (Levine and Vaz, 1970a). Like the mice, most people respond well using high doses of allergen (particularly when alumina is used as the adjuvant), but only certain genetically predisposed individuals respond to the limiting doses of allergen encountered under natural exposure conditions.

Several workers in the past (e.g., Richter *et al.*, 1958) have suggested that allergic individuals receiving immunotherapy with allergenic extracts become sensitized toward components to which they were previously not sensitive. This suggestion is supported by the experiments in nonatopics and recent findings that ragweed-sensitive individuals immunized with ragweed allergoid (Section IV,E) tend to develop a three- to fourfold increase in sensitivity to the allergoid relative to the allergen during treatment.

VI. Genetics of Allergy

A. Historical

As far back as 1872, Wyman noted that "some families suffer more than others from Autumnal Catarrh [ragweed pollen hay fever]–[and]–that not unfrequently, while some members of a family have this disease, others have June Cold [grass pollen hay fever]–." These different allergic manifestations were strikingly apparent in his own family. He also observed that some members of allergic families were "subjects of spasmodic asthma" following exposure to pollens or nonspecific irritants such as sulfur dioxide. Although not realized at the time, his findings laid the foundation for genetic studies of allergy, and constituted one of the earlier series of documented observations in human immunogenetics. With today's hindsight, we can distinguish two separate discoveries: (1) there is a general familial predisposition toward allergies, including asthma and (2) allergically predisposed individuals often develop sensitivities to different allergenic substances present in the environment.

In a comprehensive study of the familial predisposition toward allergic rhinitis, atopic eczema, and asthma, Cooke and VanderVeer (1916) confirmed and considerably extended Wyman's observations. They found that 48.4% of a population of 504 allergic individuals had positive family histories, whereas only 14.5% of 76 nonallergics had similar positive histories. They observed that, among the allergic population, individuals with a bilateral family history of allergies usually develop allergic manifestations during childhood, those with a unilateral family history more often develop symptoms around puberty and those with asymptomatic parents usually become allergic later in life. In particular, they noted that children are not born with allergic manifestations, but inherit the tendency to become allergic equally from both parents, suggesting that the transmission is genetic and autosomal. While carefully documenting that allergic children often have quite different specific sensitivities and allergic manifestations than their parents, Cooke and VanderVeer were content to consider that a single gene governs the inheritance of all allergies. This general presumption was followed in virtually every research publication up to 1960 (for reviews, see Schwartz, 1952; Ratner and Silberman, 1953; Vaughan and Black, 1954; Sherman, 1965; Bias, 1973; Black and Marsh, 1975). The main argument centered around whether the mode of inheritance was simple Mendelian dominant or recessive. Since neither hypothesis fitted the data, Weiner *et al.* (1936) presented statistical evidence claiming that individuals who were homozygous for the allergy-controlling allele developed allergy in childhood, while only 18% of individuals with one such allele developed allergy later in life due to an "incompletely recessive gene." Using either Mendelian dominant or recessive hypotheses, various authors (Schwartz, 1952; Van Arsdel and Motulsky, 1959) suggested varying degrees of allergic manifestation in people who were heterozygous at the allergy-controlling locus. Such devices merely avoided recognizing that no "one gene hypothesis" fitted the data.

In 1954, Tips demonstrated that the inheritance of each of the three principal allergic manifestations, rhinitis, asthma, and eczema, was autosomal. He presented evidence for a "three gene hypothesis" in which each of these manifestations was controlled as a recessive trait at its own distinct locus. Tips' consideration of the three prin-

4. Allergens and the Genetics of Allergy

cipal allergic states as three distinct entities were based on their quite different manifestations, and earlier observations showing that (1) patients with allergic rhinitis are usually not afflicted with asthma and/or eczema and asthmatics are often free from eczema (Cooke and VanderVeer, 1916) and (2) it is possible for an individual to be asthmatic without evidence of any reaginic component (the so-called *intrinsic* asthmatic; Rackemann, 1918).

Besides the many family studies of allergy, two moderately large twin studies were carried out by Spaich and Ostertag (1936) and Bowen (1953). The first authors reported, for individuals aged 3–79 years, a higher concordance for hay fever, asthma, and eczema in monozygotics than dizygotics, as one would anticipate for a disease more strongly influenced by genetic than environmental factors. On the other hand, Bowen found that only 7 of 59 sets of monozygotics (aged mainly between 6 and 15 years) had similar clinical histories of allergy in both members. Unfortunately, their criteria for determining both zygosity of the twin pairs and the presence of reagin-mediated allergies were not well documented. The main difference between the two studies was in the ages of the subjects. Evaluation of allergy mainly by clinical history and the possible differential exposure to allergens in the members of Bowen's young subjects could account for his anomalous findings.

An alternate more recent approach to studying the genetics of allergy was based on the hypothesis that allergic people differ from nonallergic people in the permeability of their mucosal membranes to inhaled or ingested allergens; membranes of allergic individuals were proposed to have greater permeability. This hypothesis was extensively tested by Salvaggio and associates (Salvaggio *et al.*, 1964, 1966, 1969, 1971) and other groups (reviewed in Leskowitz *et al.*, 1972), by attempting artificially to induce IgE-mediated sensitivity in groups of unrelated allergic and nonallergic subjects using intranasal immunization with a variety of different antigens. The results were equivocal, in that certain antigens (e.g., ribonuclease) seemed to show the hypothesized difference, but in other cases (e.g., tetanus toxoid) there was no difference between allergic and nonallergic groups.

Very recently, Kontou-Karakitsos *et al.* (1975) presented data that appear to rule out the "permeability hypothesis." Sites on the backs of groups of allergic and nonallergic subjects were passively sensitized with serum containing IgE antibody against allergens to which *neither* group was sensitive. Both groups were then challenged intranasally with precisely measured doses of the allergens. No differences in the intensity of the ensuing P–K reactions (normalized for individual differences in P–K responsiveness) were observed between the two groups.

Chang and Marsh (1974) have shown that mouse strains that respond well to low doses of ribonuclease also respond well to ragweed AgE and rye grass Group I; the same appears also to be true for man in that (ragweed and grass) allergic people more readily respond to ribonuclease than nonallergic subjects. On the other hand, tetanus toxoid is a complex cross-linked antigen which will be immunogenic in a wider range of people (Section IV,D). Thus, the results of Salvaggio and co-workers may well be due to immunogenetic differences between allergic and nonallergic people.

Major problems with most of the earlier genetic studies (reviewed in detail by Black and Marsh, 1975) were that ill-defined and often questionable criteria were used to designate "allergy" and that virtually all the evidence for familial aggregation in allergy was obtained by taking histories, usually from the propositus, and often in the form of a written questionnaire. Few cases of skin testing were reported, even in the propositus. Furthermore, no tests were performed using the available purified allergens (Newell, 1941), although it had already been shown that different allergic individuals were differentially sensitive not only to different allergen complexes (e.g., different pollens, danders, etc.), but also to different fractions which could be isolated from these complexes (Section II,A). The general failure to perform any objective tests for allergies must certainly have resulted in some misdiagnoses, particularly in recognizing the less pronounced allergic conditions. This probably resulted in the researchers failing to recognize the significance of genes controlling allergic response to specific allergens (what we now refer to as immune response, or Ir, genes). Nevertheless, from these early studies, there is strong evidence that each of the major allergic manifestations are largely determined by genetic factors. Since no "one gene hypothesis" fitted the data, and in view of the observed complexity of allergic disease, the most reasonable conclusion from the early studies is that the mode of inheritance of allergy is multigenic.

B. Modern Approaches

1. Discovery of IgE and Ir Genes

Discoveries in the late 1960's revolutionized the approach toward understanding some of the specific genetic factors involved in atopic

4. Allergens and the Genetics of Allergy

allergy. The Ishizakas and their associates clearly identified immunoglobulin E (IgE) as the carrier of atopic hypersensitivity (Ishizaka et al., 1966; Ishizaka and Ishizaka, 1968). With the aid of simple synthetic polypeptide antigens developed by Sela (1969), McDevitt and associates (McDevitt and Tyan, 1968; McDevitt and Chinitz, 1969) demonstrated the existence of H-2-linked immune response (Ir) genes in inbred strains of mice. Strong confirmatory evidence for the important role of Ir genes linked to the major histocompatibility (H) type of animals came from many experiments in mice, guinea pigs, rats, and, recently, monkeys (McDevitt and Benacerraf, 1969; Benacerraf and McDevitt, 1972; McDevitt and Landy, 1972; Balner et al., 1973). It now appears that these genes primarily control T cell function. In the mouse, they are known to be distinct from the serologically defined D and K specificities of H-2. The influence of H-linked Ir genes is most clearly evident when *inbred* strains of animals are subjected to *limiting immunogenic stimulation*, as when simple synthetic polypeptides or extremely low doses of complex proteins are used as antigens.

Histocompatibility-linked Ir genes control IgE as well as IgG antibody responses of inbred mice to limiting doses (0.1 or 1.0 μg) of protein antigens (Vaz and Levine, 1970; Levine and Vaz, 1970a). In addition to the Ir genes controlling responsiveness to specific antigens, the general ability of inbred mice to produce an IgE response (of, apparently, any specificity) is under a different genetic control, not linked to H type (Levine and Vaz, 1970b). These findings show two distinct types of genetic control of IgE responsiveness: (1) antigen-specific and (2) ability to synthesize IgE of any specificity. More recently, Marsh and associates (Chang and Marsh, 1974; Patrucco and Marsh, 1974) have demonstrated association with H-2 type of the responsiveness of inbred mice to limiting doses of the rye grass Group I, ragweed AgE, and Asc-1 allergens.

2. RELEVANCE OF ANIMAL EXPERIMENTS TO MAN

In man, IgE-mediated sensitivity to inhaled pollen allergens arises due to exquisitely limiting immunogenic stimulation, probably of only nanogram quantities of each allergen per year (Section V,A). It is now well established that allergic individuals respond selectively to different, immunochemically distinct highly purified allergens that have been isolated from grass and ragweed pollens (Section IV,B,2). Furthermore, the major H complex of man, the HL-A system, closely resembles the mouse H-2 complex; both contain two major serologically defined loci, the *D* and *K* loci of H-2, and the first and second loci of HL-A. Recently, significant associations have been found between specific HL-A types and susceptibility to certain immunologically based diseases (McDevitt and Landy, 1972).

With these factors in mind, several investigators set out to study possible relationships between specific HL-A types and immune responsiveness to specific highly purified pollen allergens. Two main approaches have been used: (1) populations of unrelated, highly allergic individuals have been investigated in attempts to demonstrate statistically significant *associations* between specific HL-A types and specific IgE-mediated sensitivities; (2) studies in allergic families have tried to show *genetic linkage* between a specific familial HL-A haplotype* with specific IgE and IgG responsiveness. Due to genetic recombination, specific immune responsiveness may be linked to different serologically defined HL-A haplotypes in different families, presuming that the Ir genes are distinct entities. The finding of a particular association in a population study does not necessarily imply that the analogous linkage can be demonstrated in families, since the inheritance of specific IgE responsiveness is multigenic, and not all family members may have the full complement of genes necessary to express the specific sensitivity (Marsh *et al.*, 1973c; Marsh, 1974).

3. POPULATION STUDIES

The first breakthrough in population studies came with the availability of the low molecular weight ragweed allergen, Ra5 (Section IV,B,2; Tables III and IV). Due to its very simple structure (MW 5000) and ultralimiting dosage, it was reasoned that natural exposure to Ra5 represents an exquisitely limiting immunogenic challenge, which would favor the possibility of observing associations between specific immune response and specific HL-A type even in a population as genetically polymorphic as man.

In two related studies, Marsh and associates (1973a; Marsh, 1974) divided over a hundred highly ragweed-sensitive individuals into two groups, according to the magnitude of their Ra5/AgE skin sensitivity ratios. Sensitivity ratios, rather than absolute sensitivity to Ra5, were used since the common denominator of AgE sensitivity represents an index of the degree of ragweed exposure and of other genetic factors governing the manifestation of skin reactivity to ragweed allergens. In the second enlarged study (Table VI), statistical

---

* A haplotype is comprised of a first and a second locus HL-A specificity located on the same chromosome. Due to close genetic linkage, the two specificities are usually inherited together.

TABLE VI

Comparisons of the Frequencies of HL-A7, HL-A5, and the HL-A7 and HL-A5 Cross-Reacting Groups (Cregs), in Highly Ragweed Allergic Individuals, Who Are Either Sensitive or Insensitive to Allergen Ra5[a]

	HL-A	Ra5 sensitive	Ra5 insensitive	p
	7	14 (46.7%)	15 (19.5%)	0.009
	7 Creg	22 (73.3%)	26 (33.8%)	<0.0005
	5	4 (13.3%)	7 (9.0%)	N.S.[b]
	5 Creg	8 (26.7%)	18 (23.4%)	N.S.[b]
All 7 Creg excluded:	5 Creg	5/8 (62.5%)	13/51 (25.5%)	0.08

[a] In this analysis, a 300-fold difference in Ra5/AgE skin sensitivity weight ratio separated Ra5 sensitive from Ra5 insensitive individuals. The comparison for "all 7 Creg excluded" involves only those people who did not have an HL-A7 Creg antigen in their phenotype. Values of p were determined by chi-squared analysis, using Yates' correction. From Marsh (1974).

[b] N.S., not significant.

analysis revealed a significant elevation only in the frequency of the second locus HL-A7 specificity in 30 Ra5-sensitive relative to 77 Ra5-insensitive people ($p = 0.009$). When the combined frequencies of structurally similar H antigens comprising the HL-A7 cross-reacting group (Creg) were considered, the elevation of this group of specificities was even more significant among Ra5-sensitive individuals ($p < 0.0005$). In the same study, it was also found that 5 of 8 Ra5-sensitive people who did not have HL-A7 Creg possessed HL-A5 Creg antigens. These findings led to the suggestion that the HL-A7 Creg antigens are closely associated with Ir gene(s) which control recognition of the principal carrier determinant on the Ra5 molecule; whereas, it was tentatively speculated that Ir genes associated with HL-A5 Creg antigens may control recognition of a secondary carrier determinant. In another study, Marsh *et al.* (1973b) showed that individuals possessing IgE-mediated sensitivity to Ra5 also produce detectable levels of IgG antibody in their sera. Thus, in accord with animal experiments, the Ir genes for Ra5 appear to control production of both IgG and IgE antibodies.

4. Family Studies

In a preliminary report, Levine (1971) showed association between ragweed hay fever and the presence of a haplotype containing the first locus serotype W-28, based on the occurrence of W-28 in 7 of 8 ragweed-allergic members of a single family. In more extensive studies of 11 families having two or more allergic members and at least three children, Marsh *et al.* (1972) were unable to confirm this preliminary finding. In addition to quantitative skin testing with AgE, they tested with ragweed allergens Ra3 and Ra5, rye grass allergens of Groups I, II, III, and IV, and timothy grass AgB (Section IV,B,2). In all cases, they were unable to demonstrate linkage between familial HL-A haplotype and any specific sensitivity. They concluded that the results "strongly suggested that in man the genetic transmission of specific allergic responsiveness, and probably of immune responsiveness to limiting antigenic stimulation in general, is complex."

In a study of 7 families, selected for "expressivity" of IgE-mediated sensitivity to AgE (and ragweed hay fever), Levine *et al.* (1972) attempted to demonstrate linkage between HL-A haplotype and sensitivity to AgE within the family. Seven other families were interviewed, although not selected for study, due to the presence of ragweed allergy in only one family member. In each of the reported families, AgE skin sensitivity segregated with a particular HL-A haplotype, although this haplotype differed from family to family. In one family, four of six family members with the HL-A1,8 haplotype were highly skin sensitive to AgE; none of the seven family members with the other HL-A haplotype of the proposita responded to AgE, although one gave a weakly positive reaction. The two family members with HL-A1,8, but without skin sensitivity to AgE, were found to have trace amounts of IgG antibody to fraction D, a heterogeneous ragweed preparation that contains about 19% AgE (King *et al.*, 1964). Overall, in the seven families, 20 of 26 individuals with the putative hay fever-associated HL-A haplotype had ragweed hay fever and AgE sensitivity. None of the 20 with the other haplotypes had ragweed hay fever, although three were weakly skin sensitive to AgE. Skin tests with two different crude allergens showed no such correlation.

In the one family reported in detail, the linkage between the HL-A1,8 haplotype and responsiveness to AgE is equivocal because specific IgE-mediated skin sensitivity was not studied in all family members, including the proposita's and most other relevant spouses. Furthermore, IgG antibody was examined only in six people and was measured to *impure* AgE, which makes these results difficult to interpret. It seems quite possible that Ir gene(s) for AgE could have been inherited from family members who were not studied for IgE and/or IgG antibody responses. Results on some of the remaining six families (reported at meetings) are less persuasive since they include two or more five-member families in which IgE-mediated sensitivity

4. Allergens and the Genetics of Allergy

to AgE is expressed in just one of the parents and one child. Particularly since no IgG antibody measurements were reported in these families, it is possible to explain the transmission of reaginic sensitivity to AgE primarily by some mechanism other than a gene linked to HL-A (in particular, see discussion of the IgE-controlling gene below).

More recently, Blumenthal et al. (1974) tried to show linkage between an Ir gene for AgE (termed IrE) and the second locus of HL-A in a large three-generation family comprising 57 members. Starting with the assumption that an Ir gene for AgE is linked to the HL-A system, these authors observed that IgE-mediated skin sensitivity to AgE (and crude ragweed) was most frequently associated with a familial haplotype containing HL-A12. This led to their postulating linkage between HL-A12 and IrE. They were then faced with the problem of explaining why 12/22 members (55%) possessing HL-A12 (derived from the grandfather) did not express IgE-mediated sensitivity to AgE (tested up to a concentration of 1 μg/ml by intradermal test). People with HL-A12 who were negative to AgE were designated "transmitters of skin reaction to E," "HL-A-IrE recombinants" or "possible HL-A-IrE recombinants" in order to fit the hypothesized linkage. Two of these people, the grandfather and one of his sons, who are critical to the analysis, were classified as "transmitters," even though they had a history of seasonal allergy and, therefore, must have had most of the genes needed for the overall expression of allergy. Another problem was to explain why three blood relatives of the grandfather, who did not possess HL-A12, nevertheless were skin reactive to AgE. These people were classified as an "HL-A-IrE recombinant," a "possible HL-A-IrE recombinant," and one was assumed to have received an IrE gene from a nonallergic "transmitter" parent who was not a blood relative of the grandfather. Other points are discussed by Bias and Marsh (1975). Clearly, the authors need to provide definitive experimental evidence for their hypothesized "transmitters" and "recombinants."

In another report, Buckley et al. (1973) investigated, in three families, linkage between HL-A haplotype and skin sensitivity to several different complex mixtures of natural product antigens. Their data are presently difficult to evaluate because of the extreme complexity of the antigens studied.

In their investigation of over 25 families containing members who respond to pollen allergens, Marsh, Bias, and their associates (Marsh et al., 1972, 1974; Bias et al., 1973; Marsh, 1974) have been unable to confirm linkage between a specific familial HL-A haplotype and a specific IgE and/or IgG response to a single highly purified pollen allergen so far studied. Responsiveness to the ragweed allergens, AgE, Ra3, and Ra5, and rye Group I has been studied in detail and responsiveness to other highly purified allergens (cf. Fig. 9) less completely. In studies of ten large families, Black et al. (1974) were unable to demonstrate genetic linkage between familial HL-A haplotype and immune responsiveness to any one of the four extensively studied allergens, even when antigen-induced lymphocyte proliferation (determined by cellular incorporation of [^{3}H]thymidine *in vitro*) was used in addition to measurement of IgE-mediated skin sensitivity and serum IgG antibody as indices of specific immune responsiveness.

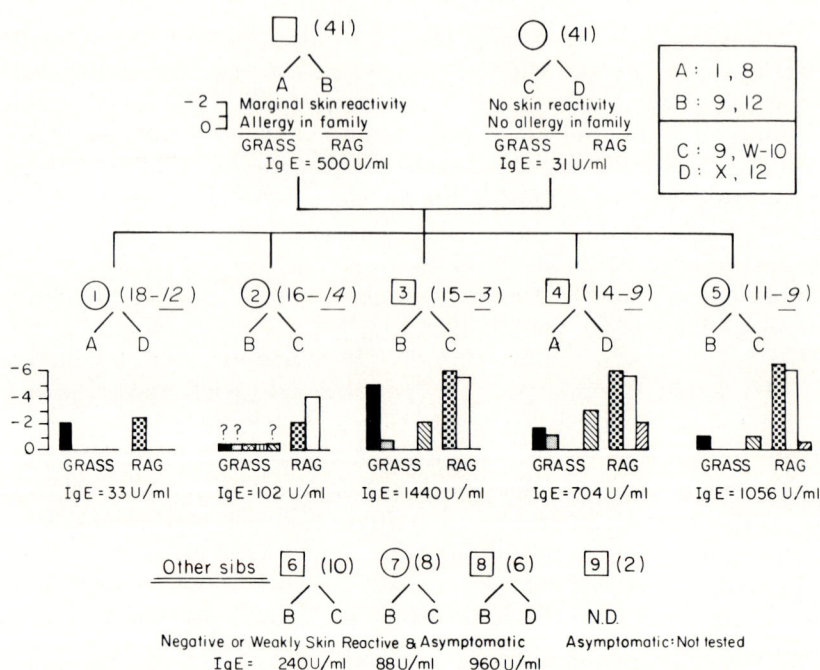

Fig. 9. Distribution of specific IgE-mediated skin sensitivities, HL-A haplotype and total serum IgE level in one family. Sibs are numbered 1 through 9; their ages and the ages of onset of allergic rhinitis (italicized) in allergic sibs are given in parentheses. Vertical bars represent quantitative skin titrations, results being expressed as the log$_{10}$ (allergen concentration in μg/ml) which elicit 2-plus reactions. Designations for the allergens are as follows: ■ Group I, ▨ Group II, ▨ Group III, ▥ Group IV, ▨ AgB, ▨ AgE, □ Ra3 and ▨ Ra5. (From Marsh et al., 1974.)

Nevertheless, in view of all the genetic data from animal experiments, and the marked associations seen in unrelated allergic populations between specific second locus HL-A type and specific IgE response, the hypothesized linkage is almost certainly correct. However, there is presently insufficient evidence to support this view. The problem is that HL-A linked Ir genes represent only one level of control (presumptively the T cell level, McDevitt and Landy, 1972) which, in itself, seems to be genetically complex (cf. Black *et al.*, 1974). Other levels of genetic control of the immune response and immunopharmacologic processes governing IgE-mediated sensitivity are also important (cf. Marsh *et al.*, 1973c). One such gene, controlling total IgE level, is discussed in detail below.

5. Genetic Control of Basal Serum IgE Levels

As previously mentioned, the ability to produce IgE antibody (of any specificity) in mice appears to be under genetic control. Family and twin studies by Bazaral *et al.* (1971) and Hamburger *et al.* (1973) strongly suggested that the basal level of IgE is under a fairly simple genetic control, the mechanism of which was not elucidated. Preliminary family studies by Marsh *et al.* (1973d) indicated that high IgE levels were inherited as a simple Mendelian recessive trait. In a later study (Marsh *et al.*, 1974), the distribution frequencies of IgE levels in populations of unrelated allergic and nonallergic subjects were used to determine the cut-off point between high and low IgE levels. This was taken to be the concentration at which the sum of the percentages of allergics with atypically low IgE levels and nonallergics with atypically high IgE levels was minimized. The cut-off point, occurring at 95 ± 5 U/ml, was used in more extensive studies of 28 families. The results strongly supported simple recessive inheritance of high IgE levels. The proposed dominant "R" (IgE regulator) allele was found to have a gene frequency of 0.48 in the general population. It is of interest to note that results of genetic experiments in atopic dogs (Schwartzman *et al.*, 1971) are also consistent with the proposed recessive inheritance of high IgE levels.

The IgE-regulating gene was found to have a profound influence over specific IgE responses, apparently masking the effects of Ir genes in family studies (Marsh *et al.*, 1974). Figure 9 shows one large family in which specific skin sensitivities of allergic sibs to eight highly purified pollen allergens correlate much more closely with serum IgE levels than with HL-A haplotypes (with which there is no apparent correlation). This family also shows a definite failure to transmit allergy as a single dominant trait. In seven other families, there was no correlation between HL-A haplotype and overall patterns of specific IgE-mediated skin sensitivities. There was, however, a marked effect of the IgE-regulating gene. Sib pairs with both members having high IgE levels showed significantly higher concordance for specific sensitivities than did sib pairs with widely different IgE levels ($p = 0.001$).

While family studies emphasize the importance of the IgE-regulating gene over HL-A-linked Ir genes in the inheritance of allergy, population studies point to the interrelationship between the two types of genetic control.

6. Interrelationship of IgE-Regulating Gene and HL-A Associated Immune Response Genes

The specific IgE-mediated sensitivities in 205 highly allergic subjects were measured to the allergens rye grass Group I (Rye I) and ragweed AgE (Marsh, 1974; Marsh and Bias, 1974). Individuals sensitive to Rye I with or without AgE sensitivity were compared with those sensitive to AgE but not Rye I. In this large population, both HL-A8 and the HL-A8 Creg (8 and W-14) were found to be significantly elevated in the Rye I-*sensitive* group relative to the Rye I-*insensitive* group ($p = 0.005$ for HL-A8 and 0.006 for HL-A8 Creg). However, the overall percentage of Rye I-sensitive individuals possessing HL-A8 Creg antigens was not impressive (39%). Each of the two groups was then divided into quartiles on the basis of IgE level, and the frequency of HL-A8 Creg compared in the respective quartiles (Fig. 10). The most important finding was a significant elevation in the frequency of the HL-A8 Creg in the first, relative to the fourth, quartile of the Rye I-sensitive group. Also, there was a highly significant difference in the frequency of the HL-A8 Creg between the first quartiles of the two groups. Additionally, mirror image curves (on either side of the general population frequency of the HL-A8 Creg) can be seen in the frequency distributions of HL-A8 Creg for the two groups. This probably results from HL-A8 Creg antigens being allelic with other second locus HL-A antigens, some of which are presumptively associated with Ir genes for AgE.

These results demonstrate the interrelationship of the two types of control of immune responses. Sensitivity to Rye I is seen to be most closely associated with the possession of HL-A8 Creg in people with genetically determined limiting low IgE levels; at high IgE levels, this association is no longer apparent. A plausible interpretation of these results is that "high quality" recognition of the Rye I molecule is required only under the most limiting circumstances; this probably

4. Allergens and the Genetics of Allergy

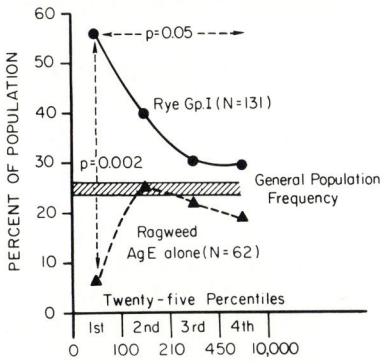

Fig. 10. Distribution frequency of HL-A8 Creg in sub-populations of *Group C* (sensitive to Rye I ± AgE, solid line) and *Group D* (sensitive only to AgE, dashed line), plotted against total basal serum IgE level. Total IgE levels were mainly determined on samples collected in the winter; twenty-five percentile divisions were obtained by dividing the whole allergenic population studied. The frequencies of HL-A8 Creg in unselected Caucasian populations (limits of shaded area) were calculated from the data of Dausset and Hors (1971) and Terasaki (1971). (Data taken from Marsh, 1974, by permission of copyright owners.)

occurs by strong interaction, at the cellular level, of an immunodominant carrier determinant of Rye I with product(s) of Ir gene(s) frequently associated with HL-A8 Creg antigens. On the other hand, for people with high IgE levels, the requirement for high quality allergenic recognition seems to be less crucial.

D. G. Marsh and W. B. Bias (unpublished observations) have investigated, in more detail, the interrelation between HL-A8 Creg antigens and total IgE level in a population of 134 Rye I-sensitive Caucasians. They confirmed the interrelation between the frequency of HL-A8 Creg and IgE level. In addition, they showed that similar interrelations exist between each of the separate 8 Creg specificities (8 and W-14) and IgE level. Marsh and Bias also investigated the interrelation between IgE level and frequency of HL-A type in 180 AgE-sensitive Caucasians, but were not able to detect a significant association with any HL-A type or HL-A Creg, even at limiting low IgE levels. This is probably due to the marked immunogenicity of the AgE molecule and to the presence of at least two other complex allergens, AgK and BPA-R, in ragweed which cross-react with AgE (Section IV,B,2). These findings suggest that AgE is a poor choice for studies of man's genetic ability to respond to a specific allergen. On the other hand, it is very useful as a control for ragweed exposure and ragweed allergy in studies such as those performed with Ra5, due to the pronounced genetic complexity of responsiveness to AgE and related molecules.

Preliminary analysis of 30 Ra5-sensitive Caucasians (unpublished) shows that the frequency of HL-A7 Creg is markedly elevated at all IgE levels (60–11,000 U/ml). In this highly limiting situation H-associated Ir gene recognition appears to be the overriding factor independent of IgE level.

In a very recent study Marsh et al. (1975b) investigated the interrelation between total IgE level and specific HL-A type in ragweed-allergic Caucasians who were either sensitive or insensitive to Ra3. This ragweed allergen has a molecular weight of 11,000 daltons, intermediate between Ra5 (MW 5000) and Rye I (MW 27,000). Specificities HL-A2 and 12 were both found to be elevated 1.4-fold in 65 Ra3-sensitive versus 43 Ra3-insensitive subjects. In the sensitive group the proportions of HL-A2, HL-A12, and HL-A2 + 12 in the phenotype were markedly higher in the lowest versus the highest IgE quartiles (cf. the data on Rye I). For individuals with IgE levels in the lowest quartile (≤ 130 U/ml), HL-A frequencies for the Ra3-sensitive versus the Ra3-insensitive groups were as follows: HL-A2, 13/14 versus 4/15 ($p = 0.001$); HL-A12, 9/14 versus 4/15 ($p = 0.09$); and HL-A2 + 12, 8/14 versus 1/15 ($p = 0.005$). The only person in the Ra3-sensitive group without HL-A2 possessed HL-A12. This finding, together with arguments based on the "linkage disequilibrium" within the HL-A system (see below), led the authors to suggest that the most probable location for a major Ir gene for Ra3 is between the 2 and 12 loci of HL-A2,12, one of the most commonly found haplotypes among Caucasians (cf. Terasaki, 1971). This interesting observation is being further investigated in families.

The above experiments provide evidence that both IgE-regulating and H-associated Ir genes play important roles in the development of IgE-mediated responses to allergens and that different effects can be seen depending on the complexity of the immunogen and of the host's genetic capacities to recognize specific antigens and to synthesize IgE.

7. DISCUSSION

We have seen how useful highly purified grass and ragweed pollen allergens can be in helping to solve the complex genetics of immune responsiveness in man. The critical factor is that immunogenic stimulation by naturally inhaled allergens is highly limiting. Two types of genetic control have been demonstrated: (1) specific histocompatibility-associated immune response genes controlling responses to particular antigens; and (2) a gene that controls IgE biosynthesis to any antigen. By analogy with work in experimental animals, we may postulate that HL-A-associated Ir genes control some function of T cells, possibly the recognition process. Despite the finding of close association between specific HL-A type (or group of types) and specific IgE-mediated sensitivity and IgG antibody response, family studies have so far failed to demonstrate *genetic linkage* convincingly. This arises from the polygenic nature of these responses and the probability that multiple alleles control specific immune recognition at certain of these levels (Marsh *et al.*, 1973c).

The immune responses to allergens tend to be associated with the second locus of HL-A, analogous to findings of association and linkage between specific immune responses and the *K* locus of H-2 in the mouse (reviewed in McDevitt and Landy, 1972). Furthermore, in man and the mouse, susceptibility or resistance to certain immunologically based diseases are also mainly associated with particular second and *K* locus specificities. The principal mouse Ir genes have been mapped near the major *MLC* locus. Due to the aforementioned analogies between HL-A and H-2, this finding has led to a general speculation that man's Ir locus is close to his major *MLC* locus. However, the relative map position of the major *MLC* locus differs in the two species; it lies *between* the serologically defined *D* and *K* loci of the mouse, but *outside* the region between the first and second loci of man (beyond the second locus). These species differences have been partially resolved by analysis of *MLC* data that suggest the presence of a second *MLC* locus between man's first and second HL-A loci (Bodmer, 1973a). Further definition of the relative map positions of Ir and *MLC* loci in the major histocompatibility regions of the two species awaits further experiment and analysis.

An important characteristic of the HL-A system is the existence of "linkage disequilibrium" between particular alleles of its component genes (Bodmer, 1973a). For example, in unrelated Caucasian populations the gene coding for the first locus specificity, HL-A1, is found on the same chromosome as the gene for second locus antigen, HL-A8, 3–6 times more frequently than predicted from the separate population frequencies of these two antigens. (For example, Terasaki, 1971, reports a frequency of HL-A1,8 5.6 times higher than predicted, although this varies from population to population.) The establishment of this linkage disequilibrium between HL-A1 and HL-A8 has evidently arisen due to some selective advantage of possessing the HL-A1,8 haplotype. The existence of further linkage disequilibria between certain disease susceptibility (DS-A) and second locus specificities has been postulated (Bodmer, 1973b and in McDevitt and Landy, 1972) to explain associations between susceptibility to certain diseases and HL-A type, such as Hodgkin's Disease and HL-A5 Creg. It is presently not clear whether such disease susceptibility arises from the possession of particular Ir genes, although this is a good possibility. In any case, linkage disequilibrium effects most probably account for the association between specific Ir genes and HL-A (such as an Ra5-Ir gene and HL-A7), as well as for the recently observed remarkably high (around 80–90%) association between HL-A serotype W-27 and susceptibility to ankylosing spondylitis and to Reiter's syndrome (Schlosstein et al., 1973; Brewerton et al., 1973a,b; Morris et al., 1974).

Many of the genes within an animal's major histocompatibility complex play important roles in immune function (McDevitt and Landy, 1972). Thus it does not seem unreasonable to postulate that linkage disequilibria between certain Ir and HL-A alleles have arisen due to their combination selectively *improving* immune function. In such cases the HL-A antigens themselves may well functionally interact with Ir gene products in determining the overall ability of the host to respond immunologically. The hypothesized placement of an important Ra3-Ir gene within the common Caucasian HL-A2,12 haplotype (see above) is of considerable interest in this regard.

The recently discovered IgE-regulating gene is a further important factor determining the expression of specific IgE-mediated sensitivity in man, as shown both by family and population studies. A simple hypothesis is that the product of the dominant R allele of this gene regulates IgE biosynthesis. Other explanations include genetic control of secretion of IgE, removal of IgE from the circulation, regulation of the IgE response (perhaps by T cells; Tada et al., 1973), or regulation of the differentiation of plasma cells from B cell precursors. Whatever the mechanism, this gene appears to modulate the expression of specific immune response genes differentially, according to whether the individual has a high or low total IgE level. Complex protein allergens, such as rye Group I, undoubtedly possess many structural regions recognized at T cells; these are referred to as carrier determinants. The limiting dosage of Rye I presumably restricts their number to a few immunodominant regions, the recognition of which may be controlled by different Ir genes linked to different HL-A types. If a further limitation is imposed, in terms of the ability to produce IgE (reflected in a low total serum

IgE level), recognition of Rye I appears to be narrowed down mainly to one determinant, controlled by the possession of Ir gene(s) associated with HL-A8 Creg. Based on these considerations, it is not difficult to understand why individuals with very high IgE levels tend to have multiple allergies and those with low levels have relatively few sensitivities, usually to complex "major" allergens.

In addition to the gene regulating IgE level, genes controlling other steps of the immune response process and the immunopharmacologic release of chemical mediators from mast cells and basophils await to be discovered. In particular, it seems reasonable to postulate from animal experiments that allotype-linked Ir genes are likely to be important in controlling antigenic recognition at B cells (McDevitt and Landy, 1972). Genetic control of macrophage function, suggested by Santilli *et al.* (1973), could be a further important factor. Also, the results of kidney transplants (Kissmeyer-Nielsen *et al.*, 1971) suggest that the HL-A1,8 haplotype in Caucasians may be associated with a generalized (non-antigen specific) enhanced immune responsiveness, since kidney recipients bearing this haplotype more readily reject mismatched kidneys than other people. This finding suggests the possibility that gene(s) controlling generalized immune responsiveness may also be associated with HL-A. One might anticipate that any one of the aforementioned genes might interfere with the expression of specific IgE-mediated sensitivity and, therefore, of detection of genetic linkage between a specific HL-A type and specific response in families (Marsh *et al.*, 1973c; Marsh, 1974).

To date, experiments measuring IgE-mediated skin sensitivity or serum antibody levels have sought to demonstrate genetic expressivity several steps removed from the T cell. In order to minimize the effects of non-H-linked genes, studies currently in progress will measure T cell function more directly by antigenic stimulation of peripheral lymphocytes *in vitro*. In this regard, further studies using low molecular weight allergens such as Ra5 should be particularly useful.

VII. Practical Considerations

Since 1911, when Noon discovered that treatment of patients with allergenic extracts was useful in the therapy of allergic disease, extracts for testing and immunization purposes have generally been prepared without proper immunologic standardization. Solutions of extracts have usually been prepared on a weight per volume (gm pollen/100 ml extracting fluid) or a protein nitrogen unit (PNU) per ml basis. Of these, the current PNU does not properly measure *protein* nitrogen, since the phosphotungstic acid used in the precipitation step precipitates a wide variety of low molecular weight peptides in addition to protein. In either case, it is only fortuitous if the immunologic potency of an extract prepared by one manufacturer is identical in potency with a similar extract (expressed in the same unitage) prepared by another. Fortunately, this situation is now changing, albeit slowly (Aas and Belin, 1972; Baer, 1974).

The concentrations of allergenic components antigen E and grass Group I have been shown to correlate closely with the biologic activities or ragweed and certain grass pollens, respectively (Baer *et al.*, 1970, 1974). As a first step toward full immunologic standardization, therefore, it is appropriate to base the potencies of crude extracts on the concentrations of these purified allergens. For both well and less well characterized extracts, the radioallergosorbent test (RAST) can readily be adapted for allergen standardization (Foucard *et al.*, 1972; Gleich *et al.*, 1974). The test employs a standard preparation of insolubilized cellulose–crude allergen conjugate and a standard serum pool from allergic individuals. The abilities of unknown and standard allergen extracts to inhibit binding of serum IgE antibody to the insoluble allergen complex are then compared in the RAST system. As an adjunct to the immunologic analyses, it is appropriate to confirm the biologic activity as allergenic materials using quantitative skin tests or histamine release assay.

These tests investigate the question of allergenic reactivity rather than immunogenic potency; the latter is particularly important to establish in the case of modified allergens such as allergoids. Methods based on the immunization of laboratory animals have been used as the criterion for immunogenicity (Marsh *et al.*, 1970b). This is very time consuming and generally not practicable for the investigation of large numbers of allergenic extracts, so other methods will have to be developed in the future. In order to improve further the solutions used in the testing and treatment of allergic individuals, it will also be necessary to perform more detailed antigenic analysis. The method of choice would be the Laurell crossed immunoelectrophoresis technique (Section IV,A).

Having standardized an allergen preparation, it is necessary to insure that biologic potency is maintained over long periods of time. Storage of extracts at 4° in the lyophilized state or in 50% glycerin has been found to prolong shelf life. The dilute allergen solutions used by the allergist for treatment and testing rapidly lose their biologic potency if not properly stabilized, due to surface adsorption and denaturation effects. This problem has recently been investigated by P. S. Norman and D. G. Marsh (unpublished observations) who compared the adsorption of radioactive allergen onto glass with the concomitant loss of biologic activity. In order to combat this problem, Hjorth (1958) recommended adding a small quantity of a nonionic detergent such as Tween 80 to the allergen solution; other workers (e.g., Malley et al., 1962) have used siliconized glassware. A further alternative is to dilute the allergen in a buffer containing a large excess of nonallergenic nonantigenic protein, such as 0.03% human serum albumin (King et al., 1964; Norman et al., 1973). In analyzing conditions of storage, Norman and Marsh concluded that the simplest approach is probably to incorporate 0.005% Tween 80 into the buffer used for dilution of the allergens.

VIII. Concluding Remarks

There appears to be an almost limitless array of substances which man encounters in his environment and toward which he may develop IgE-mediated sensitivity; these substances have generally been termed "allergens." Each allergically predisposed person develops a characteristic "sensitivity spectrum" to the immunochemically distinct allergens to which he is exposed. On the one hand, the factors that govern whether a particular substance will induce an IgE antibody response in man include the degree of immunogenicity of the allergen, its dosage, frequency, and route of administration (Sections IV,C; V,A). For inhaled or ingested allergens, there appears to be a limit on the molecular size (40,000–60,000 daltons) determined by the relative lack of mucosal membrane permeability toward macromolecules of higher molecular weight. On the other hand, a most important consideration determining whether a particular person will develop IgE-mediated allergies is the genetic predisposition of the individual (Section VI). Two distinct genetic factors have so far been discovered but not yet fully elucidated; these are the capacity to regulate total IgE level, and the ability to respond to specific allergenic stimulation (probably at the T cell level), controlled by specific Ir genes associated with HL-A type. Genes controlling other processes in the highly complex series of events which leads to IgE-mediated sensitivity remain to be defined.

Allergens have generally been found to be proteins or glycoproteins of widely different compositions, although carbohydrate allergens are also known. There seems to be no distinct chemical features that characterize allergens as apart from other antigens. Like most antigenic determinants, the major (*immunodominant*) allergenic determinants of protein allergens appear to comprise regions of the three-dimensional structure of the molecule exposed to the outer surface under physiological conditions. The possibility that some determinants are made up of portions of the primary structure should, however, be seriously considered in view of recent observations that some antigens possess such determinants (Benjamini *et al.*, 1972).

Future understanding of the physical and chemical structure of immunodominant determinants on allergens will allow for solution of a number of difficult problems presently facing immunologists interested in reaginic hypersensitivity. These problems include determination of (1) the molecular basis of allergen–IgE antibody interaction occurring on basophilic leukocyte and mast cell membranes; this will allow understanding of the way in which the cell receives the signal to release pharmacologically active mediators such as histamine; and (2) the detailed structural and immunogenetic basis for immune recognition of allergenic/antigenic determinants on the allergen molecule. Particularly in immunogenetic studies, the allergens should be prepared in an ultra pure ($>$ 99.9% pure) state (Section IV,A). Utilization of allergens of relatively simple structure, such as Ra5 (Section IV,B,2b), should greatly facilitate the elucidation of these problems.

One unexpected offshoot of research into the chemistry of pollen allergens may be improved knowledge of the components involved in pollen-stigma recognition systems required for plant fertilization (Section V,B). If interspecies cross-fertilization can be completely overcome, hybrids having superior food production capacities may well be developed. This will help to alleviate the growing world food shortage.

Development of chemically modified allergens (allergoids, Section IV,E), suitable for high dosage immunization of allergic humans without provoking anaphylaxis, should lead to better modes of treatment and improved understanding of the mechanism of immunotherapy. Areas now only vaguely understood, such as allergic reactions to foods, can now be approached due to recent knowledge of the structure of certain good allergens, in particular codfish allergen M (Section IV,B,3). Growing knowledge of the allergens in venoms should soon greatly improve treatment of the life-threatening sensitivity to stinging insects. Two further important areas of allergic disease, namely, atopic asthma and eczema are presently only barely understood. The allergens provoking these diseases need to be defined more precisely and the biochemical and immunologic aberrations that lead to disease expression need further extensive investigation.

As the dosage of allergen is increased, or as it becomes molecularly more complex (and, thus, more immunogenic), a greater percentage of the human population is able to develop specific IgE-mediated sensitivity to the allergen. This appears to be due primarily to a relaxation of the requirement for a specific genetic constitution for IgE responsiveness to each specific allergen. Thus, allergens of simple structure inhaled in ultralimiting dosage tend to be of relatively minor importance (e.g., ragweed Ra5), since the genetic requirements for allergen recognition at all levels of immune response are highly restrictive. Conversely, the more complex allergens inhaled in somewhat high dosages (e.g., grass Group I) are generally of major importance, since the limitations on immune recognition are less severe. If a complex allergen is administered parenterally in a relatively high, nonimmunogenically limiting, dosage (particularly if adsorbed to alumina adjuvant), the genetic differences separating atopic from nonatopic people are overcome, and most nonatopics develop pronounced IgE-mediated sensitivity. Unlike naturally induced allergy, this artificially induced sensitivity is usually transient and does not give rise to clinical symptomatology. The reasons for these differences are presently obscure but are no doubt fundamental to our understanding of the nature of allergic responsiveness.

Investigation of the genetic basis of allergy in man promises to be a rapidly expanding area, keeping pace with the current explosion in knowledge of the genetic control of immune responsiveness in animals. Because of the extreme molecular diversity of allergens which man encounters in his environment, and their generally immunogenically limiting dosage, study of man's immune responsiveness to these substances at every level will offer the possibility of mapping man's genetic responsiveness to foreign macromolecules. This will lead to a clearer understanding of the genetic basis of many diseases and, thereby, of improved prognosis and prophylaxis of each disorder. For these exciting prospects, detailed structural studies of many different allergens—particularly those of relatively simple structure—will be essential.

Acknowledgments

The work in this chapter was supported by U. S. Public Health Service Grant No. R01 AI 09565 and Research Career Development Award No. 5K4 AI 50304 and Food and Drug Administration Contract No. FDA-73-156. This review is Publication No. 132 from the O'Neill Laboratories at The Good Samaritan Hospital.

It is a pleasure to thank my colleagues, Wilma B. Bias, Paul L. Black, Lawrence Goodfriend, Lawrence M. Lichtenstein, and Philip S. Norman, for discussion of some of the ideas expressed in this review. I also wish to thank Jeanne E. Marsh and Te Piao King for reading and improving the text and Margaret Askey for typing the manuscript through several revisions.

References

Aas, K. (1967). *Int. Arch. Allergy Appl. Immunol.* **31**, 239.
Aas, K. (1974). *Allergol. Proc. Int. Congr., 8th 1973*, pp. 400–402. Excerpta Medica, Amsterdam.
Aas, K., and Belin, L. (1972). *Acta Allergol.* **27**, 439.
Aas, K., and Elsayed, S. M. (1969). *J. Allergy* **44**, 333.
Abramson, H. A., Moore, D. H., and Gettner, H. H. (1942). *J. Phys. Chem.* **46**, 192.
Ambler, J., and Orr, T. S. C. (1972). *Immunochemistry* **9**, 263.
Andrews, P. (1964). *Biochem. J.* **91**, 222.
Attallah, N. A., and Sehon, A. H. (1969). *Immunochemistry* **6**, 609.
Augustin, R. (1952). *Quart. Rev. Allergy Appl. Immunol.* **6**, 290.
Augustin, R. (1959a). *Immunology* **2**, 148.
Augustin, R. (1959b). *Immunology* **2**, 230.
Augustin, R., and Hayward, B. J. (1962). *Immunology* **5**, 424.
Axelson, N. H. (1971). *Infec. Immunity* **4**, 525.
Baer, H. (1974). *Allergol. Proc. Int. Congr., 8th, 1973*, pp. 379–380. Excerpta Medica, Amsterdam.
Baer, H., Godfrey, H., Maloney, C. J., Norman, P. S., and Lichtenstein, L. M. (1970). *J. Allergy* **45**, 347.
Baer, H., Maloney, C. J., Norman, P. S., and Marsh, D. G. (1974). *J. Allergy Clin. Immunol.* **54**, 157.
Balner, H., Dorf, M. E., de Groot, M. L., and Benacerraf, B. (1973). *Transplant. Proc.* **5**, 1555.
Barker, S. A., Cruickshank, C. N. D., and Morris, J. H. (1967). *Biochim. Biophys. Acta* **74**, 239.
Batchelor, F. R., and Dewdney, J. M. (1968). *Proc. Roy. Soc. Med.* **61**, 897.
Bazaral, M., Orgel, H. A., and Hamburger, R. N. (1971). *J. Immunol.* **107**, 794.
Belin, L. (1972a). *Int. Arch. Allergy Appl. Immunol.* **42**, 300.
Belin, L. (1972b). *Int. Arch. Allergy Appl. Immunol.* **42**, 329.
Belin, L., and Norman, P. S. (1974). *J. Allergy Clin. Immunol.* **53**, 329 (abstr.).
Belin, L., and Rowley, J. R. (1971). *Int. Arch. Allergy Appl. Immunol.* **40**, 754.
Belin, L., Hoborn, J., Falsen, E., and André, J. (1970). *Lancet* **2**, 1153.
Benacerraf, B., and McDevitt, H. O. (1972). *Science* **175**, 273.
Benjamini, E., Scibienski, R., and Thompson, K. (1972). *Contemp. Top. Immunochem.* **1**, 49.

4. Allergens and the Genetics of Allergy 351

Bennich, H., and Johansson, S. G. O. (1971). *Advan. Immunol.* **13**, 1.
Bernstein, I. L., and Safferman, R. S. (1966). *J. Allergy* **38**, 166.
Bernton, H. S. (1949). *Ann. Allergy* **7**, 13.
Berrens, L. (1971). *In* "The Chemistry of Atopic Allergens." Karger, Basel.
Berrens, L. (1974). *Ann. N. Y. Acad. Sci.* **221**, 183.
Bias, W. B. (1973). *In* "Asthma: Physiology, Immunopharmacology, and Treatment" (K. F. Austen and L. M. Lichtenstein, eds.), pp. 39–53. Academic Press, New York.
Bias, W. B., and Marsh, D. G. (1975). *Science* (in press).
Bias, W. B., Marsh, D. G., and Ishizaka, K. (1973). *Amer. J. Hum. Genet.* **25**, 16A.
Black, P. L., and Marsh, D. G. (1975). *In* "Bronchial Asthma: Mechanisms and Therapeutics" (M. S. Segal and E. B. Weiss, eds.) Little, Brown, Boston, Massachusetts (in press).
Black, P. L., Marsh, D. G., Jarrett, E., Delespesse, G. J., and Bias, W. B. (1974). *Int. Leuk. Cong., 9th*, Abstr. No. 25, p. 23.
Blackley, C. H. (1873). "Experiments and Researches on the Causes and Nature of *Catarrhus Aestivus.*" Ballière, London.
Bleumink, E., and Young, E. (1969). *Int. Arch. Allergy Appl. Immunol.* **35**, 1.
Bleumink, E., and Young, E. (1971). *Int. Arch. Allergy Appl. Immunol.* **40**, 72.
Bloch, K. J. (1967). *Progr. Allergy* **10**, 84.
Blumenthal, M. N., Amos, D. B., Noreen, H., Mendell, N. R., and Yunis, E. J. (1974). *Science* **184**, 1301.
Bodmer, W. F. (1973a). *In* "Histocompatibility Testing, 1972" (J. Dausset and J. Colombani, eds.), pp. 611–617. Munksgaard, Copenhagen.
Bodmer, W. F. (1973b). *Nat. Cancer Inst. Monogr.* **36**, 127.
Bonilla-Soto, O. (1969). *J. Allergy* **43**, 125.
Borek, F. (1972). *In* "Immunogenicity" (F. Borek, ed.), pp. 45–86. North-Holland Publ., Amsterdam.
Bostock, J. (1828). *Med.-Chir. Trans.* **14**, 437.
Bowen, R. (1953). *J. Allergy* **24**, 236.
Bradbury, S. M., Percy, D. H., and Strejan, G. H. (1974). *Int. Arch. Allergy Appl. Immunol.* **46**, 498.
Brandt, R., Ponterius, G., and Yman, L. (1973). *Int. Arch. Allergy Appl. Immunol.* **45**, 447.
Brewerton, D. A., Hart, F. D., Nicholls, A., Caffrey, M., James, D. C. O., and Sturrock, R. D. (1973a). *Lancet* **1**, 904.
Brewerton, D. A., Caffrey, M., Nicholls, A., Walters, D., and James, D. C. O. (1973b). *Lancet* **2**, 966.
Bridger, G. P., and Proctor, D. F. (1971). *Ann. Otol., Rhinol., Laryngol.* **80**, 445.
Britton, C. J. C., Coombs, R. R. A., Johnson, P., and Thorne, H. V. (1958). *Int. Arch. Allergy Appl. Immunol.* **13**, 305.
Bruce, C. A., Rosenthal, R. R., Lichtenstein, L. M., and Norman, P. S. (1974). *J. Allergy Clin. Immunol.* **53**, 230.
Brunner, M. (1934). *J. Allergy* **5**, 257.
Buckley, C. E., Dorsey, F. C., Corley, R. B., Ralph, W. B., Woodbury, M. A., and Amos, D. B. (1973). *Proc. Nat. Acad. Sci. U. S.* **70**, 2157.
Busse, W. W., Reed, C. E., and Hoehne, J. H. (1972). *J. Allergy Clin. Immunol.* **50**, 289.
Callaghan, O. H., and Goldfarb, A. R. (1962). *J. Immunol.* **89**, 612.
Campbell, D. H., Luescher, E., and Lerman, L. S. (1951). *Proc. Nat. Acad. Sci. U. S.* **37**, 575.
Caulfield, A. H. W. (1925). *Proc. Soc. Exp. Biol. Med.* **23**, 38.

Ceska, M., Eriksson, R., and Varga, J. M. (1972). *Int. Arch. Allergy Appl. Immunol.* **42**, 430.
Chang, E. B., and Marsh, D. G. (1974). *J. Allergy Clin. Immunol.* **53**, 65 (abstr.).
Coca, A. F. (1922). *J. Immunol.* **7**, 163.
Coca, A. F., and Cooke, R. A. (1923). *J. Immunol.* **8**, 163.
Coca, A. F., and Grove, E. (1925). *J. Immunol.* **10**, 445.
Connell, J. T. (1969). *J. Allergy* **43**, 33.
Cooke, R. A., and VanderVeer, A. (1916). *J. Immunol.* **1**, 201.
Craig, L. C., and King, T. P. (1962). *Methods Biochem. Anal.* **10**, 175.
Crifó, S., and Iannetti, G. (1969). *Acta Allergol.* **24**, 294.
Cuatrecasas, P. (1970). *J. Biol. Chem.* **12**, 3059.
Dausset, J., and Hors, J. (1971). *Transplant. Proc.* **3**, 1004.
Davidson, A. G., Baron, B., and Walzer, M. (1947). *J. Allergy* **18**, 359.
Davis, B. J. (1964). *Ann. N. Y. Acad. Sci.* **121**, 404.
Deutsch, H. F., and Morton, J. J. (1961). *Arch. Biochem. Biophys.* **93**, 654.
de Weck, A. L. (1971). *Int. Arch. Allergy Appl. Immunol.* **41**, 393.
de Weck, A. L. (1974). *Allergol. Proc. Int. Congr., 8th, 1973*, pp. 347–355. Excerpta Medica, Amsterdam.
de Weck, A. L., Schneider, C. H., Spengler, H., Toffler, O., and Lazary, S. (1973). *In* "Mechanisms in Allergy. Reagin-mediated Hypersensitivity" (L. Goodfriend, A. H. Sehon, and R. P. Orange, eds.), pp. 323–338. Dekker, New York.
Dietrich, F. M. (1966). *Int. Arch. Allergy Appl. Immunol.* **30**, 497.
Dische, Z. (1955). *Methods Biochem. Anal.* **2**, 313.
Elliott, W. B., Shepherd, G. W., and Arbesman, C. E. (1974). *J. Allergy Clin. Immunol.* **53**, 103 (abstr.).
Elsayed, S. M., and Aas, K. (1970). *Int. Arch. Allergy Appl. Immunol.* **38**, 536.
Elsayed, S. M., and Aas, K. (1971a). *Int. Arch. Allergy Appl. Immunol.* **40**, 428.
Elsayed, S. M., and Aas, K. (1971b). *J. Allergy Clin. Immunol.* **47**, 283.
Elsayed, S. M., Aas, K., and Christensen, T. (1971). *Int. Arch. Allergy Appl. Immunol.* **40**, 439.
Feigen, G. A., Sanz, E., Meyers, R. L., and Campbell, D. H. (1967). *Int. Arch. Allergy Appl. Immunol.* **32**, 174.
Feinberg, J. G. (1960). *Int. Arch. Allergy Appl. Immunol.* **16**, 1.
Feinberg, S. M. (1946). *In* "Allergy in Practice," p. 216. Yearbook Publ., Chicago, Illinois.
Foucard, T., Johansson, S. G. O., Bennich, H., and Berg, T. (1972). *Int. Arch. Allergy Appl. Immunol.* **43**, 360.
Fox, I., Knight, W. B., and Bayona, I. G. (1963). *J. Allergy* **34**, 196.
Fraefel, W., and Acher, R. (1968). *Biochim. Biophys. Acta* **154**, 615.
Francis, T. (1934). *Proc. Soc. Exp. Biol. Med.* **31**, 493.
Freedman, S. O., Krupey, J., and Sehon, A. H. (1961). *Nature (London)* **192**, 241.
Fries, J. H., and Lightstone, A. C. (1962). *Ann. Allergy* **20**, 351.
Gay, L. N. (1926). *J. Immunol.* **11**, 371.
Gell, P. G. H., and Coombs, R. R. A., eds. (1968). "Clinical Aspects of Immunology," 2nd ed. Blackwell, Oxford.
Gill, T. J. (1972). *In* "Immunogenicity" (F. Borek, ed.), pp. 5–44. North-Holland Publ., Amsterdam.
Gleich, G. J., Averbeck, A. K., and Swedlund, H. A. (1971). *J. Lab. Clin. Med.* **77**, 690.
Gleich, G. J., Larson, J. B., Jones, R. T., and Baer, H. (1974). *J. Allergy Clin. Immunol.* **53**, 158.

4. Allergens and the Genetics of Allergy

Gold, W. M. (1973) In "Asthma: Physiology, Immunopharmacology, and Treatment" (K. F. Austen and L. M. Lichtenstein, eds.), pp. 169–184. Academic Press, New York.
Goldfarb, A. R. (1964). *J. Asthma Res.* **2**, 7.
Goldfarb, A. R. (1968). *J. Immunol.* **100**, 902.
Goldfarb, A. R. (1972). *J. Asthma Res.* **9**, 139.
Goldfarb, A. R., Moore, D. H., Rappaport, H. G., Sklarofsky, B., Gettner, H. H., and Abramson, H. A. (1954). *Proc. Soc. Exp. Biol. Med.* **85**, 255.
Goodfriend, L., and Lapkoff, C. (1972). *Fed. Proc. Fed. Amer. Soc. Exp. Biol.* **31**, 757 (abstr.).
Gottschalk, A. (1966). "Glycoproteins." Elsevier, New York.
Grabar, P., and Burtin, P. (1960). "L'analyse immunoélectrophorétique; Ses applications aux liquides biologiques humains." Masson, Paris.
Greenert, S., Bernstein, I. L., and Michael, J. G. (1971). *Lancet* **2**, 1121.
Griffiths, B. W. (1972). *J. Chromatogr.* **69**, 391.
Griffiths, B. W., and Brunet, R. (1971). *Can. J. Biochem.* **49**, 396.
Grove, E. F., and Coca, A. F. (1925). *J. Immunol.* **10**, 471.
Gussoni, C. (1966). *Int. Arch. Allergy Appl. Immunol.* **29**, 591.
Habermann, E. (1972). *Science* **177**, 314.
Hackman, R. H., and Goldberg, M. (1958). *J. Insect Physiol.* **2**, 221.
Haddad, Z. H., Marsh, D. G., and Campbell, D. H. (1972). *J. Allergy Clin. Immunol.* **49**, 197.
Hamburger, R. N., Orgel, H. A., and Bazaral, M. (1973). In "Mechanisms in Allergy. Reagin-mediated Hypersensitivity" (L. Goodfriend, A. H. Sehon, and R. P. Orange, eds.), pp. 131–139. Dekker, New York.
Herbertson, S., Porath, J., and Colldahl, H. (1958). *Acta Chem. Scand.* **12**, 737.
Hirs, C. H. W., and Timasheff, S. N., eds. (1972). "Methods in Enzymology" Vol. 25 Academic Press, New York.
Hitchcock, A. S. (1950). "Manual of the Grasses of the United States," 2nd ed. U. S. Govt. Printing Office, Washington, D. C. (Also in two vols., Dover, New York, 1971.)
Hjorth, N. (1958). *Acta Allergol.* **12**, 316.
Hogarth-Scott, R. S., Watt, B. J., Ogilvie, B. M., and Rothwell, T. L. W. (1973). *Int. J. Parasitol.* **3**, 735.
Hussain, R., Bradbury, S. M., and Strejan, G. (1973). *J. Immunol.* **111**, 260.
Ishizaka, K. (1973). In "The Antigens" (M. Sela, ed.), Vol. I, pp. 479–528. Academic Press, New York.
Ishizaka, K., and Ishizaka, T. (1968). *J. Allergy* **42**, 330.
Ishizaka, K., and Ishizaka, T. (1969). *J. Immunol.* **103**, 589.
Ishizaka, K., Ishizaka, T., and Hornbrook, M. M. (1966). *J. Immunol.* **97**, 75.
Ishizaka, K., Tomioka, H., and Ishizaka, T. (1970). *J. Immunol.* **105**, 1459.
Johansson, S. G. O. (1972). *Scand. J. Clin. Lab. Invest.* **29**, 7.
Johansson, S. G. O., and Bennich, H. (1967). *Immunology* **13**, 381.
Johansson, S. G. O., Bennich, H., and Wide, L. (1968). *Immunology* **14**, 265.
Johnson, P., and Marsh, D. G. (1965a). *Eur. Poly. J.* **1**, 63.
Johnson, P., and Marsh, D. G. (1965b). *Nature (London)* **206**, 935.
Johnson, P., and Marsh, D. G. (1966a). *Immunochemistry* **3**, 91.
Johnson, P., and Marsh, D. G. (1966b). *Immunochemistry* **3**, 101.
Johnson, P., and Padley, P. J. (1959). *Int. Arch. Allergy Appl. Immunol.* **15**, 321.
Johnson, P., and Thorne, H. V. (1958). *Int. Arch. Allergy Appl. Immunol.* **13**, 257.

Jyo, T., Komoto, K., Tsuboi, S., Katsutani, T., and Otsuka, T. (1973). *Allergol. Proc. Int. Congr., 8th, 1973* Abstract No. 253.
Kabat, E. A., Turino, G. M., Tarrow, A. B., and Maurer, P. H. (1957). *J. Clin. Invest.* **36**, 1160.
Kailin, E. W., Rossbach, E. A., and Walzer, M. (1950). *J. Allergy* **21**, 225.
Kammann, O. (1904). *Beitr, Chem. Physiol. Pathol.* **5**, 346.
Kammann, O. (1912). *Biochem. Z.* **46**, 151.
Kaufman, W. (1958). *Int. Arch. Allergy Appl. Immunol.* **13**, 68.
Kawai, T., Marsh, D. G., Lichtenstein, L. M., and Norman, P. S. (1972). *J. Allergy Clin. Immunol.* **50**, 117.
Kern, F., Sobotka, A. K., Valentine, M. D., and Lichtenstein, L. M. (1974). *J. Allergy Clin. Immunol.* **53**, 111 (abstr.).
Kilburn, K. H., ed. (1974). "Pulmonary Reactions to Organic Materials," *Ann. N. Y. Acad. Sci.* **221**.
King, T. P. (1972). *Biochemistry* **11**, 367.
King, T. P. (1974). *Allergol. Proc. Int. Congr., 8th, 1973*, pp. 394–399. Excerpta Medica, Amsterdam.
King, T. P., and Norman, P. S. (1962). *Biochemistry* **1**, 709.
King, T. P., Norman, P. S., and Connell, J. T. (1964). *Biochemistry* **3**, 458.
King, T. P., Norman, P. S., and Lichtenstein, L. M. (1967a). *Biochemistry* **6**, 1992.
King, T. P., Norman, P. S., and Lichtenstein, L. M. (1967b). *Ann. Allergy* **25**, 541.
King, T. P., Norman, P. S., and Tao, N. (1974). *Immunochemistry* **11**, 83.
Kissmeyer-Nielsen, F. *et al.* (35 others). (1971). *Transplant. Proc.* **3**, 1019.
Knox, R. B., and Heslop-Harrison, J. (1971). *J. Cell Sci.* **9**, 239.
Knox, R. B., Willing, R. R., and Ashford, A. E. (1972). *Nature (London)* **237**, 381.
Koessler, K. K. (1914). *In* "Forchheimer's Therapeusis of Internal Diseases," Vol. V, p. 671. Appleton, New York.
Kojis, F. E. (1942). *Amer. J. Dis. Child.* **64**, 91.
Kontou-Karakitsos, K., Salvaggio, J. E., and Mathews, K. P. (1975). *J. Allergy Clin. Immunol.* (in press).
Lapkoff, C. B., and Goodfriend, L. (1974). *Int. Arch. Allergy Appl. Immunol.* **46**, 215.
Laurell, C.-B. (1972). *Scand. J. Clin. Lab. Invest.* **29**, 21.
Layton, L. L., Greene, F. C., Panzani, R., and Corse, J. W. (1965). *J. Allergy* **36**, 84.
Layton, L. L., Panzani, R., and Corse, J. W. (1966). *J. Allergy* **38**, 268.
Leskowitz, S., Salvaggio, J. E., and Schwartz, H. J. (1972). *Clin. Allergy* **2**, 237.
Levine, B. B. (1966). *N. Engl. J. Med.* **275**, 1115.
Levine, B. B. (1971). John Sheldon Memorial Lecture presented at the 27th Annual Meeting of the American Academy of Allergy. Quoted by Levine *et al.*, 1972.
Levine, B. B., and Vaz, N. M. (1970a). *Int. Arch. Allergy Appl. Immunol.* **39**, 156.
Levine, B. B., and Vaz, N. M. (1970b). *J. Clin. Invest.* **49**, 58 (abstr.).
Levine, B. B., Stember, R. H., and Fotino, M. (1972). *Science* **178**, 1201.
Levy, D. A., and Osler, A. G. (1966). *J. Immunol.* **97**, 203.
Lichtenstein, L. M. (1972). *In* "Clinical Immunobiology" (F. H. Bach and R. A. Good, eds.), Vol. 1, pp. 243–269. Academic Press, New York.
Lichtenstein, L. M., and Osler, A. G. (1964). *J. Exp. Med.* **120**, 507.
Lichtenstein, L. M., Marsh, D. G., and Campbell, D. H. (1969). *J. Allergy* **44**, 307.
Lichtenstein, L. M., Roebber, M., and Goodfriend, L. (1973a). *J. Allergy Clin. Immunol.* **51**, 285.
Lichtenstein, L. M., Ishizaka, K., Norman, P. S., Sobotka, A., and Hill, B. M. (1973b). *J. Clin. Invest.* **52**, 472.
McDevitt, H. O., and Benacerraf, B. (1969). *Advan. Immunol.* **11**, 31.

4. Allergens and the Genetics of Allergy

McDevitt, H. O., and Chinitz, A. (1969). *Science* **163,** 1207.
McDevitt, H. O., and Landy, M., eds. (1972). "Genetic Control of Immune Responsiveness." Academic Press, New York.
McDevitt, H. O., and Tyan, M. L. (1968). *J. Exp. Med.* **128,** 1.
Malley, A., and Dobson, R. L. (1966). *Fed. Proc., Fed. Amer. Soc. Exp. Biol.* **25,** 729 (abstr.).
Malley, A., and Harris, R. L. (1967). *J. Immunol.* **99,** 825.
Malley, A., Reed, C. E., and Lietze, A. (1962). *J. Allergy* **33,** 84.
Malley, A., Campbell, D. H., and Heimlich, E. M. (1964a). *J. Immunol.* **93,** 420.
Malley, A., Saha, A., and Campbell, D. H. (1964b). *Immunochemistry* **1,** 237.
Malley, A., Crossley, G., Baecher, L., Wilson, B. J., Perlman, F., and Burger, D. (1973). *In* "Mechanisms in Allergy. Reagin-mediated Hypersensitivity" (L. Goodfriend, A. H. Sehon, and R. P. Orange, eds.), pp. 83–96. Dekker, New York.
Mancini, G., Carbonara, A. O., and Heremans, J. F. (1964). *Immunochemistry* **2,** 235.
Marsh, D. G. (1971). *Int. Arch. Allergy Appl. Immunol.* **41,** 199.
Marsh, D. G. (1973). *In* "Asthma: Physiology, Immunopharmacology, and Treatment" (K. F. Austen and L. M. Lichtenstein, eds.), pp. 50 and 308. Academic Press, New York.
Marsh, D. G. (1974). *Allergol. Proc. Int. Congr., 8th, 1973,* pp. 381–393. Excerpta Medica, Amsterdam.
Marsh, D. G. (1975a). In preparation.
Marsh, D. G. (1975b). In preparation.
Marsh, D. G., and Bias, W. B. (1974). *Fed. Proc., Fed. Amer. Soc. Exp. Biol.* **33,** 774 (abstr.).
Marsh, D. G., and Bias, W. B. (1975). Submitted for publication.
Marsh, D. G., and Haddad, Z. H. (1968). *Fed. Proc., Fed. Amer. Soc. Exp. Biol.* **27,** 368 (abstr.).
Marsh, D. G., and Lichtenstein, L. M. (1975). In preparation.
Marsh, D. G., and Norman, P. S. (1974). In preparation.
Marsh, D. G., Milner, F. H., and Johnson, P. (1966). *Int. Arch. Allergy Appl. Immunol.* **29,** 521.
Marsh, D. G., Haddad, Z. H., and Campbell, D. H. (1970a). *J. Allergy* **46,** 107.
Marsh, D. G., Lichtenstein, L. M., and Campbell, D. H. (1970b). *Immunology* **18,** 705.
Marsh, D. G., Lichtenstein, L. M., and Norman, P. S. (1972). *Immunology* **22,** 1013.
Marsh, D. G., Bias, W. B., Hsu, S. H., and Goodfriend, L. (1973a). *Science* **179,** 691.
Marsh, D. G., Bias, W. B., Goodfriend, L., and Ishizaka, K. (1973b). *Fed. Proc., Fed. Amer. Soc. Exp. Biol.* **32,** 1000 (abstr.).
Marsh, D. G., Bias, W. B., Hsu, S. H., and Goodfriend, L. (1973c). *In* "Mechanisms in Allergy. Reagin-mediated Hypersensitivity" (L. Goodfriend, A. H. Sehon, and R. P. Orange, eds.), pp. 113–129. Dekker, New York.
Marsh, D. G., Hsu, S. H., and Bias, W. B. (1973d). *Hosp. Prac.,* p. 41.
Marsh, D. G., Bias, W. B., and Ishizaka, K. (1974). *Proc. Nat. Acad. Sci. U. S.* **71,** 3588.
Marsh, D. G., Belin, L., Bruce, C. A., and Lichtenstein, L. M. (1975a). Submitted.
Marsh, D. G., Chase G. A., and Bias, W. B. (1975b). *Fed. Proc., Fed. Amer. Soc. Exp. Biol.* **34,** 980.
Maunsell, K., Wraith, D. G., and Cunnington, A. M. (1968). *Lancet* **1,** 1267.
May, C. D., Lyman, M., Alberto, R., and Cheng, J. (1970). *J. Allergy* **46,** 12.
Metzger, H. (1973). *In* "Mechanisms in Allergy. Reagin-mediated Hypersensitivity" (L. Goodfriend, A. H. Sehon, and R. P. Orange, eds.), pp. 301–311. Dekker, New York.
Milford, E. L. (1930). *J. Allergy* **1,** 331.

Minchin Clarke, H. G., and Freeman, T. (1966). *Protides Biol. Fluids, Proc. Colloq.* **14**, 503.
Miyamoto, T. (1974). *Allergol. Proc. Int. Congr.*, 8th, 1973, pp. 403-410. Excerpta Medica, Amsterdam.
Miyamoto, T., Oshima, S., Ishizaki, T., and Sato, S. (1968). *J. Allergy* **42**, 14.
Mole, L. E., Goodfriend, L., Lapkoff, C. B., Kehoe, J. M., and Capra, J. D. (1974). *Fed. Proc., Fed. Amer. Soc. Exp. Biol.* **33**, 751 (abstr.); *Biochemistry* (in press).
Moore, M. B., Cromwell, H. W., and Moore, E. E. (1930). *J. Allergy* **2**, 6.
Morris, J. H., Berrens, L., and Young, E. (1965). *Clin. Chim. Acta* **12**, 407.
Morris, R., Metzger, A. L., Bluestone, R., and Terasaki, P. I. (1974). *N. Engl. J. Med.* **290**, 554.
Nadel, J. A. (1973). *In* "Asthma: Physiology, Immunopharmacology, and Treatment" (K. F. Austen and L. M. Lichtenstein, eds.), pp. 29-38. Academic Press, New York.
Naterman, H. L. (1957). *J. Allergy* **28**, 76.
Naterman, H. L. (1965). *J. Allergy* **36**, 226.
Neumann, W., and Habermann, E. (1954). *Arch. Exp. Pathol. Pharmakol.* **222**, 367.
Newell, J. M. (1941). *J. Allergy* **13**, 177.
Noon, L. (1911). *Lancet* **1**, 1572.
Norman, P. S. (1969). *J. Allergy* **44**, 129.
Norman, P. S. (1973). *In* "Asthma: Physiology, Immunopharmacology, and Treatment" (K. F. Austen and L. M. Lichtenstein, eds.), pp. 211-219. Academic Press, New York.
Norman, P. S., and Lichtenstein, L. M. (1973). *J. Allergy* **52**, 94.
Norman, P. S., Marsh, D. G., and Lichtenstein, L. M. (1972). *J. Allergy* **49**, 114.
Norman, P. S., Lichtenstein, L. M., and Ishizaka, K. (1973). *J. Allergy Clin. Immunol.* **52**, 210.
Norman, P. S., Marsh, D. G., Lichtenstein, L. M., and Ishizaka, K. (1975). *J. Allergy Clin. Immunol.* **55**, 78.
Ohman, J. L., Jr., Lowell, F. C., and Bloch, K. J. (1973). *J. Allergy Clin. Immunol.* **52**, 231.
Orange, R. P., and Austen, K. F. (1969). *Advan. Immunol.* **10**, 105.
Ornstein, L. (1964). *Ann. N. Y. Acad. Sci.* **121**, 321.
Osler, A. G., Lichtenstein, L. M., and Levy, D. A. (1968). *Advan. Immunol.* **8**, 183.
O'Sullivan, S. (1968). Ph.D. Thesis, University of Liverpool.
Ovary, Z., and Taranta, A. (1963). *Science* **140**, 193.
Palmstierna, H., Ende, H. A., and Ripe, E. (1962). *Sci. Tools.* **9**, 25.
Parish, W. E. (1973). *In* "Asthma: Physiology, Immunopharmacology, and Treatment" (K. F. Austen and L. M. Lichtenstein, eds.), pp. 71-90. Academic Press, New York.
Patrucco, R., and Marsh, D. G. (1974). *J. Allergy Clin. Immunol.* **53**, 65.
Patterson, R., Suszko, I. M., and McIntire, F. C. (1973a). *J. Immunol.* **110**, 1402.
Patterson, R., Suszko, I. M., Pruzansky, J. J., and Zeiss, C. R. (1973b). *J. Immunol.* **110**, 1413.
Pepys, J. (1969). "Hypersensitivity Disease of the Lungs Due to Fungi and Organic Dusts." Karger, Basel.
Pepys, J. (1973). *In* "Asthma: Physiology, Immunopharmacology, and Treatment" (K. F. Austen and L. M. Lichtenstein, eds.), pp. 279-294. Academic Press, New York.
Pepys, J., Hargreaves, F. E., Longbottom, J. L., and Faux, J. (1969). *Lancet* **1**, 1181.
Perlman, F. (1958). *J. Allergy* **29**, 302.
Peterson, E. A., and Sober, H. A. (1956). *J. Amer. Chem. Soc.* **78**, 751.

Phillips, E. W. (1939). *J. Allergy* **11**, 28.
Phills, J. A., Harrold, A. J., Whiteman, G. B., and Perelmutter, L. (1972). *N. Engl. J. Med.* **286**, 965.
Porath, J., and Flodin, P. (1959). *Nature (London)* **183**, 1657.
Prausnitz, C., and Küstner, H. (1921). *Zentralbl. Bakteriol., Parasitenk., Infektionskr. Hyg., Abt. 1: Orig.* **86**, 160.
Proctor, D. F., Swift, D. L., Quinlan, M., Salman, S., Takagi, Y., and Evering, S. (1969). *Arch. Environ. Health* **18**, 671.
Pulaski, E. J., Baker, H. J., Tarrow, A. B., and Amspacher, W. H. (1951). Report to National Research Council Committee on Shock (cited in Kabat *et al.*, 1957).
Rackemann, F. M. (1918). *Arch. Intern. Med.* **22**, 552.
Rackemann, F. M., and Stevens, A. H. J. (1927). *J. Immunol.* **13**, 389.
Rackemann, F. M., and Wagner, H. C. (1936). *J. Allergy* **7**, 319.
Radola, B. J. (1973). *Ann. N. Y. Acad. Sci.* **209**, 127.
Raffel, S. (1973). *In* "Mechanisms in Allergy. Reagin-Mediated Hypersensitivity" (L. Goodfriend, A. H. Sehon, and R. P. Orange, eds.), pp. 313–321. Dekker, New York.
Ratner, B., and Silberman, D. E. (1953). *J. Allergy* **24**, 371.
Ricci, M. (1974). *Allergol. Proc. Int. Congr., 8th, 1973*, pp. 411–416. Excerpta Medica, Amsterdam.
Richter, M., Sehon, A. H., Gordon, J., Grégoire, C., and Rose, B. (1958). *J. Allergy* **29**, 287.
Robbins, K. C., Wu, H., and Hsieh, B. (1966). *Immunochemistry* **3**, 71.
Roebber, M., and Goodfriend, L. (1970). *Fed. Proc., Fed. Amer. Soc. Exp. Biol.* **29**, 576 (abstr.).
Roebber, M., Marsh, D. G., and Goodfriend, L. (1975). Submitted for publication.
Salvaggio, J., Cavanaugh, J. J. A., Lowell, F. C., and Leskowitz, S. (1964). *J. Allergy* **35**, 62.
Salvaggio, J., Kayman, H., and Leskowitz, S. (1966). *J. Allergy* **38**, 31.
Salvaggio, J., Castro-Murillo, E., and Kundur, V. (1969). *J. Allergy* **44**, 344.
Salvaggio, J., Waldman, R., Arquembourg, P., and Johnson, J. (1971). *J. Allergy Clin. Immunol.* **47**, 117 (abstr.).
Santilli, J., Sverak, L., Marsh, D. G., Lichtenstein, L. M., and Bellanti, J. A. (1973). *J. Allergy Clin. Immunol.* **51**, 115 (abstr.).
Schachman, H. K. (1959). "Ultracentrifugation in Biochemistry." Academic Press, New York.
Schlosstein, L., Terasaki, P. I., Bluestone, R., and Pearson, C. M. (1973). *N. Engl. J. Med.* **288**, 704.
Schneeberger, E. E. (1974). *Ann. N. Y. Acad. Sci.* **221**, 238.
Schwartz, M. (1952). "Heredity in Bronchial Asthma." Munksgaard, Copenhagen.
Schwartzman, R. M., Rockey, J. H., and Halliwell, R. E. (1971). *Clin. Exp. Immunol.* **9**, 549.
Seabury, J., Salvaggio, J., Domer, J., Fink, J., and Kawai, T. (1973). *J. Allergy* **51**, 161.
Segal, A. T., Kemp, J. P., and Frick, O. L. (1970). *J. Allergy* **45**, 120.
Sela, M. (1969). *Science* **166**, 1365.
Shapiro, A. L., Vinuela, E., and Maizel, J. V. (1967). *Biochem. Biophys. Res. Commun.* **28**, 815.
Sherman, W. B. (1959). *Annu. Rev. Med.* **10**, 207.
Sherman, W. B. (1965). *Med. Clin. N. Amer.* **49**, 1597.
Sherman, W. B. (1968). "Hypersensitivity. Mechanisms and Management," Saunders, Philadelphia, Pennsylvania.

Shipolini, R. A., Callewart, G. L., Cottrell, R. C., Doonan, S., Vernon, C. A., and Banks, B. E. C. (1971a). *Eur. J. Biochem.* **20**, 459.
Shipolini, R. A., Callewart, G. L., Cottrell, R. C., and Vernon, C. A. (1971b). *Fed. Eur. Biochem. Soc. Lett.* **17**, 39.
Shulman, S. (1968). *Progr. Allergy* **12**, 246.
Siraganian, R. P., Schenkein, I., and Levine, B. B. (1973). *J. Allergy Clin. Immunol.* **51**, 102 (abstr.).
Smithies, O. (1959). *Advan. Protein Chem.* **14**, 65.
Sobotka, A. K., Valentine, M. D., Benton, A. W., and Lichtenstein, L. M. (1974a). *J. Allergy Clin. Immunol.* **53**, 170.
Sobotka, A. K., Franklin, R., Valentine, M., Adkinson, N. F., Jr., and Lichtenstein, L. M. (1974b). *J. Allergy Clin. Immunol.* **53**, 103 (abstr.).
Soulsby, E. J. L. (1968). In "Clinical Aspects of Immunology" (P. G. H. Gell and R. R. A. Coombs, eds.), 2nd ed., pp. 167–168. Davis, Philadelphia, Pennsylvania.
Spaich, D., and Ostertag, M. (1936). *Z. Ges. Anat., Abt. 2* **19**, 731.
Spieksma, F. T. M., and Voorhorst, R. (1969). *Acta Allergol.* **24**, 124.
Spies, J. R. (1973). *J. Milk Food Technol.* **36**, 225.
Spies, J. R. (1974a). *J. Agr. Food Chem.* **22**, 30.
Spies, J. R., and Coulson, E. J. (1943). *J. Amer. Chem. Soc.* **65**, 1720.
Spies, J. R., and Coulson, E. J. (1964). *J. Biol. Chem.* **239**, 1818.
Spies, J. R., and Umberger, E. J. (1942). *J. Amer. Chem. Soc.* **64**, 1889.
Spies, J. R., Coulson, E. J., Bernton, H. S., and Stevens, H. (1940). *J. Amer. Chem. Soc.* **62**, 1420.
Spies, J. R., Coulson, E. J., Chambers, D. C., Bernton, H. S., and Stevens, H. (1944). *J. Amer. Chem. Soc.* **66**, 748.
Spies, J. R., Stevan, M. A., Stein, W. J., and Gordon, W. G. (1974). *Int. Arch. Allergy Appl. Immunol.* (in press).
Squire, J. R. (1950). *Clin. Sci.* **9**, 127.
Stanworth, D. R. (1957). *Biochem. J.* **65**, 582.
Stanworth, D. R. (1963). *Advan. Immunol.* **3**, 181.
Stanworth, D. R. (1973). "Immediate Hypersensitivity." North-Holland Publ., Amsterdam.
Sternberger, L. A., Feinberg, A. R., Feinberg, S. M., Clarke, M., Benaim, C., and Warren, S. A. (1956). *J. Allergy* **27**, 16.
Strejan, G. H., Hussain, R., and Bradbury, S. (1973). In "Mechanisms in Allergy. Reagin-mediated Hypersensitivity" (L. Goodfriend, A. H. Sehon, and R. P. Orange, eds.), pp. 33–42. Dekker, New York.
Stull, A., Chobot, R., and Cooke, R. A. (1930). *J. Allergy* **1**, 470.
Stull, A., Cooke, R. A., and Chobot, R. (1931). *J. Biol. Chem.* **92**, 569.
Stull, A., Cooke, R. A., Sherman, W. B., Hebald, S., and Hampton, S. F. (1940). *J. Allergy* **11**, 439.
Sutherland, C. (1945). *Med. J. Aust.* **32**, 584.
Tada, T., and Ishizaka, K. (1970). *J. Immunol.* **104**, 377.
Tada, T., Okumura, K., and Taniguchi, M. (1973). In "Mechanisms in Allergy. Reagin-mediated Hypersensitivity" (L. Goodfriend, A. H. Sehon, and R. P. Orange, eds.), pp. 43–61. Dekker, New York.
Terasaki, P. I. (1971). *Dis.a-Mon.* **12**, 10.
Tips, R. L. (1954). *Amer. J. Hum. Genet.* **6**, 328.
Underdown, B. J., and Goodfriend, L. (1969). *Biochemistry* **8**, 980.
Unger, L., Cromwell, H. W., and Moore, M. B. (1932). *J. Allergy* **3**, 253.
Van Arsdel, P. P., and Molulsky, A. G. (1959). *Acta Genet.* **9**, 101.

4. Allergens and the Genetics of Allergy 359

Van Holde, K. E., and Baldwin, R. L. (1958). *J. Phys. Chem.* **62**, 734.
Vannier, W. E., and Campbell, D. H. (1959). *J. Allergy* **30**, 198.
Vaughan, W. T., and Black, J. H. (1954). "Practice of Allergy," 3rd ed., p. 74. Mosby, St. Louis, Missouri.
Vaz, N. M., and Levine, B. B. (1970). *Science* **168**, 852.
Vesterberg, O. (1972). *Biochim. Biophys. Acta* **257**, 11.
Vesterberg, O. (1973). *N. Y. Acad. Sci.* **209**, 23.
von Pirquet, C. (1906). *Muenchen. Med. Wochenschr.* **53**, 1457.
Voorhorst, R. (1958). *In* "Occupational Allergy" (H. E. Stenfert Kroese, ed.), p. 260. H. E. Stenfert Kroese, Leiden.
Voorhorst, R., Spieksma, F. T. M., Varekamp, H., Leupen, M. J., and Lyklema, A. W. (1967). *J. Allergy* **39**, 325.
Walzer, M. (1939). *J. Allergy* **10**, 72.
Waterhouse, A. T. (1914). *Lancet* **2**, 946.
Weiner, A., Zieve, I., and Fries, J. (1936). *Ann. Eugen.* **7**, 141.
Wide, L., Bennich, H., and Johansson, S. G. O. (1967). *Lancet* **2**, 1105.
Williams, C. A., and Chase, M. W., eds. (1967). "Methods in Immunology and Immunochemistry," Vols. 1 and 2. Academic Press, New York.
Williams, C. A., and Chase, M. W., eds. (1970). "Methods in Immunology and Immunochemistry," Vol. 3. Academic Press, New York.
Williams, C. A., and Chase, M. W., eds. (1970). "Methods in Immunology and Immunochemistry," Vol. 4. Academic Press, New York.
Wilson, A. F., Novey, H. S., Berke, R. A., and Surprenant, E. L. (1973). *N. Engl. J. Med.* **288**, 1056.
Wodehouse, R. P. (1954). *Int. Arch. Allergy Appl. Immunol.* **5**, 337.
Wodehouse, R. P. (1955). *Int. Arch. Allergy Appl. Immunol.* **6**, 65.
Wodehouse, R. P. (1957). *Ann. Allergy* **15**, 527.
Wodehouse, R. P. (1971). "Hayfever Plants," 2nd ed. Hafner, New York.
Wright, G. L. T., and Clifford, H. T. (1965). *Med. J. Aust.* **2**, 74.
Wright, G. P., and Hopkins, S. J. (1941). *J. Pathol. Bacteriol.* **53**, 243.
Wyman, M. (1872). "Autumnal Catarrh (Hay Fever)," p. 82. Hurd & Houghton, Cambridge, Massachusetts.
Yunginger, J. W., and Gleich, G. J. (1972). *J. Allergy Clin. Immunol.* **50**, 326.

CHAPTER 5

A Biologic and Chemical Profile of Histocompatibility Antigens

S. FERRONE, M. A. PELLEGRINO, AND R. A. REISFELD

I. Introduction	362
II. History	362
Histocompatibility Antigens of Other Species.	365
III. Genetics	368
A. The H-2 System	368
B. The HL-A System	369
IV. Serologic Detection of H Antigens	371
A. The Lymphocytotoxicity Assay	372
B. Platelet-Complement Fixation	383
C. Serologic Evaluation of Soluble HL-A Antigens	383
V. Cell Surface Expression of H Antigens	385
A. Tissue Distribution	385
B. Arrangement of H Antigens on Cell Membranes	388
C. Expression of H Antigens during the Cell Cycle	392
D. Effect of Inhibitors of Macromolecular Synthesis	395
VI. Cross-Reactivity of H Antigens.	398
A. Cross-Reactivity within the HL-A System.	398
B. Cross-Reactivity between H Antigens of Different Species	400
VII. Extraction, Purification, and Biologic Activity of Soluble H Antigens	402
A. Antigen Source Material	402
B. Extraction of Soluble H Antigens	407
C. Purification of H Antigens	414
D. Biologic Reactivity of Soluble H Antigens.	416
VIII. Chemical and Molecular Nature of HL-A Antigens	418
A. Physical Properties	418
B. Chemical Properties	418
C. β_2 Microglobulin and HL-A Antigens.	420
D. Molecular Nature.	430
IX. Perspectives	431
References.	435

I. Introduction

A study of histocompatibility (H) antigens is a challenging task dealing with an intriguing biologic and chemical phenomenon—the uniqueness of the individual. H antigens are genetically segregating cell surface structures which differ among individuals. These antigens can be defined since grafts exchanged between individuals who differ with respect to these antigens are rejected by the immune system of the recipient. Transplantation systems thus make it possible to study gene systems which determine histocompatibility as well as their gene products represented by a set of chemical markers. The clarification of the chemical and molecular nature of H antigens will further facilitate their use as genetically determined markers with which to study cell membrane cytoarchitecture and to gain insight into those membrane functions that determine antigenic recognition and immune responsiveness.

Several recent reviews have adequately dealt with the enormous amount of literature dealing with H antigens which has accumulated over the last 30 years (Nathenson, 1970; Ceppellini, 1971; Mann and Fahey, 1971; Walford et al., 1971; Albert and Terasaki, 1972; Batchelor and Brent, 1972; Kahan and Reisfeld, 1973; Dausset, 1973; Yunis et al., 1973). Rather than duplicate these efforts, we chose to focus on some aspects of H antigens investigated in our laboratory. References to the work of others in these same areas of research are incomplete as they were only used to implement the discussion of our experimental data.

II. History

Transplantation antigens of inbred strains of mice were first described by Gorer (1936) who discovered four blood group antigens, one of which, antigen II, was also found in tissues and affected the survival of tumor transplants. After Snell (1948) suggested that these antigens involved in transplantation should be called histocompatibility (H) antigens, antigen II was designated H-2. Little and Johnson (1922), Loeb (1930), and Snell (1948) demonstrated the role of H antigens in the genetic relationship between donor and host when grafts exchanged between members of the same inbred strain survived indefinitely, while those between members of different strains were quickly rejected. Then, Medawar (1944) concluded that

5. Histocompatibility Antigens: Biology and Chemistry

grafts caused the release of antigens which induced a destructive, immune response by the host resulting in graft rejection. Although these antigens were found initially in tissues of experimental animals, examination of their blood disclosed that H antigens were also on leukocytes (Medawar, 1944). In each species investigated (Palm, 1964; Snell and Stimpfling, 1966; Rapaport et al., 1970; Balner et al., 1971; Klein and Shreffler, 1971) these antigens were considered to be the products of a strong transplantation locus and of several weaker loci on a single chromosomal region. Once H antigens had been observed on leukocytes, many serologic investigations were launched to characterize them. Amos (1953) studied leukocyte agglutinins formed in mice given allogeneic skin grafts. Afterwards, Dausset (1954) and Miescher and Fauconnet (1954) showed that formation of alloimmune leukoagglutinins was induced by blood transfusion. Somewhat later, Payne and Rolfs (1958) and van Rood et al. (1958) independently found that alloantibodies against leukocytes may be formed during pregnancy. Dausset (1958) then characterized the first human white cell antigen "Mac," which was detected in 60% of the French volunteers whom he surveyed, and he demonstrated that these antigens were genetically determined since cells from monozygotic twins reacted identically in the leukagglutination test. These latter data were strengthened by several family studies (Payne and Rolfs, 1958; van Rood et al., 1958). van Rood (1962) introduced computer analysis of sera and could thus examine a large number of blood samples from pregnant women. van Rood (1962) identified the first example of a leukocyte group with at least two specificities, 4a and 4b, controlled by alleles. A second set of allelic leukocyte antigens, designated LA, was characterized by Payne et al. (1964). Walford's (1965) introduction of rabbit complement for lymphocytotoxicity testing and the miniaturization of this method by Terasaki and McClelland (1964) were subsequent improvements in the methodology of histocompatibility typing. When Terasaki and his colleagues (1965) observed a correlation between matching of human histocompatibility antigens (HL-A) and survival of kidney transplants, extensive characterization of this antigenic system appeared to be a solution to human allograft rejection. However, after the initial enthusiasm it appeared that, although HL-A typing was a useful tool for the selection of donor–recipient combinations among siblings, it did not fulfill this role among unrelated individuals (Mickey et al., 1971). This apparent contradiction was at first explained on the basis of: (1) HL-A typing is limited because of technical errors and disparities, (2) HL-A determinants have a latent heterogeneity, and (3) the most important determinants evoke only weak humoral but strong cellular immunity.

More recent data suggest a major involvement of other antigenic systems that control reactivity in the mixed lymphocyte (MLC) reaction since graft survival correlates with the results of the MLC reaction in vitro (Bach et al., 1970; Hamburger et al., 1971; Cochrum et al., 1973; van Rood et al., 1973). However, the HL-A system still plays a key role in transplantation when production of a recipient's humoral antibodies has been evoked by previous immunization, e.g., by pregnancy or blood transfusion (Terasaki et al., 1971; van Rood, 1971; van Rood et al., 1973).

Rapid progress in the serologic and genetic characterization of HL-A antigens was facilitated by the organization of several international Histocompatibility Workshops. At the first in 1964 (Russell and Winn, 1965) serologic methods in tissue typing were compared; at the second in 1965 (Amos and van Rood, 1966) correspondence of H antigenic groups was studied, and at the third in 1967 (Curtoni et al., 1967) data from family studies established the concept of a single H locus, which in man was termed HL-A. In 1968, a WHO committee on international nomenclature designated 6 HL-A antigens, then in 1970 and 1972 added 4 and 5 more HL-A antigens, respectively. The fourth Histocompatibility Workshop in 1970 (Terasaki, 1970) confirmed the concept of the 2 HL-A segregant series, while the fifth Workshop in 1972 (Dausset and Colombani, 1973) showed that the HL-A specificities thus far named were largely valid only for Caucasian populations. Because non-Caucasian populations had other unknown specificities, possibly their antibodies might be highly useful in the further characterization of HL-A antigens in Caucasians. Practical applications for results of studies in the H antigen field were extended by the report that HL-A antigens were associated with diseases in man, e.g., Hodgkin's disease (Amiel et al., 1967), glomerulonephritis (Patel et al., 1969; Mickey et al., 1970), leukemia (Thorsby et al., 1969; Walford et al., 1970). Then, chemical characterizations of H antigens began with efforts to solubilize H-2 antigens (Kandutsch, 1960; Nathenson and Davies, 1966; Manson and Palm, 1968) so that allograft survival could be prolonged (Billingham et al., 1956). Solubilization of HL-A antigens was also attempted by a variety of methods largely to study their physicochemical nature and antigenic reactivity in vitro (Bruning et al., 1967; Metzgar et al., 1967; Kahan et al., 1968; Mann et al., 1968; Sanderson and Batchelor, 1968). Presently, many investigators are clarifying the role of these genetically segregating cell surface markers in cell economy aside from the man-made transplantation phenomena. Because of their

5. Histocompatibility Antigens: Biology and Chemistry

strategic locations on plasma cell membranes, H antigens can be used in future investigations of the cytological architecture and metabolism of cell membranes in normal and pathological conditions. The likely involvement of cell membranes and their receptors in neoplasia further emphasizes the necessity for their complete characterization.

Histocompatibility Antigens of Other Species

The recognition that genetic constitution plays a major role in determining the fate of tissue grafts (Little and Johnson, 1922; Loeb, 1930; Snell, 1948) led to numerous investigations showing that in each species studied there is a single, strong histocompatibility locus.

1. MOUSE

Of the major histocompatibility systems studied, the H-2 system of the inbred laboratory mouse has been most extensively investigated. Following the pioneer work of Gorer (1936) and of Snell (1948), there has been an immense amount of work which cannot be adequately reviewed here. Only a brief description of the genetics of the H-2 system is reported below.

The genetic organization of the H-2 complex has been extensively reviewed by Klein and Shreffler (1971) and by Klein (1973). Generally speaking, the H-2 complex consists of 19 known H-2 chromosomes of which 8 or 9 are suspected to be derived from other H-2 chromosomes by recombination. The two major regions of the H-2 complex, H-2K and H-2D, contain 10 and 11 different alleles, respectively. A more realistic estimate of the H-2 complexity, i.e., its extensive polymorphism, has been achieved through a study of wild mice (Klein and Park, 1973). Among 150 wild mice from 25 different localities, more than 30 different phenotypes were found from which 30 H-2 chromosomes were isolated (Klein, 1971a). There have also been extensive studies dealing with the solubilization of H-2 antigens from cell membranes and with the chemical and molecular characterization of these antigens. Again the volume of this work is too extensive to permit its adequate review here.

2. RAT

Next to the H-2 and HL-A histocompatibility systems, the H-1 (Ag-B) system in inbred rats has been most extensively investigated

(Palm, 1964; Stark et al., 1968). At least 16 autosomal histocompatibility loci have been detected in rats (Silvers and Billingham, 1970; Mullen and Hildemann, 1971). Some 22 antigenic specificities have been associated with 10 alleles of the major H-1 (Ag-B) system in 39 inbred and 6 congenic strains of rats (Stark et al., 1970; Palm, 1971). The maternal fetal histoincompatibilities which confer survival advantages on fetuses possessing H antigens absent in the mother are believed to bring about selection pressure in favor of heterozygotes, thus maintaining alloantigenic polymorphism (Palm, 1970). Rat histocompatibility antigens have been solubilized and partially characterized by chemical means (Stroehmann and DeWitt, 1972), and recently the species antigens and major Ag-B alloantigens were physically separated and characterized to be two separate molecules (Callahan et al., 1974).

3. Dog

In dogs at least 6 cellular antigenic systems have been identified (Swisher et al., 1962; Storb et al., 1970). The major histocompatibility system in the dog, the DL-A system, was found to be extremely polymorphic and consists of two series of multiple alleles (Vriesendorp et al., 1971). The recombination frequency between the two series is similar (0.007 and 0.008) (Svejgaard et al., 1971).

4. Pig

In the pig a major histocompatibility locus has been demonstrated. This locus segregates in a simple Mendelian fashion and has been demonstrated by the use of lymphocytotoxic antisera. The locus segregates independently of the major blood group systems and was found linked to a locus controlling stimulation in mixed lymphocyte cultures (*MLC*). This locus was shown to be important in the rejection of skin and kidney allografts (White et al., 1973).

5. Rhesus Monkey

In the rhesus monkey a major histocompatibility system similar to that found in man has been described. This RhL-A system is highly polymorphic and controlled by two closely linked series of alleles. Products of ~50% of the genes of each series have thus far been identified serologically. Recombination frequency within the RhL-A region is 1–2%, similar to that found in man. Intersib skin grafting established the relevance of RhL-A to histocompatibility. Similar to man, genetic disparity at RhL-A is correlated with stimulation in

MLC, suggesting close linkage between RhL-A and the system controlling MLC reactivity (Balner et al., 1973).

6. GUINEA PIG

There have been several investigations dealing with histocompatibility antigens of guinea pigs. In early studies it was estimated that inbred strains 2 and 13 differ by at least 4–6 histocompatibility antigens (Bauer, 1960). More recently cross-immunization with leukocytes in an outbred guinea pig colony led to the serologic identification (microlymphocytotoxicity) of several leukocyte antigens which behave as alleles of a single locus (GPL-A). The significant prolongation of skin graft survival achieved in pairs of animals matched according to these leukocyte antigens indicated a system of transplantation antigens (de Weck et al., 1971). Extensive studies have been carried out on the solubilization and biologic and chemical characterization of histocompatibility antigens isolated from spleen cells of strain 2 and 13 guinea pigs. Briefly, H antigens could be solubilized by low frequency sound and purified by ion-exchange chromatography, gel exclusion chromatography, and acrylamide gel electrophoresis. This antigenic material (1) induced the accelerated rejection of test allografts, (2) elicited specific delayed-type hypersensitivity reactions upon intradermal challenge of allogeneic hosts that had been presensitized with donor-type grafts, (3) participated with sensitized cells in third-party local passive transfer reactions in transformation of lymphocytes in vitro. This study has been extensively reviewed (Reisfeld and Kahan, 1970). Chemically, the purified antigens were shown to be electrophoretically homogeneous at pH 9.4. The antigenic component isolated from strain 2 guinea pigs proved immunogenic as its injection (1–3 μg) into allogeneic strain 13 hosts accelerated the rejection of donor-type strain 2 grafts but not of strain 13 isografts. The antigenic activity of this electrophoretically homogeneous component was also demonstrated by elicitation of a specific delayed-type hypersensitivity response by intradermal injection of presensitized allogeneic hosts with 0.1 μg of antigen. The purified antigen thus induced a state of transplantation immunity and elicited expression of delayed type hypersensitivity following the induction of immunity by skin grafts. The purified strain 2 and strain 13 antigens showed molecular weights of 15,000 daltons as ascertained by sedimentation equilibrium techniques and gel filtration in the presence of 5 M guanidine. Neither lipid nor carbohydrate could be detected in the antigen at levels exceeding 1%. Strain 2 and strain 13 antigens showed limited and reproducible differences in amino acid composition. These data suggested that the two transplantation antigens possess allotypic specificities related to protein structure (Kahan and Reisfeld, 1968).

III. Genetics

There are several extensive and up-to-date reviews and discussions dealing with the genetics of H-2 antigens (Klein and Shreffler, 1971; Snell *et al.*, 1971) and HL-A antigens (Kissmeyer-Nielsen and Thorsby, 1970; Ceppellini, 1971). The following is just a brief discussion of some of the major findings concerning the genetics of H antigens.

A. *The H-2 System*

The H-2 complex of the mouse is located on chromosome no. 17 and is approximately 0.5 map unit long (Shreffler, 1970) and 15 map units distant from the centromere (Klein, 1971a). The H-2 complex can be divided into 6 regions. Starting from the centromere, they are K, Ir, Ss-Slp, X, D, and TL. The K region consists of a single gene (H-2K) or possibly a gene cluster, the products of which can be detected by serologic and transplantation methods. The Ir region, which is known to control immune responses to a variety of thymus (T)-dependent antigens, consists of more than one gene. It has been postulated that Ir gene products are cell surface receptors for different antigens (McDevitt and Benacerraf, 1969; Benacerraf and McDevitt, 1972). For this to occur the Ir genes should be expressed in only one particular cell type, i.e., most likely T lymphocytes. In addition, each clone of T lymphocytes would express only one or possibly a few Ir genes while different clones would express different genes (Klein and Park, 1973).

The Ss-Slp region most likely consists of at least two genes. The Ss gene controls a substance found in high concentration in some sera of some strains and low concentration in that of others (Shreffler, 1965). The Slp gene controls a sex-linked protein present in sera of males of some inbred strains (Passmore and Shreffler, 1970). The Ss region seems thus far to be functionally unrelated to the H-2 complex, but in a still undefined way is related to the complement system (Hinzová *et al.*, 1972; Démant *et al.*, 1973).

The X or unknown region is a chromosomal segment between the

5. Histocompatibility Antigens: Biology and Chemistry

Ss-Slp and D regions. As many as 21 recombinants of the 34 mapped intra-H-2 recombinants are located in this region which thus most likely consists of many genes. The function of the X region and its relationship to the rest of the H-2 complex are unknown (Klein and Park, 1973). The D region, similar to the K region, consists of a gene (H-2D) or a gene cluster controlling serologically detectable transplantation antigens.

Although the TL region has not been considered to be part of the H-2 complex, the TLa gene, which is within one map unit of H-2D, codes for membrane alloantigens detectable only on thymocytes and some leukemic cells (Boyse et al., 1966). There is, however, recent evidence that differences in the TL region can cause skin graft rejection (Boyse et al., 1972). These data suggest either that H genes are closely linked to the TLa gene or that the latter cannot be detected serologically as it is expressed on skin cells. The above structure of the H-2 complex is based upon analyses of a limited number of inbred strains most of which were related in origin. A better analogy to the HL-A system with its outbred population and consequent great polymorphism is the occurrence of H-2 loci in wild mice. When natural mouse populations were analyzed with anti-H-2 reagents obtained by cross-immunization of inbred strains, 2 major antigen categories were designated: public and private (Klein, 1971b). Inbred-derived public H-2 antigens have a high frequency in wild mice, whereas inbred-derived private antigens occur extremely rarely. Since inbred-derived H-2 reagents are of no value in defining new H-2 chromosomes, Klein (1973) produced antisera against wild-derived H-2 antigens to differentiate wild-derived H-2 chromosomes. In these studies it became apparent that the H-2 system was enormously polymorphic in wild mice collected in a small geographical area of Michigan. Klein proposed two alternative explanations for the extensive polymorphism of the H-2 system. The first assumes evolutionary neutrality of the H-2 system. Thus, cell mutants survive and reproduce normally in contrast to other genetic systems where most mutations are lethal. The second alternative ascribes a high selective advantage to the H-2 polymorphism, e.g., in susceptibility or resistance to disease and in immune surveillance.

B. The HL-A System

Knowledge of the development of the genetics and serology of the HL-A system is closely linked with facts learned from experiments on the H-2 system in inbred mouse strains. Thus, the HL-A system is described as a bipartite locus containing two segregant series. The system thus far is known to contain at least 14 specificities in the first or LA series and 27 in the second or FOUR series resulting in a minimum of 378 haplotypes. When the chromosome is inherited, specificities determined by the two series are usually inherited together suggesting that the two loci are closely linked. A given chromosome will have one specificity of the first and one of the second, but never two from within one series. Thus, any individual has two chromosomes that determine his or her HL-A type, one inherited from the father and one from the mother. The phenotype is made up of the two chromosomes or haplotypes. When two individuals have a child, one or another of the haplotypes from each parent is inherited by the offspring. Crossovers between the first and second segregant series have been observed suggesting that two separate loci exist. All HL-A antigens tested thus far appear to be codominant. The HL-A system seems to be one of the most polymorphic systems in man (Cavalli-Sforza and Bodmer, 1971). Preliminary data on recombinants between the two segregant series show a recombinant fraction of 0.5 to 1% (Svejgaard et al., 1971); thus one can assume that there are many genes between the two subloci. In fact, it is uncertain at this time whether the antigens are products of single or multiple structural cistrons or whether HL-A biosynthesis is affected by other genes.

It should be pointed out, however, that the simplistic two subloci concept is not completely consistent with all available data. Thus, sometimes individuals form alloantibodies against antigenic specificities not present on the sensitizing leukocyte preparation, and at times the antibodies are directed against specificities present on the cells of the recipient (Amos, 1970). In addition, some alloantibodies have broad reactivities that cannot be accounted for within the HL-A system which is basically held to be one of "private" specificities. On some occasions, broad antibodies reflecting "public" specificities have been disregarded. On other occasions, broad antibodies are considered to be associated in so-called inclusion groups. This inclusion phenomenon is explained by unidirectional cross-reactivity of the corresponding antibodies.

A number of studies suggest a general homology between the HL-A and the H-2 systems. Although there are some parallels between the two systems, some important differences also exist. Thus, in the mouse a single chromosome determines more than two antigens, i.e., in some cases (H-2[a]) up to 19 antigens (Klein and Shreffler, 1971). In addition, only private antigens controlled by the

5. Histocompatibility Antigens: Biology and Chemistry

two H-2 complexes are mutually exclusive (Snell et al., 1971). Moreover, these antigens are quite rare in the mouse population, and the limited studies have not proved whether or not they are controlled by allelic series. In general, the HL-A system seems to be serologically and genetically simpler than the H-2 system. However, as pointed out by Klein and Shreffler (1971) a different interpretation may account for discrepancies between the serologies of the two systems. Thus, according to Hirschfeld (1965), any immunogenetic system can be interpreted in two ways: the simple-complex and the complex-simple models. In the simple-complex system antibodies are simple because they react with a single antigenic determinant. On the other hand, antigens are complex because each molecule carries several antigenic determinants. The H-2 system has essentially been interpreted on the basis of this model. In the complex-simple system, antibodies are complex cross-reacting with more than one antigenic determinant, whereas the antigens are simple with each molecule possessing only one antigenic determinant. The HL-A system has been traditionally interpreted according to this model. Both systems are idealized and thus false in that they assume either simple specific antibodies or simple antigens with only one kind of antigenic determinant. It seems indeed most difficult to draw any meaningful conclusions as to which of the two models is more realistic until the chemical basis for the antigenic differences in these two complicated immunogenetic systems is better known. As pointed out by Shreffler (1967), no matter what the mode of interpretation, it seems difficult if not impossible to relate serologic properties to the molecular structure of gene products and to the properties of the controlling genes.

IV. Serologic Detection of H Antigens

Because they are simple, rapid, precise, and specific, serologic methods have been extensively utilized for the characterization of histocompatibility antigens. Among several techniques with many modifications employed to increase the sensitivity of the test and the reproducibility of the results, two have been the most instrumental in accumulating our knowledge of HL-A antigens. Leukoagglutination proved effective in delineating the first 10 well-defined HL-A antigens, because with this relatively insensitive technique many alloantisera reacted as if they were monospecific. Since then the poor reproducibility of results, the low incidence of leukoagglutinins, the great influence of physiological variations in leukocyte donors, and the necessity of considering the ABO groups of cell and sera donors have all greatly reduced the usefulness of this method for characterization of HL-A antigens. At present it is employed to study antigens that are detectable only by leukoagglutination: a classic example is the granulocytic specific antigen which may cause granulocytopenia of the newborn (Lalezari and Bernard, 1966; Lalezari et al., 1970, 1971; van der Weerdt and Lalezari, 1972).

A. The Lymphocytotoxicity Assay

Lymphocytotoxicity, now the most commonly used test for histocompatibility, relies upon alterations in permeability of the cell membrane induced by the action of complement on target lymphocytes which have been exposed to cytotoxic antibodies. Scanning electron microscopy has shown that human lymphocytes exposed to HL-A alloantisera and complement have abnormal shapes and irregular craters with cracked surfaces (Lambertenghi-Deliliers et al., 1971). Under transmission, electron microscope (Claesson et al., 1971; Lambertenghi-Deliliers et al., 1971) the cytoplasmic membrane has no projections but presents perforations that are larger than those observed in sheep red blood cell membranes exposed to antibody and complement (Borsos et al., 1964). Lesions that progress with prolonged exposure of the cells to antibodies and complement are observed in the cytoplasm and nuclei. Early in the cytotoxic reaction, the number of free ribosomes increases causing increased density of the cytoplasm; the mitochondria exhibit varying degrees of degeneration; in the nucleus heterochromatin is condensed and euchromatin disappears. Late in the cytotoxic reaction, all advanced lymphoid cell decay is manifested in the cytoplasm by hydropic swelling and the appearance of numerous intracellular vacuoles. The nucleus shows a predominant heterochromatin substance condensed into a compact mass. In the euchromatic part of the chromatin a fibrillar material is often seen. The perinuclear cisterna is sometimes dilated and contains an electron dense material, but the perinuclear membrane is without perforations and seems fairly well preserved even in the most advanced stages of lysis.

It is noteworthy that all these lesions, which may be considered to represent a pyknotic type of cell necrosis, are not characteristic of the damage induced by HL-A antibody and complement. They have in fact also been observed in nonimmunologic reactions (Zucker-

TABLE I

The Microcytotoxicity Test

Target cells:	Human peripheral lymphocytes or human cultured lymphoid cells.
HL-A alloantisera:	Alloantisera from multiparous women or from subjects immunized with blood transfusions or transplants.
Complement:	Selected rabbit serum for peripheral lymphocytes. Absorbed or suitably diluted rabbit serum for cultured human lymphoid cells.
Procedure:	Sera (2 µl) + cells (2000) are incubated under mineral oil for 30 minutes at room temperature. Rabbit complement (3 µl) is added and the incubation is continued for 60 minutes at room temperature. Eosin 5% (2 µl) is added and after 2 minutes the reaction is stopped by the addition of 2 µl of formalin 33%. The percentage of dead cells is determined under phase contrast microscopy.

Franklin, 1965; Walford *et al.*, 1966; Lucas and Peakman, 1969), thus they may actually be a general consequence of injury to cytoplasmic membranes rather than a specific effect of cytotoxic HL-A alloantibody (Glick *et al.*, 1970; Claesson *et al.*, 1971).

The principal steps in the lymphocytotoxic test as utilized in this laboratory are summarized in Table I; this microtest is a modification of a technique originated by Terasaki and McClelland (1964) who designed a microtest to save HL-A alloantisera.

1. TARGET CELLS

Lymphocytes can be prepared by a variety of techniques that are based on differential centrifugation (Greenwalt *et al.*, 1962; Weisbart *et al.*, 1972), on density gradients (Boyum, 1968; Perper *et al.*, 1968) and/or the adhesive and phagocytic properties of granulocytes (Levine, 1956; Johnson and Garvin, 1959). Cultured lymphoid cells may be used as targets in the cytotoxic test, and they may constitute a useful tool in the characterization of HL-A antigens and of HL-A alloantisera, since they retain HL-A antigens after prolonged periods of tissue culture (Papermaster *et al.*, 1969; Rogentine and Gerber, 1969, 1970). However, since HL-A determinants are denser on cultured lymphocytes than on autologous peripheral lymphocytes (Rogentine and Gerber, 1970; Pellegrino *et al.*, 1972a), the former are more sensitive in the cytotoxic test, as indicated by increased titers with HL-A alloantisera (Bernoco *et al.*, 1969; Papermaster *et al.*, 1972) and by the greater lytic efficiency of human complement (Ferrone *et al.*, 1971a) which is usually poorly effective in the cytotoxic test with peripheral lymphocytes. With the latter cells, HL-A antibodies, which are believed to be IgG, are too sparsely spaced on the cell surface to initiate complement fixation, since attachment of two continuous IgG molecules are required to fix complement for cell lysis and histocompatibility antigens are separated from each other by several thousand angstroms (Davis and Silverman, 1968; Karnovsky et al., 1972).

2. Sources of HL-A Alloantisera

HL-A alloantisera are obtained from subjects previously immunized against HL-A antigens. Parous women are the most common source of monospecific HL-A alloantisera; however, the limited incidence of lymphocytotoxic antibodies among pregnant women, i.e., about 20% (Ferrone et al., 1968), requires screening of many sera to obtain reagents suitable for HL-A typing. Moreover, lymphocytotoxic antibodies usually remain for a short time in the circulation so that only a few bleedings can be performed. Sera from polytransfused or transplanted patients are seldom monospecific because of the exposure of the patients to a large number of HL-A antigens, but may be used after suitable dilution or absorption. Planned immunization of volunteers with repeated skin grafts, with injection of purified leukocytes and platelet suspensions, or with transfusions of blood has yielded valuable antisera, especially for the identification of new HL-A specificities. HL-A alloantisera produced in these ways have low titer because if immunization is continued after the formation of cytotoxic antibodies, other antibodies develop first to antigens which cross-react with the principal antigen, then against other determinants.

Although no major inconvenience to volunteers has been reported from these immunizations, it should be stressed that sensitization of healthy subjects to strong transplantation antigens might jeopardize the success of subsequent allografts, if required.

To overcome the limited supply of HL-A alloantisera and to obtain reagents of high titer and affinity, Batchelor (1969), Einstein et al. (1971a), Ferrone et al. (1972a, 1973a), and Metzgar and Miller (1972) have attempted to produce HL-A heteroantisera by immunizing different species with whole cells or with soluble HL-A antigens. Heteroantibodies may even have a higher resolution capacity than the average human antiserum (van Rood et al., 1972). In fact man may have an innate cellular immunity against all but his own HL-A antigens which, in turn, may "confuse" the production of HL-A antibodies during the immunization process. By appropriate dilutions or absorptions, monospecific HL-A heteroantisera have occasionally been obtained, suggesting that production of HL-A heteroantisera is possible, although optimal experimental conditions have yet to be devised.

As pointed out by Walford et al. (1967), HL-A alloantisera are only operationally monospecific since most of them contain additional weak HL-A antibodies which become apparent when the sensitivity of the cytotoxic test is increased. This limitation should be kept in mind when one is reacting HL-A alloantisera with cells that may have increased concentrations of HL-A antigens on their surfaces (e.g., cultured human lymphoid cells) or whose structures may have been altered by pathological conditions or by treatment *in vitro* with proteolytic enzymes or sulfhydryl compounds. These phenomena may be important causes of spurious correlations between HL-A typing and some diseases which modify lymphocytes and may explain why a number of HL-A typing sera show increased incidences of reactivity with chronic lymphocytic leukemia cells, but other antisera of the same HL-A specificity do not (Walford et al., 1971). The limited specificity of HL-A alloantisera may account for the bizarre HL-A phenotype described in patients with abnormalities of lymphocytes, such as leukemia and immunodeficiency, or observed in cultured human lymphoid cells. In the course of HL-A direct typing of human cultured lymphoid cell lines by the dye exclusion cytotoxic test, Ferrone et al. (1972b) observed that some cell lines had more than two HL-A determinants within each segregating series. However, in some instances, these cells could not absorb typing antibodies from the alloantisera, although they could react positively in the direct cytotoxic test. These results suggest that positive reactions are caused by HL-A antibodies other than those already defined.

3. Role and Pathway of Activation of the Complement System

Rabbit serum is the most efficient source of complement in the cytotoxic reaction (Walford et al., 1964) (Fig. 1), despite its relatively low content of complement components in the conventional hemolytic test with sensitized sheep erythrocytes (Nelson and Biro, 1968). When human peripheral lymphocytes are utilized as target cells, rabbit serum which lacks any spontaneous cytotoxic activity must be selected as the source of complement. When cultured lymphoid cells are the targets, rabbit serum must be either absorbed (McDonald *et al.*, 1970) or suitably diluted (Rogentine and Gerber, 1969; Ferrone *et al.*, 1971a) to eliminate its direct cytotoxic effect on these cells.

The superior effectiveness of rabbit serum as a source of comple-

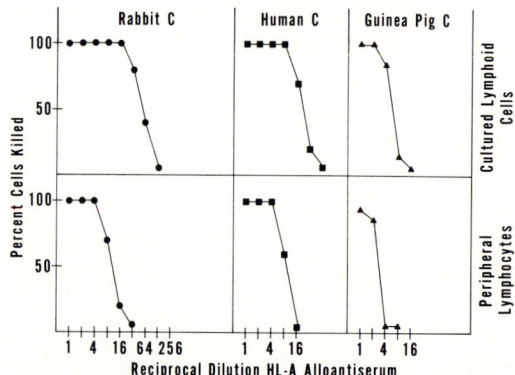

Fig. 1. Efficiency of rabbit, human, and guinea pig complement in the cytotoxic test with HL-A alloantisera and cultured human lymphoid cells or peripheral lymphocytes.

ment depends on the supply to the cytotoxic reaction of complement components and natural antibodies (Ferrone et al., 1971b) directed against a polymorphic antigenic system present on human lymphoid cells (Mittal et al., 1973a). These natural antibodies are apparently of the IgM class, since they are sensitive to mercaptoethanol treatment, behave like macroglobulins on gel filtration, and react with monospecific antisera to rabbit IgM (Ferrone et al., 1974c) (Fig. 2). Natural rabbit antibodies display different specificities; when 49 normal rabbit sera were analyzed against a large panel of human lymphocytes from random individuals and members of families, at least four specificities were identified that appeared to be unrelated to any known HL-A specificity or ABO group (Mittal et al., 1973a). The antigenic receptors for natural rabbit antibodies are more dense on cultured human lymphoid cells than on human peripheral lymphocytes (Ferrone et al., 1971a); treatment of lymphoid cells with neuraminidase (Yunis et al., 1970) or with the sulfhydryl compound 2-aminoethylisotiouronium bromide (AET) (Sirchia and Ferrone, 1971) increases their reactivity. Neuraminidase exposes new cell surface structures that react with these antibodies, but researchers have not determined yet whether AET uncovers new antigenic sites or only increases the sensitivity of the cell membrane to the lytic action of complement.

The role of natural antibodies in rabbit serum is clearly indicated by the inefficient cytotoxicity of rabbit complement absorbed with peripheral lymphocytes or with human cultured lymphoid cells. After such absorption, the cytotoxic titer of the alloantiserum is

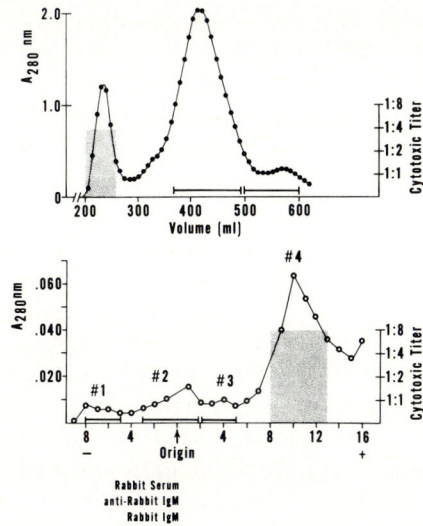

Fig. 2. Isolation of natural rabbit antibodies by ammonium sulfate precipitation, Sephadex G-200 filtration (upper part) and Pevikon block electrophoresis (central part). Reactivity of purified rabbit IgM with anti-rabbit IgM serum on immunoelectrophoresis (lower part).

reduced and with some alloantisera false negative reactions occur (Ferrone *et al.*, 1971a). Not only is rabbit serum with a low level of natural antibodies poorly effective as a source of complement in the lymphocytotoxic test, but also increased quantities of natural rabbit antibodies directed against antigens present in the lymphoid tissue greatly improve its sensitivity (Ferrone and Pellegrino, 1973).

Complement-antibody mediated lysis of cells depends on a critical concentration of complement accumulating at the cell surface. This level cannot be reached even with a large excess of antibody and complement if antigen receptors are too few (Linscott, 1970). The relatively low density of histocompatibility antigens on cell surfaces which are separated from each other by large empty areas (Karnovsky *et al.*, 1972) may bind insufficient complement to interact with HL-A antibodies and ultimately to effect cell lysis. Therefore, human complement is poorly cytolytic on human peripheral lymphocytes reacted with anti-HL-A alloantisera. This view is reinforced by the fact that human complement is more cytolytic against cultured human lymphoid cells, which have a high concentration of HL-A antigens on their surfaces, than against peripheral lymphocytes which do not (Ferrone *et al.*, 1971b).

In this regard, activation of the late complement components can be mediated through two pathways (Sandberg et al., 1970; Frank et al., 1971; Götze and Müller-Eberhard, 1971): one, the classical pathway, begins with C1, C4, C2 while the other, the alternate pathway, bypasses these first components, starts with a still unidentified component, and proceeds with C3 proactivator. Both pathways converge at the step where C3 becomes involved. The pathway can be identified by several means such as: (1) the ability of antibodies to mediate lysis when the complement selected is lacking in components essential for one of the two pathways, (2) the cytolytic activity of antibodies when the complement used is deprived of calcium but not of magnesium, the former being required for activation of the classical but not of the alternate pathway (Fine et al., 1972), (3) the quantitation of consumption of early complement components by cells sensitized with antibodies, and (4) the quantitation of uptake of labeled complement components by cells sensitized with antibodies, when one of the pathways is shut off.

When human serum is the source of complement, some HL-A alloantisera activate only the alternate pathway since heating of complement at 50°C for 20 minutes, which destroys C3PA (a component of the alternate pathway) (Götze and Müller-Eberhard, 1971), or depletion of C3PA by immunoabsorbent completely eliminate lymphocytotoxicity (Ferrone et al., 1973c). Cytolytic potential and the ability to bind radiolabeled complement components are fully restored when highly purified C3PA is added to the heated complement (Ferrone et al., 1973c). Treatment of the human complement source with EGTA, which chelates calcium and inhibits the classical pathway, or the use of C2 deficient complement does not significantly reduce the ability of the complement in conjunction with the alloantisera to mediate cytolysis (Ferrone et al., 1973c) (Fig. 3). Other HL-A alloantisera activate only the classical pathway of human complement, as treatment with EGTA or the use of C2 deficient complement completely prevents cytolysis; this is restored when purified C2 is added to the C2 deficient complement (Ferrone et al., 1973c). With these alloantisera heating of the complement source at 50°C for 20 minutes has no influence on the cytolytic potential (Fig. 4). Still other HL-A alloantisera can activate both complement pathways. With these sera lysis is prevented only by the simultaneous blocking of the classical and alternate pathways, i.e., by treatment of human complement with EDTA which chelates magnesium, essential for the two pathways (Ferrone et al., 1973c) (Fig. 5). HL-A alloantisera that activate the classical pathway consume more C4 than alloantisera that activate the alternate pathway or both pathways (Ferrone et al., 1973c).

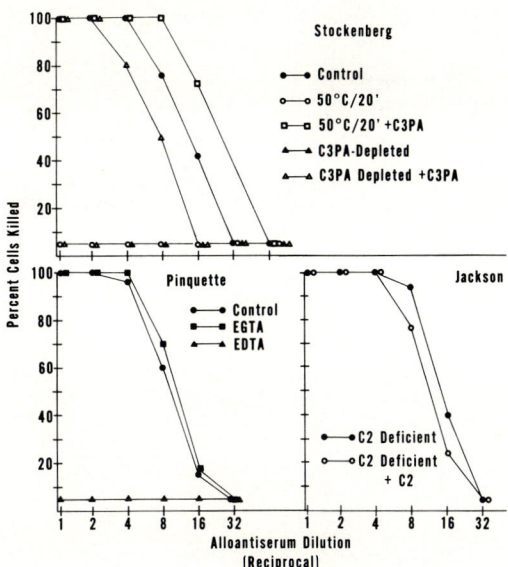

Fig. 3. Cytolytic activity of some HL-A alloantisera against human lymphoid cells (WI-L2 or RPMI 8866) in conjunction with human complement inhibited in the classic and/or alternate pathway.

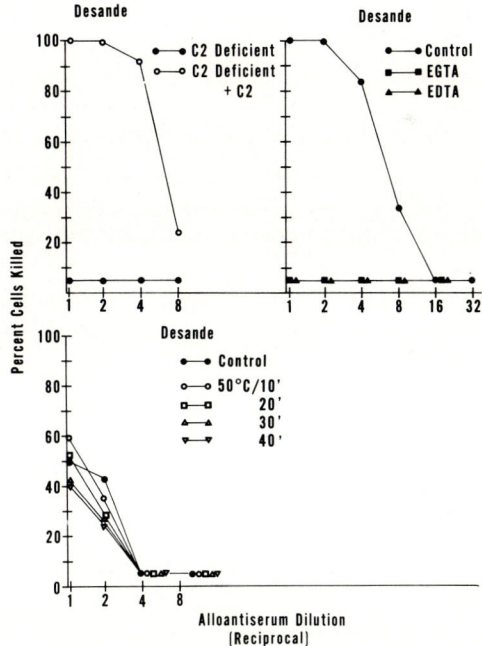

Fig. 4. Cytolytic activity of HL-A alloantisera (Desande) against human cultured lymphoid cells (WI-L2) in conjunction with human complement inhibited in the classic and/or alternate pathway.

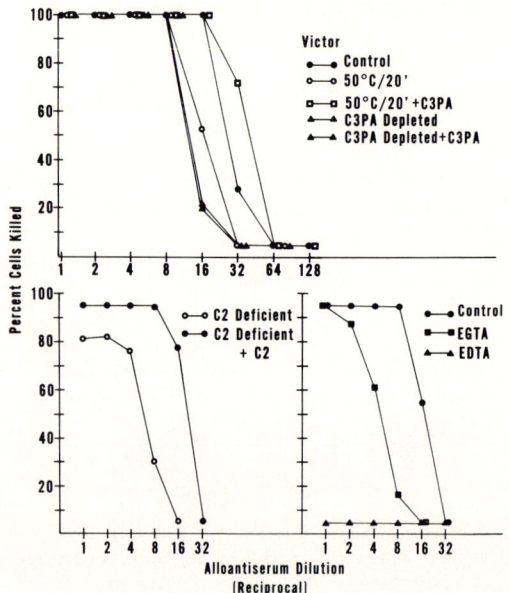

Fig. 5. Cytolytic activity of HL-A alloantisera (Victor) against human cultured lymphoid cells (WI-L2) in conjunction with human complement inhibited in the classic and/or alternate pathway.

When rabbit serum containing natural antibodies is the source of complement in the cytotoxic reaction with HL-A alloantisera, the complement system is activated only through the classical pathway (Ferrone et al., 1974b), since lympholysis is prevented by using C2 deficient complement and restored by addition of purified C2 (Ferrone et al., 1974b). Furthermore, treatment of complement with EGTA completely blocks the lytic process, whereas heating the complement for 30 minutes at 50°C does not reduce its cytolytic activity (Ferrone et al., 1974b).

4. INDICATOR SYSTEMS

Several indicator systems are available to measure cell death. Dye exclusion has gained widespread acceptance for detecting human leukocyte antigens in HL-A typing: supravital dyes, such as eosin (Terasaki et al., 1967) or trypan blue (Walford et al., 1964; Amos, 1966), are excluded by viable cells but penetrate the membranes and stain dead cells, making their recognition easy with the aid of an inverted phase microscope. Morphological studies (Terasaki and McClelland, 1964) are based on the loss of refractibility of dead lymphocytes under a phase contrast microscope; whereas living cells have poorly resolved nuclei in the cytoplasm, killed cells are dark, slightly enlarged, and exhibit clearly distinguishable nuclei within the cytoplasm. In the fluorochromasia test (Bodmer et al., 1967; Celada and Rotman, 1967; Tosi et al., 1967; Takasugi, 1971) target lymphoid cells are labeled with a fluorescing material prior to testing; the cytotoxic effects of HL-A alloantisera and complement on the target cells are assessed by determining the number of fluorescing cells remaining after the cytotoxic reaction. The dead cells having leaked out the accumulated fluorescein do not fluoresce when exposed to ultraviolet light; this test may offer the advantage of automatically recording the results. A combination of dye exclusion and fluorochromatic technique has been recently described as useful for typing lymphocyte samples with a high background of killed cells (Fong and Kissmeyer-Nielsen, 1972). The cytotoxic action of alloantisera can also be detected by the loss of intracellular isotopic markers from dead cells. Thus, lymphocytes labeled with sodium dichromate ^{51}Cr are exposed to antisera and complement, and the amount of radiochromium released in the supernatant is measured (Rogentine, 1967; Sanderson and Batchelor, 1967).

5. Limitations of the Lymphocytotoxicity Assay

The most important limitation of the lymphocytotoxic test is the occurrence of CYNAP (cytotoxic negative-absorption positive) (Ferrone et al., 1967) reactions that indicate a negative cytotoxic reaction even though antigen on the target cells can be demonstrated by absorption. Several mechanisms can be responsible for the occurrence of CYNAP reactions which essentially reflect an insufficient activity of complement to lyse target cells. Perhaps the HL-A antigenic determinants on the cell surface may be too sparse for the critical concentration of complement to be reached; in fact, variations in the number of HL-A antigenic determinants available to react with alloantisera have been shown in human peripheral lymphocytes (Pellegrino et al., 1972a) and in cultured human lymphoid cells (Pellegrino et al., 1973a). Some HL-A antigens can interfere with the expression of others or can affect the reactivity of target cells with certain HL-A alloantisera, since most HL-A alloantisera are only operationally monospecific and contain sublytic amounts of antibodies directed against other HL-A specificities. The antigenic determinants against which natural antibodies present in rabbit serum are directed are expressed variably on cell membranes of lymphocytes from different subjects (Mittal et al., 1973a). This variability as well as the relationship of these determinants to HL-A antigens may account for different reactivities by human lymphocytes in the cytotoxic test with HL-A alloantisera and rabbit complement. Anticomplementary activity of sera is a well-known phenomenon that may disturb all complement requiring reactions; possible mechanisms have been described such as presence of γ-globulin aggregates (Davis et al., 1944; Olhagen, 1945; Ishizaka and Ishizaka, 1959), complementoid (Polley and Mollison, 1961), and bacterial contamination (Kabat and Mayer, 1961). In the cytotoxic test for HL-A typing, human IgM present in HL-A alloantisera can interact with natural rabbit antibodies (Herberman, 1970) reducing the amount of the latter antibodies available to react with the target cells and deviating complement. The physiological and metabolic state of the cell may play a role, since changes in configuration, charge, or structure of the plasma membrane can render it resistant to cytotoxicity as well as alter its ability to repair damage to the plasma membrane. In this regard, leukemia cells, induced in mice injected with Moloney virus and sensitized by anti-Moloney virus antibodies, activate the complement system at like levels throughout their growth cycles, but are sensitive to lysis only in the G_1 phase (Lerner et al., 1971). Furthermore, treatment in vitro of target cells with sulfhydryl compounds or with trypsin does not appear to increase the number of antigenic determinants reacting with HL-A alloantisera (Ferrone and Pellegrino, 1973; Brautbar et al., 1973) but significantly enhances the reactivity of target cells in the cytotoxic reaction (Sirchia and Ferrone, 1971; Gibofsky and Terasaki, 1972).

Several attempts have been made to increase the sensitivity of cytotoxic testing in order to improve the accuracy of HL-A typing and to detect antibodies in the sera of recipients of grafts; cytotoxic antibodies present in the recipient's serum and directed against donor's antigens can cause rejection of the graft (Kissmeyer-Nielsen et al., 1966; Terasaki et al., 1968; Patel et al., 1969).

The reactivity of human peripheral lymphocytes in the cytotoxic reaction can be increased by treatment in vitro with enzymes or sulfhydryl compounds (Mittal et al., 1968, 1969; Sirchia and Ferrone, 1971; Yunis et al., 1970; Grothaus et al., 1971; Mercuriali et al., 1971; Gibofsky and Terasaki, 1972). Sublytic amounts of anti-human lymphocyte serum added to the reaction mixture detect antibodies in sera nonreactive in the regular test and increase the potency of some antibodies weakly detected by the standard method (Nelken et al., 1970; Ting et al., 1973). Finally, addition of antiglobulin reagent to the reaction mixture has been reported to increase the cytotoxic

5. Histocompatibility Antigens: Biology and Chemistry

activity of HL-A alloantibodies (Colombani et al., 1964; Dos Reis et al., 1973).

Thus, increasing the test's sensitivity by these approaches as well as by prolonging the incubation time of the reaction may augment information on HL-A antigens and antibodies and facilitate lymphocyte alloantibody detection before kidney transplantation.

B. Platelet-Complement Fixation

The amount of complement fixed by the platelet antigen–antibody reaction can be measured by quantitating lysis of sheep red blood cells sensitized by hemolytic antibodies (Aster et al., 1964; Shulman et al., 1964; Colombani et al., 1967). Microtechniques have been developed (Colombani et al., 1970; D'Amaro et al., 1970; Gabb and Bodmer, 1970; Smith and Walford, 1970), and results may be scored automatically with a microscope densitometer (Bruning et al., 1972). However, the complement fixation test is only approximately 1/20 as sensitive as the microcytotoxicity test (Svejgaard et al., 1967), and good typing reagents for complement fixation are more difficult to find than for microcytotoxicity. Platelet-complement fixation testing for the time being seems to be confined to special studies such as quantitative expression of HL-A determinants on the cell surface. Investigations of gene-dose effects (Svejgaard, 1969) have shown that on an average homozygous platelets have twice as many antigenic sites as heterozygous ones. In addition since platelets can be stored at 4°C for long periods, the same sample can be tested repeatedly.

C. Serologic Evaluation of Soluble HL-A Antigens

1. THE BLOCKING TEST

These assays are based on the ability of soluble HL-A antigens to combine specifically with HL-A antibodies and to prevent subsequent antibody activity as measured by the killing of target cells in the lymphocytotoxic test. By this simple, rapid, and sensitive means the activity of as little as 0.001 μg of soluble HL-A antigen can readily be detected (Pellegrino et al., 1973b). The validity of this serologic test is also indicated by the fact that antigenic preparations found inactive by it do not elicit the production of lymphocytotoxic antibodies in rabbits (Pellegrino et al., 1973b). However, it should be pointed out that the results of the lymphocytotoxic test can be influenced by several variables such as: (1) time of incubation of soluble HL-A alloantigen with HL-A alloantisera, (2) diluent used for the antigenic preparation, (3) sequence of incubation of the antigen preparation with target cell and HL-A alloantisera, and (4) different combinations of antisera and target cells (Etheredge *et al.*, 1971; Pellegrino *et al.*, 1973f).

In order to compare data from different experiments and from different antigen preparations, the following parameters have proven to be extremely useful (Kahan *et al.*, 1971; Pellegrino *et al.*, 1973f): (1) inhibition dose and (2) specificity ratio.

The inhibition dose (ID_{50}) represents the amount of soluble HL-A antigen required to halve the cytotoxic activity of operationally monospecific alloantisera. The specificity ratio (SR) (Sanderson, 1968) is the relationship between the amount of soluble HL-A antigen preparation required for 50% inhibition of the cytotoxic activity of an alloantiserum (indifferent antiserum) directed against HL-A determinants not detected in the phenotype of cells used for the extraction and the amount required to inhibit an alloantiserum directed against HL-A determinants present in the phenotype of the source of soluble antigen. While ID_{50} indicates the serologic potency of soluble HL-A alloantigens, SR reflects their immunologic specificity.

2. The Absorption Test

The absorption test can detect both false negative reactions (CYNAP) (Ferrone *et al.*, 1967), which may occur when HL-A typing is done serologically by direct cytotoxic testing of cells, and false positive reactions, which may frequently occur in direct HL-A typing of human cultured lymphoid cells (Ferrone *et al.*, 1972b).

Quantitative absorptions can determine the relative amounts of HL-A antigenic determinants available on the cell surface to react with HL-A alloantisera. An economical quantitative microabsorption technique has been developed in this laboratory (Pellegrino *et al.*, 1972a) and is performed as follows: HL-A alloantisera are diluted to twice the minimal amount required to lyse 95% of selected target cells. Five µl of alloantisera are incubated with 5 µl of serial two-fold dilutions of absorbing cell suspensions for 60 minutes at room temperature in Beckman tubes and mixed every 10 minutes. At the end of the incubation period, the mixture is centrifuged for 5 minutes at room temperature at 13,000 g in a Beckman microfuge. The supernatant fluid is tested for residual cytotoxic activity against selected target cells. The 50% absorption dosage (AD_{50}) (the number of cells required to reduce by 50% the cytotoxicity of a selected alloantiserum) is used as a criterion for comparing results of various quantitative absorptions.

V. Cell Surface Expression of H Antigens

A. Tissue Distribution

Histocompatibility alloantigens are present in nearly all tissues, suggesting that their function is associated with the general physiology of the cells rather than with any particular function of a differentiated tissue. The tissues vary with respect to the relative amount of alloantigens present, and the amount changes with the age of the organism. In the mouse high concentrations of H-2 alloantigens are found in spleen, liver, and lymphoid tissue, whereas kidney, lung, adrenal, and gastrointestinal tract contain intermediate amounts, and heart, skeletal muscle, and brain contain very little (Pizarro et al., 1961). In man, HL-A antigens are most highly concentrated in the spleen, with lesser amounts in lung, liver, kidney, intestine, heart, aorta, and brain (Berah et al., 1970). Human fetal kidneys appear to contain more HL-A antigens than do spleens and lungs, at least as judged by the amount that can be extracted in soluble form (Pellegrino et al., 1970).

The question as to whether histocompatibility antigens occur on spermatozoa is not definitely resolved yet, although many researchers believe that they are present. After the negative results by Barth and Russell (1964), who by means of immunofluorescence could not detect H-2 antigens on mouse spermatozoa, Vojtiskova (1969) and Vojtiskova et al. (1969), utilizing the techniques of immunogenicity, antibody-absorption, and indirect immunofluorescence, reported them to be present. Similar results were achieved with cytotoxic tests of both human and murine spermatozoa (Fellous and Dausset, 1970; Goldberg et al., 1970, 1971; Fellous, 1971; Johnson and Edidin, 1972). However, Johnson and Edidin (1972) could detect H-2 antigens with the cytotoxic test but not with immunofluorescence. Furthermore, Seigler and Metzgar (1970) did not succeed in absorbing HL-A leukoagglutinins with human spermatozoa. Each test has its own limitations, and these conflicting results may reflect the different sensitivities of the techniques. Immunogenicity and absorption, which detect histocompatibility antigens in a suspension of spermatozoa without identifying the cell type carrying the antigen, are subject to the criticism that nonspermatozoa contaminant cells or secretions may account for all the antigenic activity. In the case of negative absorptions, the number of spermatozoa utilized may have been insufficient, especially if the ratio between the antigenicity of spermatozoa and lymphocytes is low as observed with murine cells. In the cytotoxic test, natural cytotoxic antibodies for spermatozoa have been found in normal mouse sera (Johnson and Edidin, 1972). In addition the expression of histocompatibility antigens on spermatozoa varies according to the H-2 type, as H-2^b antigens on spermatozoa give a weaker immunofluorescent reaction than H-2^d (Vojtiskova et al., 1969). With all these limitations it seems hazardous to conclude that two antigenically distinct types of spermatozoa exist as suggested by Fellous and Dausset (1970) on the basis of: (1) higher proportion of spermatozoa killed by a single HL-A alloantiserum in homozygotes than in heterozygotes and (2) higher percentage of spermatozoa killed by a mixture of antisera against two HL-A specificities, when the genetic determinants are in trans rather than in cis configuration.

Histocompatibility antigens are not detected on trophoblast cells, but are expressed in most tissues of early embryos and increase progressively toward the approach of delivery. Serologic tests indicate that antigen concentrations of spleen cells and erythrocytes in mice increase rapidly soon after birth and reach adult reactivity during the first two weeks of life (Edidin, 1973; Seigler and Metzgar, 1973).

Histocompatibility antigens are in an unusual configuration or are bound differently in some tissues as is suggested when treatment with EDTA releases detectable amounts of H-2 antigens from tissues of 9- to 10½-day murine embryos, but is ineffective on older embryonic, newborn, or adult tissues (Edidin, 1966, 1967).

The cell surface expression of HL-A antigens is also influenced by the degree of cellular maturity. Thus, in the erythroid series, reticulocytes have been reported to contain HL-A antigens, whereas mature erythrocytes lack them altogether (Harris and Zervas, 1969; Silvestre et al., 1970); in lymphoid tissues the ratio of the absorbing capacity for HL-A alloantisera between human cultured lymphoid cells and peripheral lymphocytes ranges from 2 to 5.2 (Rogentine and Gerber, 1970; Pellegrino et al., 1972a). The amount of histocompatibility antigens is also influenced by the development of new antigens or by variation in content of other antigens.

Evidence has accumulated that transformation of normal cells to malignant cells may be accompanied by qualitative and/or quantitative changes in their histocompatibility antigenic makeup. H-2 antigens are decreased in H-2 homozygous murine tumor cells (Amos, 1956; Hoecker and Hauschka, 1956), and H-2 heterozygous tumors may irreversibly lose antigens controlled from one of the two H-2 alleles (see Hellström and Möller, 1965, for review). In chemically or virus induced mouse lymphoblastic leukemias (Ting and Herberman, 1971; Cikes *et al.*, 1973; Motta and Bruley, 1973) general reduction of all the H-2 specificities or decrease of some H-2 specificities with the concomitant increase of others has been reported. Knowledge of the mechanisms underlying these changes is only speculative: mucopolysaccharides may coat malignant cells more thickly than normal cells or new antigens may rearrange the membrane architecture and account for the general decrease of H-2 antigens.

In TL leukemia cells a reciprocal relationship between the thymus-leukemia (TL) and H-2 antigens has been described. The phenotypic expression of TL antigens reduces the demonstrable amount of certain H-2 antigens on the cell surface (Boyse *et al.*, 1967), while the decrease of TL antigens caused by a modulation phenomenon evokes a compensatory increase in H-2 antigen expression (Old *et al.*, 1968).

Similar results have been reported in man, obtained mainly with the direct cytotoxic test. Therefore, unfortunately one cannot exclude the possibilities that negative responses may be CYNAP reactions, and extrapositive responses may be false positive reactions caused by an increased sensitivity of the cells to the lytic process. Decrease or loss of HL-A antigens have been reported during some malignancies (Bertrams *et al.*, 1971; Seigler *et al.*, 1971; van Rood and van Leeuwen, 1971), whereas in others reactivity of leukemic cells has increased with some HL-A alloantisera (Schlesinger and Amos, 1971; Walford *et al.*, 1971; Harris, 1973), probably reflecting heightened expression of HL-A antigens. In some patients suffering from acute leukemia, changes in the HL-A profiles paralleled the activity of the disease as new HL-A antigens appeared during the acute phase of the disease, disappeared during remission, and reappeared during relapse (Pegrum *et al.*, 1971).

Infection of cells with virus has various effects on the expression of histocompatibility antigens, possibly related to the maturation properties of the virus; murine cells infected with vesicular stomatitis viruses that mature at the cell surface show greater than 70% reduction in the expression of histocompatibility antigens (Hecht and Summers, 1972). The pathogenic mechanism of this reduction is not fully understood; it is caused neither by perturbation of protein synthesis in infected cells, nor by masking of antigenic sites by the virus. Decreased H-2 expression may be caused by configurational changes in the cell surface during insertion of viral proteins into the host membrane *in vivo*. Infection of cells with SV40 increases the number of H-2 antigenic sites on murine fibroblasts (Tsakraklides *et* al., 1973) but does not detectably change the cell surface expression of HL-A antigens (Kersey et al., 1973). However, changes in the cell membrane structure and architecture caused by the viral infection confer to the cells the ability to absorb some of the alloantisera directed against certain HL-A specificities (M. A. Pellegrino and S. Ferrone, unpublished results).

Cells infected with feline leukemia virus acquire an increased reactivity with HL-A alloantisera in the complement dependent cytotoxic test, but retain unchanged their ability to absorb HL-A alloantibodies, suggesting that the viral infection does not affect the expression of histocompatibility antigens, but changes the reactivity of the membrane (M. A. Pellegrino and S. Ferrone, unpublished results). This hypothesis is supported by the observation that the spontaneous cytotoxicity of normal rabbit complement is greater against infected cells than noninfected cells (S. Ferrone and M. A. Pellegrino, unpublished results).

B. Arrangement of H Antigens on Cell Membranes

A large body of evidence indicates that histocompatibility antigens are arrayed on cell surface membranes. After the early observation that alloantibodies could specifically agglutinate or lyse intact lymphoid cells in the presence of complement, histocompatibility antigens were visually located on cell membranes by immunofluorescence (Möller, 1961; Barth and Russell, 1964; Cerottini and Brunner, 1967; Gervais, 1968; Pellegrino et al., 1972b) and by electron microscopy (Davis and Silverman, 1968; Hammerling et al., 1968; Aoki et al., 1969; Kourilsky et al., 1971; Willingham et al., 1971). No definite evidence exists to mark the subcellular distribution of histocompatibility antigens, although they have been described in endoplasmic reticulum and in lysosomes.

In fact, disrupted murine cells were reported to be more immunogenic for H-2 antigens than whole cells, suggesting the presence of histocompatibility antigens inside the cells (Manson et al., 1968). Yet, whole cell homogenates are as effective as intact lymphoid cells in absorbing cytotoxic H-2 antibodies from immune sera (Haughton, 1966); if internal histocompatibility antigens were present, one would expect a large increase in antibody binding activity following the breakage of the cell. However, enhanced immunogenicity does not necessarily reflect increases of histocompatibility antigens, and the possible destruction of histocompatibility antigens during the cell disruption process cannot be ruled out. Furthermore, from the work by Evans and Bruning (1970) comparison of H-2 antigen distribution in particulate cell fractions, in order to be meaningful, requires the fractions to be in identical physical states and composed of particles equivalent in size and equally dispersed in the test reaction.

According to the fluid mosaic model proposed by Singer and Nicolson (1972), the protein components of the cell membrane are floating in the lipid bilayer as globular molecules that can be rearranged and displaced under special circumstances without disrupting the basic structure. There is growing evidence that this proposal is valid for histocompatibility antigens that are permanently in a dynamic state and subjected to active membrane turnover. The movement of histocompatibility antigens on the cell membrane is suggested by the early and elegant experiments of Frye and Edidin (1970), who reported rapid intermixing of H-2 antigens and human heterologous antigens at the surfaces of human-mouse hybrid cells formed by virus-induced cell fusion. Mobilization of histocompatibility antigens on the cell surface can be caused by the corresponding antibodies. Binding of HL-A or H-2 antisera to the membranes of living human or murine lymphoid cells induces rearrangement of the once evenly distributed histocompatibility determinants into discrete spots irregularly distributed over the entire area (Bernoco et al., 1971; Kourilsky et al., 1972; Neauport-Sautes et al., 1973a,b). In contrast with immunoglobulins and θ antigens (Taylor et al., 1971), which are easily agglomerated into caps after the addition of the corresponding antibodies, histocompatibility antigens are easily agglomerated in caps when anti-γ-globulin antibodies are added to the reaction mixture (Kourilsky et al., 1972; Unanue et al., 1972; Bernoco et al., 1973). It has been suggested that the cause for the different movement properties of histocompatibility antigens and immunoglobulins lies in the density of these determinants and in their degree of anchoring in the cell membrane; histocompatibility antigens are separated from each other by large empty areas on the cell surface (Davis and Silverman, 1968), while Ig receptors are close together (Karnovsky et al., 1972). Aggregation seems to be induced by multivalent binding of antibodies, but the spacing among histocompatibility antigenic determinants is beyond the reach of the corresponding antibodies. Whether or not metabolism is required for rearrangement of histocompatibility antigens is controversial: actinomycin D and mitomycin C as well as puromycin and cycloheximide are not inhibitory suggesting that DNA and protein metabolism are not primarily involved in the rapid membrane changes (Kourilsky et al., 1972). On the contrary, incubation at low temperature or treatment with sodium azide and potassium cyanide inhibits spot and cap formation, suggesting active metabolic participation of the cell in the antibody-induced redistribution of histocompatibility antigens (Kourilsky et al., 1972); however, it is not possible to rule out cold as an inhibitor of movement by changing the physical properties of the cell membrane (Kourilsky et al., 1972). Sodium azide and potassium cyanide are effective at concentrations very close to those inducing direct cytotoxic effects on living cells so that a nonspecific action of these inhibitors on the cell membrane also cannot be excluded (Kourilsky et al., 1972).

The fate of the histocompatibility antigen–antibody complex on a cell is not completely clear. Some complexes have been shown to be interiorized into the cells by endocytosis, but the suggestion has also been put forward that the antigen–antibody complex is released into the growth medium (Amos et al., 1970; Bernoco et al., 1971; Loor et al., 1972; Miyajima et al., 1972), since this can inhibit the mixed lymphocyte reaction more efficiently than the corresponding amount of the original alloantiserum (Bernoco et al., 1971).

The biologic significance of the antibody-induced redistribution of histocompatibility antigens is not known; it seems to be responsible for decreased sensitivity to the lytic action of complement of lymphoid cells presensitized with anti-H-2 (Amos et al., 1970; Takahashi, 1971) or anti-HL-A (Bernoco et al., 1971; Miyajima et al., 1972) antisera and incubated at 37°C. Loss of sensitivity of lymphoid cells to complement occurs over a range of time (between 1 and 12 hours) which depends on the HL-A specificity, on the concentration of antiserum and on the physiological state of the lymphocytes (Miyajima et al., 1972). In fact, escape from sensitization occurs more rapidly to HL-A9 than to HL-A1, HL-A2, or HL-A7; low concentrations of antibodies as well as the addition of anti-Ig antibodies induce resistance to lysis earlier than high concentration of antibodies (Miyajima et al., 1972, Bernoco et al., 1973). Anti-Ig antibodies might be the key to understanding the conflicting results when anti-Ig is added to sensitized cells before exposing them to complement as a means of boosting cytotoxic reactions in the antiglobulin microcytotoxic test (Colombani et al., 1964; Mittal et al., 1968; Miggiano et al., 1970; Johnson et al., 1972; Dos Reis et al., 1973). In these experiments the cytotoxicity of alloantisera is unpredictably augmented or diminished by this procedure. Finally cells aged by storage for 1 day at 5°C have sharply impaired abilities to escape sensitization (Miyajima et al., 1972). Mechanisms of this phenomenon seem to be multiple: antibodies have been eluted from the surfaces of sensitized cells in antibody free medium, but this does not account entirely for the escape from sensitization since inhibition of the metabolic activities of cells prevents them from escaping sensitization (Miyajima *et al.*, 1972; Schlesinger and Chaouat, 1972). Furthermore, resistance to the lytic action of complement occurs long before the disappearance of antibodies from the cell surface, as if aggregation of antigenic determinants alone may be sufficient to cause this resistance in spite of the binding of the complement to the cells (Bernoco *et al.*, 1973).

The escape from antibody sensitization is different from the antigenic modulation phenomenon described for TL antigens (Old *et al.*, 1968); in the latter, which is a phenotypic suppression of TL antigens occurring when TL+ cells are exposed to TL antibodies, incubation of cells with fresh anti-TL sera and complement does not bring about lysis (Old *et al.*, 1968), while cells that have escaped sensitization are killed by the addition of fresh alloantisera and complement (Bernoco *et al.*, 1971; Miyajima *et al.*, 1972). Modulation of histocompatibility antigens does not occur with lymphoid cells but has been reported with murine peritoneal cells (Schlesinger and Chaouat, 1972).

If these mechanisms observed *in vitro* are shown to have counterparts *in vivo*, they may play a decisive role in the immunobiology of grafts and tumors, since allografts or cancer cells could thus escape immunologic attacks.

Contrasting views have been reported on the mode of distribution of histocompatibility antigens; Winn (1962), using a complement-consumption assay system, inferred that H-2 antigens are discontinuously distributed on cell membranes. A similar conclusion was reached with the aid of an immunofluorescent staining technique (Cerottini and Brunner, 1967; Kourilsky *et al.*, 1972; Pellegrino *et al.*, 1972b). These data were substantiated by indirect electron microscopy of labeled ferritin conjugated antibodies or hybrid antibodies with activity directed against globulin and against either ferritin or virus (Hammerling *et al.*, 1968; Davis *et al.*, 1971; Kourilsky *et al.*, 1971; Willingham *et al.*, 1971; Neauport-Sautes *et al.*, 1972); histocompatibility antigens formed patches without periodicity separated by intervals free of staining. On the contrary, studies performed with the direct ferritin antibody conjugated technique (Davis *et al.*, 1971) indicated a continuous distribution of histocompatibility antigens, suggesting that results obtained by indirect labeling techniques were artifacts caused when antigenic determinants were rearranged by the corresponding antibodies. However, when lymphocytes are reacted with HL-A antibodies at 0°C (a temperature at which no capping occurs), staining of the cells is even and appears as a ring by immunofluorescence (Kourilsky et al., 1972; Bernoco et al., 1973); in contradistinction, if cells sensitized with HL-A alloantisera are stained with ferritin-coupled rabbit anti-human IgG in the cold and then observed under an electron microscope, the circumference of lymphocyte sections reveals a discontinuous distribution of ferritin grains with zones of labeling separated by unlabeled areas.

Mapping histocompatibility antigenic determinants on the cell surface has been attempted by interference of antibody bound to one antigenic site with antibody binding to other sites. D and K end H-2 antigens have been found to occupy distinct and relatively remote sites on the cell surface (Boyse et al., 1968; Cresswell and Sanderson, 1968; Kristofova et al., 1970). In man histocompatibility specificities that are adjacent when determined by genes in the cis position occupy remote areas on the cell membrane when determined by genes in the trans position (Legrand and Dausset, 1971). Histocompatibility antigens appear to be located on different molecules than immunoglobulin determinants in the membrane mosaic as capping of the latter does not affect the distribution of histocompatibility antigens (Taylor et al., 1971; Loor et al., 1972; Preud'homme et al., 1972; Bernoco et al., 1973). Similar approaches hint that the products of the four recognized HL-A genes are carried by different molecules (Bernoco et al., 1973; Neauport-Sautes et al., 1973b), a conclusion that, however, still requires chemical proof.

C. Expression of H Antigens during the Cell Cycle

The progression of cells through the mitotic cycle is characterized by ordered temporal changes in macromolecular synthesis. Changes in cell membrane structure are of particular interest, since many lines of evidence indicate that they play a major role in regulating cell proliferation. Critical alterations of the cell surface are believed to be among the major causes for the disordered proliferation of malignant cells. Expression of histocompatibility antigens has been investigated both in human and murine cultured lymphoid cells at different stages of their growth cycles; the results of these studies are conflicting.

In murine tumor cells the expression of H-2 antigens varies during the cell cycle, being maximal in G_1 and decreasing during the G_1-S period, as judged by their sensitivity in the complement-dependent lymphocytotoxic test (Fig. 6), by indirect immunofluorescent studies

5. Histocompatibility Antigens: Biology and Chemistry

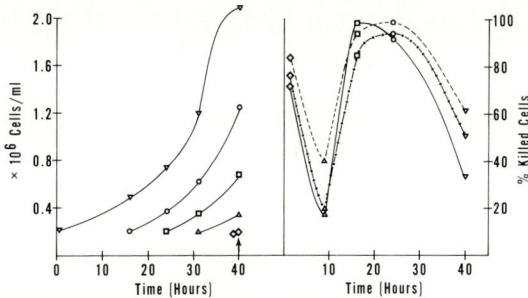

Fig. 6. Relationship between cell growth of L1210 cells (left) and sensitivity in the complement dependent cytotoxic test (right) as indicated by the percentage of killed cells caused by anti-H-2.4 (----), anti-H-2.28 (–·–·), and anti-H-2.31 (—) sera. Cells derived from five cultures grown for different times were harvested on the same day (indicated by the arrow). The sera were used at a dilution effecting 95% killing of the most sensitive cells (in mid-log phase).

and by quantitative absorption experiments (Cikes and Friberg, 1971; Pasternak *et al.*, 1971; Cikes *et al.*, 1972; Götze *et al.*, 1972b). Therefore, the H-2 antigen character of the cell surface does not reflect the increased amount of other membrane constituents, since its expression decreases when most macromolecular synthesis is maximal (Warmsley and Pasternak, 1970). Besides cyclical changes in the number of antigenic determinants available to react with H-2 alloantisera, there may be changes in the sensitivity of the membrane to the lytic action of complement since variations in absorbing capacity do not parallel variations of the sensitivity of the cells at every phase of the cell growth in the complement dependent cytotoxic test (Götze *et al.*, 1972b).

The amount of H-2 antigens solubilized by 3 M KCl or by freezing and thawing methods from cells in different stages of their growth parallels the expression of histocompatibility antigens on the corresponding intact living cells (Cikes and Klein, 1972b; Götze *et al.*, 1972b), suggesting that the varying expression of H-2 antigens is not caused by masking of cell-surface antigens during some growth phases.

In human cell lines, expression of HL-A antigens during the cell cycle appears to depend upon the source of the cells: those derived from a Burkitt lymphoma express HL-A antigens maximally in G_1 phase (Cikes, 1971), when cells RPMI 8866 derived from a leukemic patient have a reduced sensitivity to the lytic action of complement activated by HL-A antibodies (Reisfeld *et al.*, 1974) (Fig. 7). In cultured lymphoid cells (WI-L2) derived from a donor free of malig-

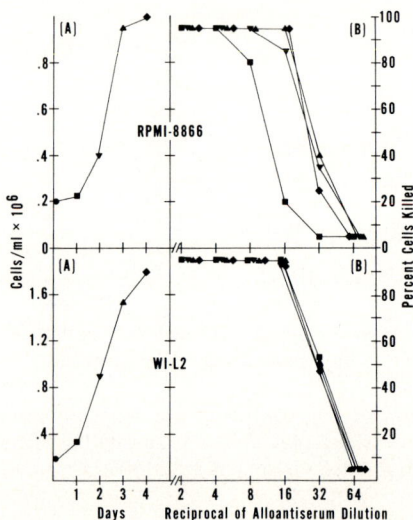

Fig. 7. Susceptibility of cultured human lymphoid cells RPMI 8866 and WI-L2 during different stages of their growth cycle to the lytic action of HL-A alloantisera and complement in the microcytotoxic test. Panel A depicts the respective growth curves of the cell lines. Panel B illustrates their respective titration curves: the growth phase of the cells is indicated by the corresponding symbol in the growth curve (Panel A).

nancy, no change was detected in the expression of histocompatibility antigens throughout the growth cycle, as judged by the cytotoxic test, by their absorbing capacity, by the activation of the complement system (Fig. 8), and by the uptake of radiolabeled complement components when the cultured lymphoid cells were sensitized with HL-A alloantisera (Pellegrino *et al.*, 1972b, 1973c; Ferrone *et al.*, 1973b). It is worthwhile emphasizing that the results obtained

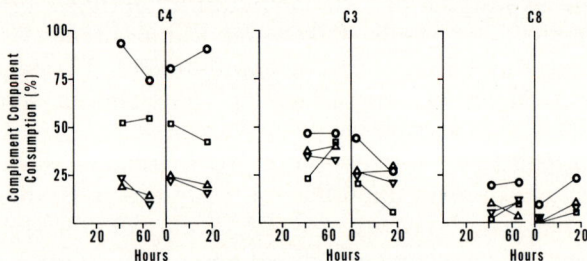

Fig. 8. Consumption of complement component in serum exposed to cultured human lymphoid cells WI-L2 in different stages of their growth cycle. Sensitized with rabbit anti-human lymphocyte serum (○—○), anti-HL-A1 (□—□), anti-HL-A2 (∇—∇), or anti-HL-A5 (△—△).

from various cell lines do not reflect technical artifacts, since in this laboratory different results were also obtained with various cell lines when the same techniques were employed. On the contrary, it is tempting to speculate that the variability in the expression of surface antigens observed in some cell lines may reflect a specific defect of these cells in the regulation of either synthesis or shedding of cell surface markers.

The variable expression of histocompatibility antigens during the growth cycle is similar to that of other antigens such as blood groups H and AB (Kuhns and Bramson, 1968; Kuhns et al., 1969) and virus receptors on cultured cells (Cikes, 1970; Lerner et al., 1971); furthermore, the amount of total immunoglobulin detected on cell membrane (Lerner et al., 1972) as well as the rate of synthesis vary during the cell cycle (Buell and Fahey, 1969; Lerner and Hodge, 1971).

The continuous expression of histocompatibility antigen throughout the growth cycle of cultured cells suggests that these cell surface markers are an essential part of membrane cytoarchitecture or are critical for the normal function of the cell membrane. This view is reinforced by the presence of histocompatibility antigens on almost all the tissues and by their persistence on murine (Klein et al., 1970) and human (Papermaster et al., 1969; Rogentine and Gerber, 1969, 1970) lymphoid cells, even after long-term culture, although other antigens have been lost (Högman, 1959; Chessin et al., 1965). Similarly, human diploid fibroblasts, which have a finite life span in vitro, change morphologically, metabolically, and functionally during senescence, but their surface expression of HL-A antigens remains practically unchanged throughout (Brautbar et al., 1972, 1973).

D. Effect of Inhibitors of Macromolecular Synthesis

Inhibitors of macromolecular synthesis affect the cell surface expression of HL-A antigens and are under investigation; although subject to limitations, such studies can contribute to understanding the biosynthesis of histocompatibility antigens. Actinomycin D enhances the cell surface expression of histocompatibility antigens in murine tumor cells induced by Moloney leukemia virus, and this superinductive effect is blocked by inhibitors of protein synthesis (Cikes and Klein, 1972a). However, this drug reduces the absorbing capacity for HL-A alloantisera of Raji cells, but does not affect that of cultured cells WI-L2 derived from a donor free of malignancy (Ferrone et al., 1972c, 1974a). The varying effects of actinomycin D on the surface expression of histocompatibility antigens on different cell lines is analogous to the effect of the drug on the production of proteins in different tissues; while in murine tumor cells the synthesis of the myeloma globulin is stable only for a few hours after the addition of actinomycin D (Shutt and Krueger, 1972), in several differentiated and specialized tissues, the protein-synthesizing machinery is stabilized so that it is not subjected to inhibition by actinomycin D (Marks *et al.*, 1962; Scott and Bell, 1964; Moscona and Kirk, 1965; Wessels and Wilt, 1965; Stewart and Papaconstantinou, 1967; Fantoni *et al.*, 1968). There is no clear rationale for the differential effect of actinomycin D on different cell lines. Assuming that such inhibitor studies provide a fairly direct measurement of mRNA half-life in lymphoid cells, the following possibilities must be considered: (1) some cell lines may derive from precursors in which the changeover from unstable to stable mRNA has not occurred yet and (2) the mRNA instability may be correlated with the neoplastic condition of the cell line. Alternatively one might assume that actinomycin D affects only the production of a substance(s) that regulates antigen expression either by interfering mechanically with the binding of specific antibodies to the antigenic determinants on the cell surface or by inhibiting the synthesis and/or the assembly of subunits of antigenic determinants in the cell membranes. The metabolism of such postulated substance(s) may vary in different cell lines. No experimental data are available to help us choose among these possibilities.

5-Bromodeoxyuridine, ethidium bromide, rifampicin, and chloramphenicol do not affect the cell surface expression of HL-A antigens during periods up to 18–24 hours of incubation at 37°C (Ferrone *et al.*, 1972c). In contrast, puromycin reduces the capacity of cultured lymphoid cells to absorb anti-HL-A alloantisera specifically directed against antigenic determinants of the first and second segregant series (Ferrone *et al.*, 1972c). The effects of this drug on the expression of HL-A antigens and on protein synthesis depend on the length of incubation as well as on the dose (Ferrone *et al.*, 1972c). After extensive treatment with puromycin, 95% of protein synthesis is inhibited, while about 30% of HL-A antigens persist on the membrane; this may be attributable to the release of HL-A antigens from "reserve pools," i.e., HL-A determinants not readily accessible to anti-HL-A antibodies such as "masked" antigenic determinants as well as those not located on the plasma membrane surface per se (Ferrone *et al.*, 1972c). Interpretating results from the direct cytotoxic test with puromycin-treated cells is rather complex because of the interplay between a decrease of HL-A determinants on the cell surface and an increased sensitivity of cell membrane to the lytic action of complement caused by the injurious action of the drug (Ferrone et al., 1974a). It has not yet been determined whether puromycin affects HL-A antigen expression by inhibiting the synthesis and/or the assembly of subunits of antigenic determinants in the cell membrane or by changing the configuration of membrane proteins, thus interfering with the binding of specific HL-A antibody to the antigenic determinants. Puromycin does not affect the capacity of the cell to absorb HL-A antisera by steric hindrance since analogues of puromycin that do not affect protein synthesis do not cause any detectable change in absorbing capacities of the cells (Pellegrino et al., 1973d). The effects of puromycin on the expression of HL-A antigens are reversible (Fig. 9); in fact, cells partially depleted of HL-A antigens by treatment with puromycin, once washed and incubated in fresh medium, again acquire a full expression of HL-A antigens within 5 hours (Ferrone et al., 1972c). Actinomycin D does not affect the reexpression of HL-A antigens, whereas puromycin completely blocks it (Ferrone et al., 1972c). The time span for regeneration of HL-A antigens on puromycin treated cells is similar to that observed with murine or human cells from which histocompatibility antigens have been stripped *in vitro* by treatment with papain (Schwartz and Nathenson, 1971; Chapel and Welsh, 1972; Turner et al., 1972) or by incubation with HL-A alloantisera and anti-human Ig (Bernoco et al., 1973).

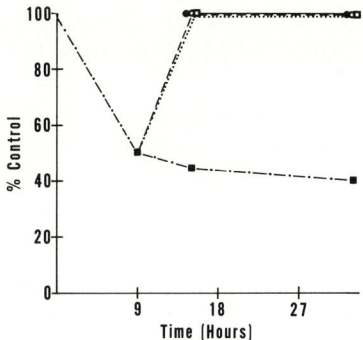

Fig. 9. Effect of actinomycin D and puromycin on the reexpression of HL-A antigens on WI-L2 cells initially treated with puromycin (50 µg/ml) for 9 hours (■-·-■). Cells were washed thoroughly and then reincubated in medium (1) without any further addition of inhibitors (●---●), (2) with puromycin (50 µg/ml) (■-··-■), (3) with actinomycin D (5 µg/ml) (○····○), and (4) with cycloheximide (100 µg/ml) (□---□).

Cycloheximide, like puromycin, interferes with the normal function of the translational complex, but by a different mechanism. Thus, puromycin, an analogue of aminoacyl-tRNA, accepts a growing polypeptide chain and then dissociates from the polyribosomes, whereas cycloheximide inhibits peptide chain initiation as well as elongation. This drug, although inhibiting the incorporation of [^{14}C]leucine into protein by at least 95% (i.e., at a level similar to that obtained with puromycin), does not significantly change the capacity of human and murine lymphoid cells to absorb histocompatibility alloantisera for periods up to 24 hours at a dose of 100 µg/ml (Ferrone et al., 1972c).

Galper and Darnell (1971) have shown that protein synthesis in the mitochondrial fractions of HeLa cells is sensitive to puromycin but not to cycloheximide. Ashwell and Work (1968) have found that this insensitivity is not the result of a permeability barrier. The different effects of puromycin and cycloheximide thus suggest that the mechanism(s) for the biosynthesis of HL-A antigens is similar to that for protein synthesis in mitochondria. Although this hypothesis is attractive to explain the differences observed in cells treated with puromycin or with cycloheximide, the possibility that these differences may result from secondary effects of these drugs cannot be ignored.

VI. Cross-Reactivity of H Antigens

A. Cross-Reactivity within the HL-A System

Cross-reactivity among HL-A determinants has been documented by a variety of experiments. Human peripheral lymphocytes (Svejgaard and Kissmeyer-Nielsen, 1968; Thorsby et al., 1970), cultured lymphoid cells (Pellegrino et al., 1973a), platelets (Dausset et al., 1968; Svejgaard and Kissmeyer-Nielsen, 1968; Colombani et al., 1970; Mittal and Terasaki, 1972; Mittal et al., 1973a,b; Pellegrino et al., 1974b), or soluble HL-A (Ferrone et al., 1972d) antigens bearing a given HL-A specificity can absorb or inhibit operationally monospecific alloantisera directed against other HL-A determinants. In this case, the number of cells (Pellegrino et al., 1973a, 1974b) or the amount of soluble HL-A antigens (Ferrone et al., 1972d) is greater than that required to absorb or inhibit a homologous HL-A alloantiserum, but significantly less than that necessary to absorb or inhibit antisera directed against unrelated HL-A specificities. This observation suggests that the affinity of HL-A antibodies is greater for the specific determinant than for cross-reacting specificities and correlates with results from direct cytotoxic testing where cross-reacting antibodies kill target cells when their reactivity is increased *in vitro* by treatment with sulfhydryl compounds (Mercuriali *et al.*, 1971) or with proteolytic enzymes (Braun *et al.*, 1972).

Women immunized by pregnancies (Thorsby *et al.*, 1970), subjects immunized by planned transfusions (Legrand *et al.*, 1971; Thorsby and Kissmeyer-Nielsen, 1970) or skin allografts (Legrand *et al.*, 1971), or rabbits injected with soluble HL-A antigen (Ferrone *et al.*, 1972a) may produce antibodies against antigens cross-reacting with those present on the immunogen. This cross-reactivity has clinical relevance since the probability of sensitization due to HL-A incompatibility is reduced, and skin grafts (Dausset *et al.*, 1970; Dausset, 1971) and kidney transplants (Dausset, 1971) survive longer when the mismatched antigen is within cross-reacting groups. According to some investigators, groups or families of cross-reacting HL-A specificities can be identified within each segregant series (Colombani *et al.*, 1970; Dausset and Hors, 1971), whereas others find that cross-reacting groups do not form isolated clusters but are interconnected (Mittal and Terasaki, 1972). The data so far available clearly indicate that cross-reactivity occurs only between allelic gene products of a single HL-A segregant series and not between those of the two different series (Svejgaard and Kissmeyer-Nielsen, 1968, Colombani *et al.*, 1970; Mittal and Terasaki, 1972), although, when the joint occurrence of antibodies directed against different specificities in sera from parous women was studied, in a few cases antibodies occurred jointly for pairs of specificities belonging to the two segregant series more frequently than expected (Albert *et al.*, 1973). On the contrary, in mice cross-reactivity has been observed between the determinants of the D and K end of the H-2 system (David *et al.*, 1973).

Two nonmutally exclusive explanations of cross-reactivity have been given. The first assumes that the same population of antibodies is capable of reacting with determinants that are slightly different from one another; the second interpretation assumes that HL-A specificities differ one from another by at least one determinant but share the same configuration in some parts of the molecules, hence, share other determinants. In the latter case cross-reacting antigens may be products of allelic genes derived from an ancestor gene that has undergone duplications and mutations. These mutations would be sufficiently limited to maintain the general structure of the antigen which would be the common structure. This conception is in agreement with the idea that histocompatibility antigens play an important role in cell economy and therefore even with their polymorphism keep their fundamental structure to exert their biologic function.

B. Cross-Reactivity between H Antigens of Different Species

Sharing of antigenic determinants by widely separated phylogenic groups has been investigated extensively and may characterize the evolutionary development of antigenic systems. Common antigens retained throughout phylogeny may very well represent structures required for the performance of functions essential to cell survival. The rapidly accumulating evidence of the fundamental role of the cell membrane in conditioning host reactions to the internal and external environment has prompted a number of studies on cross-reactions between cell membrane antigens of different species with histocompatibility antigens used as markers. These approaches in turn will help to better define the heterogeneity of antigenic specificities of histocompatibility systems.

Several lines of evidence suggest cross-reactivity between HL-A or H-2 antigens and bacterial antigens. The cytotoxic activity of HL-A or H-2 alloantisera can be inhibited by bacterial cell membrane components (Davies, 1968; Hirata and Terasaki, 1970; Hirata et al., 1970, 1973; Mittal et al., 1973c). Conversely, HL-A alloantisera or heteroantisera can prevent the DNA synthesis stimulation induced in human lymphocytes by streptococcal M1 proteins (Pellegrino et al., 1972c). Furthermore, group A streptococci are able to induce a state of allograft sensitivity in mice (Rapaport et al., 1966). Cross-reactivity has been reported between mouse, rabbit, and rat histocompatibility systems (Abeyounis and Milgrom, 1969; Sachs et al., 1971). Similarly, humans and rabbits share histocompatibility antigen determinants, as rabbits immunized with homologous histocompatibility antigens may produce antibodies capable of detecting antigens related to the HL-A system (Albert et al., 1969). The counterpart of this observation is that human subjects sensitized with allogeneic histocompatibility antigens (leukocytes, skin, or kidney allografts) may develop immunoglobulins directed against antigens present on the

5. Histocompatibility Antigens: Biology and Chemistry

surface of rat, sheep, and guinea pig erythrocytes (Iwasaki et al., 1967; Rapaport et al., 1967; 1968; McDonald and Mukherjee, 1973). Detection and titration of these antibodies to predict the outcome of kidney allografts has also been investigated (McDonald and Mukherjee, 1973). Data are clearer, however, concerning cross-reactivity between HL-A and ChL-A, the main histocompatibility system in chimpanzees; chimpanzee alloantisera can specifically detect HL-A1, HL-A11, 4a, and 4b in the human population, while human HL-A1, HL-A11, 4a, and 4b antisera give similar reaction patterns with chimpanzee antisera (Metzgar and Seigler, 1973). Sharing of antigens between human and murine histocompatibility systems is indicated by the following experiments: sera from rabbits immunized with soluble HL-A antigens extracted from human lymphoid cells react in the cytotoxic test not only with human lymphocytes but also with murine lymphocytes from different strains (Götze et al., 1972a). H-2 antigens solubilized from murine lymphoid cells L1210 ($H-2^d$) by the 3 M KCl method can specifically inhibit the cytotoxic activity of immune rabbit heteroantisera with a similar level of activity as that shown in the inhibition test with monospecific H-2 alloantisera. The specificity of the reaction is indicated by the lack of inhibitory activity of antigen solubilized from murine lymphoid cells which do not react with the immune rabbit serum either in the direct cytotoxic assay or in the absorption test. These results only seem to disagree with findings by Einstein et al. (1971b), who could not show any activity of sera from rabbits immunized with partially purified, papain-solubilized cell membrane components bearing HL-A activity against murine lymphoid cells in the lymphocytotoxic test. However, the cultured lymphoid cells used as a source of soluble HL-A antigen had a different phenotype from those used in the prior experiment, and the immune rabbit sera were tested only against cells of one mouse strain (Einstein et al., 1971b). The specific cross-reactivity between human and murine histocompatibility systems could very well explain the negative findings by Einstein et al. (1971b). There is no conclusive evidence for an HL-A type specific reaction pattern of mono- or oligospecific mouse anti-H-2 sera, as the majority of mouse alloantisera react with 60–100% of a panel of human lymphocytes (Ivasková et al., 1972; Pellegrino et al., 1974a). Serologic cross-reactivity between HL-A and H-2 systems seems relevant to transplantation, since mice sensitized with soluble HL-A antigens reject the skin from mice strains sharing antigens with the immunogen in an accelerated fashion (Götze et al., 1973).

VII. Extraction, Purification, and Biologic Activity of Soluble H Antigens

The elucidation of the molecular nature and chemical structure of antigenic markers on mammalian cell surfaces is one of the more challenging research problems in immunology. The solution of this problem requires unique technical advances with, first and foremost, the development of separation and isolation methods that can unravel the complex hydrophobic network of mammalian cell surface membranes. It will be evident from the following discussion that, although some progress has been made in a few areas, the major problems in discovering the chemical nature of cell surface markers still remain.

Interest in the molecular and chemical nature of soluble histocompatibility antigens was largely stimulated by Medawar's (1963) discovery that nonparticulate H antigens induced a degree of immunologic unresponsiveness resulting in prolonged allograft survival. Recent and intense interest in the cytoarchitecture and in antigen receptors of mammalian cells has redoubled investigations into the chemical composition of these cell surface markers.

However, clarification of the molecular structures and chemistry of H antigens has progressed more slowly than anticipated for a variety of reasons: (1) inadequate amounts of antigen from genetically uniform sources, (2) nonselective and inefficient procedures for extracting antigen, and (3) an overly complex antigen assay system lacking standard parameters as well as characterized monospecific alloantisera to assess H antigenic potency *in vitro*.

A. Antigen Source Material

Although the use of inbred animals such as mice and guinea pigs has been essential for studying transplantation antigens, insufficient amounts of H antigens have been extracted from these sources to permit thorough chemical characterizations. One guinea pig spleen yielded only 1 μg of highly purified transplantation antigen (Reisfeld and Kahan, 1970), while a single mouse spleen yielded 0.35 μg of highly purified H-2 antigen (Shimada and Nathenson, 1969). In dealing with human beings, the situation was even worse, because HL-A determinants are extremely polymorphic in this outbred population. The spleen of an individual donor yielded at best 1–2 mg of antigen (Kahan *et al.*, 1968; Sanderson, 1968; Davies, 1969).

1. HL-A Antigens from Cultured Cells

Finally, the difficulty of attaining a large, uniform source for the extraction of HL-A antigens was overcome when lymphoid cells in long-term culture proved an excellent supply (Mann et al., 1968; Reisfeld et al., 1970). Lymphoid cell lines derived both from healthy human donors and from those with lymphoid malignancies were first cultured in suspensions on a large scale by Moore et al. (1967). At present numerous investigators have such lines in continuous culture; however, even this seemingly ideal source has disadvantages. First, to grow large number of cells in continuous culture requires considerable technical as well as financial efforts. In addition, only a limited selection of HL-A phenotypes are available from this source. Second, all lymphoid cell lines contain part of the EB-viral genome (P. Gerber, personal communication), and many lines are contaminated with mycoplasma. In fact, human cells go into suspension culture only if the donor has had a recent viral infection, e.g., influenza or infectious mononucleosis, or if "EB-viral filtrate" is added to the cells (G. E. Moore, personal communication). Thus, most if not all cultured human lymphoid cell lines carry a foreign genetic load (zur Hausen et al., 1972), a finding that is somewhat difficult to assess at present. However, it is of interest that even though EB virus could be detected readily in RPMI 1788 cells used for antigen extraction, antigens extracted from them with KCl were devoid of it (P. Gerber, personal communication).

2. HL-A Antigens from Spent Culture Media

Fluid from spent culture media subjected to extensive ultracentrifugation (164,000 g, 6 hours) contained no soluble HL-A antigens; however, HL-A antigens were released from the sediment either by low intensity sound or more effectively with 3 M KCl (16 hours, 4°C) (Pellegrino et al., 1973e). Recovery of HL-A2 (ID_{50} units) from the particulate matter ranged from 20–75% compared to that from whole cultured cells which ranged from 70–100% (Pellegrino et al., 1973e). 3 M KCl solubilization of HL-A antigen from the particulate matter of spent culture media does not alter the ratio among different HL-A specificities expressed on the same cell indicating that with this procedure there is no preferential solubilization or destruction of certain HL-A specificities (Pellegrino et al., 1973e). The ID_{50} units of HL-A2 antigenic activity recovered from 1 liter of exhausted media compared favorably in 7 out of 27 preparations with the average number of these units recovered from the cultured cells (10^9) which

TABLE II

Recovery of ID_{50} Units from Exhausted Culture Media

Number of preparations[a]	ID_{50}	Total ID_{50}/liter[b]
5	0.03[c]	660,000
2	0.10	200,000
3	0.15	133,000
6	0.25	80,000
6	0.35	56,000
5	0.60	34,000

[a] All 27 preparations were obtained from cell line RPMI 1788.
[b] Total ID_{50} units/liter of medium = mg protein per liter medium/ID_{50}.
[c] Average of ID_{50} values of HL-A2 specificity.

were originally perpetuated in 1 liter of media (Pellegrino et al., 1973e). Table II shows, however, that this yield varied considerably among the 27 different preparations analyzed.

Among the advantages of utilizing spent culture media as a source for HL-A antigen extraction is the lack of nucleic acid and nucleoprotein contaminants which considerably complicate the purification of these antigens from 3 M KCl extracts of whole cultured cells. Practically speaking, since it is important to obtain the greatest possible yield from cultured cells, which are expensive to propagate in large numbers, exhausted media offer an additional source of antigen at no additional cost.

3. Peripheral Leukocytes

Attempts were made to solubilize antigens from this source (Etheredge et al., 1973) as well as from splenocytes (Etheredge and Najarian, 1971). However, the low yield as well as preferential solubilization of only certain HL-A specificities and poor stability in storage at −20°C made this particular source unprofitable.

4. HL-A Antigens from Platelets

When HL-A antigens were solubilized from platelets by 3 M KCl extraction, recovery ranged between 50–100% (Table III). HL-A antigen thus solubilized specifically inhibited the cytotoxic activity of alloantisera directed against specificities on the donor's cells and cross-reacting determinants, but did not affect that directed against unrelated specificities (Pellegrino et al., 1974b). However, the total

TABLE III

Soluble Antigen (SPL-Ag) Yields from Platelets (PL) for Different HL-A Specificities

Donor no. HL-A phenotype	Protein (mg/1 × 10⁹ platelets)	ID$_{50}$ units/ 1 × 10⁹ platelets and % recovery[a]	First segregant series				Second segregant series			
			1	2	3	9	5	7	8	12
3 (3,9,5,12)	0.9	PL	—	—	6,666	20,000	25,000	—	—	—
		SPL-Ag	—	—	6,000	15,000	22,500	—	—	—
		% recovery	—	—	90	75	90	—	—	—
4 (1,7,8)	1.0	PL	16,000	—	—	—	—	20,000	5,000	—
		SPL-Ag	10,000	—	—	—	—	10,000	4,000	—
		% recovery	60	—	—	—	—	50	80	—
1 (2,66,50,58)	1.2	PL	—	20,000	13,333	—	—	—	—	—
		SPL-Ag	—	12,000	12,000	—	—	—	—	—
		% recovery	—	60	90	—	—	—	—	—
5 (1,2,12)	1.0	PL	11,111	25,000	—	—	—	—	—	10,000
		SPL-Ag	10,000	10,000	—	—	—	—	—	8,333
		% recovery	90	40	—	—	—	—	—	83
2 (2,3,5,12)	1.2	PL	—	12,500	20,000	—	16,666	—	—	—
		SPL-Ag	—	8,000	10,000	—	10,000	—	—	—
		% recovery	—	64	50	—	60	—	—	—

[a] Percent recovery = 100 × (SPL-Ag ID$_{50}$units/10⁹ platelets)/(PL ID$_{50}$ units/10⁹ platelets).

amount of antigen obtained from platelets was relatively low, i.e., only 1 mg of protein is recoverable from 10^9 platelets (Pellegrino et al., 1974b). HL-A antigens solubilized from platelets appear to be relatively unstable upon storage at $-20°C$ as were antigens solubilized from splenocytes (M. A. Pellegrino, unpublished results). Although methods have been developed to obtain large numbers of platelets (up to 10^9) from blood donors (Graw et al., 1971; Borberg et al., 1972), the low yield and poor stability of antigens recovered limit the usefulness of this source for the isolation of materials suitable for chemical studies. However, HL-A antigens from platelets are most suitable for biologic studies, e.g., treatment of allograft recipients with the donor's soluble antigen to achieve some degree of immunologic unresponsiveness resulting in the prolongation of allograft survival.

5. HL-A Antigens in Serum

An early observation indicated that human serum inhibited the cytotoxic activity of HL-A alloantisera (Ferrone et al., 1967). This was thought to reflect incompatibility between human and rabbit complement in the lymphocytotoxic test. Later the use of better defined HL-A alloantisera made it possible for van Rood et al. (1970a,b) to detect soluble HL-A antigens in human serum, a finding that was questionable because this activity was lost after ultracentrifugation at 100,000 g. More recently the presence of soluble HL-A antigens in serum has been clearly established by several investigators (Charlton and Zmijewski, 1970; Miyajima et al., 1972; Schultz and Shreffler, 1972; Miyakawa et al., 1973a; Billing and Terasaki, 1974; Billing et al., 1973) as well as in our laboratory (Pellegrino et al., 1974b; Oh et al., 1974). The immunologic nature of this material is indicated by its ability to affect graft survival (van Rood et al., 1970b) and to elicit monospecific cytotoxic antibodies in rabbits (Billing and Terasaki, 1974; Ferrone et al., 1974c). Interestingly enough, soluble H-2 antigens could not be detected serologically in sera from B10.D2 (H-2^d) mice (S. Ferrone, unpublished results).

Although detailed and quantitative information as to the actual yields of antigens is as yet incomplete, some preliminary data (Oh et al., 1974) indicate that from 0.5 to 1.5 mg of crude antigenic material and up to 32,000 ID$_{50}$ units can be obtained from 1 ml of serum.

It is not known whether this HL-A antigenic material in human serum consists of antigen shed from lymphocytes or of antigen secreted in soluble form by these cells. What seems likely from preliminary work in our laboratory (Oh et al., 1974) is that this HL-A-like material is associated with one or several serum components and that its isolation in a chemically pure and defined state may be a fairly formidable task.

B. Extraction of Soluble H Antigens

During the last decade an array of extraction procedures was developed to solubilize H antigens from their sites on the plasma cell membrane. These methods utilized detergents (for review, see Metzgar et al., 1973), proteases (for review, see Nathenson, 1970; Mann and Fahey, 1971; Sanderson and Welsh, 1973), low frequency sound (Kahan and Reisfeld, 1971), as well as complex (Mann, 1973 and simple salts (Reisfeld et al., 1971a; Reisfeld and Pellegrino, 1973). It is now fairly evident that none of these procedures has been optimally effective because they are all quite nonselective, i.e., they solubilize relatively small amounts of antigen together with vast quantities of contaminants. Most of the effective methods for isolating naturally soluble serum proteins or enzymes proved to be inadequate for solubilizing H antigens which most likely are embedded in a sea of hydrophobic materials on the cell membrane, e.g., lipids and complex glycolipids. The above mentioned procedures have, however, all yielded H antigenic substances that, although varying somewhat in molecular size and charge, were capable of evoking humoral and/or cellular immune responses characteristic of H or transplantation antigens.

The choice of a method for H antigen extraction depends largely on one's objectives. For example, if it is desirable, especially for biologic evaluations, to "solubilize" H antigens together with at least some of their membrane attachments and neighboring components, the utilization of detergents seems most profitable. This is especially true if precautions are taken to avoid any proteolytic enzyme activation as has been observed during detergent treatment of lymphoid cells (L. A. Manson, personal communication). Although the antigens may not be simple, water-soluble moieties but rather complex micelles, they may, nevertheless, be quite adequate for biologic studies. All the other extraction procedures most likely solubilize a portion of that H antigen molecule which may naturally exist in or on the membrane. It is quite feasible that the antigenic portion of this molecule may be relatively intact, at least as determined by the known humoral and cellular immune responses which it can evoke. In other words, ultimately it may be feasible to use these approaches to isolate small, functional antigenic fragments with meaningful biologically reactivities.

1. SALT EXTRACTION OF H ANTIGENS

After the effective use of low frequency sound to isolate guinea pig transplantation antigens (Kahan and Reisfeld, 1967) and HL-A antigen mainly from spleen cells (Kahan et al., 1968) and from cultured lymphoid cells (Reisfeld et al., 1970), we progressed to using a simple hypertonic salt (3 M KCl) extraction method. Thus, HL-A antigens were isolated from cultured human lymphoid cells (Reisfeld et al., 1971a), spent culture media (Pellegrino et al., 1973e), and platelets (Uhlenbruck et al., 1973; Pellegrino et al., 1974b); H-2 antigens were isolated from murine splenocytes (Götze and Reisfeld, 1972) and L1210 murine leukemia cells (Götze and Reisfeld, 1972). This method has now found wide application to solubilization of human tumor-associated antigens, including malignant melanoma and sarcoma (W. Winters, personal communication), colonic carcinoma, and leukemia antigens (Gutterman et al., 1972). We selected this procedure mainly because of its simplicity, reproducibility, and relative high efficiency. Specifically, the most efficient extractions were achieved with 3 M KCl for 16 hours at 4°C. Cells were dispersed routinely in phosphate-buffered saline, pH 7.4, containing 3 M KCl (20 ml/10^9 cells), and the cell suspension was gently agitated on a rotary shaker. The resulting viscous extract was centrifuged overnight at 163,000 g, lipid layers were siphoned off, and the supernatant was dialyzed against 3 changes of 200 volumes each of isotonic saline. A gelatinous material, which was comprised largely of DNA, could be removed by centrifugation at 1500 g for 20 minutes. DNA could not be detected in significant amounts in the supernatant by the diphenylamine test of a hot trichloroacetic acid extract or by radiolabeling experiments. Thus, the 1500 g extract antigen from 2 generations of WI-L2 lymphoid cells, which had been uniformly labeled with [2-^{14}C]thymidine, contained less than 1% DNA (Reisfeld et al., 1971a).

2. MODE OF ACTION OF KCl

KCl most likely solubilizes H antigens chaotropically by dissociating hydrophobic attractions which are the most important stabilizing forces of native cell membrane structures. This is attributable to the fact that van der Waals attractions between apolar groups are weak, and hydrogen bonds of the C=O · · · N and C=O · · · H—O type are thermodynamically unstable if not protected from water (Klotz and Farnham, 1968). Apolar groups form hydrophobic bonds largely because of this fact. In addition, the transfer of an apolar molecule from a lipophilic surrounding to water is accompanied by a decrease in entropy, which is in essence due to the highly ordered structure of water. Any disorder in the water structure can reduce this negative entropy change. This can be achieved by certain inorganic anions, e.g., SCN^-, ClO_4^-, I^-, Br^-, or Cl^-, which have relatively large positive entropies due to their structure breaking effects on water. These anions also reduce the polarity of the surrounding water making it more lipophilic. Thus, hydrophobic attractions largely responsible for native membrane structure are weakened, and the entry of apolar molecules into the aqueous phase is greatly enhanced (Kauzman, 1959). Because of these characteristics, such anions which break the ordered water structure are referred to as chaotropic agents (Hamaguchi and Geiduschek, 1962). Chaotropes are less effective in salting out globular proteins, because they trigger dissociation and unfolding, than ions which cause folding, coiling, and association and thus are highly effective protein precipitants (Hofmeister, 1888). We believe that KCl, although it is a relatively weak chaotropic agent, functions as described above to solubilize H antigens from cell membrane surfaces. In addition, we have evidence that this solubilizing process is not triggered by intracellular proteases (Oh et al., 1973). Specifically, during KCl extraction, aliquots of HL-A antigens from cultured human lymphoid cells showed little or no proteolytic activity when tested against acid denatured hemoglobin at 37°C (Table IV). Essentially the same results were obtained with other substrates such as casein, azocasein and N,N^1-[^{14}C]dimethylcasein. When self digestion was measured in the extract, values were

TABLE IV

Time Course Study of Protease Activity[a] during the 3 M KCl Extraction of Cultured Lymphocytes

Cell lines	Protein digested (%) at (Time of assay)			
	1/2 hr	2 hr	8 hr	20 hr
WI-L2	0.3	1.0	0.9	0.7
RPMI 4098	2.4	1.3	0	0

[a] 0.5% acid-denatured hemoglobulin was used as substrate. Activity was checked after 1 hour incubation at 37°C at each time point. Under actual extraction conditions, i.e., 3 M KCl, 4°C, 20 hours, only 0.45% of the substrate was digested.

essentially the same as those depicted in Table IV. There was no correlation between antigen yield and reactivity and proteolytic activity, since during the early phase of extraction (½–2 hours) when proteolytic activity was maximal (2.4% of substrate digested), antigen yield was minimal, i.e., only 10% of that achieved at 16–20 hours when proteolytic activity was negligible (0.07% of substrate digested).

In addition, when antigen extracts remained in 3 M KCl at 4°C for several weeks, there was no measurable decrease in antigenic activity (Oh et al., 1973). Whether native lipolytic or glycolytic enzymes are present or have any effect on the solubilization of H antigens by KCl is unknown; however, it is generally known that such enzymes act minimally if at all in the presence of salt exceeding concentrations of 0.5 M.

It is, of course, difficult if not impossible to rule out some proteolytic cleavage in any extract of materials from cells or tissues, i.e., a single "nick" in an exposed polypeptide chain. For this reason alone it is difficult to assert that truly "native" structures are isolated from cell membranes by any method. The distinction is a matter of degree, i.e., (1) from maximizing the covalent peptide bond cleavage by the addition of large amounts (E/S ranging from 1:1 to 1:150) of extracellular proteases, (2) from using detergents that optimize the action of intracellular enzymes, or (3) from adding a mild chaotrope such as KCl which minimizes the action of intracellular proteases. From our data, KCl seems to solubilize H antigens largely if not entirely by its chaotropic effects rather than by activation of native cellular proteases.

3. Yield of KCl-Solubilized H Antigens

Most of the cultured cells utilized for antigen extraction must be viable in order to obtain maximal yields. Cells with less than 50% viability yielded only about 10% soluble HL-A antigen recovery with relatively poor immunologic potency in contrast with 50–80% recovery when the cells were from 95–100% viable (Reisfeld et al., 1971a). As shown in Table V, extracts from the same cell line on different occasions contained some variability in total protein content, in immunologic potency, and, consequently, in total amount of antigenic units recovered. However, even when extractions are carried out separately, the ratio of antigen yield between phenotypic HL-A specificities of a given cultured cell line remains essentially constant, independent of the overall antigen yield. This indicates that neither preferential extraction nor selective destruction of HL-A

TABLE V
Soluble Antigen Yields from Different Human Cultured Cell Lines

Cell line	Antigen batch no.	HL-A1 ID$_{50}$ units/ 10^9 cells	HL-A1 Recovery (%)[a]	HL-A2 ID$_{50}$ units/ 10^9 cells	HL-A2 Recovery (%)	HL-A3 ID$_{50}$ units/ 10^9 cells	HL-A3 Recovery (%)	HL-A5 ID$_{50}$ units/ 10^9 cells	HL-A5 Recovery (%)	HL-A7 ID$_{50}$ units/ 10^9 cells	HL-A7 Recovery (%)
RPMI 1788	1	—	—	620,000	51	—	—	—	—	165,000	30
	2	—	—	920,000	85	—	—	—	—	341,000	64
	3	—	—	462,000	38	—	—	—	—	170,000	31
	4	—	—	450,000	37	—	—	—	—	162,000	29
WI-L2	1	—	—	2,785,712	91	—	—	793,912	81	—	—
	2	—	—	1,800,000	60	—	—	521,371	53	—	—
RPMI 4098	1	—	—	—	—	1,666,666	100	—	—	—	—
	2	—	—	—	—	1,666,666	100	—	—	—	—
	3	—	—	—	—	833,333	50	—	—	—	—
RPMI 7249	1	350,000	17	350,000	28	—	—	—	—	35,000	12
	2	350,000	17	350,000	28	—	—	—	—	35,000	12

[a] Percent recovery = 100 × (ID$_{50}$ units/10^9 cells)/(AD$_{50}$ units/10^9 cells).

specificities takes place during KCl extraction. There also is no direct relationship between the relative density of HL-A determinants on lymphoid cell surfaces and the serologic activity of solubilized HL-A antigens (Pellegrino et al., 1973a). Thus, as also shown in Table VI, two cultured cell lines, i.e., RPMI 1788 and RPMI 7249, while sharing an essentially equal density of HL-A2 determinants, yielded vastly different recoveries of this specificity on the solubilized antigen. It is, of course, possible that antigenic determinants may be masked and undetectable by quantitative absorption analyses yet extractable by 3 M KCl, thus yields of antigen are higher than anticipated from antigen density determinations.

A similar mechanism may explain why the amount of soluble antigen extractable from cultured cells varies considerably with the stage of their growth cycle. Thus, more active antigenic preparations were obtained from cultures in late log or resting phases than from those in early log phase (Pellegrino et al., 1973c). Yet the density of HL-A determinants on the cell surface does not contribute to the yield, since these determinants are almost equally dense throughout the growth cycle (Pellegrino et al., 1972b; Ferrone et al., 1973b).

It is of some interest that only small yields (3–8%) of soluble HL-A antigen could be obtained by KCl extraction from lyophilized cells or from crude cell membrane preparations obtained by repeated freezing and thawing. Furthermore, once 3 M KCl extraction was utilized on membranes prepared according to Mann et al. (1968) or alternatively prepared by detergent (NP 40) or zinc fixation (Warren et al., 1966), yields of HL-A antigens were uniformly poor (1–3%) (M. A. Pellegrino and R. A. Reisfeld, unpublished). Marked changes on cell surfaces induced by these treatments seems to decrease the solubilizing capability of 3 M KCl. For example, "toughening" of the membranes such as that induced by isopropanol (10^{-3} M) reduces the solubilizing capacity of KCl (Oh et al., 1973). These observations support the hypothesis that the mechanism of KCl extraction is largely independent of the action of any intracellular proteases but does depend on chaotropic dissociation of hydrophobic interaction on the intact, unaltered cell surface. In addition, when materials from spent culture media were judged to be membranes after electron microscopy and were extracted with 3 M KCl, recovery of serologic activity was as much as 76% (Pellegrino et al., 1973e).

KCl has also proven useful for the solubilization of H-2 antigens from cultured cells and from splenocytes (Götze and Reisfeld, 1972; Götze et al., 1972b). H-2 antigens were extracted by 3 M KCl from cultured murine cells (L1210) derived from a lymphoid tumor in as-

TABLE VI

ID_{50} ($\mu g/\mu l$) of Soluble HL-A Antigens for Different HL-A Specificities[a]

Soluble HL-A antigens	First segregant series						Second segregant series			
	HL-A1	HL-A2	HL-A3	HL-A9	HL-A10	HL-A5	HL-A7	HL-A8	W14
127-103[b] RPMI 1788 (HL-A2,10,7, W14)	3.0	0.025	3.0	1.0	1.5	2.5	0.09	1.2	0.15
155-103[b] RPMI 4098 (HL-A3, Te 63)	>3.0	>3.0	0.01	>3.0	>3.0	>3.0	>3.0	>3.0	>3.0
179-103[b] WI-L2 (HL-A1,2,5, Te 57)	0.2	0.016	1.0	1.0	>5.0	0.047	4.8	4.5	>5.0
107-103[b] RPMI 7249 (HL-A1,2,7,8)	0.1	0.1	>10	1.0	>10.0	>10	1.0	0.1	>10.0

[a] For these experiments we selected the combination of target cells and antisera which proved most sensitive in the assay method employed.
[b] Each number denotes a single preparation of soluble alloantigen.

cites form from DBA/2(H-2^d) mice. These cells, possessing a doubling time of 11–13 hours at 36.5°C, were harvested for antigen extraction during their log growth phase. Yields of antigen quantities (8 to 15 mg protein/10^9 cells) and antigenic activities (9,000–11,000 ID_{50}/mg protein) were optimal when cultures were harvested during mid-log growth (Götze et al., 1972b). In contrast to HL-A antigens, quantities of H-2 antigens from cells in late log growth and in resting phase were low (Götze et al., 1972b). The specific activity per microgram protein of H-2 antigen extracted by KCl was about the same as that of the H-2 antigen obtained by papain; however, the amount of total antigenic activity extracted per 10^9 cells was two- to three-fold greater when 3 M KCl was used (Götze and Reisfeld, 1972).

C. Purification of H Antigens

Rigorous purification of cell surface antigens to the point where their chemical and molecular nature can be assessed critically has, for the reasons cited above, proved to be rather formidable. Thus, the nonselectivity of available extraction procedures solubilizing tiny amounts of antigen (often 1% or less) in a sea of contaminants is only part of the overall problem. In addition, an antigenic principle with soluble and relatively stable biologic activity can become less soluble and/or biologically less potent, whenever its initial milieu is drastically altered during purification. Thus, even electrophoretically purified HL-A antigens increased in their inhibitory capacity toward cytotoxic alloantibody at best only 20- to 25-fold (Reisfeld et al., 1971a). It is relevant to point out that the lack of truly monospecific HL-A alloantisera as well as their low titer and affinity may also play a role, especially since purified H-2 alloantigens when tested against monospecific H-2 alloantibody increased in their inhibitory capacity up to 700-fold (Shimada and Nathenson, 1969). In this case, even though antigenic activity was markedly potentiated, ~ 98% of total activity units were actually lost during the purification process. This formidable loss could be, at least in part, owing to changes in the relative solubility of these cell-membrane associated antigens during purification.

As far as purification strategy is concerned, reasonably one should apply as many fractionation principles and procedures as possible. Such an approach seems especially warranted if one considers the large body of evidence accumulated during the purification of naturally soluble serum proteins and enzymes. However, our experience with HL-A antigens dictated another approach since we observed

5. Histocompatibility Antigens: Biology and Chemistry

marked losses of specific activity and yield during extensive manipulation of these substances. Thus, the best strategy seemed to us the application of a limited number of purification steps.

To this end, the KCl extract, suitably centrifuged and dialyzed (see above), was salted out with ammonium sulfate (0.5 saturation), then dialyzed against 0.1 M Tris-HCl buffer, pH 7.8, and passed over a concanavalin A (con A)-Sepharose column. HL-A antigens were eluted with 0.1 M Tris-HCl, 0.15 M NaCl, pH 7.0, as they were not bound since they lacked the necessary carbohydrates, i.e., those possessing D-mannopyranose and D-glucopyranose rings (see below). However, substantial amounts (~30–40%) of contaminating glycoproteins were bound to this adsorbent. They, in turn, could be eluted with a 0.1 M solution of α-D-methylmannoside but were found to lack any HL-A antigenic activity as judged by serologic assays. Both purification steps resulted in from 5- to 10-fold purification of the serologic activity of HL-A antigens and a removal of ~70% of the original proteins present in the KCl extract. Aside from ~10–15% handling losses, the total HL-A antigenic activity present in the original extract could be recovered in the eluate which was not bound to con A-Sepharose.

Extracts containing HL-A antigenic activity were concentrated against a 50% sucrose solution to contain ~10–20 mg protein/ml and as much as 100 mg protein and then subjected to preparative polyacrylamide gel electrophoresis (PAGE) on a Polyprep 100 column (Buchler Instruments, Fort Lee, N. J.). Electrophoresis was performed at 0°C in system "B" of Rodbard and Chrambach (1971) (pH 10.2, 7½% acrylamide gel; 50 ml lower gel, 30 ml upper gel) at a constant current of 35 mA. Electrophoretic resolution of HL-A antigenic extracts was optimal under these conditions as determined by analytical PAGE at different pH values (pH 3.56, 6.96, 7.35, 7.67, and 10.2). Fractions were collected at a flow rate of 0.8 ml/minute with a Tris-HCl elution buffer (0.138 M Tris, 0.18 M HCl, pH 8.2 containing 5% sucrose). Fractions eluting at R_f 0.78–0.80 exhibited specific antigenic activity. Figure 10 depicts a typical elution diagram. Reelectrophoresis of this fraction in the same preparative PAGE system showed that under these conditions the antigenic moiety consisted of a single electrophoretic component (Fig. 11).

Protein yield and antigenic activity recovered from PAGE were assessed by utilizing a radiolabeling method and micro-Kjeldahl nitrogen analyses (Reisfeld et al., 1971a). For this purpose 1×10^9 cells in log growth phase (2×10^7 cells/ml) were incubated (4 hours) with a mixture of ^{3}H-labeled amino acids in Eagle's minimal essential medium containing only 1% of its normal amino acid content.

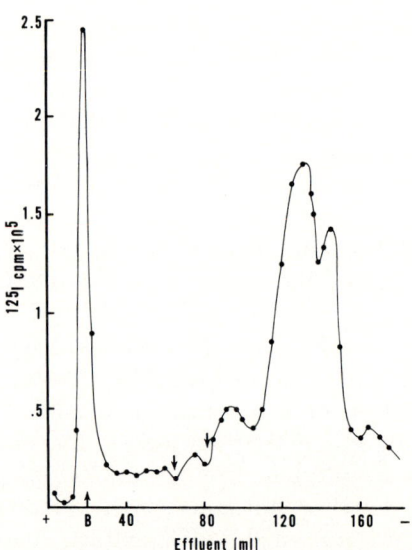

Fig. 10. Effluent diagram following PAGE of KCl extract obtained from cell line RPMI 1788. The area enclosed by the arrows contains the HL-A antigenic activity.

Approximately 15% of the radiolabel was incorporated into the cells, while 2% was found in the ultracentrifugal KCl supernate and 0.04% in the electrophoretically purified antigen. As far as the yield and activity of the purified antigen were concerned, 2% of the nitrogen and from 45–60% of the total antigenic activity applied to the column were recovered in the purified component, whereas ID_{50} units/mg nitrogen were increased 20-fold over those in the unpurified material (Reisfeld and Pellegrino, 1973).

D. Biologic Reactivity of Soluble H Antigens

Are soluble H antigens biologically relevant and useful reagents? Relatively crude extracts containing HL-A antigens solubilized with 3 M KCl elicited a humoral immune response, i.e., the production of cytotoxic antibodies in rabbits directed against all the HL-A determinants present on the immunogen (Ferrone *et al.*, 1972a). In addition these KCl-solubilized HL-A antigens also evoked a cellular immune response in humans. Nephrectomized patients sensitized by foreign grafts were shown to possess specific cellular and humoral reactivity toward donor-type soluble antigens. Only donor-type antigens could elicit direct delayed-type skin reactions, analogous to

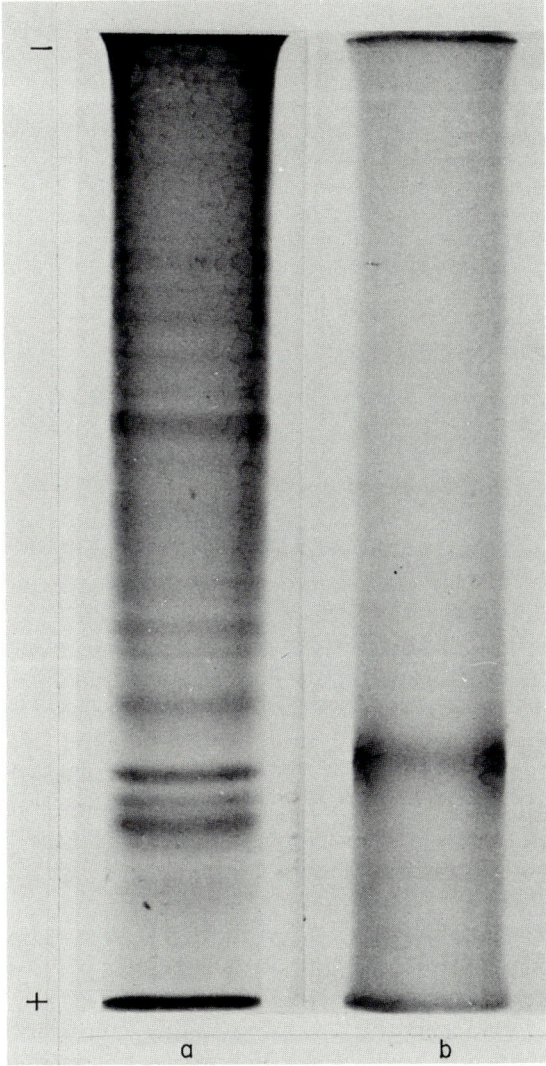

Fig. 11. Electrophoretic profile of (a) KCl extract and (b) antigen preparation obtained following reelectrophoresis of the PAGE fraction with relative mobility of 0.78–0.80.

tuberculin reactions, in patients who had previously rejected grafts. The soluble antigen also specifically blocked the cytotoxic action of antibodies produced by patients after nephrectomy and transplantation. Thus, KCl-solubilized HL-A antigens possessed specific determinants which interacted with immune components from hosts sensitized by renal allografts possessing the corresponding HL-A type (Kahan et al., 1973).

Recent work in our laboratory with H-2^d antigens solubilized with 3 M KCl from cultured murine leukemia (L1210) cells indicated that these materials elicited humoral unresponsiveness in the presence of cellular immunity (Götze and Reisfeld, 1974). This same phenomenon had also been observed with soluble H-2^d antigens (Law et al., 1972). These same antigens were active as transplantation antigens, since they specifically accelerated the rejection of allografts.

VIII. Chemical and Molecular Nature of HL-A Antigens

A. Physical Properties

HL-A antigens extracted by either low frequency sound or 3 M KCl and purified by PAGE are homogeneous in molecular size (Kahan et al., 1968; Reisfeld et al., 1971a). Thus, the molecular weight of antigen solubilized by low frequency sound was 34,600 daltons by Yphantis sedimentation equilibrium analyses assuming a partial specific volume of 0.72. The material was 94% monodisperse containing a 6% aggregated moiety with a molecular weight of 150,000 (Kahan and Reisfeld, 1969a). The KCl-solubilized antigen was essentially monodisperse and had a sedimentation coefficient $s_{20,w}$ of 2.3 and a molecular weight of 31,000 daltons by Archibald sedimentation equilibrium analyses, assuming a partial specific volume of 0.72.

The electrophoretically purified antigen preparation also possessed electrophoretic homogeneity at varying pH values and gel porosity. A certain degree of structural homogeneity was suggested by the amino acid composition approaching whole integer residue values and by tryptic peptide maps showing the number of peptides (24) expected from the arginine (5) and tyrosine (18) residues found upon amino acid analysis (Reisfeld and Kahan, 1972).

B. Chemical Properties

Largely due to a lack of adequate methods for rigorous purification, H antigens have in the past been reported to consist of substances as diverse as DNA, lipid, carbohydrate, and protein and its

5. Histocompatibility Antigens: Biology and Chemistry

various conjugated forms (for review, see Kahan and Reisfeld, 1969b; Reisfeld and Kahan, 1970). However, by general consensus, the H antigenic principle is now considered to be essentially polypeptide in nature. Available chemical data strongly support this contention. Thus, antigenic activity is irreversibly destroyed by extensive digestion with proteases, protein denaturants, extreme pH values (above 11 and below 4), temperatures greater than 50°C, or detergents and complex salts in concentrations sufficient to affect protein conformation (for reviews, see Kahan and Reisfeld, 1969b; Reisfeld and Kahan, 1970).

There have been numerous postulates that carbohydrate moieties are responsible for antigenic activity; however, there is little evidence, although papain-solubilized H-2 and HL-A antigens were reported to contain from 3–8% neutral carbohydrates (Sanderson et al., 1971). In fact, digestion of these antigens with carbohydrases, which split off much of the neutral carbohydrates and hexosamines, or with neuraminidase, which cleaves off the neuraminic acid residues, essentially had no detectable effect on the antigenic activity of H-2 antigens as assessed by serologic tests (Muramatsu and Nathenson, 1971). Also, neither highly purified guinea pig antigens nor HL-A antigens solubilized by low frequency sound and 3 M KCl extraction contained more than 1% lipid or neutral carbohydrates (Kahan and Reisfeld, 1968, 1969a; Reisfeld et al., 1971a,b). Thus, guinea pig antigen (MW 15,000 daltons, Kahan and Reisfeld, 1969a) and HL-A antigen (MW 31,000 daltons, Reisfeld and Kahan, 1973) have at best one or two carbohydrate residues, respectively.

Reproducible and significant differences found among the amino acid compositions of H antigens extracted from cells derived from histoincompatible individuals support the contention that H antigenic determinants are mainly protein in nature. Thus, differences in the content of serine, alanine, valine, leucine, and isoleucine were detected between antigens derived from strains 2 and 13 of histoincompatible guinea pigs (Kahan and Reisfeld, 1968). In addition, amino acid analyses of highly purified HL-A antigens solubilized by low frequency sound from cell lines and possessing different alloantigenic specificities showed differences in content of aspartic acid, serine, proline, alanine, and tyrosine (Reisfeld and Kahan, 1971). The remaining amino acids were present in strikingly similar amounts. Thus, it seems reasonable that, as with immunoglobulin light and heavy chains of different allotypic specificities, these HL-A antigens also possess genetically segregating alloantigenic specificities which are expressed by polypeptide structures.

The amino acid composition of HL-A antigens solubilized by 3 M KCl contain 4 residues of cysteic acid and 3.6 residues of S-carboxymethylcysteine, respectively, indicating the presence of 4 half-cystine groups (Reisfeld and Kahan, 1972).

C. β_2 Microglobulin and HL-A Antigens

Recent work by several investigators has raised some interesting questions concerning the molecular nature of HL-A antigens, i.e., specifically its polypeptide chain structure. Thus, it has been postulated that β_2 microglobulin (β_2-μ) may be a subunit of HL-A antigens (Nakamuro et al., 1973; Grey et al., 1973; Peterson et al., 1974). Briefly, β_2-μ was first isolated by Berggard and Bearn (1968) from the urine of patients with tubular proteinurias. This molecule was found to have a molecular weight of 11,600 daltons, containing no carbohydrate, no free sulfhydryl groups, and according to amino acid analyses two half-cystines involved in a disulfide bond. This same protein was also found in small amounts in serum (~1.8 mg/liter), cerebrospinal fluid (~1.7 mg/liter), and urine (0.1 mg/24 hour volume) of normal individuals. In contrast, urine from patients with proteinurias contained as much as 89 mg/24 hour volume. Immunochemical analyses ruled out that β_2-μ might be a subunit of a larger plasma protein (Berggard and Bearn, 1968). When investigating stromal protein antigens Bron and Poulik (1971) found some glycoproteins antigenically related to red cell membranes in the urine. This finding led Poulik and Motwani (1972) to look for β_2-μ bound to lymphoid cell membranes. They found these molecules in or on the membranes of normal peripheral human lymphocytes and on lymphocytes from patients with chronic lymphocytic leukemia. Simultaneously Bernier and Fanger (1972) demonstrated the β_2-μ on the surface of 18 established lymphocyte cell lines and also in the spent medium of these cultures. Poulik (1973) also was able to demonstrate that both B and T cells carry β_2-μ in their membranes. In addition, Poulik (1973) found antisera against β_2-μ to be cytotoxic in the presence of complement to normal and tissue culture lymphocytes.

As far as the chemical structure of β_2-μ is concerned, Smithies and Poulik (1972a) determined the partial amino acid sequence of this globulin and found that 24 of the first 46 amino acid residues were homologous with the amino acid sequence of parts of the heavy chain of the G-1 myeloma protein suggesting a structural relationship between β_2-μ and the constant region of human IgG immunoglobulins. In spite of this structural relatedness, specific antisera against all known immunoglobulin chains did not react with this protein. Peterson et al. (1972) then published the partial amino acid sequence of β_2-μ and found 28 amino acid residues of the 100 residues comprising β_2-μ to be homologous with the C_H3 domain of the myeloma protein. The complete amino acid sequence was subsequently published by Cunningham et al. (1973). β_2-μ was suggested to be a free immunoglobulin domain possibly serving an effector function similar to that of the C_H3 domain of γ-1 chains of immunoglobulin G (Peterson et al., 1972). It was also suggested from the complete sequence data that the gene coding for β_2-μ evolved directly from a primitive precursor gene for immunoglobulins (Cunningham et al., 1973). A homologous protein was also isolated from the dog and its partial amino acid sequence established and related to human β_2-μ (Smithies and Poulik, 1972b).

The link between β_2-μ and HL-A antigens was first made by Nakamuro et al. (1973) who found that an 11,000 dalton fragment isolated from spent culture medium of cell line RPMI 1788 had essentially the identical amino acid composition as urinary β_2-μ. This fragment was, in turn, found to be identical in electrophoretic mobility and isoelectric point to a molecule of equal size derived from papain-solubilized HL-A antigens by acid degradation procedures. This 11,000 dalton fragment was previously found in HL-A antigen preparations derived from blood plasma (Miyakawa et al., 1973b). This fragment, although devoid of any HL-A antigenic activity, was, however, considered to possess "HL-A common antigenic activity" since in a radioimmunoassay it reacted consistently in HL-A antigen preparations of different phenotype with an ALS, i.e., a rabbit anti-human lymphoid cell antiserum (Miyakawa et al., 1973b). This "HL-A common portion fragment" was found to be identical with human β_2-μ both antigenically and by electrophoretic criteria. In addition, the amino acid sequence of this "HL-A common portion fragment" determined for the first 24 amino acid residues of a preparation isolated from spent culture medium was found to be identical with that reported for β_2-μ (Tanigaki et al., 1973).

Peterson et al. (1974) solubilized HL-A antigen by treating a crude spleen cell membrane fraction with papain and purified the antigen preparation by chromatography on carboxymethyl cellulose and gel filtration on Sephadex G-200. Material with HL-A antigenic activity eluted in a molecular weight region of 40,000–50,000 coincident with the elution portion for the first of two β_2-μ peaks. The second β_2-μ appeared in the same elution position as urinary β_2-μ. Immune complexes of purified radiolabeled HL-A antigens obtained by indirect precipitation with specific HL-A alloantisera resolved into two peaks upon SDS-acrylamide gel electrophoresis with approximate molecular weights of 33,000 and 12,000, respectively. When HL-A antigen preparations were reacted with rabbit anti-human β_2-μ antisera, only β_2-μ appeared upon SDS-acrylamide gel electrophoresis. Peterson et al. (1974) explained this finding by the assumption that only free β_2-μ reacts with the antiserum. On the basis of this assumption, it is difficult to see why the authors can utilize the same antiserum to detect by solid phase radioimmunoassay the β_2-μ's which are associated with the HL-A antigenic moiety following gel filtration. Furthermore, this finding contrasts with the ability of anti-β_2-μ sera to cocap the HL-A determinants on the surface of human lymphocytes and to induce resistance to lysis by HL-A alloantisera in conjunction with rabbit complement on lymphocytes coated in vitro with anti-β_2-μ sera for a suitable incubation period (Poulik et al., 1973). The latter experimental results are indeed suggestive of an association of β_2-μ and HL-A molecules although they should be confirmed by absorption experiments in view of the complexity of the direct cytotoxic test and of the effects that inhibitors of protein synthesis utilized in the experiments discussed have on the susceptibility to lysis.

In an attempt to show that only the large (MW 33,000) polypeptide chain carries HL-A antigenic activity, Peterson et al. (1974) subjected a radiolabeled, purified HL-A antigen preparation to gel chromatography on Sephadex G-100 in the presence of 4 M urea and 1 M acetic acid (pH 2.4). When the two radioactive peaks were reacted with specific HL-A alloantisera about 28% of the radioactivity of the larger polypeptide chain (MW ~33,000) was recovered in the immune complex following an indirect precipitation with rabbit antihuman L-chain antibody. In contrast, the smaller polypeptide chain (MW ~12,000) did not produce any immune complex formation. Since the authors claim that β_2-μ can be dissociated with 3 M KCl at neutral pH, it is difficult to see why they did not utilize this procedure in this experiment as most likely less denaturation of the HL-A antigen would have occurred than at pH 2.4 in the presence of 4 M urea. These data would have been more convincing if more than 28% of the radioactivity had precipitated as was the case when HL-A antigen was denatured by acid-urea treatment.

Grey et al. (1973) presented evidence to show by immunologic techniques that the 11,000 dalton peptide found on HL-A antigen preparations and β_2-μ's are identical. These investigators surface labeled thoracic duct lymphocytes obtained from patients with chronic lymphatic leukemia with ^{125}I by the lactoperoxidase method and prepared cell lysates with 0.5% Nonidet P40. Immunoprecipitates of the cell lysate with rabbit anti-human β_2-μ serum could only be obtained indirectly by using goat anti-rabbit γ-globulin as a coprecipitating agent. Immune precipitates thus obtained when completely reduced and alkylated yielded two radioactive peaks upon SDS-acrylamide gel electrophoresis with relative molecular weights of 45,000 and 11,000, respectively. In contrast, when radioactive papain digests of radiolabeled cultured human lymphoid cells were directly precipitated with turkey anti-human β_2-μ sera, SDS-acrylamide gel electrophoresis resulted in two size moieties of 34,000 and 11,000, respectively. This SDS-gel pattern appeared quite similar when superimposed on one obtained previously by some of the authors (Cresswell et al., 1973) when utilizing one HL-A alloantiserum (anti-HL-A7). Grey et al. (1973) do not explain why indirect precipitation with rabbit anti-β_2-μ of an NP 40 lysate of thoracic duct lymphocytes results in molecular size fragments of 45,000 and 11,000, whereas either direct precipitation of a purified papain digest of cultured human lymphoid cells with turkey anti-human β_2-μ antiserum or indirect precipitation with an anti-HL-A7 alloantiserum results upon SDS-acrylamide gel electrophoresis in the resolution of fragments with molecular size of 34,000 and 11,000, respectively.

Cresswell et al. (1973) also reported that papain-solubilized HL-A antigens from cultured human lymphocytes contained two major size classes of peptide fragments, i.e., 34,000 and 11,000. They labeled RPMI 4265 cultured cells in situ with either [^{3}H]glucosamine, [^{3}H]mannose, a mixture of [^{3}H]amino acids, or [^{14}C]amino acids. After Sephadex G-150 gel filtration, fractions were pooled which contained HL-A antigenic activity as determined by the ^{51}Cr release blocking assay. The pooled and concentrated fractions were allowed to form soluble immune complexes with anti-HL-A2 and anti-HL-A7 alloantisera, as determined by their gel filtration on the same Sephadex G-150 columns. The fraction in the inclusion volume of the gel after removal of the HL-A2 complex was treated with anti-HL-A7 alloantiserum and again produced an immune complex in the exclusion volume of the column. Yet reincubation of this sample with anti-HL-A2 alloantiserum produced little or no complex formation. The authors believe their data indicate that HL-A2 and HL-A7 determinants are on different fragments after solubilization by papain.

Cresswell et al. (1973) used still different procedures, all under protein-denaturing conditions, which resulted in separating peptides of two major size classes from the immune complexes composed of papain-solubilized HL-A alloantigens and HL-A alloantisera. These molecules were, respectively, 32,000 and 13,000 MW by Sephadex G-200 filtration on 1% dodecyl sulfate, 29,000 and 11,000 MW by agarose (A-5m) filtration in 6 M guanidine–hydrochloride, and 34,000 and 11,000 MW by SDS-polyacrylamide gel electrophoresis. Due to the strong protein denaturing conditions used it was impossible to determine which of these peptide size classes carried the HL-A specificity or whether both of them were required for HL-A antigenic expression. The ratio of molecular weights of the two peptide size classes was 2.6:1, whereas the ratio of radioactivity ([^{14}C]amino acid) was found to be 1.9:1. From the similarity of these ratios Cresswell *et al.* (1973) concluded that the fragments are present in a 1:1 molar ratio.

In an extension of the work described by Grey *et al.* (1973), Cresswell *et al.* (1974) showed by immunologic techniques virtually total identity between a small subunit of HL-A, derived by either papain or detergent solubilization, and β_2-μ. Initially, these investigators solubilized RPMI 4265 lymphoblastoid cells with papain and showed that the purified HL-A7,12 antigens from them contained β_2-μ as determined by a specific radioimmunoassay in which purified ^{125}I-labeled urinary β_2-μ and anti-β_2-μ antiserum were used. From the inhibition curves, it appeared that 8.75 ng of HL-A7,12 as compared to 2.06 ng of unlabeled β_2-μ were needed to obtain 50% inhibition. On the basis of these data Cresswell *et al.* (1974) calculated that 23% of the protein of HL-A7,12 was β_2-μ.

In order to prove that the 12,000 molecular size material associated with HL-A antigens is indeed β_2-μ and not a closely related polypeptide cross-reacting with β_2-μ, Cresswell *et al.* (1974) sought to inhibit lysis of human lymphocytes by β_2-μ antiserum. Since they found that normal peripheral human lymphocytes could be lysed by rabbit anti-β_2-μ antiserum in the presence of rabbit complement, these investigators studied the capacity of soluble HL-A and purified β_2-μ to inhibit the cytotoxic reaction of rabbit anti-β_2-μ antiserum against peripheral human lymphocytes. From the results, they estimated that for papain-solubilized products 30% of an HL-A 2 antigen preparation or 39% of an HL-A 7,12 antigen preparation was composed of material cross-reactive with β_2-μ. In a similar experiment with detergent solubilized HL-A2,7,12, which was estimated to be about 50% pure, only 12% of the inhibitory capacity of purified β_2-μ was obtained. In a previous report Cresswell *et al.* (1973) assumed that a

12,000 MW peptide represented 35% of the weight of papain solubilized HL-A antigens based on the ratio of [^{3}H]amino acids in the two polypeptides. Since from 23–93% of the solubilized HL-A antigen preparations was cross-reactive with β_2-μ, the 12,000 MW moiety associated with HL-A antigen preparations evidently was β_2-μ and not a closely related protein. Cresswell et al. (1974) also showed the relationship of purified β_2-μ and the 12,000 MW fraction associated with HL-A antigens by electrophoresis in SDS and SDS-urea gels. On isoelectric focusing (pH 4–6) both moieties showed a single band having a pI of 5.2.

Poulik et al. (1974) used yet another approach to elucidate the nature and possibly the function of the association between β_2-μ and HL-A molecules. In this case HL-A antigens prepared by 3 M KCl extraction of cultured human lymphoid cells (Reisfeld et al., 1971a), naturally soluble HL-A antigens and β_2-μ available in serum were used. Rather than characterizing HL-A and β_2-μ mainly by molecular size utilizing SDS gel electrophoresis of radiolabeled cell surface materials solubilized with either detergents or papain, these investigators assessed the components primarily by serologic and immunochemical means. They also attempted to study the nature of the interaction between anti-β_2-μ antibodies coupled to solid phase adsorbents and antigenically well-characterized HL-A preparations and to determine the feasibility of purifying HL-A alloantigens with anti-β_2-μ immunoadsorbents. Poulik et al. (1974) utilized these immunoadsorbents to avoid the use of a second antibody needed to obtain immune precipitates with anti-β_2-μ antisera and HL-A antigens. They found that immunoadsorbents prepared by covalently coupling β_2-μ antibodies to CNBr activated Sepharose 4B could indeed remove all detectable HL-A antigenic activity from 3 M KCl extracts of several cultured human lymphoid cell lines.

From several experiments of these same investigators with a variety of anti-β_2-μ immunoadsorbents it also became apparent that antihuman β_2-μ xenoantibodies produced in different animals and coupled to solid state immunoadsorbents varied considerably in their capacities to bind β_2-μ. Although most of these immunoadsorbents were reported to contain from 7 to 9 mg protein/ml, their capacity to bind β_2-μ varied from 7 ng β_2-μ per μg for coupled rabbit and goat antibody to as little as 0.5 ng for coupled pig and sheep antibody. When coupled to the Sepharose 4B immunoadsorbent, turkey anti-β_2-μ seemed to have the lowest capacity since it bound only 0.05 ng β_2-μ/μg protein.

Poulik et al. (1974) also found the adsorption of HL-A antigenic activity to anti-β_2-μ antibody sites on Sepharose 4B to be quite specific. In other words, if the immunoadsorbent was first reacted with varying amounts of β_2-μ, essentially no HL-A antigenic activity was bound, most likely since the β_2-μ occupied all the available anti-β_2-μ binding sites on the adsorbent. However, addition of nonspecific antigens to the adsorbent, e.g., human serum albumin, did not prevent adsorption of HL-A antigenic activity on the anti-β_2-μ immunoadsorbent.

Since these observations led to the conclusion that there was a close association between β_2-μ and molecules with HL-A antigenic activity, it was indeed somewhat surprising that Poulik et al. (1974) found that HL-A antigenic activity present in some 3 M KCl extracts obtained from three different cell lines (WI-L2, RPMI 6410 and 8866) could not be adsorbed to anti-β_2-μ immunoadsorbents. This phenomenon could not be explained based on the actual amount of β_2-μ detectable in such antigenic extracts. Preparations from which HL-A activity could be adsorbed were found to contain essentially the same amount of β_2-μ as those from which no antigenic activity could be removed by the immunoadsorbent. It appears that in some HL-A preparations obtained by 3 M KCl extraction few, if any, β_2-μ molecules are associated with HL-A molecules. This phenomenon is not limited to HL-A antigen preparations obtained by 3 M KCl extraction. As mentioned above, Peterson et al. (1974) also found that when papain derived HL-A antigens were reacted with rabbit anti-β_2-μ antiserum and anti-human light chain only β_2-μ molecules devoid of HL-A molecules were detected in the immunoprecipitate. Poulik et al. (1974) also reported that several HL-A antigen preparations obtained by either detergent (NP 40, Bris 96/98, Lubrol) or papain treatment of cultured human lymphoid cells behaved in a similar manner when reacted with anti-β_2-μ immunoadsorbents. It would thus appear that, irrespective of the mode of solubilization, some HL-A antigen molecules are not associated with β_2-μ molecules. The latter apparently exist as monomers or aggregates and may even be associated with other molecular species.

Even so, there is now a considerable body of evidence indicating that β_2-μ molecules co-isolate with HL-A molecules in a noncovalent association, and it seems appropriate to raise the question whether such an association is indeed specific. In other words, is β_2-μ really a molecular subunit of the HL-A molecule representing a "common antigenic region," i.e., a noncovalently associated light polypeptide chain? An even more important question is whether or not β_2-μ is a subunit of HL-A antigens, and whether it does indeed exert an important function in modulating HL-A antigenic activity. Poulik et al. (1974) have shown that β_2-μ certainly is not necessary for HL-A antigens to react with HL-A alloantibody in the blocking test. In this regard, efforts are being made to determine the immunogenicity of HL-A xenoantibody. In one case, monospecific anti-W24 xenoantibody was produced in rabbits (Ferrone et al., 1974c) by an immunogen that consisted of partially purified HL-A antigen isolated from serum, but apparently contained little, if any, β_2-μ. Judging from these data, there is no compelling evidence that β_2-μ molecules are indeed needed for the expression of HL-A antigenic activity. If this finding is indeed substantiated by additional studies, then the question as to what biologic function β_2-μ serves as far as HL-A is concerned becomes even more critical.

Concerning this possible biologic function of β_2-μ, it is of interest to review briefly information pertaining to HL-A antigens in human serum. Its importance lies in the facts that both β_2-μ and HL-A molecules are present in serum, most likely due to shedding from cell surfaces, and that no stringent extractive procedures that could break their noncovalent association(s) are needed to isolate them. During some of the experiments in which human sera were reacted with rabbit or goat anti-β_2-μ antibodies coupled to immunoadsorbents, all the detectable HL-A activity could be bound to the immunoadsorbent (Poulik et al., 1974). These sera contained from 18 to 36 ng β_2-μ/mg of protein which compares well with the published figures of 1.3–2.5 mg/liter of serum (Berggard and Bearn, 1968). It should be pointed out that a number of sera with HL-A and β_2-μ antigenic activity could not be bound to the immunoadsorbent much as some cell extracts mentioned above would not bind. Furthermore, when HL-A serum antigens were purified extensively by fractional precipitation with ammonium sulfate, gel filtration, ion-exchange chromatography, and preparative acrylamide gel electrophoresis, it was found that the β_2-μ content decreased at each step (Reisfeld, unpublished observations). In fact, as determined by sensitive radioimmunoassays, highly purified, immunologically potent HL-A antigens isolated from serum contained absolutely no β_2-μ (Poulik et al., 1974). Since one could argue that the radioimmunoassay relies strictly on an antigen site(s), which is in no way hindered from reacting with antibody, Poulik et al. (1974) also determined the absence of β_2-μ by chemical means. Although no 11,000 MW moiety was detectable by SDS-acrylamide gel electrophoresis of highly purified HL-A antigens isolated from serum and possessing a molecular weight of 33,000, these investigators were not satisfied by the sensitivity of their method. Therefore, they examined the amino acid composition of such purified HL-A antigens. It was of considerable interest that the major electrophoretic component which possessed excellent HL-A antigenic activity had only one residue of isoleucine per molecule of 33,000 MW. Clearly, β_2-μ was not present since its amino acid sequence analysis revealed 5 residues of isoleucine distributed throughout the major portion of the molecule. This finding also destroyed the notion, at least for HL-A serum antigens, that β_2-μ could be a more integral part of the HL-A molecule, e.g., a peptide bond-linked portion of the HL-A polypeptide chain per se, than previously believed. All experimental data thus far strongly suggest that whatever association exists between the two molecules is of a noncovalent nature.

Poulik et al. (1974) also tried to determine whether anti-β_2-μ immunoadsorbents are a practical and useful tool for isolating and purifying HL-A antigens. Detergents (NP 40, Brij 96/98, Lubrol, and sodium dodecyl sulfate) and chaotropic agents (KCl, KI, KBr, $NaClO_4$, NaSCN, and trichloracetate) were found to vary considerably in their efficacy in desorbing HL-A and β_2-μ molecules, i.e., eluting from 10–70% of adsorbed HL-A antigenic activity. Preliminary observations indicate that 3 M KBr (pH 7.0) is optimal for the elution of HL-A antigens from anti-β_2-μ immunoadsorbents (Reisfeld, 1974, unpublished observations).

Although elution of HL-A antigens specifically bound to anti-β_2-μ immunoadsorbents seems to have considerable potential as a means of purification, the "state of the art" is such that conditions have not yet evolved which permit the application of crude cell extracts and the subsequent elution of essentially pure HL-A and/or β_2-μ antigen molecules from these adsorbents. While it is often feasible to reduce the heterogenicity of molecular size classes by this type of approach, it is far more difficult to obtain an electrophoretically homogeneous molecular species. Specifically, after interacting HL-A antigen extracts with anti-β_2-μ immunoadsorbent Poulik et al. (1974) used detergents and/or chaotropic agents to obtain eluates which possessed HL-A antigenic activity and which contained one major molecular size class of 33,000 when analyzed by SDS-polyacrylamide gel electrophoresis. However, when these eluates were analyzed by using polyacrylamide gel electrophoresis in the presence of 8 M urea, it was apparent that several molecular species with different charge properties were present although their molecular sizes were essentially the same. This is, of course, not too surprising since it is well known that electrophoretic charge is a far more sensitive parameter than molecular size to identify different molecular species.

BIOLOGIC ROLE OF β_2 MICROGLOBULIN

In view of the varied and interesting pieces of information suggesting an association of HL-A and β_2-μ at the molecular level, it is relevant to seek answers concerning the biologic function of β_2-μ at least as far as HL-A antigenic expression is concerned. However, there seems to be little or no proof thus far that β_2-μ modulates HL-A antigenic expression.

Several biologic functions have been suggested for β_2-μ or for a possible subunit consisting of HL-A and β_2-μ molecules. Thus, because anti-β_2-μ antiserum is able to inhibit the MLC reaction, β_2-μ could be involved in the recognition phase of the immune response (Bach et al., 1973; Poulik et al., 1973). In addition, because of the structural homology between β_2-μ and the C_H3 region of immunoglobulin heavy chains, it was proposed that β_2-μ might indeed represent a free immunoglobulin domain functioning much like the C_H3 domain and serving as a link between histocompatibility and immune response loci (Peterson et al., 1972; Cunningham et al., 1974).

Poulik et al. (1974) have observed that some HL-A antigens from serum and from cell extracts do not bind to β_2-μ immunoadsorbents regardless of the method of solubilization. Now the question arises whether this is a fortuitous technical artifact or whether it reflects a much more complex phenomenon. One could speculate that either β_2-μ is antigenically polymorphic or that it varies in its capacity to bind molecules bearing different HL-A phenotypes. Furthermore, it is intriguing to consider whether the latter possibility influences the heterogeneity of HL-A specificities or the difference in immunogenicity of various soluble HL-A antigens in rabbits. From experiments in progress (Ferrone et al., 1974c), HL-A antigens isolated from serum that are serologically reactive and have a wide range of HL-A specificities vary considerably in their abilities to elicit the formation of specific HL-A xenoantibody in rabbits. The functional relationship between HL-A and β_2-μ may become better defined once it is known whether the large amount of excess β_2-μ *not* associated with HL-A could be linked to other cell surface molecules. In fact, it has been reported that there are 10^7 β_2-μ sites versus only 10^3 HL-A sites on the surface of human peripheral lymphocytes (Peterson et al., 1972; Sanderson and Welsh, 1973).

Defining the structural association between HL-A and β_2-μ seems less complicated than explaining their mutual biologic interactions. Thus, it appears that HL-A molecules can be antigenically active although no β_2-μ is detectable, yet some HL-A molecules certainly are associated with molecules of β_2-μ. If such an association does not reflect a coincidental affinity of two completely unrelated molecules, then the noncovalent nature of the binding between the HL-A determinant expressed on one 33,000 MW fragment and β_2-μ indicates a multichain structure of the HL-A molecule.

D. Molecular Nature

The gene product of the H loci must be resolved in soluble form from an array of complex hydrophobic lipoprotein lattices without drastically altering the molecular arrangement of its antigenic determinants. This is a relatively complicated task, especially since the traditional static cell membrane model of Danielli and Davson (1935) is now considered less relevant than the dynamic fluid mosaic model. According to the traditional model, cellular membrane structure was postulated to consist of phosphatide bilayers with surfaces coated by membrane proteins linked to lipid head groups by ionic and/or hydrogen bonds. Singer and Nicolson (1972) on the basis of their data as well as that of Frye and Edidin (1970) extended this concept and proposed a fluid mosaic model. Globular proteins were thought to be partially embedded in a phospholipid matrix, which, in turn, was considered to be a discontinuous fluid bilayer. Accordingly, this fluid mosaic was postulated to be "analogous to a two-dimensional oriented solution of integral protein (or lipoproteins) in the viscous phospholipid bilayer solvent." Based largely on the work of Frye and Edidin (1970), Singer and Nicolson (1972) proposed that the fluid mosaic model of membrane structure was "the result of the free diffusion and intermixing of the lipids and the proteins (or lipoproteins) within the fluid lipid matrix." Although the fluid mosaic model seems to be quite useful to establish membrane-antigen models, if such a dynamic situation actually exists on the cell membrane, it complicates the assessment of the molecular nature and expression of H antigens.

Among the questions posed that received considerable attention was whether the antigenic specificities of the 2-segregant series of the HL-A locus were represented on one or two different molecular species. The first answer to this question did not come from chemical studies but rather from genetic and serologic analyses. First in studies of inbred mice and then of a limited number of human families, the recombination fraction of determinants of the two segregant series K and D and LA and FOUR ranged from 0.2–0.8% (Klein and Shreffler, 1971; Svejgaard et al., 1971). Thus, it seems reasonable to assume that the factors of the series both in mouse and man are con-

5. Histocompatibility Antigens: Biology and Chemistry

trolled by two separate structural cistrons. This notion is strengthened since the above recombination frequence probably corresponds to a map distance encompassing from 10^5–10^6 nucleotides, i.e., a few hundred average cistrons (Bodmer et al., 1970). Since the antigens of both the LA and FOUR segregant series are probably simple proteins, factors of the two series are most likely located on different molecules. However, even though it is relatively unlikely, one cannot rule out the existence of a polycistronic messenger RNA, e.g., intrachromosomal translocations such as those proposed to explain the joining of variable and common regions of Ig polypeptide chains. Thus, HL-A determinants of both series could actually be represented on a single polypeptide chain or on covalently linked chains providing a functional unit on the cell surface.

Some immunochemical evidence, presented first with papain-solubilized H-2 and then with HL-A antigens, suggests that at least some determinants of the two respective segregant series are present on separate peptide fragments obtained by proteolytic cleavage (Cullen et al., 1972; Cresswell et al., 1973). Furthermore, HL-A specificities of the two segregant series as well as H2K and H2D antigenic molecules are independent of each other on the cell membrane surface since they are free to migrate separately upon addition of specific antibodies (Bernoco et al., 1973; Neauport-Sautes et al., 1973a,b). In view of the difficulty of obtaining a single H antigenic unit with present extraction procedures, of proving it exists on the cell membrane, and of showing, at least in the HL-A system, the actual number of segregant series, it seems that for now a clear-cut description of the actual molecular nature of H antigens may not be forthcoming.

IX. Perspectives

Several considerations suggest that the major histocompatibility antigens have an important biologic function. First, they exist in every species so far studied. Second, the complex and extensive polymorphism of these antigens has been maintained in all mammalian species. Third, there has been a consistent, long-term expression of HL-A and H-2 antigens on cells maintained in tissue culture for prolonged periods of time, while other antigens are lost. Human fibroblasts which have a finite *in vitro* lifespan maintain HL-A antigens even in senescence although they lose other specialized features and are morphologically changed (Brautbar et al., 1972, 1973).

The extensive polymorphism of cell surface H antigens is believed to aid in preserving the integrity of the individual. The chemical differences are thought to lessen the chances of survival of one individual's cells whenever they invade the tissues of another individual. The correctness of this postulate, however, remains to be established experimentally.

The polymorphism of the HL-A system is believed to confer a selective advantage and thus to be crucial for man's survival. Data from family studies do not support the contention of selection at the time of conception. There is also no good evidence for selection to occur prior to birth even when maternal isoimmunization against alloantigens carried by the fetus has been shown. It appears that selection pressures for maintaining HL-A polymorphism occur after birth due to the biologic advantages accorded to some individuals with certain allotypic cell surface markers (Dausset, 1973).

In this regard in mice, evidence is convincing that H-2 type is associated with susceptibility to viral diseases. For instance, H-2 alleles have been reported to correlate with incidences of various mouse leukemia viruses, lymphocytic choriomeningitic virus, and autoimmune thyroiditis (Lilly et al., 1964; Lilly, 1966; Vladutin and Rose, 1971; Oldstone et al., 1973). In man, the available data are far less clear-cut, as associations between HL-A antigens and susceptibility to disease have been claimed and disclaimed. Associations between HL-A antigens and hematologic (Amiel et al., 1967; Forbes and Morris, 1970; Walford et al., 1970; Zervas et al., 1970) or renal diseases (Patel and Terasaki, 1969; Mickey et al. 1970) have been reported. Those interested in more details are referred to the review by Walford et al. (1971). In our opinion, the discrepancies among studies in man and mouse reflect mainly different experimental conditions for some of the following reasons: (1) Heterogeneous outbred human populations living in various environmental conditions are far different from inbred murine strains living under controlled laboratory conditions. It will be of interest to determine whether the correlation between H-2 and susceptibility to disease of inbred murine strains holds valid for polymorphic wild mice. (2) Some human diseases are grouped on the basis of similar histopathologies which may not reflect the same etiologic agent; correlations between histocompatibility antigens and disease may be completely obscure, if one compares the function of a particular human virus rather than comparing the clinical results of infection. Furthermore, some diseases (e.g., Hodgkin's disease) can be divided histologically into different types, and rarely has this differentiation been taken into account. (3) Experimental conditions are much better defined in mice than in man, in whom onset of disease is the end product of a series of uncontrolled variables.

Histocompatibility antigens may alter susceptibility to diseases by three principal mechanisms: (1) Histocompatibility antigens may represent specific receptor sites for the attachment of virus. The fact that human measles viruses are able to infect almost all human beings does not favor this mechanism, because a given HL-A antigenic determinant occurs so infrequently. Furthermore, no correlation has been found between the ability of cells to absorb virus and their H-2 type. (2) Histocompatibility antigens and viral or bacterial antigens may share determinants; in that case the organism would fail to react adequately to control the pathological process. In this regard, it is of interest that the reactivity of streptococcal antisera with human lymphocytes appears to be associated with the reactivity of first locus HL-A antisera, and frequencies of HL-A2 have been reported to be significantly increased in patients with glomerulonephritis (Patel et al., 1969; Mickey et al., 1970), a nonsuppurative sequela of streptococcal infection. Furthermore, streptococcal M1 protein or bacterial lipopolysaccarides can inhibit the cytotoxic activity of HL-A alloantisera (Hirata and Terasaki, 1970; Hirata et al., 1970; 1973; Mittal et al., 1973c), and conversely appropriate H-2 antisera can neutralize the B/T-L virus (Tennant, 1968). (3) Genes that control the specific immune response are linked to those governing the histocompatibility system; in mice and guinea pigs the ability to respond to each of several immunogens is determined by a gene or genes linked to the major histocompatibility locus of the species.

The threat of danger from an organism's own abnormal cells can be as serious as that from exogenous agents. Burnet (1970) envisioned H surface receptors as checkpoints for wandering recognition lymphocytes which police the immune system. New cell surface receptors are identified and deviant cells destroyed by these recognition lymphocytes, ensuring elimination of potentially neoplastic clones. Burnet also proposed that in early ontogeny H antigen receptors on cell surfaces may even have prevented malignancy from being contagious and thus have been instrumental in ensuring the survival of the species. The function of the extensive polymorphism of H loci may thus be to provide the variation required to protect the individuality of the members of a species.

Because of the close proximity of the immune response locus, Ir-I, and the H-2 locus, it seems possible that H genes may indeed influence immune responsiveness. The mechanism underlying such a phenomenon could be either (a) a closely linked gene determining the binding of antigen to the receptor sites of thymus-derived cells, (b) the combined effect of H antigens acting as receptors due to their steric complementarity, or (c) a nonspecific effect on cell surfaces (Biozzi et al., 1968). An important function of H genes may thus be their linkage to the general immune responsiveness of the host.

At the chemical level the problem remains quite complex. Analogous to immunoglobulin allotypes, this system based on immunogenetic serology must be converted into one based on structural genes and then gene products translated into amino acid sequences. Although the molecular nature and subunit structure of H antigens are far from clear, their character may eventually be defined since the extensive genetic polymorphism seems to be expressed mainly by changes in polypeptide structure rather than by an indirect mechanism, e.g., the insertion of specific carbohydrate structures by several enzymes. Thus, we may ultimately understand H antigens at the molecular level by following essentially the same route taken so successfully for the elucidation of the chemical and molecular structure of the antibody molecule. Judging from the antibody story, it seems reasonable to expect that the serology and genetics of H antigens will become simpler and more comprehensible once their chemical structure is clarified.

As far as the clinical implications of H antigens are concerned, it seems unlikely that even highly purified, soluble HL-A antigens will solve all the complex problems of organ transplantation. Although soluble antigens are more likely to induce some form of immunologic unresponsiveness than are particulate antigens, the induction of tolerance *in vivo* has yet to be attained. As pointed out by Nossal (1973), defined H antigens most likely play a role in sorting out phenomena such as enhancement and antibody-mediated tolerance, thus their full characterization will contribute ultimately to a better understanding of basic immunologic processes. Whether the HL-A system proves to be the key to controlling transplantation compatibility or not, perhaps chemically defined H antigens will comprise an excellent model for the study of cell surface receptors, interrelationships between cells, and functional aspects of cell membrane systems. The polymorphic H antigens thus serve as individuality markers which are crucial for maintaining an effective immunologic defense and recognition systems of the individual.

5. Histocompatibility Antigens: Biology and Chemistry

Acknowledgments

This is publication number 765 from the Department of Experimental Pathology, Scripps Clinic and Research Foundation, La Jolla, California. This work was supported by United States Public Health Service grants AI 07007 and AI 10180 and grant 70-615 from the American Heart Association, Inc.

References

Abeyounis, C. J., and Milgrom, F. (1969). *Transplant. Proc.* **1**, 556.
Albert, E., and Terasaki, P. I. (1972). *In* "Transplantation" (J. S. Narjarian and R. L. Simmons, eds.), p. 388. Lea & Febiger, Philadelphia, Pennsylvania.
Albert, E., Kano, K., Abeyounis, C. J., and Milgrom, F. (1969). *Transplantation* **8**, 466.
Albert, E. D., Mickey, M. R., and Terasaki, P. I. (1973). *Symp. Ser. Immunobiol. Stand.* **18**, 209.
Amiel, J. L., Mery, A. M., and Mathé, G. (1967). *Cong. Colloq. Univ. Liege* **43**, 197.
Amos, D. B. (1953). *Brit. J. Exp. Pathol.* **34**, 464.
Amos, D. B. (1956). *Ann. N. Y. Acad. Sci.* **63**, 706.
Amos, D. B. (1966). *In* "Histocompatibility Testing" (D. B. Amos and J. J. van Rood, eds.), p. 175. Williams & Wilkins, Baltimore, Maryland.
Amos, D. B. (1970). *Fed. Proc., Fed. Amer. Soc. Exp. Biol.* **29**, 2018.
Amos, D. B., and van Rood, J. J., eds. (1966). "Histocompatibility Testing." Williams & Wilkins, Baltimore, Maryland.
Amos, D. B., Cohen, I., and Klein, W. J., Jr. (1970). *Transplant. Proc.* **2**, 68.
Aoki, T., Hammerling, U., de Harven, E., Boyse, E. A., and Old, L. J. (1969). *J. Exp. Med.* **130**, 979.
Ashwell, M. A., and Work, T. S. (1968). *Biochem. Biophys. Res. Commun.* **32**, 1006.
Aster, R. H., Cooper, H. E., and Singer, D. L. (1964). *J. Lab. Clin. Med.* **63**, 161.
Bach, J. F., Debray-Sachs, M., Crosnier, J., Kreis, H., and Dormont, J. (1970). *Clin. Exp. Immunol.* **6**, 821.
Bach, M. L., Huang, S. W., Hong, R., and Poulik, M. D. (1973). *Science* **182**, 1350.
Balner, H., Gabb, B. W., Dersjant, H., van Vreeswijk, W., van Leeuwen, A., and van Rood, J. J. (1971). *In* "Comparative Genetics in Monkeys, Apes and Man" (A. B. Chiarelli, ed.), p. 97. Academic Press, New York.
Balner, H., D'Amaro, J., Tolh, E. K., Dersjant, H., and von Vreeswijk, W. (1973). *Transplant. Proc.* **5**, 323.
Barth, R. F., and Russell, P. S. (1964). *J. Immunol.* **93**, 13.
Batchelor, J. R. (1969). *Transplantation* **7**, 554.
Batchelor, J. R., and Brent, L. (1972). *In* "Immunogenicity" (F. Borek, ed.), p. 409. North-Holland Publ., Amsterdam.
Bauer, J. A. (1960). *Ann. N. Y. Acad. Sci.* **87**, 78.
Benacerraf, B., and McDevitt, H. O. (1972). *Science* **175**, 273.
Berah, M., Hors, J., and Dausset, J. (1970). *Transplantation* **9**, 185.
Berggård, I., and Bearn, A. G. (1968). *J. Biol. Chem.* **243**, 4095.
Bernier, G. M., and Fanger, M. W. (1972). *J. Immunol.* **109**, 407.

Bernoco, D., Glade, P. R., Broder, S., Miggiano, V. C., Hirschhorn, K., and Ceppellini, R. (1969). *Haematologica* **54**, 795.
Bernoco, D., Mattiuz, P. L., Miggiano, V. C., and Ceppellini, R., (1971). *G. Batteriol. Virol., Immunol. Ann. Osp. Maria Vittoria Torino* **64**, 314.
Bernoco, D., Cullen, S., Scudeller, G., Trinchieri, G., and Ceppellini, R. (1973). *In* "Histocompatibility Testing" (J. Dausset and J. Colombani, eds.), p. 527. Munksgaard, Copenhagen.
Bertrams, J., Kuwert, E., Gallmeier, W. M., Reis, H. E., and Schmidt, C. G. (1971). *Tissue Antigens* **1**, 105.
Billing, R., and Terasaki, P. I. (1974) *Transplantation* **17**, 231.
Billing, R., Mittal, K. K., and Terasaki, P. I. (1973). *Tissue Antigens* **3**, 251.
Billingham, R. E., Brent, L., and Medawar, P. B. (1956). *Nature (London)* **178**, 514.
Biozzi, G., Stiffel, C., and Mouton, D. (1968). *Ann. Inst. Pasteur, Paris* **115**, 965.
Bodmer, W. F., Tripp, M., and Bodmer, J. G. (1967). *In* "Histocompatibility Testing" (E. S. Curtoni, P. L. Mattiuz, R. M. Tosi, eds.), p. 341. Munksgaard, Copenhagen.
Bodmer, W. F., Bodmer, J. G., and Tripp, M. (1970). *In* "Histocompatibility Testing" (P. I. Terasaki, ed.), p. 187. Munksgaard, Copenhagen.
Borberg, H., Voigtmann, R., Salfner, B., Heumann, H., and Siebel, E. (1972). *Tissue Antigens* **2**, 478.
Borsos, R., Dourmashkin, R. R., and Humphrey, J. H. (1964). *Nature (London)* **202**, 251.
Boyse, E. A., Old, L. J., and Stockert, E. (1966). *Immunopathol. Int. Symp., 4th, 1965* p. 23.
Boyse, E. A., Stockert, E., and Old, L. J. (1967). *Proc. Nat. Acad. Sci. U. S.* **58**, 954.
Boyse, E. A., Old, L. J., and Stockert, E. (1968). *Proc. Nat. Acad. Sci. U.S.* **60**, 886.
Boyse, E. A., Flaherty, L., Stockert, E., and Old, L. J. (1972). *Transplantation* **13**, 431.
Boyum, A. (1968). *Scand. J. Clin. Lab. Invest.* **21S**, 97.
Braun, W. E., Grecek, D. R., and Murphy, J. J. (1972). *Transplantation* **13**, 337.
Brautbar, C., Payne, R., and Hayflick, L. (1972). *Exp. Cell Res.* **75**, 31.
Brautbar, C., Pellegrino, M. A., Ferrone, S., Payne, R., Reisfeld, R. A., and Hayflick, L. (1973). *Exp. Cell Res.* **78**, 367.
Bron, C., and Poulik, M. D. (1971). *Immunochemistry* **8**, 447.
Bruning, J. W., Masurel, M., Bent, V. D., and van Rood, J. J. (1967). *In* "Histocompatibility Testing" (E. S. Curtoni, P. L. Mattiuz, and R. M. Tosi, eds.), p. 303. Munksgaard, Copenhagen.
Bruning, J. W., Douglas, R., Scholtus, M., and van Rood, J. J. (1972). *Tissue Antigens* **2**, 473.
Buell, D. N., and Fahey, J. L. (1969). *Science* **164**, 1524.
Burnet, F. M. (1970). *Nature (London)* **226**, 123.
Callahan, G. N., Stroehmann, I., and DeWitt, C. W. (1974). *Immunology* (in press).
Cavalli-Sforza, L. L., and Bodmer, W. F. (1971). *In* "The Genetics of Human Populations." Freeman, San Francisco, California.
Celada, F., and Rotman, B. (1967). *Proc. Nat. Acad. Sci. U. S.* **57**, 630.
Ceppellini, R. (1971). *In* "Progress in Immunology" (B. Amos, ed.), p. 973. Academic Press, New York.
Cerottini, J. C., and Brunner, K. T. (1967). *Immunology* **13**, 395.
Chapel, H. M., and Welsh, K. I. (1972). *Transplantation* **13**, 347.
Charlton, R. K., and Zmijewski, C. M. (1970). *Science* **170**, 636.
Chessin, L. N., Bramson, S., Kuhns, W. J., and Hirschhorn, K. (1965). *Blood* **25**, 944.

Cikes, M. (1970). *J. Nat. Cancer Inst.* **45**, 979.
Cikes, M. (1971). *Transplant. Proc.* **3**, 1161.
Cikes, M., and Friberg, S., Jr. (1971). *Proc. Nat. Acad. Sci. U. S.* **68**, 566.
Cikes, M., and Klein, G. (1972a). *J. Nat. Cancer Inst.* **48**, 509.
Cikes, M., and Klein, G., (1972)b). *J. Nat. Cancer Inst.* **49**, 1599.
Cikes, M., Friberg, S., Jr., and Klein, G. (1972). *J. Nat. Cancer Inst.* **49**, 1607.
Cikes, M., Friberg, S., Jr., and Klein, G. (1973). *J. Nat. Cancer Inst.* **50**, 347.
Claesson, M. H., Ahrons, S., and Jørgensen, O. (1971). *Tissue Antigens* **1**, 94.
Cochrum, K. C., Perkins, H. A., Payne, R. O., Kountz, S. L., and Belzer, F. O. (1973). *Transplant. Proc.* **5**, 391.
Colombani, J., Colombani, M., and Dausset, J. (1964). *Ann. N. Y. Acad. Sci.* **120**, 307.
Colombani, J., Colombani, M., Benajam, A., and Dausset, J. (1967). In "Histocompatibility Testing" (E. S. Curtoni, P. L. Mattiuz, and R. M. Tosi, eds.), p. 413. Munksgaard, Copenhagen.
Colombani, J., Colombani, M., and Dausset, J. (1970). In "Histocompatibility Testing" (P. I. Terasaki, ed.), p. 79. Munksgaard, Copenhagen.
Cresswell, P., and Sanderson, A. R. (1968). *Transplantation* **6**, 996.
Cresswell, P., Turner, M. J., and Strominger, J. L. (1973). *Proc. Nat. Acad. Sci. U. S.* **70**, 1603.
Cresswell, P., Springer, P., Strominger, J. L., Turner, M. J., Grey, H. M., and Kubo, R. T. (1974). *Proc. Nat. Acad. Sci. U. S.* **71**, 2123.
Cullen, S. E., Schwartz, B. D., and Nathenson, S. G. (1972). *J. Immunol.* **108**, 596.
Cunningham, B. A., Wang, J. L., Berggård, I., and Peterson, P. A. (1973). *Biochemistry* **12**, 4811.
Curtoni, E. S., Mattiuz, P. L., and Tosi, R. M., eds. (1967). "Histocompatibility Testing." Munksgaard, Copenhagen.
D'Amaro, J., van Leeuwen, A., Svejgaard, A., and van Rood, J. J. (1970). In "Histocompatibility Testing" (P. I. Terasaki, ed.), p. 539. Munksgaard, Copenhagen.
Danielli, J. F., and Davson, H. (1935). *J. Cell. Comp. Physiol.* **5**, 495.
Dausset, J. (1954). *Vox Sang.* **4**, 190.
Dausset, J. (1958). *Acta Haematol.* **20**, 156.
Dausset, J. (1971). *Transplant. Proc.* **3**, 8.
Dausset, J. (1973). *Progr. Clin. Immunol.* **1**, 183.
Dausset, J., and Colombani, J., eds. (1973). "Histocompatibility Testing." Munksgaard, Copenhagen.
Dausset, J., and Hors, J. (1971). *Transplant. Proc.* **3**, 1004.
Dausset, J., Colombani, J., Legrand, L., and Feingold, N. (1968). *Nouv. Rev. Fr. Hematol.* **8**, 841.
Dausset, J., Rapaport, F. T., Legrand, L., Colombani, J., and Marcelli-Barge, A. (1970). In "Histocompatibility Testing" (P. I. Terasaki, ed.), p. 381. Munksgaard, Copenhagen.
David, C. S., Shreffler, D. C., Murphy, G. B., and Klein, J. (1973). *Transplant. Proc.* **5**, 287.
Davies, D. A. L. (1968). In "Human Transplantation" (F. T. Rapaport, and J. Dausset, eds.), p. 383. Grune & Stratton, New York.
Davies, D. A. L. (1969). *Transplantation* **8**, 51.
Davis, B. D., Kabat, E. A., Harris, A., and Moore, D. H. (1944). *J. Immunol.* **49**, 223.
Davis, W. C., and Silverman, L. (1968). *Transplantation* **6**, 536.
Davis, W. C., Alspaugh, M. A., Stimpfling, J. H., and Walford, R. L. (1971). *Tissue Antigens* **1**, 89.

Démant, P., Capková, J., Hinzová, E., and Voracová, B. (1973). *Proc. Nat. Acad. Sci. U. S.* **70**, 863.
de Weck, A. L., Polak, L., Sato, W., and Frey, J. R. (1971). *Transplant. Proc.* **3**, 192.
Dos Reis, A. P., Beutel, H., Reisner, E. G., and Amos, D. B. (1973). *Transplantation* **15**, 36.
Edidin, M. (1966). *J. Embryol. Exp. Morphol.* **16**, 519.
Edidin, M. (1967). *Proc. Nat. Acad. Sci. U. S.* **57**, 1226.
Edidin, M. (1973). *In* "Transplantation Antigens" (B. D. Kahan, and R. A. Reisfeld, eds.), p. 75. Academic Press, New York.
Einstein, A. B., Jr., Mann, D. L., Gordon, H. G., Trapani, R. J., and Fahey, J. L. (1971a). *Transplantation* **12**, 299.
Einstein, A. B., Jr., Mann, D. L., Gordon, H. G., and Fahey, J. L. (1971b). *Tissue Antigens* **1**, 209.
Etheredge, E. E., and Najarian, J. S. (1971). *Transplant. Proc.* **3**, 224.
Etheredge, E. E., Franecki, B. H., and Najarian, J. S. (1971). *Tissue Antigens* **1**, 109.
Etheredge, E. E., Shons, A. R., and Najarian, J. S. (1973). *Immunol. Commun.* **2**, 141.
Evans, W. H., and Bruning, J. W. (1970). *Immunology* **19**, 735.
Fantoni, A., de la Chapelle, A., Rifkind, R. A., and Marks, P. A. (1968). *J. Mol. Biol.* **33**, 79.
Fellous, M. (1971). Discussion. *In* "Proceedings of the Symposium on Immunogenetics of the H-2 Systems" (A. Lengerova and M. Vojtiskova, eds.), p. 274. Karger, Basel.
Fellous, M., and Dausset, J. (1970). *Nature (London)* **225**, 191.
Ferrone, S., and Pellegrino, M. A. (1973). *Contemp. Top. Mol. Immunol.* **2**, 185.
Ferrone, S., Tosi, R. M., and Centis, D. (1967). *In* "Histocompatibility Testing" (E. S. Curtoni, P. L. Mattiuz, and R. M. Tosi, eds.), p. 357. Munksgaard, Copenhagen.
Ferrone, S., Sirchia, G., Farina, C., and Dambrosio, F. (1968). *Ric. Clin. Lab.* **7**, 56.
Ferrone, S., Pellegrino, M. A., and Reisfeld, R. A. (1971a). *J. Immunol.* **107**, 613.
Ferrone, S., Cooper, N. R., Pellegrino, M. A., and Reisfeld, R. A. (1971b). *J. Immunol.* **107**, 939.
Ferrone, S., Natali, P. G., Hunter, A., Terasaki, P. I., and Reisfeld, R. A. (1972a). *J. Immunol.* **108**, 1718.
Ferrone, S., Pellegrino, M. A., and Reisfeld, R. A. (1972b). *Lancet* **1**, 1237.
Ferrone, S., Del Villano, B. C., Pellegrino, M. A., Lerner, R. A., and Reisfeld, R. A. (1972c). *Tissue Antigens* **2**, 477.
Ferrone, S., Mittal, K. K., Pellegrino, M. A., Terasaki, P. I., and Reisfeld, R. A. (1972d). *Immunol. Commun.* **1**, 77.
Ferrone, S., Pellegrino, M. A., Götze, D., Mittal, K. K., Terasaki, P. I., and Reisfeld, R. A. (1973a). *Symp. Ser. Immunobiol. Stand.* **18**, 218.
Ferrone, S., Cooper, N. R., Pellegrino, M. A., and Reisfeld, R. A. (1973b). *J. Exp. Med.* **137**, 55.
Ferrone, S., Cooper, N. R., Pellegrino, M. A., and Reisfeld, R. A. (1973c). *Proc. Nat. Acad. Sci. U. S.* **70**, 3665.
Ferrone, S., Pellegrino, M. A., Dierich, M. P., and Reisfeld, R. A. (1974a). *Tissue Antigens* **4**, 275.
Ferrone, S., Cooper, N. R., Pellegrino, M. A., and Reisfeld, R. A. (1974b). *Transplant. Proc.* **6**, 13.
Ferrone, S., Pellegrino, M. A., Billing, R., Terasaki, P. I., and Reisfeld, R. A. (1974c). *Tissue Antigens* (in press).
Fine, D. P., Marney, S. R., Jr., Cooley, D. G., Sergent, J. S., and Des Prez, R. M. (1972). *J. Immunol.* **109**, 807.

5. Histocompatibility Antigens: Biology and Chemistry 439

Fong, R., and Kissmeyer-Nielsen, F. (1972). *Tissue Antigens* **2**, 57.
Forbes, J. F., and Morris, P. J. (1970). *Lancet* **2**, 849.
Frank, M. M., May, J., Gaither, T., and Ellman, L. (1971). *J. Exp. Med.* **134**, 176.
Frye, L. D., and Edidin, M. (1970). *J. Cell Sci.* **7**, 319.
Gabb, B. W., and Bodmer, W. F. (1970). *In* "Histocompatibility Testing" (P. I. Terasaki, ed.), p. 543. Munksgaard, Copenhagen.
Galper, J. B., and Darnell, J. E. (1971). *J. Mol. Biol.* **57**, 363.
Gervais, A. G. (1968). *Transplantation* **6**, 261.
Gibofsky, A., and Terasaki, P. I. (1972). *Transplantation* **13**, 192.
Glick, A. D., Horn, R. G., Collins, R. D., and Bryant, R. E. (1970). *Exp. Mol. Pathol.* **12**, 275.
Goldberg, E. H., Aoki, T., Boyse, E. A., and Bennett, D. (1970). *Nature (London)* **228**, 570.
Goldberg, E. H., Boyse, E. A., Bennett, D., Scheid, M., and Carswell, E. A. (1971). *Nature (London)* **232**, 478.
Gorer, P. A. (1936). *Brit. J. Exp. Pathol.* **17**, 42.
Götze, D., and Reisfeld, R. A. (1972). *Fed. Proc., Fed. Amer. Soc. Exp. Biol.* **31**, 2419.
Götze, D., and Reisfeld, R. A. (1974). *J. Immunol.* **112**, 1643.
Götze, D., Ferrone, S., and Reisfeld, R. A. (1972a). *J. Immunol.* **109**, 439.
Götze, D., Pellegrino, M. A., Ferrone, S., and Reisfeld, R. A. (1972b). *Immunol. Commun.* **1**, 533.
Götze, D., Lee, S., Ferrone, S., Pellegrino, M. A., and Reisfeld, R. A. (1973). *Transplant Proc.* **5**, 467.
Götze, O., and Müller-Eberhard, H. J. (1971). *J. Exp. Med.* **134**, 90S.
Graw, R. G., Jr., Herzig, G. P., Eisel, R. J., and Perry, S. (1971). *Transfusion* **11**, 94.
Greenwalt, T. J., Gajewski, M., and McKenna, J. L. (1962). *Transfusion* **2**, 221.
Grey, H. M., Kubo, R. T., Colon, S. M., Poulik, M. D., Cresswell, P., Springer, T., Turner, M., and Strominger, J. L. (1973). *J. Exp. Med.* **138**, 1608.
Grothaus, E. A., Wayne, F. M., Yunis, E., and Amos, D. B. (1971). *Science* **173**, 542.
Gutterman, J. U., Mavligit, G., McCredie, K. B., Bodey, G. P. S., Freireich, E. J., and Hersh, E. M. (1972) *Science* **177**, 1114.
Hamaguchi, K., and Geiduschek, E. P. (1962). *J. Amer. Chem. Soc.* **84**, 1329.
Hamburger, J., Crosnier, J., Descamps, B., and Rowinska, D. (1971). *Transplant. Proc.* **3**, 1.
Hammerling, U., Aoki, T., de Harven, E., Boyse, E. A., and Old, L. J. (1968). *J. Exp. Med.* **128**, 1461.
Harris, R. (1973). *Nature (London)* **241**, 95.
Harris, R., and Zervas, J. D. (1969). *Nature (London)* **221**, 1062.
Haughton, G. (1966). *Transplantation* **4**, 238.
Hecht, T. T., and Summers, D. F. (1972). *J. Virol.* **10**, 578.
Hellström, K. E., and Möller, E. (1965). *Progr. Allergy* **9**, 158.
Herberman, R. B. (1970). *J. Immunol.* **104**, 805.
Hinzová, E., Démant, P., and Ivànyi, P. (1972). *Folia Biol. (Prague)* **18**, 237.
Hirata, A. A., and Terasaki, P. I. (1970). *Science* **168**, 1095.
Hirata, A. A., Armstrong, A. S., Kay, J. W. D., and Terasaki, P. I. (1970). *In* "Histocompatibility Testing" (P. I. Terasaki, ed.), p. 475. Munksgaard, Copenhagen.
Hirata, A. A., McIntire, F. C., Terasaki, P. I., and Mittal, K. K. (1973). *Transplantation* **15**, 441.
Hirschfeld, J. (1965). *Science* **148**, 968.
Hoecker, G., and Hauschka, T. S. (1956). *Transplant. Bull.* **3**, 134.
Hofmeister, F. (1888). *Arch. Exp. Pathol. Pharmakol.* **24**, 247.

Högman, C. (1959). *Vox Sang.* **4**, 319.
Ishizaka, T., and Ishizaka, K. (1959). *Proc. Soc. Exp. Biol. Med.* **101**, 845.
Ivasková, E., Dausset, J., and Iványi, P. (1972). *Folia Biol. (Prague)* **18**, 194.
Iwasaki, Y., Talmage, D., and Starzl, T. E. (1967). *Transplantation* **5**, 191.
Johnson, A. H., Rossen, R. D., and Butler, W. T. (1972). *Tissue Antigens* **2**, 215.
Johnson, M. H., and Edidin, M. (1972). *Transplantation* **14**, 781.
Johnson, T. M., and Garvin, J. E. (1959). *Proc. Soc. Exp. Biol. Med.* **102**, 333.
Kabat, E. A., and Mayer, M. M. (1961). "Experimental Immunochemistry," 2nd ed. Thomas, Springfield, Illinois.
Kahan, B. D., and Reisfeld, R. A. (1967). *Proc. Nat. Acad. Sci. U. S.* **58**, 1430.
Kahan, B. D., and Reisfeld, R. A. (1968). *J. Immunol.* **101**, 237.
Kahan, B. D., and Reisfeld, R. A. (1969a). *Transplant. Proc.* **1**, 483.
Kahan, B. D., and Reisfeld, R. A. (1969b). *Science* **164**, 514.
Kahan, B. D., and Reisfeld, R. A. (1971). *Bacteriol. Rev.* **35**, 59.
Kahan, B. D., and Reisfeld, R. A. (1973). "Transplantation Antigens." Academic Press, New York.
Kahan, B. D., Reisfeld, R. A., Pellegrino, M., Curtoni, E. S., Mattiuz, P. L., and Ceppellini, R. (1968). *Proc. Nat. Acad. Sci. U. S.* **61**, 897.
Kahan, B. D., Pellegrino, M. A., Papermaster, B. W., and Reisfeld, R. A. (1971). *Transplant. Proc.* **3**, 227.
Kahan, B. D., Mittal, K. K., Reisfeld, R. A., Terasaki, P. I., and Bergan, J. J. (1973). *Surgery* **74**, 153.
Kandutsch, A. A. (1960). *Cancer Res.* **20**, 262.
Karnovsky, M. J., Unanue, E. R., and Leventhal, M. (1972). *J. Exp. Med.* **136**, 907.
Kauzman, W. (1959). *Advan. Protein Chem.* **14**, 1.
Kersey, J. H., Yunis, E. J., Todaro, G. J., and Aaronson, S. A. (1973). *Proc. Soc. Exp. Biol. Med.* **143**, 453.
Kissmeyer-Nielsen, F., and Thorsby, E. (1970). *Transplant. Rev.* **4**, 1.
Kissmeyer-Nielsen, F., Olsen, S., Posborg Petersen, V., and Fjeldborg, O. (1966). *Lancet* **1**, 662.
Klein, D., Merchant, D. J., Klein, J., and Shreffler, D. C. (1970). *J. Nat. Cancer Inst.* **44**, 1149.
Klein, J. (1971a). *Proc. Nat. Acad. Sci. U. S.* **68**, 1594.
Klein, J. (1971b). *Nature (London)* **229**, 635.
Klein, J. (1973). *Symp. Ser. Immunobiol. Stand.* **18**, 250.
Klein, J., and Park, J. M. (1973). *J. Exp. Med.* **137**, 1213.
Klein, J., and Shreffler, D. C. (1971). *Transplant. Rev.* **6**, 3.
Klotz, I. M., and Farnham, S. B. (1968). *Biochemistry* **7**, 3879.
Kourilsky, F. M., Silvestre, D., Levy, J. P., Dausset, J., Nicolai, M. G., and Senik, A. (1971). *J. Immunol.* **106**, 454.
Kourilsky, F. M., Silvestre, D., Neauport-Sautes, C., Loosfelt, Y., and Dausset, J. (1972). *Eur. J. Immunol.* **2**, 249.
Kristofová, H., Lengerová, A., and Reizkoyá, J. (1970). *Folia Biol. (Prague)* **16**, 81.
Kuhns, W. J., and Bramson, S. (1968). *Nature (London)* **219**, 938.
Kuhns, W. J., Faur, Y., Bramson, S., and Friedhoff, F. (1969). *Proc. Soc. Exp. Biol. Med.* **131**, 67.
Lalezari, P., and Bernard, G. E. (1966). *J. Clin. Invest.* **45**, 1741.
Lalezari, P., Thalenfeld, B., and Weinstein, W. J. (1970). *In* "Histocompatibility Testing" (P. I. Terasaki, ed.), p. 319. Munksgaard, Copenhagen.
Lalezari, P., Murphy, G. B., and Allen, F. H., Jr. (1971). *J. Clin. Invest.* **50**, 1108.

5. Histocompatibility Antigens: Biology and Chemistry 441

Lambertenghi-Deliliers, G., Ferrone, S., Ranzi, T., and Sirchia, G. (1971). *Blood* **38**, 759.
Law, L. W., Appella, E., Strober, S., Wright, P. W., and Fischetti, T. (1972). *Proc. Nat. Acad. Sci. U. S.* **69**, 1858.
Legrand, L., and Dausset, J. (1971). *Nature (London) New Biol.* **234**, 271.
Legrand, L., Dausset, J., and Rapaport, F. T. (1971). *Transfusion* **11**, 233.
Lerner, R. A., and Hodge, L. D. (1971). *J. Cell. Physiol.* **77**, 265.
Lerner, R. A., Oldstone, M. B. A., and Cooper, N. R. (1971). *Proc. Nat. Acad. Sci. U. S.* **68**, 2584.
Lerner, R. A., McConahey, P. J., Jansen, I., and Dixon, F. J. (1972). *J. Exp. Med.* **135**, 136.
Levine, S. (1956). *Science* **123**, 185.
Lilly, F., Boyse, E. A., and Old, L. J. (1964). *Lancet* **2**, 1207.
Lilly, F. (1966). *Nat. Cancer Inst., Monogr.* **22**, 631.
Linscott, W. D. (1970). *J. Immunol.* **104**, 1307.
Little, C. C., and Johnson, B. W. (1922). *Proc. Soc. Exp. Biol. Med.* **19**, 163.
Loeb, L. (1930). *Physiol. Rev.* **10**, 547.
Loor, F., Forni, L., and Pernis, B. (1972). *Eur. J. Immunol.* **2**, 203.
Lucas, D. R. and Peakman, E. M. (1969). *J. Pathol.* **99**, 163.
McDevitt, H. O., and Benacerraf, B. (1969). *Advan. Immunol.* **11**, 31.
McDonald, J. C., and Mukherjee, G. N. (1973). *Transplant. Proc.* **5**, 481.
McDonald, J. C., Jacobbi, L., and Williams, R. W. (1970). *Transplantation* **10**, 499.
Mann, D. L. (1973). *In* "Transplantation Antigens" (B. D. Kahan and R. A. Reisfeld, eds.) p. 287. Academic Press, New York.
Mann, D. L., and Fahey, J. L. (1971). *Annu. Rev. Microbiol.* **25**, 679.
Mann, D. L., Rogentine, G. N., Fahey, J. L., and Nathenson, S. G. (1968). *Nature (London)* **217**, 1180.
Manson, L. A., and Palm, J. (1968). *Transplantation* **6**, 667.
Manson, L. A., Hickey, C. A., and Palm, J. (1968). *In* "Biological Properties of the Mammalian Surface Membrane" (L. A. Manson, ed.), p. 93. Wistar Inst. Press, Philadelphia, Pennsylvania.
Marks, P. A., Burka, E. R., and Schlessinger, D. (1962). *Proc. Nat. Acad. Sci. U. S.* **48**, 2163.
Medawar, P. B. (1944). *J. Anat.* **78**, 176.
Medawar, P. B. (1963). *Transplantation* **1**, 21.
Mercuriali, F., Richiardi, P., Mattiuz, P. L., and Sirchia, G. (1971). *Tissue Antigens* **1**, 290.
Metzgar, R. S., and Miller, J. L. (1972). *Transplantation* **13**, 467.
Metzgar, R. S., and Seigler, H. F. (1973). *In* "Transplantation Antigens" (B. D. Kahan and R. A. Reisfeld, eds.), p. 209. Academic Press, New York.
Metzgar, R. S., Flanagan, J. F., and Mendes, N. F. (1967). *In* "Histocompatibility Testing" (E. S. Curtoni, P. L. Mattiuz, and Tosi, R. M. eds.), p. 307. Munksgaard, Copenhagen.
Metzgar, R. S., Miller, J. L., and Seigler, H. F. (1973). *In* "Transplantation Antigens" (B. D. Kahan and R. A. Reisfeld, eds.), p. 299. Academic Press, New York.
Mickey, M. R., Kreisler, M., and Terasaki, P. I. (1970). *In* "Histocompatibility Testing" (P. I. Terasaki, ed.), p. 237. Munksgaard, Copenhagen.
Mickey, M. R., Kreisler, M., Albert, E. D., Tanaka, N., and Terasaki, P. I. (1971). *Tissue Antigens* **1**, 57.
Miescher, P., and Fauconnet, M. (1954). *Schweiz. Med. Wochensch.* **84**, 597.

Miggiano, V. C., Nabholtz, M., and Bodmer, W. F. (1970). In "Histocompatibility Testing" (P. I. Terasaki, ed.), p. 623. Munksgaard, Copenhagen.
Mittal, K. K., and Terasaki, P. I. (1972). *Tissue Antigens* **2**, 94.
Mittal, K. K., Mickey, M. R., Singal, D. P., and Terasaki, P. I. (1968). *Transplantation* **6**, 913.
Mittal, K. K., Mickey, M. R., and Terasaki, P. I. (1969). *Transplantation* **8**, 801.
Mittal, K. K., Ferrone, S., Mickey, M. R., Pellegrino, M. A., Reisfeld, R. A., and Terasaki, P. I. (1973a). *Tissue Antigens* **3**, 88.
Mittal, K. K., Mickey, M. R., and Terasaki, P. I. (1973b). *Symp. Ser. Immunobiol. Stand.* **18**, 165.
Mittal, K. K., Terasaki, P. I., Springer, G. F., Desai, P. R., McIntire, F. C., and Hirata, A. A. (1973c). *Transplant. Proc.* **5**, 499.
Miyajima, T., Hirata, A. A., and Terasaki, P. I. (1972). *Tissue Antigens* **2**, 64.
Miyakawa, Y., Tanigaki, N., Kreiter, V. P., Moore, G. E., and Pressman, D. (1973a). *Transplantation* **15**, 312.
Miyakawa, Y., Tanigaki, N., Yagi, Y., and Pressman, D. (1973b). *Immunology* **24**, 67.
Möller, G. (1961). *J. Exp. Med.* **114**, 415.
Moore, G. E., Gerner, R. F., and Franklin, H. A. (1967). *J. Amer. Med. Ass.* **199**, 519.
Moscona, A. A., and Kirk, D. L. (1965). *Science* **148**, 519.
Motta, R., and Bruley, M. (1973). *Transplantation* **15**, 22.
Mullen, Y., and Hildemann, W. H. (1971). *Transplant. Proc.* **3**, 669.
Muramatsu, T., and Nathenson, S. G. (1971). *Fed. Proc., Fed. Amer. Soc. Exp. Biol.* **30**, 2768.
Nakamuro, K., Tanigaki, N., and Pressman, D. (1973). *Proc. Nat. Acad. Sci. U. S.* **70**, 2863.
Nathenson, S. G. (1970). *Annu. Rev. Genet.* **4**, 69.
Nathenson, S. G., and Davies, D. A. L. (1966). *Proc. Nat. Acad. Sci. U. S.* **56**, 676.
Neauport-Sautes, C., Silvestre, D., Nicolai, M. G., Kourilsky, F. M., and Levy, J. P. (1972). *Immunology* **22**, 833.
Neauport-Sautes, C., Lilly, F., Silvestre, D., and Kourilsky, F. M. (1973a). *J. Exp. Med.* **137**, 511.
Neauport-Sautes, C., Silvestre, D., Kourilsky, F. M., and Dausset, J. (1973b). In "Histocompatibility Testing" (J. Dausset, ed.), p. 539. Munksgaard, Copenhagen.
Nelken, D., Cotten, I., and Furcaig, I. (1970). *Transplantation* **10**, 347.
Nelson, R. A., Jr., and Biro, C. E. (1968). *Immunology* **14**, 527.
Nossal, G. J. V. (1973). In "Transplantation Antigens" (B. D. Kahan and R. A. Reisfeld, eds.), p. 503. Academic Press, New York.
Oh, S. K., Pellegrino, M. A., and Reisfeld, R. A. (1973). *Fed. Proc., Fed. Amer. Soc. Exp. Biol.* **32**, 4500.
Oh, S. K., Pellegrino, M. A., Ferrone, S., Sevier, E. D., and Reisfeld, R. A. (1974). *Eur. J. Immunol.* (in press).
Old, L. J., Stockert, E., Boyse, E. A., and Kim, J. H. (1968). *J. Exp. Med.* **127**, 523.
Oldstone, M. B. A., Dixon, F. J., Mitchell, G. F., and McDevitt, H. O. (1973). *J. Exp. Med.* **137**, 1201.
Olhagen, B. (1945). *Acta Med. Scand., Suppl.* **162**, 1.
Palm, J. (1964). *Transplantation* **2**, 603.
Palm, J. (1970). *Transplant. Proc.* **2**, 162.
Palm, J. (1971). *Transplant. Proc.* **3**, 169.
Papermaster, B. W., Papermaster, V. M., Reisfeld, R. A., Pellegrino, M. A., Ferrone, S., Kahan, B. D., Terasaki, P. I., Takasugi, M., and Albert, E. A. (1972). In "Cellular Antigens" (A. Nowotny, ed.), p. 186. Springer-Verlag, New York and Berlin.

5. Histocompatibility Antigens: Biology and Chemistry

Papermaster, V. M., Papermaster, B. W., and Moore, G. E. (1969). *Fed. Proc., Fed. Amer. Soc. Exp. Biol.* **28**, 379.
Passmore, H. C., and Shreffler, D. C. (1970). *Biochem. Genet.* **4**, 351.
Pasternak, C. A., Warmsley, A. M., and Thomas, D. B. (1971). *J. Cell Biol.* **50**, 562.
Patel, R., and Terasaki, P. I. (1969). *N. Engl. J. Med.* **280**, 735.
Patel, R., Mickey, M. R., and Terasaki, P. I. (1969). *Brit. Med. J.* **2**, 424.
Payne, R., and Rolfs, M. R. (1958). *J. Clin. Invest.* **37**, 1756.
Payne, R., Tripp, M., Weigle, J., Bodmer, W., and Bodmer, J. (1964). *Cold Spring Harbor Symp. Quant. Biol.* **29**, 285.
Pegrum, G. D., Balfour, T. C., Evans, C. A., and Middleton, V. L. (1971). *Lancet* **1**, 852.
Pellegrino, M. A., Pellegrino, A., and Kahan, B. D. (1970). *Transplantation* **10**, 425.
Pellegrino, M. A., Ferrone, S., and Pellegrino, A. (1972a). *Proc. Soc. Exp. Biol. Med.* **139**, 484.
Pellegrino, M. A., Ferrone, S., Natali, P. G., Pellegrino, A., and Reisfeld, R. A. (1972b). *J. Immunol.* **108**, 573.
Pellegrino, M. A., Ferrone, S., Safford, J. W., Jr., Hirata, A. A., Terasaki, P. I., and Reisfeld, R. A. (1972c). *J. Immunol.* **109**, 97.
Pellegrino, M. A., Ferrone, S., Mittal, K. K., Pellegrino, A., and Reisfeld, R. A. (1973a). *Transplantation* **15**, 42.
Pellegrino, M. A., Ferrone, S., Pellegrino, A., and Reisfeld, R. A. (1973b). *Symp. Ser. Immunobiol. Stand.* **18**, 209.
Pellegrino, M. A., Ferrone, S., Pellegrino, A., and Reisfeld, R. A. (1973c). *Clin. Immunol. Immunopathol.* **1**, 182.
Pellegrino, M. A., Ferrone, S., Del Villano, B. C., and Reisfeld, R. A. (1973d). *Transplant. Proc.* **5**, 91.
Pellegrino, M. A., Pellegrino, A., Ferrone, S., Kahan, B. D., and Reisfeld, R. A. (1973e). *J. Immunol.* **111**, 783.
Pellegrino, M. A., Ferrone, S., and Pellegrino A. (1973f). *In* "Transplantation Antigens" (B. D. Kahan and R. A. Reisfeld, eds.), p. 433. Academic Press, New York.
Pellegrino, M. A., Ferrone, S., Mittal, K. K., Götze, D., Terasaki, P. I., and Reisfeld, R. A. (1974a). *Immunogenetics* **1**, 158.
Pellegrino, M. A., Ferrone, S., Pellegrino, A., Oh, S., and Reisfeld, R. A. (1974b). *Eur. J. Immunol.* **4**, 250.
Perper, R. J., Zee, T. W., and Mickelson, M. M. (1968). *J. Lab. Clin. Med.* **72**, 842.
Peterson, P. A., Cunningham, B. A., Berggård, I., and Edelman, G. M. (1972). *Proc. Nat. Acad. Sci. U. S.* **69**, 1697.
Peterson, P. A., Rask, L., and Lindblom, J. B. (1974). *Proc. Nat. Acad. Sci. U. S.* **71**, 35.
Pizarro, O., Hoecker, G., Rubinstein, P., and Ramos, A. (1961). *Proc. Nat. Acad. Sci. U. S.* **47**, 1900.
Polley, M. J., and Mollison, P. L. (1961). *Transfusion* **1**, 9.
Poulik, M. D. (1973). *Immunol. Commun.* **2**, 403.
Poulik, M. D., and Bloom, A. D. (1973). *J. Immunol.* **110**, 1430.
Poulik, M. D., and Motwani, N. (1972). *Clin. Res.* **20**, 795.
Poulik, M. D., Bernoco, M., Bernoco, D., and Ceppellini, R. (1973). *Science* **182**, 1352.
Poulik, M. D., Ferrone, S., Pellegrino, M. A., Sevier, E. D., Oh, S. K., and Reisfeld, R. A. (1974). *Transplant. Rev.* (in press).
Preud'homme, J. L., Neauport-Sautes, C., Piat, S., Silvestre, D., and Kourilsky, F. M. (1972). *Eur. J. Immunol.* **2**, 297.

Rapaport, F. T., Chase, R. M., Jr., and Solowey, A. C. (1966). *Ann. N. Y. Acad. Sci.* **129**, 102.
Rapaport, F. T., Dausset, J., Hamburger, J., Hume, D. M., Kano, K., Williams, G. M., and Milgrom, F. (1967). *Ann. Surg.* **166**, 596.
Rapaport, F. T., Kano, K., and Milgrom, F. (1968). *J. Clin. Invest.* **47**, 633.
Rapaport, F. T., Hanaoka, T., Shimada, T., Cannon, F. D., and Ferrebee, J. W. (1970). *J. Exp. Med.* **131**, 881.
Reisfeld, R. A., and Kahan, B. D. (1970). *Advan. Immunol.* **12**, 117.
Reisfeld, R. A., and Kahan, B. D. (1971). *Transplant. Rev.* **6**, 81.
Reisfeld, R. A., and Kahan, B. D. (1972). *Contemp. Top. Immunochem.* **1**, 51.
Reisfeld, R. A., and Kahan, B. D. (1973). *In* "Transplantation Antigens" (B. D. Kahan and R. A. Reisfeld, eds.), p. 489. Academic Press, New York.
Reisfeld, R. A., and Pellegrino, M. A. (1973). *In* "Transplantation Antigens" (B. D. Kahan and R. A. Reisfeld, eds.), p. 259. Academic Press, New York.
Reisfeld, R. A., Pelegrino, M., Papermaster, B. W., and Kahan, B. D. (1970). *J. Immunol.* **104**, 560.
Reisfeld, R. A., Pellegrino, M. A., and Kahan, B. D. (1971a). *Science* **172**, 1134.
Reisfeld, R. A., Pellegrino, M., Papermaster, B. W., and Kahan, B. D. (1971b). *Immunopathol., Int. Symp., 6th, 1970* p. 139.
Reisfeld, R. A., Pellegrino, M. A., Ferrone, S., Oh, S. K., and Götze, D. (1974). *Atti Accad. Naz. Lincei, Cl. Sci. Fis., Mat. Natur., Rend.* (in press).
Rodbard, D., and Chrambach, A. (1971). *Anal. Biochem.* **40**, 95.
Rogentine, G. N., Jr. (1967). *In* "Histocompatibility Testing" (E. S. Curtoni, P. L. Mattiuz, and R. M. Tosi, eds.), p. 371. Munksgaard, Copenhagen.
Rogentine, G. N., Jr., and Gerber, P. (1969). *Transplantation* **8**, 28.
Rogentine, G. N., Jr., and Gerber, P. (1970). *In* "Histocompatibility Testing" (P. I. Terasaki, ed.), p. 333. Munksgaard, Copenhagen.
Russell, P. S., and Winn, H. J., eds. (1965). "Histocompatibility Testing," Publ. No. 1229. Nat. Acad. Sci.—Nat. Res. Counc., Washington, D. C.
Sachs, D. H., Winn, H. J., and Russell, P. S. (1971). *Transplant. Proc.* **3**, 210.
Sandberg, A. L., Osler, A. G., Shin, H. S., and Oliveira, B. (1970). *J. Immunol.* **104**, 329.
Sanderson, A. R. (1968). *Nature (London)* **220**, 192.
Sanderson, A. R., and Batchelor, J. R. (1967). *In* "Histocompatibility Testing" (E. S. Curtoni, P. L. Mattiuz, and R. M. Tosi, eds.), p. 367. Munksgaard, Copenhagen.
Sanderson, A. R., and Batchelor, J. R. (1968). *Nature (London)* **219**, 184.
Sanderson, A. R., and Welsh, K. I. (1973). *In* "Transplantation Antigens" (B. D. Kahan and R. A. Reisfeld, eds.), p. 273. Academic Press, New York.
Sanderson, A. R., and Welsh, K. I. (1973). *Biochem. Soc. Trans.* **1**, 956.
Sanderson, A. R., Cresswell, P., and Welsh, K. I. (1971). *Nature (London) New Biol.* **230**, 8.
Schlesinger, M., and Amos, D. B. (1971). *Transplant. Proc.* **3**, 895.
Schlesinger, M., and Chaouat, M. (1972). *Tissue Antigens* **2**, 427.
Schultz, J. S., and Shreffler, D. C. (1972). *Transplantation* **13**, 186.
Schwartz, B. D., and Nathenson, S. G. (1971). *Transplant. Proc.* **3**, 180.
Scott, R. B., and Bell, E. (1964). *Science* **145**, 711.
Seigler, H. F., and Metzgar, R. S. (1970). *Transplantation* **9**, 478.
Seigler, H. F., and Metzgar, R. S. (1973). *In* "Transplantation Antigens" (B. D. Kahan and R. A. Reisfeld, eds.), p. 115. Academic Press, New York.
Seigler, H. F., Kremer, W. B., Metzgar, R. S., Ward, F. E., Taung, A. T., and Amos, D. B. (1971). *J. Nat. Cancer Inst.* **46**, 577.

5. Histocompatibility Antigens: Biology and Chemistry

Shimada, A., and Nathenson, S. G. (1969). *Biochemistry* **8**, 4048.
Shreffler, D. C. (1965). *In* "Isoantigens and Cell Interactions" (J. Palm, ed.), p. 11. Wistar Inst. Press, Philadelphia, Pennsylvania.
Shreffler, D. C. (1967). *Proc. Int. Congr. Hum. Genet., 3rd, 1966* p. 217.
Shreffler, D. C. (1970). *In* "Blood and Tissue Antigens" (D. Aminoff, ed.), p. 85. Academic Press, New York.
Shulman, N. R., Marder, V. J., Hiller, M. C., and Collier, E. M. (1964). *Progr. Hematol.* **4**, 222.
Shutt, R. H., and Krueger, R. G. (1972). *J. Immunol.* **108**, 819.
Silvers, W. K., and Billingham, R. E. (1970). *Transplant. Proc.* **2**, 152.
Silvestre, D., Kourilsky, F. M., Nicolai, M. G., and Levy, J. P. (1970). *Nature (London)* **228**, 67.
Singer, S. J., and Nicolson, G. L. (1972). *Science* **175**, 720.
Sirchia, G., and Ferrone, S. (1971). *Blood* **37**, 563.
Smith, G. S., and Walford, R. L. (1970). *In* "Histocompatibility Testing" (P. I. Terasaki, ed.), p. 549. Munksgaard, Copenhagen.
Smithies, O., and Poulik, M. D. (1972a). *Science* **175**, 187.
Smithies, O., and Poulik, M. D. (1972b). *Proc. Nat. Acad. Sci. U. S.* **69**, 2914.
Snell, G. D. (1948). *J. Genet.* **49**, 87.
Snell, G. D., and Stimpfling, J. H. (1966). *In* "Biology of the Laboratory Mouse" (E. L. Green, ed.), p. 457. McGraw-Hill, New York.
Snell, G. D., Cherry, M., and Démant, P. (1971). *Transplant. Proc.* **3**, 183.
Solheim, B. G., and Thorsby, E. (1974). *Tissue Antigens* (in press).
Stark, O., Kren, V., Frenzl, B., and Brdicka, R. (1968). *In* "Advances in Transplantation" (J. Dausset, J. Hamburger, and G. Mathé, eds.), p. 331. Williams & Wilkins, Baltimore, Maryland.
Stark, O., Krenova, D., Kren, V., and Frenzl, B. (1970). *Folia Biol. (Prague)* **16**, 1.
Stewart, J. A., and Papaconstantinou, J. (1967). *J. Mol. Biol.* **29**, 357.
Storb, R., Graham, T. C., Shiurba, R., and Thomas, E. D. (1970). *Transplantation* **10**, 165.
Stroehmann, I., and DeWitt, C. W. (1972). *Immunology* **23**, 929.
Svejgaard, A. (1969). *Vox Sang.* **17**, 112.
Svejgaard, A., and Kissmeyer-Nielsen, F. (1968). *Nature (London)* **219**, 868.
Svejgaard, A., Kjerbye, K. E., and Kissmeyer-Nielsen, F. (1967). *In* "Histocompatibility Testing" (E. S. Curtoni, P. L. Mattiuz, and R. M. Tosi, eds.), p. 385. Munksgaard, Copenhagen.
Svejgaard, A., Bratlie, A., Hedin, P. J., Högman, C., Jersild, C., Kissmeyer-Nielsen, F., Lindblom, B., Lindholm, A., Low, B., Messeter, L., Möller, E., Sandberg, L., Staub-Nielsen, L., and Thorsby, E. (1971). *Tissue Antigens* **1**, 81.
Swisher, S. N., Young, L. E., and Trabold, N. (1962). *Ann. N. Y. Acad. Sci.* **97**, 15.
Takahashi, T. (1971). *Transplant. Proc.* **3**, 1217.
Takasugi, M. (1971). *Transplantation* **12**, 148.
Tanigaki, N., Nakamuro, K., Appella, E., Poulik, M. D., and Pressman, D. (1973). *Biochem. Biophys. Res. Comm.* **55**, 1234.
Taylor, R. B., Duffus, P. H., Raff, M. C., and de Petris, S.(1971). *Nature (London) New Biol.* **233**, 225.
Tennant, J. R. (1968). *In* "Advances in Transplantation" (J. Dausset, J. Hamburger, and G. Mathé, eds.), p. 507. Munksgaard, Copenhagen.
Terasaki, P. I., ed. (1970). "Histocompatibility Testing." Munksgaard, Copenhagen.
Terasaki, P. I., and McClelland, J. D. (1964). *Nature (London)* **204**, 998.
Terasaki, P. I., Marchioro, T. L., and Starzl, T. E. (1965). *In* "Histocompatibility

Testing" (P. S. Russell and H. J. Winn, eds.), Publ. No. 1229, p. 83. Nat. Acad. Sci.—Nat. Res. Counc., Washington, D. C.
Terasaki, P. I., Vredevoe, D. L., and Mickey, M. R. (1967). *Transplantation* **5**, 1057.
Terasaki, P. I., Trasher, D. L., and Hauber, T. H. (1968). *In* "Advances in Transplantation" (J. Dausset, J. Hamburger, and G. Mathé, eds.), p. 225. Munksgaard, Copenhagen.
Terasaki, P. I., Kreisler, M., and Mickey, M. R. (1971). *Postgrad. Med. J.* **47**, 98.
Thorsby, E., and Kissmeyer-Nielsen, F. (1970). *Vox Sang.* **18**, 134.
Thorsby, E., Bratlie, A., and Lie, S. O. (1969). *Scand. J. Haematol.* **6**, 409.
Thorsby, E., Kjerbye, K. E., and Bratlie, A. (1970). *Vox Sang.* **18**, 373.
Ting, A., Hasegawa, T., Ferrone, S., and Reisfeld, R. A. (1973). *Transplant. Proc.* **5**, 813.
Ting, C. C., and Herberman, R. B. (1971). *Nature (London) New Biol.* **232**, 118.
Tosi, R. M., Pellegrino, M., Scudeller, G., and Ceppellini, R. (1967). *In* "Histocompatibility Testing" (E. S. Curtoni, P. L. Mattiuz, and R. M. Tosi, eds.), p. 350. Munksgaard, Copenhagen.
Tsakraklides, E., Kersey, J., and Good, R. A. (1973). *Fed. Proc., Fed. Amer. Soc. Exp. Biol.* **32**, 1018.
Turner, M. J., Strominger, J. L., and Sanderson, A. R. (1972). *Proc. Nat. Acad. Sci. U. S.* **69**, 200.
Uhlenbruck, G., Voigtmann, R., Salfner, B., Bube, F. W., and Seibel, E. (1973). *Symp. Ser. Immunobiol. Stand.* **18**, 218.
Unanue, E. R., Perkins, W. D., and Karnovsky, M. J. (1972). *J. Exp. Med.* **136**, 885.
van der Weerdt, C. H. M., and Lalezari, P. (1972). *Vox Sang.* **22**, 438.
van Rood, J. J. (1962). Thesis, University of Leiden.
van Rood, J. J. (1971). *In* "Progress in Immunology" (B. Amos, ed.), p. 1027. Academic Press, New York.
van Rood, J. J., and van Leeuwen, A. (1963). *J. Clin. Invest.* **42**, 1382.
van Rood, J. J., and van Leeuwen, A. (1971). *Transplant. Proc.* **3**, 1283.
van Rood, J. J., Eernisse, J. G., and van Leeuwen, A. (1958). *Nature (London)* **181**, 1735.
van Rood, J. J., van Leeuwen, A., and van Santen, M. C. (1970a). *Nature (London)* **226**, 366.
van Rood, J. J., van Leeuwen, A., Koch, C. T., and Frederiks, E. (1970b). *In* "Histocompatibility Testing" (P. I. Terasaki, ed.), p. 483. Munksgaard, Copenhagen.
van Rood, J. J., van Leeuwen, A., and Balner, H. (1972). *Transplant. Proc.* **4**, 55.
van Rood, J. J., Koch, C. T., van Hooff, J. P., van Leeuwen, A., van den Tweel, J. G., Frederiks, E., Schippers, H. M. A., Hendriks, G., and van der Steen, G. J. (1973). *Transplant. Proc.* **5**, 409.
Vladutin, A. O., and Rose, N. R. (1971). *Science* **174**, 1137.
Vojtiskova, M. (1969). *Nature (London)* **222**, 1293.
Vojtiskova, M., Polackova, M., and Pokorno, Z. (1969). *Folia Biol. (Prague)* **15**, 322.
Vriesendorp, H. M., Rothengatter, G., Bos, E., Westbrock, D. L., and van Rood, J. J. (1971). *Transplantation* **11**, 440.
Walford, R. L., Gallagher, R., and Sjaarda, J. R. (1964). *Science* **144**, 868.
Walford, R. L., Gallagher, R., and Troup, G. M. (1965). *Transplantation* **3**, 387.
Walford, R. L., Latta, H., and Troup, G. M. (1966). *Ann. N. Y. Acad. Sci.* **129**, 490.
Walford, R. L., Shanbrom, E., Troup, G. M., Zeller, E., and Ackermann, B. (1967). *In* "Histocompatibility Testing" (E. S. Curtoni, P. L. Mattiuz, and R. M. Tosi, eds.), p. 221. Munksgaard, Copenhagen.

5. Histocompatibility Antigens: Biology and Chemistry

Walford, R. L., Finkelstein, S., Neerbout, R., Konrad, P., and Shanbrom, E. (1970). *Nature (London)* **225**, 461.
Walford, R. L., Smith, G. S., and Waters, H. (1971). *Transplant. Rev.* **7**, 78.
Warmsley, A. M. H., and Pasternak, C. A. (1970). *Biochem. J.* **119**, 493.
Warren, L., Glick, M. C., and Nass, M. K. (1966). *J. Cell. Physiol.* **68**, 269.
Weisbart, R. H., Webb, W. F., Bluestone, R., and Goldberg, L. S. (1972). *Vox Sang.* **23**, 478.
Wessels, N. K., and Wilt, F. H. (1965). *J. Mol. Biol.* **13**, 767.
White, D. S. G., Bradley, B., Calne, R. Y., and Binns, R. M. (1973). *Transplant. Proc.* **5**, 317.
Willingham, M. C., Spicer, S. S., and Graber, C. D. (1971). *Lab. Invest.* **25**, 211.
Winn, H. (1962). *Ann. N. Y. Acad. Sci.* **101**, 23.
Yunis, E. J., Ward, F. E., and Amos, D. B. (1970). *In* "Histocompatibility Testing" (P. I. Terasaki, ed.), p. 351. Munksgaard, Copenhagen.
Yunis, E. J., Gatti, R. A., and Amos, D. B., eds. (1973). "Tissue Typing and Organ Transplantation." Academic Press, New York.
Zervas, J. D., Delamore, I. W., and Israëls, M. C. O. (1970). *Lancet* **2**, 634.
Zucker-Franklin, D. (1965). *Amer. J. Pathol.* **47**, 419.
zur Hausen, H., Diehl, V., Wolf, H., Schulte-Holthausen, H., and Schneider, U. (1972). *Nature (London) New Biol.* **237**, 184.

CHAPTER 6

Antigens of the Mycoplasmatales and Chlamydiae

GEORGE E. KENNY

I.	Introduction	449
II.	Classification and Nomenclature	450
III.	Biology	451
	A. Morphology	451
	B. Host–Parasite Relationships	454
	C. Biochemistry	455
IV.	Phylogenetic Relationships	456
	A. Analytical Serology of the Mycoplasmatales	456
	B. Heterogeneity of the Mycoplasmatales Compared to Homogeneity of the Chlamydiae	459
V.	Antigenic Analysis of Mycoplasmata	459
	A. Preparation of Antigens	459
	B. Preparation of Antisera	461
	C. Serologic Assay of Mycoplasmic Antigens	462
	D. Double Immunodiffusion Analysis	462
VI.	Antigenic Analysis of Chlamydiae	464
VII.	Growth Inhibition and Mycoplasmacidal Activity of Serum	464
	A. Inhibition of Colonial Growth on Agar	464
	B. Metabolic Inhibition Testing	465
	C. Mycoplasmacidal Reactions	466
VIII.	Antigenic Structure	467
	A. Carbohydrate Antigens	468
	B. Lipid Antigens	469
	C. Protein Antigens	472
	References	476

I. Introduction

The characteristics of the antigens of two groups of microorganisms, the Mycoplasmatales and the chlamydiae, are discussed together in this chapter because these two groups of organisms represent the smallest and likely the simplest prokaryotic organisms known. The organisms classified in the Mycoplasmatales are considered to be the smallest free-living organisms presently known and the chlamydiae, although present evidence indicates that they are obligate intracellular parasites, contain substantial enzymatic activity and apparently carry out their own replication processes without direct aid from the host cell. Both groups of organisms are small, about 300 μm for round forms, and are barely visible in the light microscope. Small size has important consequences for organisms (Pirie, 1969), the most relevant of which to this article is that the amount of surface area increases greatly relative to the total mass of the organism as size is reduced. Both groups of organisms have small amounts of genetic material, hence the number of potential antigens which can be synthesized should be sharply limited relative to more complex organisms. Although simplicity of the organism should have substantial virtues for antigenic analysis, simplicity also indicates limited synthetic ability with corresponding difficulties of cultivating the organisms in readily usable quantities. Thus antigenic analysis of both groups of organisms has been greatly handicapped by the complex cultivation systems required for the organisms and the low yield of organisms.

II. Classification and Nomenclature

The organisms which resembled the agent of bovine pleuropneumonia, *Mycoplasma mycoides* var. *mycoides*, were classified by Edward and Freundt (1956) into a single genus *Mycoplasma* with 15 species. Since that time, some 30 additional species have been recognized (Edward and Freundt, 1973) and a substantial number of new species will be named in the near future. Some degree of heterogeneity has been recognized since the group of species that do not require cholesterol and that grow in medium without serum have been reclassified into genus *Acholeplasma* (these species include *Acholeplasma laidlawii* and *Acholeplasma granularum* which were previously classified as species in genus *Mycoplasma* as well as a new species *Acholeplasma axanthum*). Each genus is classified into one family, Mycoplasmataceae and Acholeplasmataceae, respectively, which in turn are grouped in one order the Mycoplasmatales and which is included in a new class Mollicutes (Edward and Freundt, 1969a,b, 1970). Mycoplasmata is the trivial name for species

6. Antigens of the Mycoplasmatales and Chlamydiae   451

in genus *Mycoplasma* though the term mycoplasmas (the English common name) is used more frequently. Similarly acholeplasmata would be the trivial name for organisms in genus *Acholeplasma* though acholeplasmas is being used. No general trivial term has yet been used to describe species in the Mycoplasmatales though the term mycoplasmata or mycoplasmas may well fill that need. Earlier papers cite different terminology: the term pleuropneumonia-like organisms (PPLO) has been used to describe the entire group, and genus *Asterococcus* was used for classification prior to the reclassification by Edward and Freundt (1956).

The chlamydiae have been known by a variety of other names in the past: bedsoniae, miyagawanella, psittacosis-lymphogranuloma-trachoma (PLT) group, and trachoma-inclusion conjunctivitis (TRIC) agents. Recently these organisms have been reclassified into genus *Chlamydia* with two species *C. psittaci* and *C. trachomatis* (Page, 1966, 1968). Since the host spectrum, disease caused, and immunologic properties of the species differ widely, the number of strains is large and an extensive typing system has been proposed for *C. trachomatis* strains (Wang and Grayston, 1971). The trivial term, chlamydiae, has been well accepted.

III. Biology

A. Morphology

The organisms classified in the Mycoplasmatales are small (0.3–0.5 μm) membrane bounded organisms without morphological or chemical evidence of a cell wall. The organisms form small colonies (1–100 μm) on enriched solid medium frequently with the appearance of a "fried egg" (Fig. 1). The structure of the individual organisms has been a highly controversial subject since morphology is greatly influenced by growth conditions, methods of concentrating organisms, and fixation techniques (Rodwell, 1969; Lemcke, 1972). The term Mycoplasma refers to a filamentous shape and refers to the filamentous forms frequently seen in the type species of genus *Mycoplasma: Mycoplasma mycoides* var. *mycoides*. In spite of the controversy surrounding structure, the organisms in the Mycoplasmatales appear to show substantial heterogeneity in morphology. Generally organisms in the Mycoplasmatales appear as membrane-bounded bodies that enclose ribosomes and strands of nuclear material coursing through the cytoplasm. *Mycoplasma gallisepticum* cells

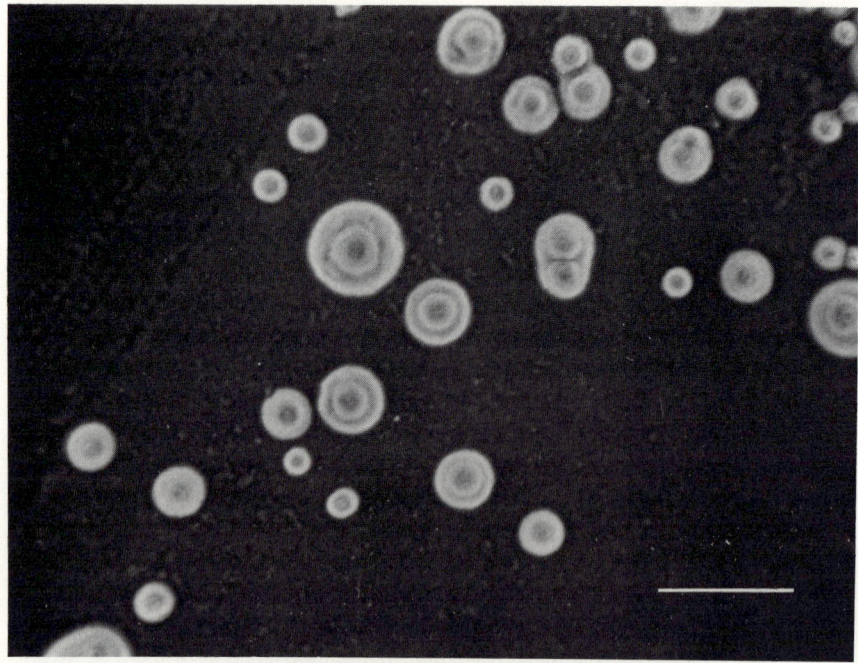

Fig. 1. Colonies of *Mycoplasma pneumoniae* growing on agar (Kenny, 1969a), 10 days incubation at 37°C. Anoptral phase contrast. The fried egg appearance can be clearly seen, though the center is not dark as in ordinary light microscopy. Bar, 100 μm.

are ovoid shaped with a terminal bleb (Maniloff and Morowitz, 1967). *Mycoplasma pneumoniae* cells possess delicate filaments in broth cultures with frequent star shapes (Boatman and Kenny, 1971a,b), whereas the organisms grown on glass coverslips frequently are tear-shaped and show motility (Bredt, 1968). A terminal body has been shown in the filaments of some *M. pneumoniae* cells (Biberfeld and Biberfeld, 1970). Cells of *Mycoplasma felis* show star shapes with shorter and broader "arms" than those of *M. pneumoniae* (Boatman and Kenny, 1970). A comparison of these three species mixed together shows that the species are readily distinguishable by their morphologies (Fig. 2). Additional studies of the Mycoplasmatales will no doubt show additional differences between species. Although the earlier literature on the Mycoplasmatales contains abundant references to "elementary bodies" (small dense bodies capable of replication), this idea has been discarded since no

6. Antigens of the Mycoplasmatales and Chlamydiae

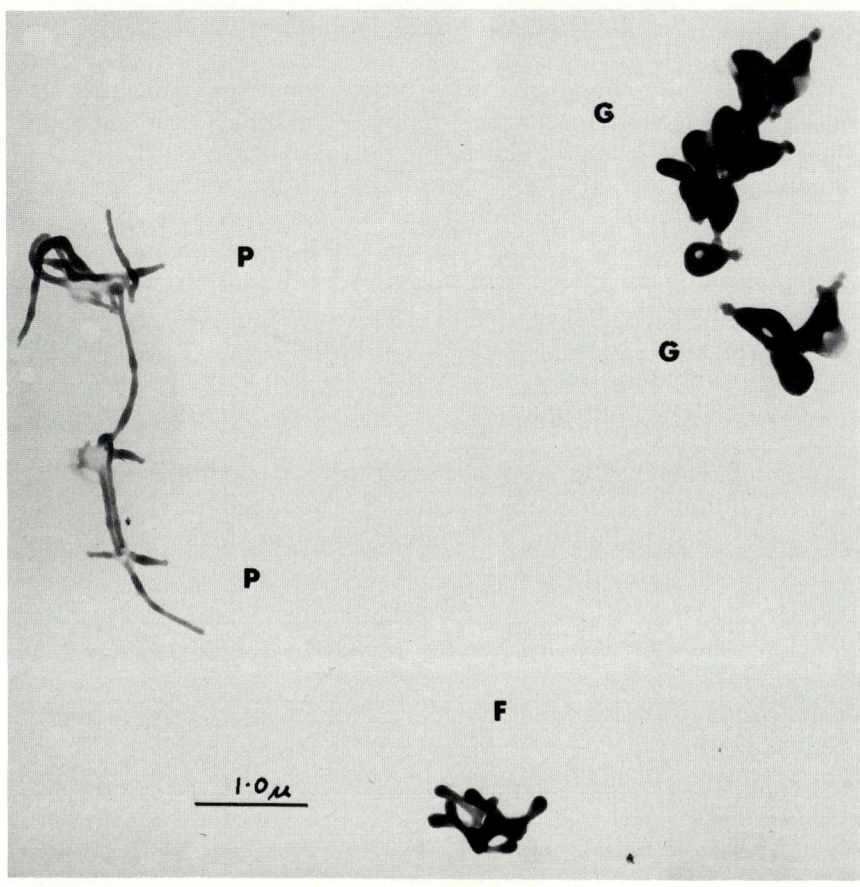

Fig. 2. Morphologies of negatively stained mycoplasmata: P, *Mycoplasma pneumoniae* strain 3546, G, *Mycoplasma gallisepticum* strain S-6, F, *Mycoplasma felis* strain B-2. Photograph courtesy of Dr. E. S. Boatman.

clear evidence exists to indicate that particles less than 0.2–0.3 μm in diameter are viable (Maniloff and Morowitz, 1972).

Chlamydiae, however, show two distinct morphological forms: the dense form (elementary body) and the reticulate body. The dense form in the infective form (about 0.3 μm in diameter) and contains a clearly defined cell wall (Jenkin, 1960; Higashi, 1965). The reticulate body is a developmental form that primarily exists intracellularly, contains a less clearly defined cell wall, and is larger (0.5–1.0 μm) than the elementary body (Tamura *et al.*, 1971).

B. Host–Parasite Relationships

The best generality that can be made about the parasitic relationships of mycoplasmata to their hosts is that they are surface parasites. In mammalian cell cultures the organisms grow on the surface of cells (see Kenny, 1973a, for a summary). Although less is known about the *in vivo* systems, it appears that the organisms appear intracellularly only in phagocytic cells (Organick *et al.*, 1966). *Mycoplasma pneumoniae* organisms grow on the surface of lung and grow in among the cilia of tracheal organ cultures (Collier, 1972). The diseases caused by mycoplasmata in their natural animal host include respiratory disease and arthritis. In man only one species is a proven pathogen, *M. pneumoniae*, though *M. hominis* appears to be an opportunist.

Although chlamydiae are recognized to be intracellular parasites, in a sense they too are surface parasites. The organism is incapable of directly penetrating the cell but is taken up in a vacuole and

TABLE I

Serologic Heterogeneity of the Mycoplasmatales as Demonstrated by Double Immunodiffusion[a]

Antigen	% G + C[b]	Antisera[c]											Identifying no.
		1	2	3	4	5	6	7	8	9	10	11	
1 *M. species* cal goat	28.9	6[d]											ATCC 15718
2 *M. bovigenitalium*	30.4		8	(1)									ATCC 19852
3 *M. edwardii*	29.2			6	2	1							ATCC 23462
4 *M. hyorhinis*	27.0	1		1	6	1							ATCC 17981
5 *M. neurolyticum*	26.2	(1)		1	1	7							ATCC 15049
6 *M. gallisepticum*	31.8						7						ATCC 15302
7 *M. pneumoniae*	39.9							7					AP-164
8 *M. laidlawii* A	33.0								9	2			ATCC 14089
9 *A. axanthum*	—								2	6			S-743
10 *M. arginini*	—										10	2	Str. 230
11 *M. gallinarum*	27.0									3	9		ATCC 15315

[a] Adapted from Kenny (1973b).

[b] % G + C, percentage of guanine plus cytosine in mycoplasmic DNA. Data are from Williams *et al.* (1969), who give a difference greater than 2.8% as significant.

[c] Antisera for organisms 1 through 9 were prepared in rabbits by use of organisms that were grown in soy peptone dialysate broth supplemented with 12% agamma calf serum. Antisera to organism 11 were prepared in dialysate broth supplemented with 12% agamma rabbit serum. Serologic test antigens were grown in the same medium supplemented with agamma horse serum.

[d] Numbers represent number of clearly visible precipitin lines. The broken squares represent groups of organisms; the solid squares indicate homologous reactions. Numbers in parentheses represent weak reactions.

replicates there (Weiss, 1971). Replication of chlamydiae is accompanied by a shutdown of host DNA synthesis followed by a slow down in host RNA and protein synthesis. Energy production continues at the same rate in the cell suggesting that energy is being diverted to the parasite (Moulder, 1970). The host cell dies in the process of the growth of chlamydiae. Although mycoplasmata can clearly cause a number of effects on cells in culture (see Kenny, 1973a, for a summary) from their external location, little is known of their effects on cells in the intact animal.

C. Biochemistry

Several features of the biochemistry of these organisms are of substantial interest to the antigenic characterization of the organisms. The genome sizes for the organisms are small: 500×10^6 daltons for mycoplasmata (Maniloff and Morowitz, 1972), and 660×10^6 for chlamydiae (Becker, 1972), whereas acholeplasmata have a genome size of approximately 1000×10^6 daltons (Maniloff and Morowitz, 1972). Thus the organisms have a limited synthetic ability, a fact that is reflected in their complex growth requirements. The percent guanine plus cytosine (% G + C) in mycoplasmic deoxyribonucleic acid (DNA) is low (Table I), ranging from 23–40% (Neimark, 1970). For chlamydiae, the % G + C is about 40 (Weiss, 1971).

The chemical composition of the mycoplasmatales is widely variable. *Mycoplasma mycoides* produces a large amount of polysaccharide during growth whereas some other species contain little detectable polysaccharide (Smith, 1971). Mycoplasmata contain large amounts of lipid (8–20% of their dry weight), which is comprised of phospholipids, cholesterol, and in some cases glycolipids (Smith, 1973). *Acholeplasma laidlawii* and *A. granularum* contain carotenoids but do not contain cholesterol (Smith, 1973).

Physiologically the Mycoplasmatales are widely variable. Acholeplasmata utilize glucose but do not require cholesterol. Three additional groups can be recognized in the sterol requiring species: (1) glycolytic organisms, (2) arginine hydrolyzing species, and (3) organisms that hydrolyze urea (the T strains). Although some glycolytic organisms hydrolyze arginine, these three properties are usually mutually exclusive in genus *Mycoplasma*.

In contrast, the chlamydiae possess a rigid cell wall in elementary bodies whereas the cell wall is less rigid in the reticulate body stage, possibly the result of poor cross-linkage because of the relatively low concentrations of cysteine and methionine (Tamura and Manire,

1967). As prokaryotic organisms, the chlamydiae are remarkable in that they apparently do not synthesize adenosine triphosphate (Weiss, 1971). In contrast, mycoplasmata have a number of energy yielding pathways (Smith, 1971).

IV. Phylogenetic Relationships

I am giving what might be considered unusual emphasis for a chapter in "The Antigens" on the phylogenetic relationships between the organisms in the Mycoplasmatales as revealed by antigenic analysis. The major reason for this emphasis is that the organisms in the Mycoplasmatales appear to be a remarkably disparate group. It appears that their common properties derive from the fact that they are small membrane-bounded prokaryotic cells and not from any fundamental close biologic relationship. In contrast, the organisms classified in the chlamydiae appear to be strongly homogeneous.

Present classification methods for the description of new species involve at least the following criteria: (1) demonstration that the organisms lack a cell wall ultrastructurally, (2) demonstration that the organisms do not revert to form typical bacterial cells or colonies, (3) demonstration that the organisms are small, (4) demonstration that the organisms do not cross-react with any known mycoplasmic or acholeplasmic species by tests involving surface antigens (growth-inhibition, metabolic inhibition, and fluorescent antibody determinations), and (5) demonstration that the organisms form typical colonies on solid medium. It is important to note that criteria (1) and (2) are negative criteria. Such features as % G + C content, genome size, and analytic serology have not been used as criteria for classification.

A. Analytical Serology of the Mycoplasmatales

Identification of *Mycoplasma* species by more sophisticated immunologic methods gives rather different results. When double immunodiffusion methods are employed with potent antiserum, most species can be clearly separated from others (Lemcke, 1965). In a comparison of ten glycolytic species, it was found that the species of the genus did not have common antigens although common antigens could be found within groups of species (Kenny, 1969a). *Mycoplasma pneumoniae* and *M. gallisepticum* were serologically

6. Antigens of the Mycoplasmatales and Chlamydiae 457

unique and showed almost no cross-reactions with other species. However, other organisms such as *Acholeplasma laidlawii* and *A. granularum* showed strong cross-reactions with each other. Similarly a group of organisms (*M. felis, M. canis, M. hyorhinis, M. neurolyticum,* and *M. fermentans*) showed cross-reactions generally throughout the group. The serologic relationships were reflected in the % G + C of the DNA of the organisms in that organisms of significantly different G + C content did not show cross-reactions whereas organisms with similar G + C frequently cross-reacted, though separation into distinct serologic groups also was seen in organisms with similar % G + C (Kenny, 1973b). Neimark (1970) divided the organisms into groups by their % G + C content of their DNA and by their glycolytic abilities; his conclusions are complementary to those shown here by serology.

I have thus far compared 21 of the some 45 known species by double immunodiffusion with potent rabbit antiserum (Table II). Six or seven groups of organisms can be identified depending upon whether more powerful antiserum to *M. bovigenitalium* or better analytical techniques (two-dimensional electrophoresis) show a relationship of that organism to group VI. It is of considerable interest to note that all of these organisms (except *M. bovigenitalium*) can be distinguished from each other by disk inhibition with specific antiserum without any evidence of cross-reactions. Although *M. mycoides* var. *mycoides* and *M. mycoides* var. *capri* cannot be studied within the United States, antiserum from the National Institutes of Health was available to these two strains which had been prepared in Dr. Freundt's laboratory in Denmark. These antisera showed strong cross-reactions with *M. species* cal goat but not with other species, suggesting that this organism is related to the type species of the genus. At least six to as many as eleven precipitin lines could be resolved in this system. The number of precipitin lines observed is shown in Table I for 11 of the 22 species which are representative of the spectrum of differences seen. Several cross-reactions were observed with antiserum to both *M. bovirhinis* and *M. species* cal goat but these reactions were not reciprocal so their present significance is unknown. The essential point of the data is that the species in the order are markedly serologically heterogeneous showing no common antigens throughout the genus, a result one would certainly expect in a bacterial genus. Thus certain species still classified in genus *Mycoplasma* may be as distant from other species in different groups as *Escherichia coli* is from *Mycobacterium tuberculosis*. A comparison of the % G + C and serologic differences seen between *M.*

TABLE II

Serologic Taxonomy of the Mycoplasmatales

	Strain	Host	Disease
Glycolytic species			
Group I *Mycoplasma* (25–28% GC)			
M. species cal goat	ATCC 15718	Goats	Arthritis
M. mycoides var. mycoides[a]	PG-1	Cattle	Pleuropneumonia
Group II *Acholeplasma* (30–32% GC)			
{A. granularum[b]	Friend	Swine	Arthritis?
{A. laidlawii	ATCC 14191	Sewage, nature	Not known
A. axanthum	S-743	Cell cultures	Not known
Group III (30.4% GC)			
M. bovigenitalium[c]	ATCC 19852	Cattle	Genital disease
Group IV (32% GC)			
M. gallisepticum	S-6	Chickens	Sinusitis
Group V (39.9% GC)			
M. pneumoniae	AP-164	Man	Pneumonia
Group VI (25–28% GC)			
M. anatis	1340	Ducks	Not known
M. bovimastitis	ATCC 25025	Cattle	Mastitis
{M. canis	ATCC 19525	Dogs	Not known
{M. edwardii	ATCC 23462	Dogs	Not known
{M. felis	B2	Cats	Not known
M. fermentans	PG-18	Man	Not known
{M. hyorhinis	ATCC 17981	Swine	Arthritis
{M. pulmonis	63	Rats, mice	Respiratory disease, arthritis
M. neurolyticum	ATCC 15049	Mice	Rolling disease
M. synoviae	WVU 1853	Chickens	Synovitis
Nonglycolytic arginine-utilizing species			
Group VII (27–29% GC)			
M. hominis		Man	Opportunist
M. gallinarum	ATCC 15315	Chickens	Not known
M. arginini	Str. 230	Goats	Not known

[a] NIH reference antisera shows a strong relationship to organisms in this group but not to other groups.

[b] Strains bracketed are more closely related to each other than to other species in the group.

[c] May have some relationship to Group VI.

pneumoniae (39.9% G + C) and *M. neurolyticum* (26.2% G + C) is indicative of the more extreme differences seen in genus *Mycoplasma* (Tables I and II). Thus the use of any one species as a model for the entire group is a hazardous venture though such a model may provide general information about membrane bounded organisms. However, the relationships provided in Tables I and II may prove useful in selecting organisms as representative models for the various groups. Interestingly, the morphologies shown in Fig. 1 are different and the organisms shown were chosen because of their serologic differences. If we consider the separation of the acholeplasmata into a separate genus as a precedent, then at least four additional families would have to be created to accommodate the diversity in order Mycoplasmatales. However, such reclassification should be delayed at least until some information is available on the nature of the antigens involved in the cross-reactions. The T strains appear markedly different physiologically and probably represent an additional group.

B. Heterogeneity of the Mycoplasmatales Compared to Homogeneity of the Chlamydiae

The antigenic heterogeneity of Mycoplasmatales stands in sharp contrast to that of the chlamydiae where common antigens appear to be the major components of the organisms and it is difficult to demonstrate type or species specific antigens by double immunodiffusion (Kuo et al., 1971). The antigenic heterogeneity of the Mycoplasmatales has been verified by measuring DNA–DNA homology between various strains. Although only limited data are available, strains that are strongly serologically related such as A. laidlawii and A. granularum show substantial homology (Pollock and Bonner, 1969; Neimark, 1970) whereas species that are not related serologically show very little homology. In contrast the studies done on the chlamydiae show very substantial genetic relationships between the strains tested (Gerloff et al., 1966), supporting the idea that the chlamydiae represent a closely related group of organisms.

V. Antigenic Analysis of Mycoplasmata

A. Preparation of Antigens

The yield of mycoplasmata from broth cultures is small: some 20 mg dry weight per liter. Additionally, the organisms require highly enriched media for growth requirements. In practice, the medium usually includes a plant or animal peptone, an extract of fresh yeast, and 5–20% animal serum. Defined media presently available do not give good yields (Smith, 1971). Most mycoplasmic media produce a substantial deposit when uninoculated but incubated cultures are centrifuged. This deposit of medium components may be substantially larger than the pellet of organisms which can be obtained. This difficulty can be circumvented in several manners. The medium can be incubated and then centrifuged or filtered to remove sedimentable medium particles. This is successful if no additional components precipitate during the growth of the organism. A practical method is to employ a dialysate medium derived from peptone and autoclaved yeast (Kenny, 1967) and to supplement this with "agamma" serum which has been pretested for ability to remain clear during incubation. Antigens grown in this manner appear to be contaminated with 1% or less horse serum protein as judged by immunologic assay (Kenny, 1969a). Since many mycoplasmic species will adhere to and grow on glass surfaces (Somerson *et al.*, 1967; Purcell *et al.*, 1970; Taylor-Robinson and Manchee, 1967), the organisms can be grown on glass surfaces under thin layers of medium, the medium decanted and the adherent cells washed before being removed from the surface by scraping (Somerson *et al.*, 1967). The surface method of cultivation has the difficulty of lessening the efficiency of handling cultures since it is a two-dimensional technique and suspension culture is a three-dimensional technique; however, the tedious centrifugation technique largely can be eliminated. Additionally, the high concentration of organisms on the glass surface requires good buffering of the medium to counteract the low local pH. Suspension culture of organisms such as *M. pneumoniae* must be grown with agitation for maximum yields because of inadequate aeration in stationary cultures (Low and Eaton, 1965) which is compounded by the fact that the organisms adhere to the bottom of the flask. *Mycoplasma pneumoniae* may represent a special case since it appears to be aerobic whereas many other species grow as well or better anaerobically. A major problem in removing medium components in organisms propagated either in glass or in suspension is that certain organisms such as *M. pneumoniae* grow as colonies (spherules) in fluid medium (Boatman and Kenny, 1971a) or colonies on glass (Biberfeld and Biberfeld, 1970) which appear to be loosely organized and likely contain medium components which cannot be removed by washing either monolayers on glass or pellets from broth culture. An additional stratagem for the preparation of concentrated organisms is the use of the dialysis culture technique whereby organisms are grown in a dialysis casing suspended in a larger container of broth (Pollock, 1965). This technique has been employed to produce high concentrations of *A. laidlawii*, an organism that does not require serum.

Assuming that a clear medium is available or can be devised, organisms are grown to the top of log phase and then harvested by centrifugation. It is important not to cultivate organisms beyond the log phase because substantial degradation of the structure of the organisms is observed in stationary phase with loss of ribosomes being a prominent feature (Boatman and Kenny, 1970). Incubation times range from 1 day for *A. laidlawii* to 7 days for *M. pneumoniae*. Control of pH during incubation is essential for both glycolytic and argininolytic strains if substantial amounts of utilizable substrates are included in the medium. The most practical buffers are HEPES (*N*-2-hydroxyethylpiperazine-*N*-2-ethanesulfonic acid) and TES [*N*-tris(hydroxymethyl)methyl-2-aminoethanesulfonic acid] (Pollack *et al.*, 1969). The immunogenicity of *M. pneumoniae* grown on glass was considerably compromised by the low pH (5.5) attained in medium supplemented with 1% glucose, a result that could be prevented by the inclusion of 50 mM HEPES at pH 7.5 (Pollack *et al.*, 1969). TES has been employed at 10 mM concentration for a variety of glycolytic mycoplasmic species (Kenny, 1969a).

Antigens after appropriate washing should be concentrated 100-5000-fold depending upon the serologic purpose for which they are intended. For most serologic tests concentrations of 1–20 mg protein per ml are satisfactory. Concentrated organisms can be stored at −20°C for several months with little apparent loss of antigenic or immunogenic activity; however, antigenic activity may be degraded upon longer storage at −20°C.

B. Preparation of Antisera

Although mycoplasmata have been commonly considered poor antigens, this is not true; the problem has primarily lain with the inability to produce sufficient masses of organisms. An additional and more pressing problem is the induction of substantial quantities of medium component antibody in the immunized animals because of the contamination of immunogens with large amounts of medium components (Section V,A). This problem can best be eliminated by growing the organism in a nonantigenic broth culture medium (a dialysate medium or a defined medium) supplemented with serum homologous to the species of animal to be immunized. Although rabbit serum is not an ideal serum supplement for growth of mycoplasmata, most strains can be grown in that serum, particularly agamma rabbit serum. The use of agamma rabbit serum has additional advantages. It has been shown that denatured homologous globulin can generate antiglobulin antibodies of rather broad specificities (Milgrom and Witebsky, 1960) which could cross-react with the globulins in the heterologous serum that the serologic test antigens are usually cultivated in because of the lower cost of horse and bovine sera. The extended incubation periods employed for cultivation of mycoplasmata provide large opportunities for denaturation of globulins. Another alternative is to propagate the immunizing antigen in a dialysate broth supplement with a different serum from that to be used to propagate the serologic test antigen. "Agamma" calf serum has been used as the medium serum supplement to propagate immunogens and horse serum used to propagate serologic test antigens. Although a small cross-reaction was observed between horse and calf serum, this procedure gave satisfactory results (Kenny, 1969a). Little information is available on the minimum quantities of immunogen and the optimum method of immunization of animals. For rabbits immunized with *M. pneumoniae*, 1–10 mg per rabbit gives optimum antibody response as measured by gel diffusion and complement fixation though as little as 16 μg per rabbit gave a measurable response (Kenny, 1971a). Approximately half of the immunogen was given intramuscularly with incomplete Freund adjuvant followed three weeks later by a series of intravenous doses of fluid immunogen. Similarly, dosages of 5–10 mg per rabbit of a variety of glycolytic and nonglycolytic species gave a good precipitin and complement-fixing antibody response (Kenny, 1969a, 1973b).

C. Serologic Assay of Mycoplasmic Antigens

The small yield of mycoplasmata and the high cost of producing organisms complicate assay of mycoplasmic antigens considerably. The cost of a 100 mg preparation of mycoplasmic protein is $25 for serum alone and the labor in preparing the medium and processing the culture easily doubles that figure to $50. Thus assay procedures and serologic comparisons need to be done with the least material possible.

D. Double Immunodiffusion Analysis

This analytical method is considerably complicated by the fact that nearly half of the organism is composed of membrane, the components of which are poorly soluble in purely aqueous systems. This difficulty may be partially resolved by the employment of short diffusion distances and agar supports of minimal concentration (greater pore size). One such system is the plastic matrix (Sharpless and LoGrippo, 1965) where the diffusion distance is 4 mm on a film of agar 0.6 mm thick. In such a system as many as 10 lines may be resolved for many different species (Kenny, 1969a, 1973b). Solubilizing of the membrane material with the nonionic detergent Triton X-100 has been shown by Hollingdale and Lemcke (1969) to greatly improve detection and resolution of membrane components for *M. hominis*. In the microsystem, the degree of improvement of both intensity and number of precipitin lines varies with species when organisms are solubilized with Triton (G. E. Kenny, unpublished data), some organisms showing no improvement. The shorter diffusion system in the microsystem may account for a portion of this difference, or the heterogeneity of the Mycoplasmatales may be a major factor. Although sodium dodecyl sulfate solubilizes membranes very

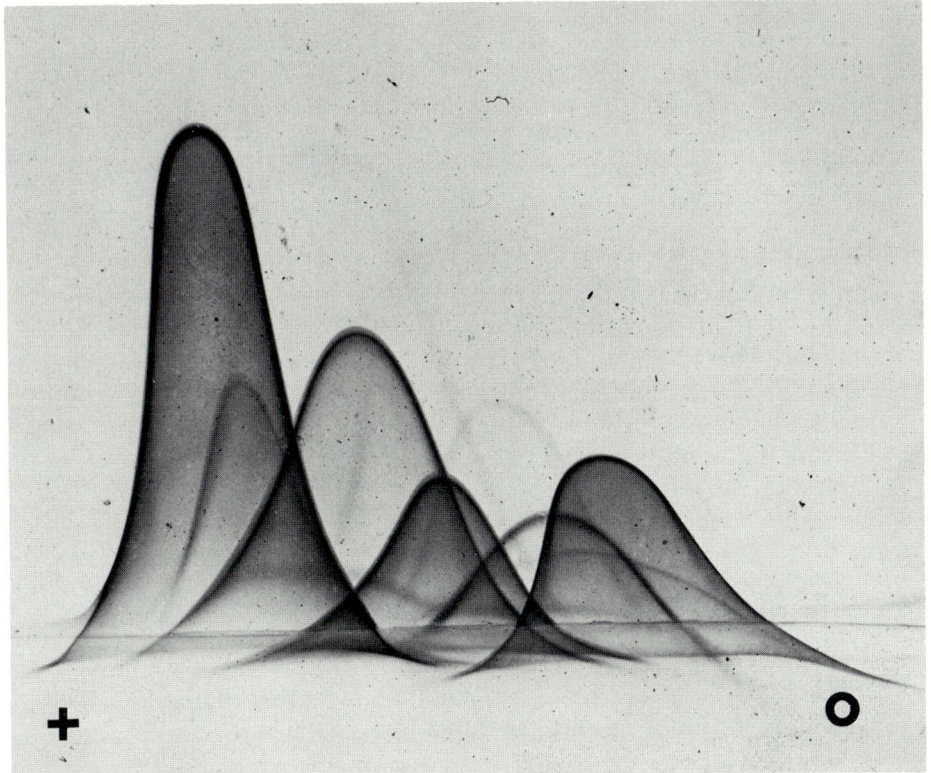

Fig. 3. Two-dimensional electrophoresis profile of *Mycoplasma arginini* antigen (50 µg protein) against homologous antiserum. 0, Point of sample application for first phase electrophoresis; +, Anode.

well, it both decreases the antigenicity of the preparations and may produce spurious precipitin lines by itself with serum proteins (Hollingdale and Lemcke, 1969).

Immunoelectrophoresis permits further characterization of the nature of the materials in the precipitin lines. The two-dimensional electrophoretic method of Laurell (1965) appears to have great promise because it not only permits detection of more antigenic determinants but more important it permits quantitative comparison of specific antigens. Ten components can be readily recognized in Fig. 3 (Thirkill and Kenny, 1974). Results in both of these methods are greatly improved by the use of nonionic detergents.

VI. Antigenic Analysis of Chlamydiae

Chlamydiae present an even greater problem in antigenic analysis than mycoplasmata. The yields of organism are smaller and the organisms are very difficult to free from contamination with host cells. Thus it is nearly impossible to prepare antiserum to the organisms without substantial amounts of host cell antibody. This difficulty can be circumvented in a manner similar to that used with mycoplasmata by growing the organisms in two immunologically unrelated host systems. Kuo *et al.* (1971) used as serologic test antigens, organisms grown in human heteroploid, (HeLa) cell cultures and used antisera prepared from purified organisms cultivated in the chick embryo yolk sac. This test system did not show cross-reactions in double immunodiffusion even though the antisera contained antibodies to yolk sac. An additional problem with chlamydiae is the difficulty in solubilizing the agent because of the presence of the cell wall. Extensive sonication is required to produce precipitin lines in double immunodiffusion (Kuo *et al.*, 1971).

VII. Growth Inhibition and Mycoplasmacidal Activity of Serum

The Mycoplasmatales are unique among prokaryotic cells in that their growth can be readily inhibited by specific antiserum.

A. *Inhibition of Colonial Growth on Agar*

Edward and Fitzgerald (1954) showed that growth of colonies on agar could be inhibited by antiserum and that this inhibition was species-specific. Clyde (1964) modified and popularized the method of Huijmans-Evers and Ruys (1956) and demonstrated that the organisms could readily be separated and identified as to species by inhibition of colonial growth on agar plates by paper disks impregnated with antiserum. The zones of inhibition resemble those observed in antibiotic sensitivity testing. The method was insensitive since large amounts of antibody were required for production of measurable zones. Early antibody produced poor zones of inhibition with *M. pneumoniae* though the sera produced precipitin lines and had high titers of complement-fixing antibody against lipid antigen (Kenny, 1971a). Late antibody appears generally to be required for most strains (Clyde, personal communication). Nevertheless, the insensitivity of the method may be advantageous since it masks small differences between strains and species. Inhibition does not require heat-labile factors in serum. This method has been employed to roughly quantitate the different species of organisms present in mixed cultures (Engel and Kenny, 1970).

B. Metabolic Inhibition Testing

Since some mycoplasmic species can reduce tetrazolium salts, the reduction of tetrazolium in broth cultures was used to measure antibody against *M. pneumoniae* (Senterfit and Jensen, 1966). Dilutions of antibody were mixed with fixed quantities of organisms in a medium containing tetrazolium and the most dilute antibody concentration which still prevented the changes in color (i.e., inhibited the metabolism of the organism) was chosen as the end point.

Metabolic inhibition methodologies have been devised for use with many mycoplasmic species using other metabolic indicators. Most species produce either an acid or alkaline reaction from an appropriate substrate (Aluotto *et al.*, 1970) which may be observed visually with an appropriate pH indicator. Glucose was used as the substrate for glycolytic species, arginine for argininolytic species, and urea for T strains (Purcell *et al.*, 1969). The end point of the test is taken as the greatest dilution of antibody which will prevent a change in color in the pH indicator which would normally occur with growth of the organism in the absence of antibody. This test is highly sensitive to the inoculum size as is inhibition of colonial growth on agar with the disk method. Fernald *et al.* (1967) altered the end point for *M. pneumoniae* and used the number of colony forming units of organism inhibited by a given dilution of serum as the end point of their assay. Complement is ordinarily not required in this test for most species though this point is controversial (Purcell *et al.*, 1969). Fernald *et al.* (1967) found that complement (heat-labile factors) enhanced inhibition of *M. pneumoniae* though some inhibition occurred in the absence of complement. The interaction with complement is difficult to establish since the test requires prolonged incubation in mycoplasmic medium which probably contains a number of anti-complementary factors. The same remarkable species specificity is observed with this test as is observed with disk inhibition on agar with few cross-reactions being observed between species (Purcell *et al.*, 1969). This method has additional advantages in that anti-medium antibody does not appear to give false positives. On the other hand, the presence of antibiotics in serum (which is likely in patients being treated for *M. pneumoniae* infections) may produce spurious inhibition of growth particularly with erythromycin.

C. Mycoplasmacidal Reactions

In both of the preceding assays, killing of the mycoplasmic cells is not essential for demonstration of the effects; inhibition of growth is all that is necessary. Barker and Patt (1967) showed that *M. gallisepticum* organisms could be eliminated from broth cultures by addition of antibody, a reaction that was dependent upon the presence of a heat-labile factor in immune serum or in normal guinea pig serum. The reaction was rapid, over 90% of the organisms being eliminated in 10 minutes or less. The heat-labile factor of guinea pig serum had a number of characteristics of complement in that it could be inhibited by chelating agents, absorbed by unrelated antigen antibody complexes, was temperature dependent and could not be removed by absorption of the guinea pig serum with organisms.

Mycoplasma pneumoniae was also demonstrated to be killed by antibody and complement (Gale and Kenny, 1970). Killing and not inhibition of organisms was judged to have occurred because the reaction could be stopped by dilution since it was much more dependent on complement concentration than on antibody concentration. Similar evidence for the heat-labile factor being complement was shown for this system as for *M. gallisepticum*. The reaction was profoundly temperature dependent since reaction mixtures could be held overnight in the cold without measurable killing occurring but killing was immediate when the reaction mixtures subsequently were incubated at 37°C. Substantial killing occurred with guinea pig serum alone, a phenomenon also noted by Fernald *et al.* (1967) in a metabolic inhibition type experiment and unheated guinea pig serum was also observed to release labeled DNA from organisms treated with complement (Coleman and Lynn, 1972). It is likely that the inhibitor in guinea pig serum is antibody. Similarly, unimmunized rabbits also had killing antibody to *M. pneumoniae*. Although this widespread evidence of antibody in laboratory animals may be somewhat alarming to considerations of specificity of this reaction, this antibody activity may be a result of antibody to glycolipids (see Section VII,B). Morphological evidence of destruction of *M. pneumoniae* by antibody and heat-labile factors was first noted by Bredt (1969) and has been shown ultrastructurally by Brunner *et al.* (1971).

Killing reactions mediated by heat-labile factors have been shown in a number of other species: *M. canis* (Tachibana *et al.*, 1970), *M. arthritidis* (Cole and Ward, 1973), *M. meleagridis* (Matsumoto and Yamamoto, 1973), and T strains (Lin and Kass, 1970). *Mycoplasma mycoides* is inactivated slowly by antibody and heat-labile factors (Gourlay and Domermuth, 1967). Thus the present evidence suggests that because a number of different species from different serotaxonomic groups are inactivated by antibody and complement, complement-mediated killing may be a general phenomenon in the Mycoplasmatales. This generalization may extend eventually to most membrane-bounded cells.

Neutralization of infectivity has been difficult to demonstrate with the chlamydiae (Jenkin *et al.*, 1961); a likely result of the fact that the cell membrane in the dense form is protected by the cell wall (Matsumoto and Manire, 1970). Neutralization of infectivity of *C. psittaci* can be greatly enhanced by the inclusion of anti-IgG into the neutralization mixture (Williams and Hahon, 1970).

VIII. Antigenic Structure

The information on the antigenic structure of both the chlamydiae and mycoplasmata is still strikingly limited in comparison to information on other microorganisms summarized in these volumes. However, although data on mycoplasmic antigens are still few, large advances have been made in the last several years [compare with earlier reviews by Kenny (1969b) and Lemcke (1969)]. The principle difficulties in mycoplasmic serology are the extraordinary heterogeneity observed in this group which precludes the use of any one species as a model system for fractionation of given types of antigens and the small amounts of material which can be produced. Similar problems exist with the chlamydiae, though the relatively greater antigenic similarity of the strains and species may simplify such studies though the ability to produce sufficient antigen for studies is even more difficult than with mycoplasmata.

A. Carbohydrate Antigens

A major antigenic component of *Mycoplasma mycoides* var. *mycoides* is a galactan (Plackett and Buttery, 1958). This antigenic component is remarkable in that the galactose residues are present in the antigen in furanose configuration (Plackett et al., 1963). The galactan may be located on the surface of the organisms particularly in "thread phase growth" (under certain conditions the organisms grow in culture as grossly visible filaments) where the material can be made more visible in the electron microscope by treatment with antiserum and resembles a capsule (Gourlay and Thrower, 1968). The galactan is best recognized serologically by the precipitin reaction, and it apparently fixes complement poorly (Cottew, 1960). In cattle, antigenemia has long been recognized and it is likely that some of the precipitin lines observed represent galactan though other antigens may be present (Gourlay, 1964).

Polysaccharides have also been isolated from bovine arthritis strains (Plackett et al., 1963) in the form of glucans. Recently a glucosamine-containing polymer has been recovered from *A. laidlawii* membranes and this component is apparently antigenic (Terry and Zupnik, 1973).

For other mycoplasmic species the existence of polysaccharide antigens is much less certain. Circumstantial evidence for a polysaccharide antigen in *M. pulmonis* has been described (Deeb and Kenny, 1967); a periodate labile, pronase stable component was described as a common antigen between subtypes of the species. Other species such as *M. gallisepticum* (Morowitz et al., 1962) and *M. hominis* (Hollingdale and Lemcke, 1969) appear to contain little, if any, polysaccharides, which would appear to affirm the fundamental heterogeneity of the Mycoplasmatales.

The group antigen of the chlamydiae, a lipid containing polysaccharide, is poorly soluble in water (Dhir et al., 1971) in contrast to the water solubility of bacterial lipopolysaccharides. This antigen is best detected by complement fixation. A polysaccharide hapten can be obtained by alkaline hydrolysis which is reactive in precipitation reactions, does not fix complement, but will inhibit complement fixation by untreated group antigen (Dhir et al., 1971). The major immunodominant group of this antigen appeared to be analogous but not identical to 2-keto-3-deoxyoctanoic acid from polysaccharides of salmonellae (Dhir *et al.*, 1972). The relationship of this antigen to the cell wall antigens demonstrated by Jenkin *et al.* (1961) is presently unknown. The cell wall antigen showed greater specificity after extraction with deoxycholate (which would presumably remove the lipopolysaccharide antigen) in that it reacted only with antiserum to the homologous strain and not the heterologous strain (meningopneumonitis and feline pneumonitis agents were compared). The group activity was also labile to periodate but the specific activity was stable (Jenkin *et al.*, 1961).

B. Lipid Antigens

1. *Mycoplasma pneumoniae*

The major antigen of *M. pneumoniae* was found in the lipid fraction of the organism (Kenny and Grayston, 1965). Antisera from humans naturally infected and from rabbits hyperimmunized with *M. pneumoniae* reacted strongly with the lipid fraction; in fact, the lipid fraction was a better serodiagnostic antigen than the whole organism. Serologically active lipid fractions were found to contain glucose and galactose when fractionated on silicic acid columns (Beckman and Kenny, 1968), though all serologically active fractions contained more than one glycolipid component. Further evidence for glycolipid structure was the fact that serologic activity could be destroyed by a mixture of carbohydrases and by periodate (Lemcke *et al.*, 1967). Upon more intensive fractionation a family of glyceroglycolipids was recovered including digalactosyl and trigalactosyl diglycerides and several other fractions which contained both glucose and galactose (Plackett *et al.*, 1969). The glycolipids were synthesized by the organisms, since radioactive glucose could be shown to be incorporated in the lipid fractions. A total of seven components were shown to be serologically active, some of which did not contain carbohydrate. Further analysis of the glycolipids of *M. pneumoniae* (strain AP-164) by gas–liquid chromatography of deacylated glycolipids indicates that five distinct components can be recognized (G. E. Kenny, unpublished data): one monoglycosyl compound (1/10 of total lipid), one diglycosyl compound (1/2), two triglycosyl compounds (1/3), and one tetraglycosyl compound (trace). The trigalactosyl fraction appeared to have the greatest serologic activity on a molar basis (Plackett *et al.*, 1969); the activity of tetraglycosyl compound has not been tested. Remarkable cross-reactions were observed with glycolipids from other sources: digalactosyl diglyceride from spinach showed a strong reaction with rabbit antiserum to *M. pneumoniae* as did diglucosyl diglyceride from *Streptococcus* MG (Plackett et al., 1969). These cross-reactions were further investigated by Kenny and Newton (1973). Although the digalactosyl diglyceride isolated from spinach reacted with some human sera, about half of the sera showed no reaction. A trace component was observed in the spinach glycolipids which had migration characteristics on thin-layer chromatography similar to the triglycosyl fraction from *M. pneumoniae*. Fractionation of spinach glycolipids by column chromatography on both silicic acid and DEAE-cellulose yielded a fraction that appeared to be a trigalactosyl diglyceride as judged by the retention time on gas–liquid chromatography of the deacylated glycolipids. Two components were observed in the trigalactosyl fraction, one of which had the same retention time as one of the triglycosyl compounds in *M. pneumoniae* (G. E. Kenny, unpublished data). When human sera were tested with the spinach triglycosyl fraction, nearly the same frequency of positives and the same height of antibody titers were observed as with crude *M. pneumoniae* lipid fractions (Kenny and Newton, 1973). The trigalactosyl fraction was at least 100 times more active than digalactosyl diglyceride when compared on a molar basis in a variety of complexing mixtures. Thus these data would tend to identify a major lipid antigen of *M. pneumoniae* as trigalactosyl diglyceride. Although digalactosyl diglyceride is broadly distributed in nature in chloroplasts of green plants (Benson, 1964), it is not presently known whether the trigalactosyl components have an equally broad distribution. Similarly, it will be of considerable interest to determine whether both of the spinach triglycosyl components are serologically active. The availability of an inexpensive source of glycolipid will do much to further efforts at determining the structure of this serologically active glycolipid.

Additional serologic cross-reactions have been observed with *M. pneumoniae* lipids. A reciprocal cross-reaction was observed between lipids of *M. pneumoniae* and *M. neurolyticum* (Kenny, 1971b). In fact *M. pneumoniae* infections could be diagnosed by use of *M. neurolyticum* lipids. It is interesting to note that this cross-reaction was only in the lipid fraction since the organisms appeared to share no immunoprecipitin lines (Kenny, 1969a). The nature of the cross-reacting lipids is presently unknown, though *M. neurolyticum* contains several glycolipids. Approximately half of human patients with *M. pneumoniae* pneumonia have antibody detectable with *Streptococcus* MG diglucosyl diglyceride (Kenny and Newton, 1973). It is interesting to note that diglucosyl diglyceride was not detected in *M. pneumoniae* by Plackett *et al.* (1969). Diglucosyl diglyceride (*Streptococcus* MG) and spinach digalactosyl diglycerides appear to represent different specificities, both of which appear to be different from the specificity of the spinach trigalactosyl fraction (Kenny and Newton, 1973). Biberfeld (1971) showed that persons infected with *M. pneumoniae* frequently had antibody to brain and more important to lipid fraction of brain and a variety of other tissues. This cross-reacting antibody could be reduced by absorption with *M. pneumoniae*. Possibly these antibodies are against glycolipid determinants, since monogalactosyl diglyceride has been recognized in brain, possibly indicating the presence of other glycolipids with longer carbohydrate chains.

A major problem for evaluating the significance of the various cross-reactions lies in the fact that it is very difficult to totally purify the glycolipids. Thus glycolipid fractions may be contaminated by trace amounts of other lipids which in fact are the serologically active components (Plackett *et al.*, 1969). For example, the much greater serologic activity of the trigalactosyl fraction compared to the digalactosyl fraction (Kenny and Newton, 1973) makes it difficult to rule out contamination by the digalactosyl fraction with the trigalactosyl fraction. Gas–liquid chromatography of deacylated glycolipids appears to be an excellent technique with which to examine the purity of glycolipids.

The purification of *M. pneumoniae* glycolipids was considerably complicated by the requirement for auxiliary lipids for demonstration of serologic activity. As glycolipids are purified away from natural glycolipids, serologic activity is lost unless auxiliary lipids such as lecithin and cholesterol are added (Plackett *et al.*, 1969). This problem was compounded by the fact that it has proved difficult to separate the glycolipids from the phospholipids (Beckman and Kenny, 1968; Razin *et al.*, 1970), thus some of the serologically active fractions tended to be regarded as phospholipids or glycophospholipids. Phosphatidyl glycerol was thought to be the serologically active component, but it was later found that the serologic activity was due to glycolipids but that phosphatidyl glycerol was an excellent auxiliary lipid (Razin *et al.*, 1970).

2. LIPID ANTIGENS IN OTHER MYCOPLASMIC SPECIES

The major complement-fixing antigen of *M. fermentans* is also found in the lipid fraction (Kenny, 1967, 1971b). That component appears to be a glycophospholipid with an apparent composition of 2 fatty acids, 1 phosphorus, 1 glucose, and 1 glycerol (G. E. Kenny, unpublished data). This conclusion has to be taken with considerable caution because of the possibility that the purified fraction may be an unresolved mixture of glycolipids and phospholipids. This fraction appears serologically unique among the *Mycoplasma* species thus far tested (Kenny, 1971b) though a comparison has not been made with the increasing number of bacterial glycophospholipids. This fraction is serologically active only when complexed with auxiliary lipid.

Diglucosyl diglyceride from *A. laidlawii* is serologically active and cross reacts with diglucosyl diglyceride from *Streptococcus* MG which is not surprising because it has the same structure (Plackett and Shaw, 1967). Since the lipid fraction of both *A. laidlawii* and closely related *A. granularum* represent only a minor portion of the serologic activity, it is likely that components other than lipid are the major antigens (Kenny, 1971b). *Acholeplasma laidlawii* also contains other glycolipids including monoglucosyl diglyceride and two glycophospholipids: glycerophosphoryl diglucosyl diglyceride (Shaw *et al.*, 1970) and phosphatidyl diglucosyl diglyceride (Smith, 1972). It is not known whether any of these compounds contribute to the serologic activity of lipids of *A. laidlawii*.

Although the preceding information may give the impression that lipid antigens might be characteristic of the Mycoplasmatales, such is not the case. Some limited surveys have been made and a number of species were found not to contain serologically active lipids or had only minor serologic activity in the lipid fractions (Kenny, 1967, 1971b). Those species were *M. pulmonis, M. hominis, M. pharyngis* (orale type 1), *M. orale* type II, *M. gallisepticum, M. canis, M. felis,* and *M. hyorhinis*. Little glycolipid was detected in those glycolytic strains which did not have serologically active lipids which would further verify that these organisms do not have major lipid antigens (G. E. Kenny, unpublished data) and which would stress the heterogeneity of the Mycoplasmatales.

3. LIPID ANTIGENS OF THE CHLAMYDIAE

The group antigen of the chlamydiae has lipid properties but was discussed in Section VIII,A because the lipid is more in the form of a lipopolysaccharide.

C. Protein Antigens

Although both mycoplasmata and chlamydiae are composed mostly of protein, very little information is available on defined protein an-

6. Antigens of the Mycoplasmatales and Chlamydiae

tigens in contrast to the more abundant, though still limited, information of lipids and carbohydrates. Antigenic studies of protein antigens have been handicapped in several areas: (1) only small amounts of material can be obtained, (2) the protein antigens are labile in contrast to the stability of carbohydrates and glycolipids, and (3) a major portion of the antigenic proteins in mycoplasmata is associated with the cell membrane which is hydrophobic and poorly separable. Similar conditions exist in the chlamydiae.

1. MEMBRANE ANTIGENS

The mycoplasmic cell has proved to be an excellent model for the study of membranes; since the organism has only one membrane, the external cell membrane and this membrane may account for 40% of cell protein. It is likely that organisms with thin filaments such as *M. pneumoniae* may have an even larger proportion of membrane protein. For antigenic analysis, however, the membranes have proved difficult to fractionate because of the hydrophobic nature of the membrane proteins and their consequent poor solubility. Solubilization with detergents gives an increasing risk of denaturation of the protein (Razin *et al.*, 1972).

However, progress has been made at fractionating membrane proteins, Ne'eman *et al.* (1972) showed that membrane antigens of *A. laidlawii* could be separated by gel filtration (Sephadex G-200) provided that the membranes were solubilized in deoxycholate and that the eluting solvent contained the same concentration of deoxycholate. When antisera were prepared in rabbits against equivalent concentrations of their four major components, only one of the fractions gave rise to antibody that inhibited the growth of the organisms on agar. The same fraction gave rise to maximum titers of antibody measurable by the metabolic inhibition test. All four fractions gave rise to equivalent amounts of antibody as detected by complement-fixation with membrane antigens. The antigens in the four fractions were also separable when tested by double immunodiffusion against membrane antibody.

Hollingdale and Lemcke (1969) prepared membrane and soluble fractions of *M. hominis*. The membrane fraction was responsible for induction of antibody measurable by metabolic inhibition testing whereas the cytoplasmic fraction had little activity. The serologic activity of the soluble fraction was also separable from that of the membrane fraction by double immunodiffusion reactions. Precipitin lines were only produced when detergents (Triton X-100 was considered best) were used for solubilization of membranes. Various strains of *M. hominis* could be differentiated in double immunodiffusion when membrane fractions were tested but not when soluble fractions were employed (Hollingdale and Lemcke, 1970). Four components were recognized in purified membranes by double immunodiffusion (Hollingdale and Lemcke, 1972). When the membranes were fractionated by polyacrylamide electrophoresis employing SDS for solubilization, 12 to 15 protein bands were observed. Antiserum was prepared to proteins eluted sections of the gel, and sera were obtained which were monospecific to two of the fractions, thus verifying the serologic differences shown by double immunodiffusion (Hollingdale and Lemcke, 1972). Pollack et al. (1970) prepared membrane and soluble fractions of M. pneumoniae by hypotonic lysis followed by differential centrifugation. Two components were recognized in the membrane fraction by double immunodiffusion against human convalescent serum. An additional component was recognized in the soluble fraction. The membrane fraction gave rise to antibody detectable by complement fixation with lipid antigen and metabolic inhibition testing. The soluble fraction gave rise to antibody that only reacted with phenol-treated antigen of Chanock et al. (1962).

2. MEMBRANE ROLE IN MYCOPLASMACIDAL AND GROWTH INHIBITION REACTIONS

The types of membrane antigens involved in mycoplasmacidal reactions have attracted substantial interest because the relevance of such antibodies toward immunity. Additionally, from the biologic viewpoint, the mycoplasmacidal activity of antibody may be used as a probe to detect surface antigens on the organism. It is clear that the rapidity of the complement-mediated killing reaction of mycoplasmata indicates clearly that a surface reaction is involved. It has also been assumed that metabolic inhibition testing reveals surface antigens; however, it is not as clear that growth inhibition on agar also demonstrates surface antigens.

The fact that the major antigens of M. pneumoniae are lipid and that lipids were strongly associated with mycoplasmic membranes prompted a study of the role of lipid in mycoplasmacidal and metabolic inhibition reactions. Antibody titers in both human and animal antisera measured by complement fixation with crude lipid antigen correlated strongly with antibody levels measured by the complement-mediated killing test (Gale and Kenny, 1970). Similarly antibody titers in human serum measured by complement fixation with lipid correlated well with titers measured by metabolic inhibition (Senterfit et al., 1973). Razin et al. (1970, 1971) demonstrated conclusively that lipids were sites for metabolic inhibition activity of antibody. They prepared antiserum by reaggregating glycolipids of *M. pneumoniae* with defatted membranes of *A. laidlawii*. These two organisms show little or no serologic cross-reaction (Kenny, 1969a). Antiserum against the hybridized material produced metabolic inhibition with *M. pneumoniae*, whereas antibody to *A. laidlawii* membranes did not inhibit. Immunization with glycolipids alone did not give rise to antibody measurable in any test. Thus these results indicate the glycolipids may be a major or perhaps the major surface determinant of *M. pneumoniae*. Since many other *Mycoplasma* species do not have lipid antigens (Kenny, 1971b), their antigenic determinants for metabolic inhibition testing can hardly be lipid. Although *A. laidlawii* possesses some minor serologic activity which is found in the lipid fraction, the immunogen responsible for inducing antibodies measurable by metabolic inhibition tests appears to be protein (Razin *et al.*, 1972). Similarly protein appears to be the immunogen for induction of metabolism-inhibiting antibody against *M. hominis* (Hollingdale and Lemcke, 1972). The major complement-fixing antigens of *M. pulmonis* appear to be heat-stable proteins that have subspecies specificities (Deeb and Kenny, 1967). These antigens do not appear to be responsible for disk inhibition on agar, but could have some role in the antigenic heterogeneity seen in that group by metabolic-inhibition testing (Haller *et al.*, 1973).

3. Cytoplasmic Antigens

Little progress has been made at the separation of cytoplasmic constituents from the organism. The principle difficulty lies in the fact that membrane fragments of widely varying size are produced during most efforts at breaking the organism, and these fragments cause extensive contamination of cytoplasmic components. Additionally, the membrane appears to be the most immunogenic portion of the organism (Kenny, 1971a). Antibody has been induced against a cytoplasmic enzyme, arginine deiminase (Gill and Pan, 1970); the arginine deiminase from *M. gallinarum* could be differentiated serologically from arginine deiminase of *M. hominis* and *M. arginini* (Hahn and Kenny, 1974).

Acknowledgments

Some of the studies cited in this chapter were supported in part by grants AI-06720, AI-09586, AI 10695, and AI-10743 from the National Institute of Allergy and Infectious Diseases, National Institutes of Health and were supported in part by the U. S. Army Medical Research and Development Command, Department of the Army under research contract No. DA-49-193-MD-2294.

References

Aluotto, B. B., Wittler, R. G., Williams, C. O., and Faber, J. E. (1970). *Int. J. Syst. Bacteriol.* **20**, 35.
Barker, L. F., and Patt, J. K. (1967). *J. Bacteriol.* **94**, 403.
Becker, Y. (1972). *Isr. J. Med. Sci.* **8**, 1134.
Beckman, B. L., and Kenny, G. E. (1968). *J. Bacteriol.* **96**, 1171.
Benson, A. A. (1964). *Annu. Rev. Plant Physiol.* **15**, 1.
Biberfeld, G. (1971). *Clin. Exp. Immunol.* **8**, 319.
Biberfeld, G., and Biberfeld, P. (1970). *J. Bacteriol.* **102**, 855.
Boatman, E. S., and Kenny, G. E. (1970). *J. Bacteriol.* **101**, 262.
Boatman, E. S., and Kenny, G. E. (1971a). *J. Bacteriol.* **106**, 1005.
Boatman, E. S., and Kenny, G. E. (1971b). *Proc. Electron Microsc. Soc. Amer.* **29**, 258.
Bredt, W. (1968). *Pathol. Microbiol.* **32**, 321.
Bredt, W. (1969). *Experientia* **25**, 436.
Brunner, H., Razin, S., Kalica, A. R., and Chanock, R. M. (1971). *J. Immunol.* **104**, 907.
Chanock, R. M., James, W. D., Fox, H. H., Turner, H. C., Mufson, M. A., and Hayflick, L. (1962). *Proc. Soc. Exp. Biol. Med.* **110**, 884.
Clyde, W. A. (1964). *J. Immunol.* **92**, 958.
Cole, B. C., and Ward, J. R. (1973). *Infec. Immunity* **8**, 199.
Coleman, L. H., and Lynn, R. J. (1972). *Proc. Soc. Exp. Biol. Med.* **140**, 383.
Collier, A. M. (1972). *In* "Pathogenic Mycoplasmas," pp. 307–319. Elsevier, Amsterdam.
Cottew, G. S. (1960). *Aust. Vet. J.* **36**, 54.
Deeb, B. J., and Kenny, G. E. (1967). *J. Bacteriol.* **93**, 1425.
Dhir, S. P., Kenny, G. E., and Grayston, J. T. (1971). *Infec. Immunity* **4**, 725.
Dhir, S. P., Hakomori, S. I., Kenny, G. E., and Grayston, J. T. (1972). *J. Immunol.* **109**, 116.
Edward, D. G. ff., and Fitzgerald, W. A. (1954). *J. Pathol. Bacteriol.* **68**, 23.
Edward, D. G. ff., and Freundt, E. A. (1956). *J. Gen. Microbiol.* **14**, 197.
Edward, D. G. ff., and Freundt, E. A. (1969a). *In* "The Mycoplasmatales and L-phase of Bacteria" (L. Hayflick, ed.), pp. 147–200. Appleton, New York.
Edward, D. G. ff., and Freundt, E. A. (1969b). *J. Gen. Microbiol.* **57**, 391.
Edward, D. G. ff., and Freundt, E. A. (1970). *J. Gen. Microbiol.* **62**, 1.
Edward, D. G. ff., and Freundt, E. A. (1973). *Int. J. Syst. Bacteriol.* **23**, 55.
Engel, L. D., and Kenny, G. E. (1970). *J. Peridontal Res.* **5**, 163.
Fernald, G. W., Clyde, W. A., and Denny, F. W. (1967). *Proc. Soc. Exp. Biol. Med.* **126**, 161.
Gale, J. L., and Kenny, G. E. (1970). *J. Immunol.* **104**, 1175.
Gerloff, R. K., Ritter, D. B., and Watson, R. O. (1966). *J. Infec. Dis.* **116**, 1966.
Gill, P., and Pan, J. (1970). *Can. J. Microbiol.* **16**, 415.
Gourlay, R. N. (1964). *Res. Vet. Sci.* **5**, 473.
Gourlay, R. N., and Domermuth, C. H. (1967). *Ann. N. Y. Acad. Sci.* **143**, 325.

6. Antigens of the Mycoplasmatales and Chlamydiae 477

Gourlay, R. N., and Thrower, K. J. (1968). *J. Gen. Microbiol.* **54**, 155.
Hahn, R. G., and Kenny, G. E. (1974). *J. Bacteriol.* **117**, 611.
Haller, G. J., Boiarski, K. W., and Somerson, N. L. (1973). *J. Infec. Dis.* **127**, S38.
Higashi, N. (1965). *Exp. Mol. Pathol.* **4**, 24.
Hollingdale, M. R., and Lemcke, R. M. (1969). *J. Hyg.* **67**, 585.
Hollingdale, M. R., and Lemcke, R. M. (1970). *J. Hyg.* **68**, 469.
Hollingdale, M. R., and Lemcke, R. M. (1972). *J. Hyg.* **70**, 85.
Huijmans-Evers, A. G. M., and Ruys, A. C. (1956). *Antonie van Leeuwenhoek; J. Microbiol. Serol.* **22**, 377.
Jenkin, H. M. (1960). *J. Bacteriol.* **80**, 639.
Jenkin, H. M., Ross, M. R., and Moulder, J. W. (1961). *J. Immunol.* **86**, 123.
Kenny, G. E. (1967). *Ann. N. Y. Acad. Sci.* **143**, 676.
Kenny, G. E. (1969a). *J. Bacteriol.* **98**, 1044.
Kenny, G. E. (1969b). *In* "Analytic Serology of Microorganisms" (J. B. G. Kwapinski, ed.), Vol. I, pp. 185–202. Wiley, New York.
Kenny, G. E. (1971a). *Infec. Immunity*, 3, 510.
Kenny, G. E. (1971b). *Infec. Immunity*, 4, 149.
Kenny, G. E. (1973a). *In* "Contamination in Tissue Culture" (J. Fogh, ed.), pp. 107–129. Academic Press, New York.
Kenny, G. E. (1973b). *J. Infec. Dis.* **127**, S2.
Kenny, G. E., and Grayston, J. T. (1965). *J. Immunol.* **95**, 19.
Kenny, G. E., and Newton, R. M. (1973). *Ann. N. Y. Acad. Sci.* **225**, 54.
Kuo, C. C., Kenny, G. E., and Wang, S. P. (1971). *In* "Trachoma and Related Disorders" (R. L. Nichols, ed.), pp. 112–123. Excerpta Med. Found., Amsterdam.
Laurell, C. B. (1965). *Anal. Biochem.* **10**, 358.
Lemcke, R. M. (1965). *J. Gen. Microbiol.* **38**, 91.
Lemcke, R. M. (1969). *In* "The Mycoplasmatales and L-phase of Bacteria" (L. Hayflick, ed.), pp. 265–281. Appleton, New York.
Lemcke, R. M. (1972). *J. Bacteriol.* **110**, 1154.
Lemcke, R. M., Marmion, B. P., and Plackett, P. (1967). *Ann. N. Y. Acad. Sci.* **143**, 691.
Lin, J. S., and Kass, E. H. (1970). *J. Infec. Dis.* **122**, 93.
Low, I. E., and Eaton, M. D. (1965). *J. Bacteriol.* **89**, 725.
Maniloff, J., and Morowitz, H. J. (1967). *Ann. N. Y. Acad. Sci.* **143**, 59.
Maniloff, J., and Morowitz, H. J. (1972). *Bacteriol. Rev.* **36**, 263.
Matsumoto, A., and Manire, G. P. (1970). *J. Bacteriol.* **101**, 278.
Matsumoto, M., and Yamamoto, R. (1973). *J. Infec. Dis.* **127**, S43.
Milgrom, F., and Witebsky, E. (1960). *J. Amer. Med. Ass.* **174**, 56.
Morowitz, H. J., Tourtellotte, M. E., Guild, W. R., Castro, E., and Woese, C. (1962). *J. Mol. Biol.* **4**, 93.
Moulder, J. W. (1970). *J. Bacteriol.* **104**, 1189.
Ne'eman, Z., Kahane, I., Kovartovsky, J., and Razin, S. (1972). *Biochim. Biophys. Acta* **266**, 255.
Neimark, H. C. (1970). *J. Gen. Microbiol.* **63**, 249.
Organick, A. B., Siegesmund, K. A., and Lutsky, I. I. (1966). *J. Bacteriol.* **92**, 1164.
Page, L. A. (1966). *Int. J. Syst. Bacteriol.* **16**, 223.
Page, L. A. (1968). *Int. J. Syst. Bacteriol.* **18**, 51.
Pirie, N. W. (1969). *In* "The Mycoplasmatales and L-phase of Bacteria" (L. Hayflick, ed.), pp. 3–14. Appleton, New York.
Plackett, P., and Buttery, S. H. (1958). *Nature (London)* **182**, 1236.

Plackett, P., and Shaw, E. J. (1967). *Biochem. J.* **104**, 61c.
Plackett, P., Buttery, S. H., and Cottew, G. S. (1963). *In* "Recent Progress in Microbiology" (N. E. Gibbons, ed.), pp. 535–547, Univ. of Toronto Press, Toronto.
Plackett, P., Marmion, B. P., Shaw, E. J., and Lemcke, R. M. (1969). *Aust. J. Exp. Biol. Med. Sci.* **47**, 171.
Pollack, J. D., Somerson, N. L., and Senterfit, L. B. (1969). *J. Bacteriol.* **97**, 612.
Pollack, J. D., Somerson, N. L., and Senterfit, L. B. (1970). *Infec. Immunity* **2**, 326.
Pollock, M. E. (1965). *J. Bacteriol.* **90**, 1682.
Pollock, M. E., and Bonner, S. V. (1969). *Bacteriol. Proc.*, p. 32.
Purcell, R. H., Chanock, R. M., and Taylor-Robinson, D. (1969). *In* "The Mycoplasmatales and L-phase of Bacteria" (L. Hayflick, ed.), pp. 221–264. Appleton, New York.
Purcell, R. H., Valdesuso, J. R., Cline, W. L., James, W. D., and Chanock, R. M. (1970). *Appl. Microbiol.* **21**, 288.
Razin, S., Prescott, B., Caldes, G., James, W. D., and Chanock, R. M. (1970). *Infec. Immunity*, **1**, 408.
Razin, S., Prescott, B., James, W. D., Caldes, G., Valdesuso, J., and Chanock, R. M. (1971). *Infec. Immunity*, **3**, 420.
Razin, S., Kahane, I., and Kovartovsky, J. (1972). *In* "Pathogenic Mycoplasmas," pp. 93–122. Elsevier, Amsterdam.
Rodwell, A. (1969). *In* "The Mycoplasmatales and L-phase of Bacteria" (L. Hayflick, ed.), pp. 413–449. Appleton, New York.
Senterfit, L. B., and Jensen, K. E. (1966). *Proc. Soc. Exp. Biol. Med.* **122**, 786.
Senterfit, L. B., Pollack, J. D., and Somerson, N. L. (1973). *Proc. Soc. Exp. Biol. Med.* **140**, 1294.
Sharpless, N. S., and LoGrippo, G. A. (1965). *Henry Ford Hosp. Med. Bull.* **13**, 55.
Shaw, N., Smith, P. F., and Verheij, H. M. (1970). *Biochem. J.* **120**, 439.
Smith, P. F. (1971). "The Biology of Mycoplasmas," pp. 1–232. Academic Press, New York.
Smith, P. F. (1972). *Biochim. Biophys. Acta* **280**, 375.
Smith, P. F. (1973). *J. Infec. Dis.* **127**, S8.
Somerson, N. L., James, W. D., Walls, B. B., and Chanock, R. M. (1967). *Ann. N. Y. Acad. Sci.* **143**, 384.
Tachibana, D. K., Hayflick, L., and Rosenberg, L. T. (1970). *J. Infec. Dis.* **121**, 541.
Tamura, A., and Manire, G. P. (1967). *J. Bacteriol.* **94**, 1184.
Tamura, A., Matsumoto, A., Manire, G. P., and Higashi, N. (1971). *J. Bacteriol.* **105**, 355.
Taylor-Robinson, D., and Manchee, R. J. (1967). *J. Bacteriol.* **94**, 1781.
Terry, T. M., and Zupnik, J. S. (1973). *Biochim. Biophys. Acta* **291**, 144.
Thirkill, C. E., and Kenny, G. E. (1974). *Infec. Immunity* **10**, 624.
Wang, S. P., and Grayston, J. T. (1971). *In* "Trachoma and Related Disorders" (R. L. Nichols, ed.), pp. 305–321. Excerpta Med. Found., Amsterdam.
Weiss, E. (1971). *In* "Trachoma and Related Disorders" (R. L. Nichols, ed.), pp. 3–12. Excerpta Med. Found., Amsterdam.
Williams, C. O., Wittler, R. G., and Burris, C. (1969). *J. Bacteriol.* **99**, 341.
Williams, T. D., and Hahon, N. (1970). *Infec. Immunity* **2**, 7.

CHAPTER 7

Virus Infections and the Immune Responses They Elicit

WILLIAM H. BURNS AND
ANTHONY C. ALLISON

I.	Introduction	480
II.	Viral Antigens	483
	A. Introduction	483
	B. Herpesviruses	484
	C. Adenoviruses	485
	D. Orthomyxoviruses	489
	E. Paramyxoviruses	494
	F. Togaviruses	495
	G. Rhabdoviruses	496
	H. Murine Leukemogenic Viruses	498
III.	Humoral Responses	500
	A. Sequence of IgM and IgG Responses	500
	B. Elicitation of Specific Immunoglobulin Classes	504
	C. Genetic Control of Antiviral Antibody Responses	505
	D. Genetic Control of Virus-Induced Diseases	505
IV.	Secretory Antibody Responses	506
V.	Thymus Dependence of Viral Antigens	507
VI.	B Lymphocyte Memory and "Original Antigenic Sin"	510
VII.	Neutralization	512
	A. Mechanisms of Neutralization	512
	B. Complement-Dependent Neutralization	515
	C. Infectious Complexes and Antiglobulin Neutralization	517
VIII.	Capacity of Macrophages to Support Virus Replication	519
IX.	Ontogeny of Macrophage Resistance to Viral Infections	522
X.	Surface Changes of Virus-Infected Cells	524
	A. Virus-Coded Antigens	524
	B. Alteration of Host Antigens or Receptors	528
	C. Capping of Viral Antigens	530
	D. Antigenic Modulation	531

E. Possible Combinations of Host and Viral Antigenic Determinants	531
XI. Evidence for Cell-Mediated Immunity to Viral Antigens	532
A. Introduction	532
B. Poxviruses	533
C. Herpesviruses	535
D. Myxoviruses	536
E. Paramyxoviruses	536
F. Murine Leukemogenic Viruses	538
G. Togaviruses	539
H. Arenaviruses	540
XII. Persistence of Immunity to Viruses	541
XIII. Tolerance to Viral Antigens	543
XIV. Cooperative Effects of Viral Antigens on Immunogenicity	546
XV. Influences of Virus Infections on Immune Responses	549
XVI. Concluding Remarks	557
References	559

I. Introduction

The immune responses elicited by animal viruses are of historical interest as well as current practical importance. The science of immunology can be said to have been founded by Edward Jenner, who in his well known "An enquiry into the causes and effects of the variolae vaccinia," published in 1798, described the inoculation of variolous matter into the arm of Mary Barge, who had previously had cow pox. He noted: "It is remarkable that variolous matter, when the system is disposed to reject it, should excite inflammation more speedily than when it produces the Small Pox." This is the first description of delayed hypersensitivity, and reactions to vaccination and rashes produced by virus infections were taken as examples of allergic reactions by von Pirquet (1907) in his pioneering study of allergy.

Since most virus infections cannot yet be treated by chemotherapy, immunoprophylaxis and isolation of cases have been the only effective ways to control virus diseases. The important epidemiologic consequences of the use of vaccines against smallpox, yellow fever, and poliovirus are well known, and it seems likely that vaccines against measles and rubella virus will also reduce the incidence of these diseases. In the veterinary field, vaccines against canine distemper, canine hepatitis, hog cholera, and Newcastle disease and Marek's disease of chickens have been highly effective. Thus, the immunogenicity of animal viruses is of considerable practical impor-

7. Virus Infections and Immune Responses

tance, and an enormous amount of information has accumulated on antibody formation in a wide range of animal forms inoculated with viruses or virus vaccines.

As expected, small viruses with low contents of nucleic acid and relatively simple structures have few antigens while large viruses, with greater contents of nucleic acid and complex structures, such as herpesviruses and poxviruses, have many antigens. With small viruses and viruses of intermediate size, such as adenoviruses or myxoviruses, the relationship between major antigens and the subunits assembled into intact virions is better understood. In this chapter only a few representative examples can be selected for discussion, to illustrate certain general principles concerning the immunogenicity of animal viruses and in what way they resemble or differ from responses to other antigens. Brief descriptions of the structures and known antigens of selected viruses will be followed by an account of the humoral and secretory responses elicited by them.

Unexpected results were obtained in the course of studies of immune responses to influenza viruses sharing some antigens but differing in others. It was found that following exposure to one such virus, infection by the second virus often elicited a stronger immune response against the first virus than the second. This phenomenon of "original antigenic sin" was one of the first examples of immunologic memory to be studied systematically, and only recently has the underlying cellular mechanism been investigated. The problem of memory formation in T and B lymphocytes to thymus-dependent and thymus-independent antigens is currently under vigorous investigation and observations on the sequential responses to cross-reacting viral antigens may be pertinent to this problem. The thymus dependence of viral antigens is also under study and results will be presented.

The most commonly studied immune responses to viruses are neutralizing antibodies in serum. The high sensitivity and precision of assays based on neutralization of plaque-forming viruses make this an excellent model system, and much information of general interest has emerged from its use. Neutralization itself has proved to be a complex phenomenon which is not yet fully understood. Among the features that have been studied and will be described are the sequence of appearance and neutralizing capacity of different classes of immunoglobulins, the avidity of antibodies, the additional effects of complement components, and the existence of infectious complexes of viruses and antibody.

Macrophages are implicated at many points in immune responses, especially in antigen processing and presentation and possibly in B and T lymphocyte interactions. They can interact directly with viruses and microorganisms and can mediate cytotoxic reactions against tumor cells and cells infected with viruses or intracellular parasites. The capacity of macrophages to support virus replication and thus spread infection, or to degrade virus and aid in recovery from infection will be discussed. The ontogeny of this virucidal capacity will be reviewed with emphasis on the influence of the thymus, either hormonally or through T lymphocytes and their products.

The interaction of sensitized lymphocytes with infected cells requires cell surface changes recognizable by the lymphocytes. Virus-induced surface changes have been described during infection for most viruses studied. Some of these represent new proteins or glycoproteins encoded in the virus genome, while others result from rearrangement of host material or derepression of host genes. The appearance of "new" host antigens or receptors (including Fc receptors) and the diminution of normally present antigens (including histocompatibility antigens) have been reported. Antigenic modulation, capping, and other phenomena previously described for nonviral cell surface antigens are also found with viral antigens and will be described.

Delayed hypersensitivity has been observed in many virus infections, and more recently *in vitro* studies have confirmed the existence of cell-mediated immune responses to viral antigens. These were regarded as little more than curiosities until children born with selective deficiencies of T cell function were found to be unduly susceptible to vaccinia virus, herpesviruses, and measles virus infections, while children with severe hypogammaglobulinemia generally are not. Observations of experimental animals confirm this importance of cell-mediated immunity in protection against certain virus infections but not others (reviewed by Allison and Burns, 1972; Allison, 1974). Thus, for some viruses, eliciting a powerful cell-mediated response is an important aspect of immunogenicity. A summary will be presented of the evidence for cell-mediated immune responses for viral antigens, particularly of observations made *in vitro*.

The fact that infections such as measles, varicella, and mumps usually occur only once had been known to medical practitioners for centuries, and when these were identified as caused by viruses it became clear that viruses are able to induce long-lasting immunity.

Two explanations have been put forward for prolonged antibody production in the absence of reinfection: persistence of virus in the host (Olitsky and Long, 1929a,b) and persistence of clones of immunocompetent cells (Burnet, 1959). Both explanations are true. The latter phenomenon is well known and evidence for virus persistence will be presented.

The observations of Traube on lymphocytic choriomeningitis infections in mice provided some of the evidence that led Burnet to postulate the existence of immunologic tolerance. In mice congenitally infected with this virus, antibody is not demonstrable in the serum, but during the last few years it has been shown that complexes of antibody and virus-specific antigen accumulate in the kidneys, giving rise to an immunopathological glomerulonephritis. Similar observations have been made with murine leukemogenic viruses. Thus the animals are not completely unresponsive to viral antigens. Cooperative phenomena, perhaps of a hapten-carrier nature and possibly responsible for some autoimmune phenomena, will be discussed.

In the same monograph in which he described reactions to vaccination and rashes produced by virus infections as allergic reactions, von Pirquet (1907) drew attention to the depression of reactions to tuberculin which occur during measles infections, the first report of suppression of an immune response by a virus. Certain virus infections (as with LDV, measles virus, the thymic agent) can dramatically affect the immune system. In addition to having important clinical consequences, these infections should be considered when interpreting laboratory studies of immune responses. Intercurrent virus infections occur in most animal colonies (especially Sendai virus, minute virus of mice, mouse pneumonitis virus). Mouse hepatitis virus can behave much like an endogenous virus, being undetectable until animals are immunosuppressed, and is frequently found in nude mice. Most passaged tumors carry LDV and other viruses. The effects of some of these virus infections on immune responses will be discussed.

II. Viral Antigens

A. Introduction

Viruses vary considerably in their structural and antigenic complexity. In a few cases their structures are known and their antigens well characterized and related to the virion structure, e.g., with adenovirus and influenza virus described below. With small viruses such as the enteroviruses, the antigenic composition is relatively simple. In each of the three types of poliovirus, for instance, two antigens are distinguishable by immunodiffusion and complement fixation (CF). Infectious virions containing RNA have a D (dense) antigen whereas noninfectious particles have a C (coreless) antigen (Hummeler et al., 1962). The D antigen can be converted to C antigen by denaturation, so that the C antigen can be regarded as a protein that has not attained or retained the D configuration brought about in the complete virion by association with the RNA-containing core. A third antigen, the S antigen, can be obtained by guanidine degradation of the virus and is probably a protein precursor of the virus coat (Scharff and Lewinton, 1963). Humans infected with poliovirus develop type-specific antibodies against C and D antigens, but only the latter neutralize the virus. In the following sections, the structures and antigens of more complicated viruses — adenovirus, influenza virus, paramyxoviruses, togaviruses, rhabdoviruses, and the herpesviruses — will be described.

B. Herpesviruses

Herpesviruses form a family of large enveloped viruses of 1800–2000 Å size with genomes of double-stranded DNA having $G + C$ contents ranging for different members from 33% to 72% (Plummer et al., 1969). The herpesviruses naturally infecting man tend to produce latent infections and focal cytopathology and are divided into four groups: (1) herpes simplex (HSV), (2) cytomegaloviruses (CMV), (3) varicellazoster (V-Z), and (4) Epstein–Barr (EB) virus. All of these viruses multiply in the cell nucleus where the naked icosohedral nucleocapsids can be seen and acquire their envelopes when budding through the inner lamella of the nuclear membrane or during their egress through the membranes of the endoplasmic reticulum. Shortly after infection, host DNA and protein synthesis cease as that of the virus commences. Viral membrane protein synthesis begins before viral DNA synthesis, and glycosylation of the virus proteins occurs in the membrane and is accomplished by host enzymes. HSV virions contain at least 24 virus-specific proteins and, although earlier studies showed HSV could be agglutinated by antisera made against the uninfected host cell (Watson and Wildy, 1963), recent studies reveal essentially no host proteins in the virion (see review by Roizman and Heine, 1972).

Most viral structural proteins, including glycoproteins, are made during the first two hours of infection before the viral DNA replication begins. Many structural proteins for HSV and EB virus, and perhaps all herpesviruses, thus represent the products of "early function" genes, and this situation differs from that usually found with bacteriophages and the papova viruses, where structural proteins are coded for by "late" genes that are transcribed after viral DNA replication. The protein portions of the membrane glycoproteins are virus-coded (Olshevsky and Becker, 1972) and genetic variants of these proteins determine such membrane phenomena as the "social behavior" of HSV, i.e., whether infected cells fuse with contiguous cells or clump. Two types of HSV are recognized and evidence has been presented for a type-specific glycoprotein, present in infected cells and on the virion surface, that can interact with antibody and result in virus neutralization (Cohen et al., 1972; Powell et al., 1974).

C. Adenoviruses

The adenoviruses are DNA viruses having icosohedral symmetry. There are at least 33 human types (Blacklow et al., 1969), and Rosen has divided them into 3 subgroups (see Table I) according to hemagglutination (HA) characteristics (Rosen, 1960). Norrby (1969a) and Schlesinger (1969) have reviewed the structure and biology of adenoviruses. About 18% of the virus protein is associated with DNA in a central nucleoid (Laver et al., 1967) which is surrounded by an outer protein coat, the capsid. The capsid contains 252 polygonal capsomeres—240 hexons forming triangular facets and 12 apices made up of pentons (Figs. 1 and 2). Each penton consists of a vertex

TABLE I

Classification of Adenoviruses

Subgroup	Serotypes	Hemagglutination	
		Rhesus	Rat
I	3,7,11,14,16,20,21,25,28	+	0
II	8,9,10,13,15,17,19,22,23,24,26,27,29,30	±	+
III	1,2,4,5,6,12,18	0	±[a]

[a] Partial agglutination, enhanced by heterotypic immune sera.

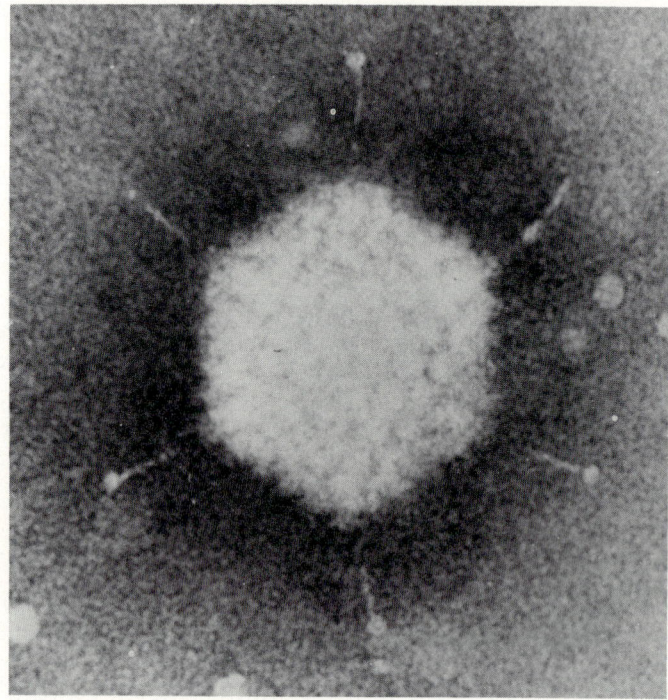

Fig. 1. Electron micrograph of adenovirus type 5, negatively stained. ×500,000. Courtesy of the late R. Valentine.

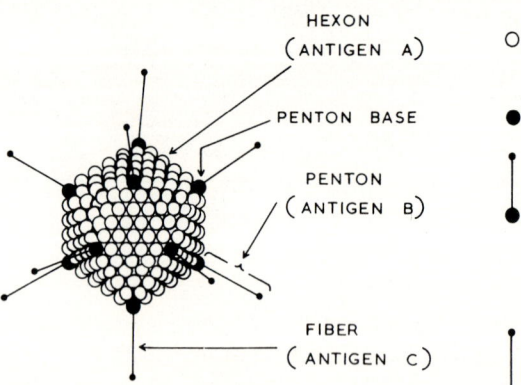

Fig. 2. Diagram of the structure of adenovirus showing the position in the virion of various components. Courtesy of H. Pereira.

capsomere (penton base) and an attached knobbed fiber. Hexons and pentons can be isolated from soluble products of infected cells or after disruption of virions. Originally, three antigens were described: a complement-fixing hexon group antigen (A antigen) common to all adenoviruses except the avian GAL virus, a penton group antigen (B antigen) toxic to cells, and a type-specific fiber antigen (C antigen).

With the awareness that antigenic sites on the intact virion may differ from some of those determined by immunization with spontaneously occurring soluble components, and that there are subpopulations of hexons of particular serotypes (Wadell, 1972), detailed analyses of adenovirus antigenic structure have been carried out using purified capsid subunits and specific antisera in absorption and HA studies. The subunits have varying capacities for HA: hexons and vertex capsomeres show no such capacity whereas all pentons and the fibers of subgroups II and III show partial HA. The latter is due to the univalency of these particles since dimers of pentons and fibers (at least in the case of subgroup III) show complete HA. Heterotypic sera, which can react with group or subgroup antigens on the fibers or vertex capsomeres can enhance HA by aggregating fibers or pentons into polyvalent complexes; this is termed the hemagglutination enhancement (HE) test. Vertex capsomeres can be identified by their ability to absorb HE antibody and thus decrease the HA normally found when a standard preparation of pentons is subsequently added; this is termed the HE antibody consumption (HEC) test.

Hexons appear to contain several antigens. The α (A) antigen is group-specific and detected in CF tests. The hexon α antigen appears to be located on the inner aspect of the capsid since antibody to it lacks HI activity and cannot be seen on ultrastructural examination (Norrby et al., 1969); moreover, processes that disrupt the virion result in increased CF activity (Smith, 1965). The presence of a type-specific antigen, ϵ, was suggested by the surprising finding that only anti-hexon sera contain neutralizing antibody (Wilcox and Ginsberg, 1963; Kjellen and Pereira, 1968). Antibody to α antigen can be absorbed with heterotypic virus or hexons, leaving homotypic (anti-ϵ) antibody which is active in hemagglutination inhibition and neutralization assays. Using negative staining, this antibody has been shown to attach to the outer surface of hexons in intact virions (Norrby et al., 1969). Agglutination of virions was prominent and might account for the HI activity of this antibody. Another possible mechanism for this HI activity is steric hindrance of the fiber hemagglutinin by antibody attached to paravertex hexons; this latter mechanism is supported by the finding that the HI activity of different anti-hexon sera was inversely related to the fiber length of the viruses tested (Norrby and Wadell, 1969). Serotypes of subgroup III, with the exception of type 4 virus, differ from those of subgroups I and II in that hexons of the latter are considerably more efficient in the induction of neutralizing antibody. Antibodies to subgroup III hexons do attach to the hexons as shown by their ability to sensitize the virus to neutralization by antiglobulin antisera (Wadell, 1972). Absorption tests suggest that hexons possess minor intrasubgroup antigens as well as α and ϵ (Norrby and Wadell, 1969).

Haase and Pereira (1972) have recently demonstrated neutralizing capacity of antibody directed against the hexon ϵ antigen of adenovirus type 2. Crystallized hexons of adenovirus type 5 were coupled to Sepharose and an immunoadsorbent column prepared. Antisera to purified hexons of adenovirus type 2 were then passed over the column to adsorb group-specific (anti-α) antibody. The unbound material possessed neutralizing ability against type 2 virus but not type 5 virus. The subsequently eluted antibody neutralized neither virus. This elegant experiment demonstrates that the type-specific (ϵ) antigen is the crucial hexon antigen involved in neutralization.

Pentons can be separated into their fibers and vertex capsomeres by guanidine treatment. Vertex capsomeres have a group-specific β (B) antigen. Toxin activity is associated with these capsomeres and its neutralization is group-specific. Absorption experiments using HEC test suggested subgroup and some intersubgroup specificity (Wadell and Norrby, 1969). Recently, studies using antiglobulin to enhance neutralization of virions sensitized with antisera to vertex capsomeres confirmed this and indicated that vertex capsomeres in intact virions have subgroup specificities not found in the monomeric soluble subunits (Norrby and Wadell, 1972).

All fibers contain a type-specific γ (C) antigen which on ultrastructural examination is located at the distal (knobbed) end (Norrby et al., 1969) and can participate in CF and HI reactions. Antibody to the fibers of all serotypes are able to sensitize the virus to neutralization by antiglobulin and perhaps to neutralize directly. Fibers of subgroups II and III also contain an intrasubgroup specific antigen, δ, located proximally; it cannot react with antibody if the vertex capsomere is attached. It is this antigen which is active in HE tests. Some intersubgroup specificity has also been detected (Wadell and Norrby, 1969).

Wigand and Fliedner (1968) observed that some adenovirus strains react differently in HI and neutralization tests, suggesting they might be intermediate strains. The two type-specific antigens, γ and ε, can be differentiated in HI tests using soluble and virion-associated hemagglutinin, respectively. Such analyses have been reported for two strains, and the HI antigen specificity was related to the fibers and the neutralization specificity to the hexons (Norrby, 1969b). The latter relationship was not complete, suggesting mutational changes in the hexon after a previous recombination between prototypes. Of practical importance, infection with such mosaic viruses might result in HI tests indicating one prototype but neutralizing antibody and protection would be against another type.

D. Orthomyxoviruses

The structures of influenza virus and the related fowl plague virus have been reviewed recently (Laver, 1973; Schulze, 1973). Orthomyxoviruses consist of a helical nucleocapsid which contains the nucleic acid (RNA), surrounded by a pleiomorphic lipid envelope with projecting spikes of glycoprotein (Figs. 3 and 4). The nucleocapsid of influenza virus is unique among myxoviruses in that it is fragmented into at least three nucleoprotein pieces which contain segments of the viral RNA. During virus infection a nonglycosylated viral protein, termed the "membrane protein" or M protein, aligns itself under the plasma membrane and viral proteins accumulate in the cell membrane above it to the exclusion of host proteins. These viral proteins thus form discrete domains on the cell membrane before budding of the virus occurs (see review by Choppin et al., 1972).

Influenza virions are 900–1100 Å in diameter and covered with two types of projecting spikes arranged in hexagonal fashion. After disruption of virus particles with lipid solvents, these spikes can be separated and the subunits of hemagglutinin and neuraminidase isolated. The hemagglutinin spikes (Fig. 5) are 40 by 140 Å rods which consist of trimers of a glycoprotein with MW 75,000–80,000 daltons. This molecule can under reducing conditions be dissociated to yield two distinct glycoproteins (HA_1 and HA_2) with molecular weights varying with the virus strain. Hemagglutinin appears to be synthesized as a single protein molecule associated with endoplasmic reticulum membranes where it is rapidly glycosylated (Taylor et al., 1969; Lazarowitz et al., 1971; Stanley and Haslam, 1971; Compans, 1973). Posttranslational cleavage of hemagglutinin differs for various virus strains, is host-dependent, and occurs in the plasma membrane (Lazarowitz et al., 1971, 1973; Klenk et al., 1972b;

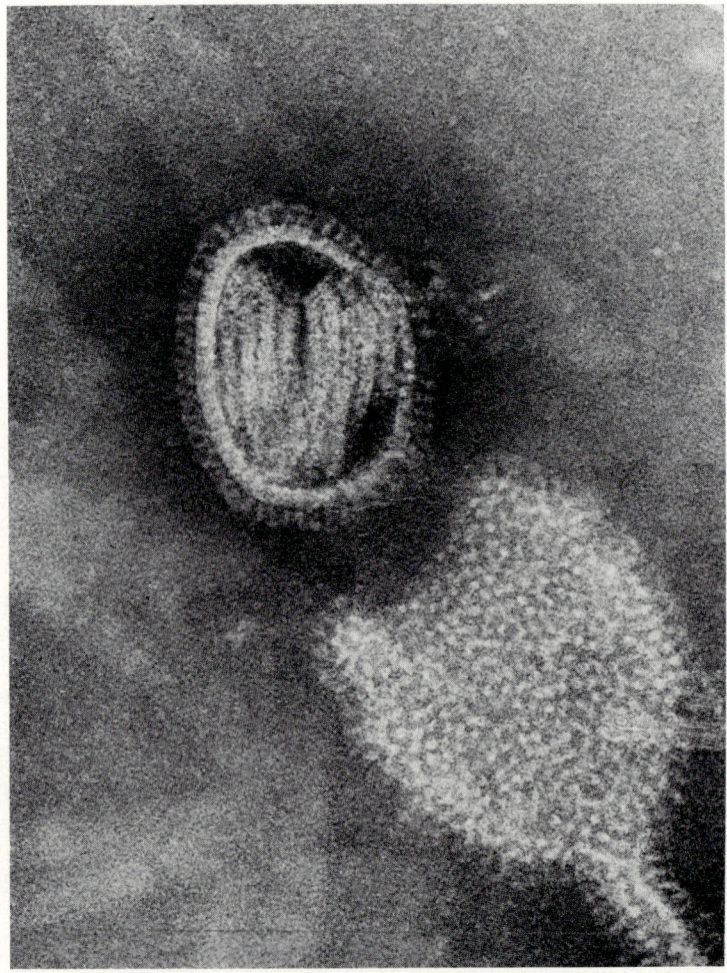

Fig. 3. Morphology of purified influenza A_2/Singapore virus particles negatively stained, showing spikes, membrane, and ribonucleoprotein. ×240,000. Courtesy of M. Nermut.

Skehel, 1972; Compans, 1973). Cleavage does not appear to affect virus infectivity or hemagglutinin titer (Stanley *et al.*, 1973). The neuraminidase spikes, shorter and distinct from the hemagglutinin spikes, consist of tetramers of subunit glycoproteins having MW 55,000–70,000 daltons (Wrigley *et al.*, 1973). The subunits of neuraminidase of some strains may consist of two polypeptides.

In contrast to the virion proteins, almost all of which are coded by

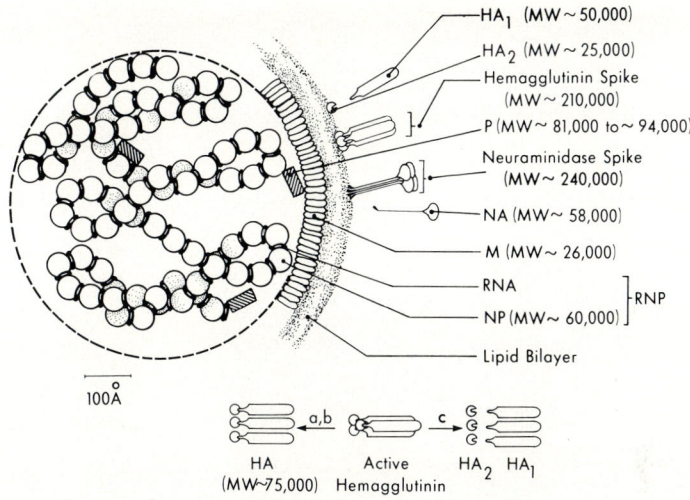

Fig. 4. Proposed model for influenza virus particle. From Schulze (1973).

the virus (Holland and Kiehn, 1970), the lipids (Kates et al., 1961) and carbohydrates (Howe et al., 1967) of the virion are host specific and the latter can alter virus antigenicity. The serologic specificities of protein-bound and lipid-bound carbohydrates are different. Treatment of virus with the proteolytic enzyme bromelin removes the spikes, leaving noninfectious, smooth-surfaced particles containing all of the virion lipid (Fig. 6) (Compans et al., 1970). Concanavalin A, a phytagglutinin from jack beans, was found to react only with intact virions whereas the phytagglutinin from *Dolichos biflorus*, which reacts with the terminal sugar of blood group A (*N*-acetylgalactosamine), reacted only with the spikeless particles, the glycolipid moieties of which were exposed by bromelin treatment (Klenk et al., 1972a). Likewise, antibody to blood group A could be absorbed with the spikeless particles but not with intact virions.

Early reports, using viral preparations probably contaminated with host cell membrane fragments, indicated that blood group antigens A and B and Forssman antigen could be detected as surface antigens on the virions if grown in cells possessing these antigens (Springer and Schuster, 1964). However, recent studies indicate that with progressive purification of the virus, Forssman antigen (a glycolipid) cannot be detected on the virion surface (Haheim and Haukenes, 1973a), but is found in the viral lipids and is accessible to antibody only after removal of the virion spikes with bromelin (Haheim and Haukenes, 1973b). A sulfated glycopeptide antigen found in the

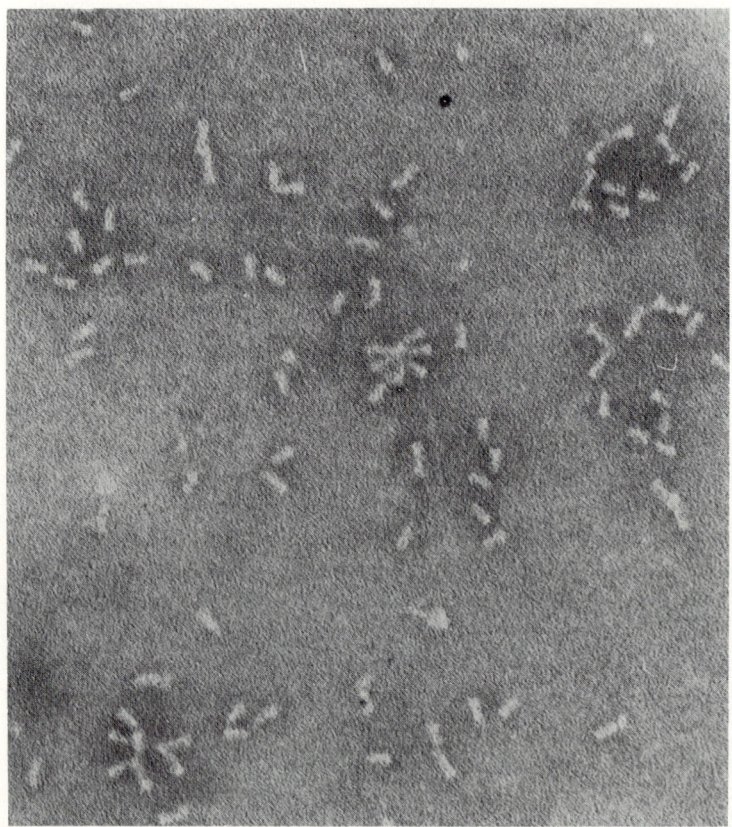

Fig. 5. Electron micrograph of negatively stained influenza virus hemagglutinin. ×250,000. Courtesy of J. Heather.

chick allantoic cavity (Haukenes *et al.*, 1966; Howe *et al.*, 1967; Lee *et al.*, 1969) and found in liver and bile of adult chickens (Harboe and Haukenes, 1966) is acquired by virus growing in the endodermal cells lining the allantoic cavity (Harboe *et al.*, 1966). Recent studies reveal this host antigen to be associated with spikes of both hemagglutinin and neuraminidase (Haheim and Haukenes, 1973b) and antibody to this host antigen reacts with the carbohydrate moieties rather than the peptide backbone of the molecule (Higginbotham *et al.*, 1971).

The virus genome determines four major antigens: hemagglutinin, neuraminidase, the membrane or M protein, and nucleoprotein. Differences in the nucleoprotein, termed the "S" (soluble) antigen,

7. Virus Infections and Immune Responses

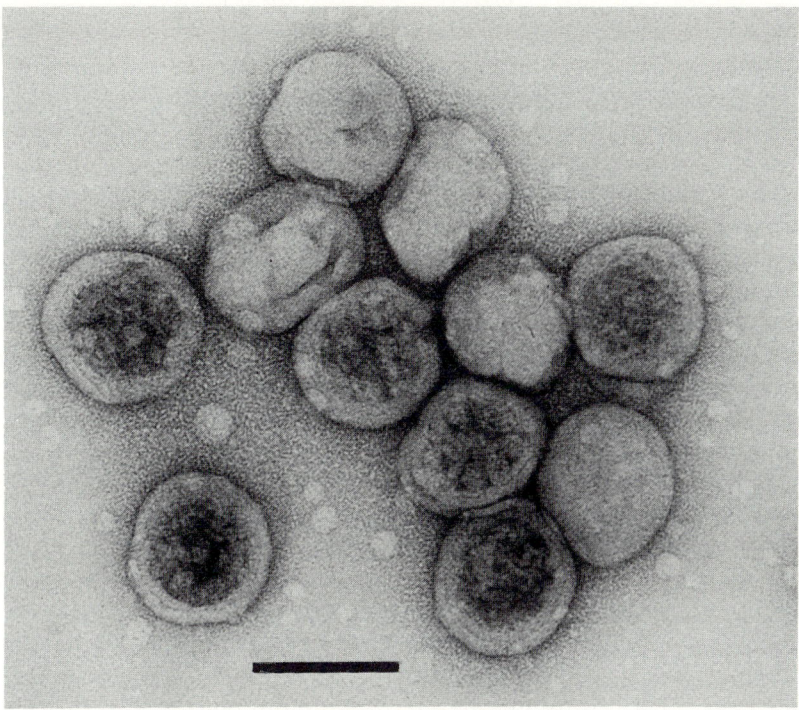

Fig. 6. Influenza A_0/WSN virions from which all glycoproteins have been removed by proteolytic treatment. Particles were negatively stained with uranyl acetate after glutaraldehyde fixation. Morphology suggestive of a double-layered wall and an internal strand is seen in some particles. ×210,000; marker = 1000 Å. From Schulze (1973).

divide influenza into three major types (A, B, and C). Although antibodies to this internal antigen and to the M protein fix complement, they have no neutralizing or hemagglutinating-inhibition (HI) activities and are probably unimportant in immunity. The hemagglutinin or "V" antigen determines strain specificity and reacts with neutralizing, CF, and HI antibody. There is great genetic stability of the internal antigens while the V antigen, exposed to immunologic selection, undergoes frequent minor changes that result in influenza epidemics. Major antigenic shifts in hemagglutinin that result in pandemics are the result of extensive changes in amino acid sequences in HA_1 and HA_2 as revealed by tryptic peptide analyses, and may involve recombination of preexisting human strains with animal strains (Laver and Webster, 1973). Neuraminidase, associated with glycoprotein spikes different from the hemagglutinin spikes, undergoes antigenic changes independently of the V antigen.

E. Paramyxoviruses

The paramyxovirus genus includes a number of common viruses which have similarities to the orthomyxoviruses as well as some interesting differences. As is true for orthomyxoviruses, host factors determine the composition of the virion lipid coat and the glycosylation of protruding protein spikes. Host glycolipid antigens (e.g., blood group antigens) may be incorporated into the virion (Isacson and Koch, 1965). However, nucleocapsids are composed of a single protein species and nonsegmented RNA, and viral nucleic acid replication occurs in the cytoplasm rather than in the nucleus.

Within the genus there are at least three distinct virus groups. The parainfluenza viruses—including Sendai virus, simian virus 5 (SV5), mumps virus, and Newcastle disease virus (NDV)—have considerable antigenic cross-reactivity and possess hemagglutinin, neuraminidase, and hemolytic and cell-fusion activities. The HA and neuraminidase activities of SV5 (Scheid et al., 1972), NDV (Scheid and Choppin, 1973), and Sendai virus (Tozawa et al., 1973; Scheid and Choppin, 1974) reside in a single glycoprotein of MW 65,000–70,000. The hemolytic and cell-fusion activities of Sendai virus have long been thought to be associated with virus protein and recent studies have confirmed this. Hosaka and Shimiza (1972) showed that isolated virus glycoprotein and virus membrane lipids were inactive separately but reconstitution of hemolytic and cell-fusion activities occurred when they were recombined. Scheid and Choppin (1974) recently demonstrated a Sendai virus glycoprotein (MW 53,000), derived from a larger precursor by natural proteolytic activity *in vivo* or by trypsinization *in vitro*, which is responsible for the hemolytic and cell-fusion activities of the virion and also influences its infectivity. Antibodies to both the hemagglutinin/neuraminidase glycoprotein and to the fusion/hemolytic glycoprotein are probably important in virus neutralization, while antibodies to the nucleocapsid protein or to the internal "M" protein are not.

The measles-rinderpest-canine distemper group of paramyxoviruses are antigenically closely related to one another and lack neuraminidase. Recent studies indicate that the measles virion contains six polypeptides, two being glycoproteins that form the projecting spikes (Hall and Martin, 1973, 1974). Norrby and co-workers have correlated certain serologic tests with structural components of measles virus (Norrby and Hammarskjold, 1972). Antibodies to nucleocapsids fix complement and antibodies that inhibit hemagglutination (HI) or hemolysis (HLI) must react with surface components. The finding that HI antibodies can block hemolysis while HLI antibodies have only slight HI activity suggests that the hemolysin represents a separate entity in the virus envelope. Following natural measles infections nucleocapsid CF antibodies predominate and neutralizing antibodies correlate better with HLI than with HI antibodies (Norrby and Gollmar, 1972). In subacute sclerosing panencephalitis (SSPE), oligoclonal IgG antibodies to the various virus components were found, especially in the CSF (Vandvik and Norrby, 1973). In one case, a population of antibodies with HLI and neutralizing but no HI activities was identified. Patients with multiple sclerosis have increased amounts of antibodies to all measles virion components in sera and CSF (Link *et al.*, 1973; Salmi *et al.*, 1973; Norrby *et al.*, 1974). The pathogenetic importance of these findings in SSPE and multiple sclerosis is uncertain.

Respiratory syncitial virus has been classed temporarily as a paramyxovirus. Although it possesses envelope spikes, it lacks hemagglutinin, neuraminidase, and hemolytic and cell-fusion activities.

F. *Togaviruses*

This large family of viruses includes what were formerly known as group A arboviruses (now alphaviruses) and group B arboviruses (now flaviviruses after its best known member, yellow fever virus), plus a small number of unclassified but structurally similar viruses, e.g., rubella virus and lactate dehydrogenase virus. There are about 20 alphaviruses and 40 flaviviruses grouped on the basis of cross-reactivity in HI tests (Casals, 1957). Complement-fixation, neutralization, and cross-protection tests are more specific but show some cross-reactions within each group. The ungrouped togaviruses are not serologically related.

Togaviruses consist of single-stranded RNA enclosed in a coat of core protein rich in lysine and arginine to form a nucleocapsid. A distinctive lipid bilayer containing some carbohydrate is applied to the nucleocapsid much as the M protein in influenza virions (Fig. 7). The peplomers, composed of one or two protein species and rich in hydrophobic amino acids to facilitate attachment, project outward from the lipid coat. The lipid and carbohydrate compositions of the virion are host-determined (Pfefferkorn and Hunter, 1963; Strauss *et al.*, 1970; Renkonen *et al.*, 1971). The peplomers can be removed

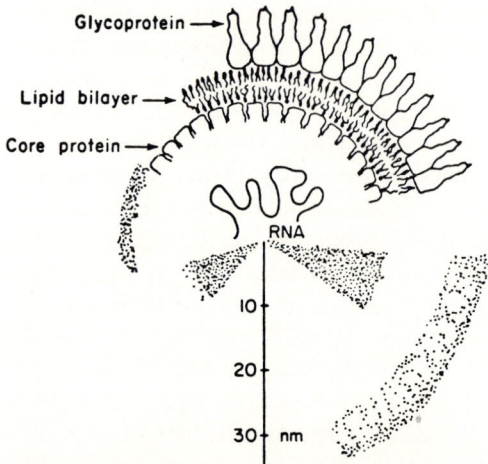

Fig. 7. Proposed structure of Sindbis virus, an alphavirus, showing the elongated glycoprotein peplomers attached to the lipid bilayer membrane and the core protein and RNA. From Harrison et al. (1971).

with proteases leaving the unchanged lipid-coated nucleocapsids (Compans, 1971). Treatment of virions with detergents yields nucleocapsids free of the lipid-glycoprotein envelope (Strauss et al., 1968). Purified peplomer glycoproteins capable of eliciting neutralizing antibodies and of blocking the neutralizing activity of convalescent sera have been isolated from Chikungunya virus (Igarashi et al., 1970, 1971), Semliki Forest virus (Appleyard et al., 1970; Kennedy, 1974), Sindbis virus (Faulkner and Dobos, 1968; Bose and Sagik, 1970), and Venezuelan equine encephalitis virus (Pedersen et al., 1973). Two distinct envelope glycoproteins isolated from Semliki Forest virus possess a common antigenic determinant (Kennedy, 1974). Excision of the carbohydrate moieties with various sugar hydrolases did not remove the antigen, which must therefore be part of the polypeptides.

G. Rhabdoviruses

Rhabdoviruses, of which vesicular stomatitis virus (VSV) and rabies virus have been particularly well studied, are bullet-shaped enveloped RNA viruses about 1700 Å long and 700 Å in diameter (Fig. 8). The single-stranded RNA of MW 4×10^6 daltons is associated with approximately 1000 capsomers of the "N" (nucleo-

7. Virus Infections and Immune Responses

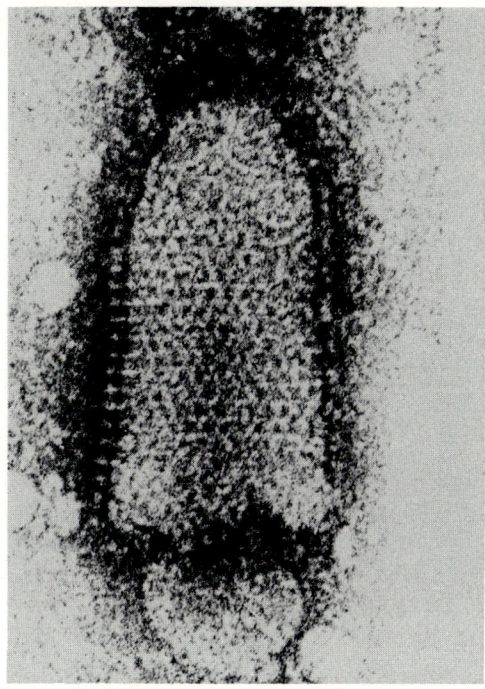

Fig. 8. Morphology of negatively stained rabies virus. On the left are well-resolved surface projections (peplomers) 60–70 Å long. ×300,000. From Hummeler *et al.* (1967).

capsid) protein and arranged in a helix of 34 turns; two other proteins, "NS" and "L," are associated with the nucleocapsid. As with influenza virus, a nonglycosylated membrane or "M" protein is closely applied to the nucleocapsid, and this protein coat is in turn surrounded by a host-derived lipid coat. The glycolipid of the virion is host-determined and thus may possess antigens of the host cell. Antisera against uninfected cells will react with highly purified virus grown in those cells, and in one study the antigen appeared to be a host hematoside incorporated into the glycolipid portion of the virion (Cartwright and Brown, 1972).

Glycoprotein peplomers (the "G" protein) of MW 69,000 daltons protrude from this lipid coat and can be removed selectively by proteases; it is the hemagglutinin and neutralizing antigen of the virion (Cartwright *et al.*, 1970; McSharry *et al.*, 1971; Kelley *et al.*, 1972). The carbohydrate portion of this glycoprotein is largely host-specified (Burge and Huang, 1970; Burge and Strauss, 1970; Grimes and Burge, 1971), and may reflect the antigenicity of the host cell membrane (Ansel, 1974). The virus glycoprotein is easily purified and thus provides a tool with which to study alterations in the glycosylation of membrane proteins induced by cell transformation (Moyer and Summers, 1974). In mixed infections of VSV and the paramyxovirus SV5, phenotypic mixing occurs and the SV5 peplomers may replace those of VSV on VSV virions without altering their overall morphology (McSharry et al., 1971); these virions can then be neutralized with antibody to SV5. It is not known if host glycoproteins can replace virus glycoprotein as peplomers. Nonionic detergents can be used sequentially to dissect the VSV or rabies virions until only the infectious ribonucleoprotein remains (Cartwright et al., 1970).

H. Murine Leukemogenic Viruses

The various murine leukemogenic viruses (MuLV) are morphologically indistinguishable from one another. They are 1200 Å in diameter and consist of a nucleoid core with an outer shell surrounded by a membrane derived during budding and possessing small surface projections. Initially, rats bearing MuLV-induced tumors were found to produce CF and precipitating antibodies against species or group-specific (gs) antigen. The first such antigen defined was named gs-1, and another shown to be an interspecies antigen was named gs-3. Both these antigens, as well as type-specific antigens for strains of MuLV from the same species, reside on the same protein, p30. This protein (MW 30,000 daltons) comprises 30% of the total virion protein and is an internal protein since neutralizing antibodies do not react with it. The gs-1 antigen is widely distributed in reticular tissues of normal mice but does not always correlate with the presence of infectious MuLV.

Virus neutralization tests detect virus envelope antigens (VEA's). Two closely related envelope glycopeptides, gp69/71, have molecular weights of 69,000 and 71,000 daltons and contain prominent group-specific (common to many or all MuLV) and type-specific (limited to a particular virus) antigens, and less easily detected interspecies determinants. Neutralization studies have led preliminarily to the classification of laboratory MuLV isolates into 5 categories (Table II). High incidence leukemia mouse strains (AKR, C58) produce MuLV serologically identical to Gross virus (with GVEA) (Hartley et al., 1969).

TABLE II

Classification of Murine Leukemogenic Viruses[a]

Subgroup	Type	Strains
1		Gross (radiation leukemia)
2	a	Friend, Graffi, Tennant, Rowson-Parr, SimLV
	b	Moloney, Abelson
	c	Rauscher, Rich, Breyere-Moloney
	d	Buffett (334C)

[a] From Lilly and Steeves, 1974.

Cell surface antigens (CSA's) of MuLV-infected cells were first defined in tumor transplantation studies. Animals rejecting such tumor grafts possess specifically cytotoxic antibodies which can (in the presence of complement) lyse tumors induced by the same virus. Most antibodies to the CSA's are not neutralizing antibodies since adsorption of virus-neutralizing activity with purified virus leaves the cytotoxic activity of the serum undiminished (Pasternak, 1967; Steeves, 1968). Also, immunoelectron microscopy studies demonstrate VEA's and CSA's in topographically separate regions of the cell surface (Aoki et al., 1970). Cross-reactive patterns with cytotoxic antibodies define two major subgroups on the basis of CSA's: Gross and Friend–Moloney–Rauscher (FMR). Type-specific CSA determinants have not been analyzed. The Gross CSA is found on many normal and preleukemic cells of high-leukemic mouse strains (AKR). In contrast, the FMR determinant is not found on normal cells. The FMR antigen appears to be an internal virion protein that differs from p30 (Friedman et al., 1974). Although they are not the principal CSA's of MuLV-infected cells, both p30 and gp69/71 are found on the surface of infected cells (Ikeda et al., 1974; Yoshiki et al., 1974a). Expression of the various genes coding for structural proteins of MuLV is regulated by many genes (Lilly and Pincus, 1973; Rowe, 1973). Multiple copies of some genes coding for virus proteins may be present in each cell and not coordinately linked (Strand et al., 1974).

Reverse transcriptase in the core of MuLV virions carries interspecies and species-specific determinants (Parks et al., 1972). The interspecies antigen of MuLV reverse transcriptase cross-reacts with that of other small mammals but not with that of primates or chickens.

III. Humoral Responses

A. Sequence of IgM and IgG Responses

The sequence of IgM and IgG responses to viral antigens is usually like that observed with nonviral antigens. Complicating factors in the humoral responses to viruses include a persisting antigenic load while infection continues, cell and tissue destruction by the virus, and influences of the virus on the immune system.

The responses of rabbits to nonreplicating viral antigens have been studied in detail with poliomyelitis type 1 (PV) (Svehag and Mandel, 1964a,b; Svehag, 1964a,b) and influenza virus (Webster, 1965, 1968a,b). In both cases with adequate antigen dose after a short inductive phase (8–12 hours in the case of PV) IgM antibodies appeared, followed later by IgG antibodies (Fig. 9). Small doses of PV produced only a transient IgM response, which after 4 days declined at a rate consistent with the metabolic decay rate of this immunoglobulin. Larger doses of PV elicited both IgM and IgG antibody responses; IgM synthesis continued for 10–14 days, whereas IgG was first detected on the third day and increased until the third week. Thereafter IgG levels remained constant for about 30 weeks and persisted at moderate titers for 2 years. This was not due to chronic infection since poliovirus does not grow in rabbit tissue and UV-irradiated virus gave the same result. Similar findings with antibodies against the bacteriophage ϕX174 in guinea pigs had been reported by Uhr and Finkelstein (1963), although the rate of an-

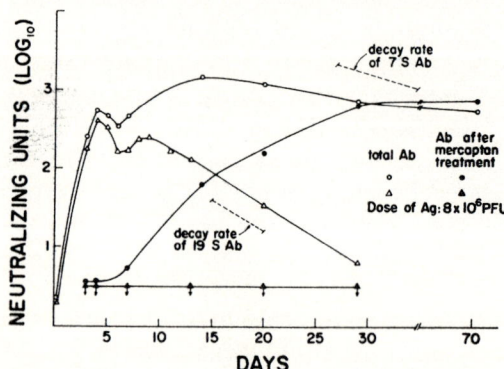

Fig. 9. Production of mercaptoethanol-sensitive (19 S) and mercaptoethanol-resistant (7 S) antibody in rabbits immunized with a large dose of poliovirus. From Svehag and Mandel (1964b).

tibody formation against the bacteriophage was less antigen-dependent than in the case of PV.

Interesting information on immunologic memory has come from the experiments with PV. With low doses of virus eliciting only IgM responses there was no detectable memory; repeated small doses of PV at monthly intervals elicited only transient and identical IgM responses (Fig. 10). However, if a second small dose of PV was administered 6 days after the first (2 days after the 19 S antibody had begun to decline), a large secondary response consisting exclusively of 19 S antibody occurred and the titer rose 100-fold. Again, this secondary response began the day after inoculation of PV and persisted for only 4 days. These results suggest that an immunologic memory of IgM antibody production does exist but is very short-lived. The early and large secondary response shows that immunocompetent cells in the primary response do not die after 4 days of antibody release but require further antigenic stimulation for continued antibody production. Similar results have been obtained with the ϕX–guinea pig system.

Studies of natural and experimental poliovirus infections of humans (using attenuated virus) have largely confirmed the findings

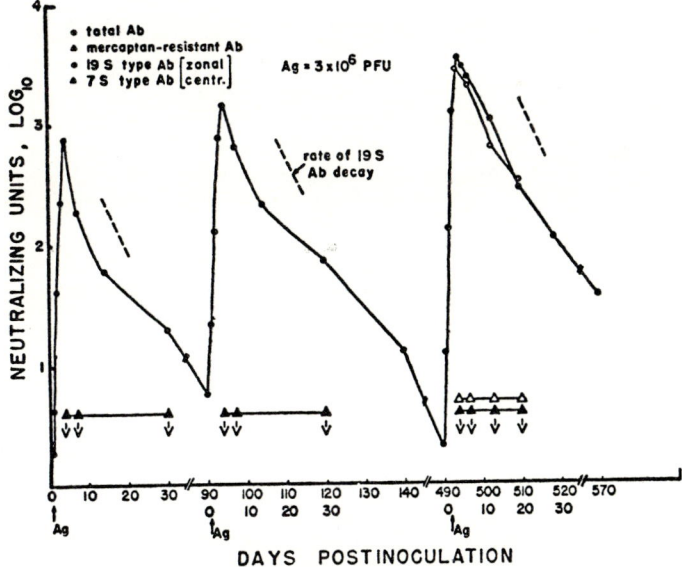

Fig. 10. Production of antibody in rabbits after repeated immunizations with small doses of poliovirus. Only 19 S antibody was produced and the responses were transient and almost identical. From Svehag and Mandel (1964b).

in rabbits previously discussed. The level of neutralizing IgM antibody rises rapidly after natural infection, reaches maximum titers in 3–4 weeks, and declines to undetectable levels by 3 months (Svehag and Mandel, 1964b; Ogra et al., 1968). IgG titers rise over a prolonged period and may not attain peak levels until after 3 months. IgA antibody is not detectable until 4–6 weeks after infection and rises for at least the ensuing 8 weeks. The early neutralizing antibody is of low avidity (Sabin, 1957). Although CF antibody (against D and C antigens) attains maximum levels after about 2 months and persists for 1–5 years, neutralizing antibody decreases to one-fourth its peak titer by 2 years and persists near that level for decades.

Ogra et al. (1968) have compared the humoral responses to live and inactivated vaccines in infants (see Figs. 11 and 12). Beginning at 2 months of age, 3 monthly doses of trivalent inactivated virus (subcutaneously), or live virus type 1 and types 2 and 3 on successive months (orally) were administered; a booster was given at 12 months of age. Poliovirus-binding antibody titers were determined by radioimmunodiffusion and neutralizing antibody assays for type 1 virus were performed on sera and secretions. Maternally derived IgG an-

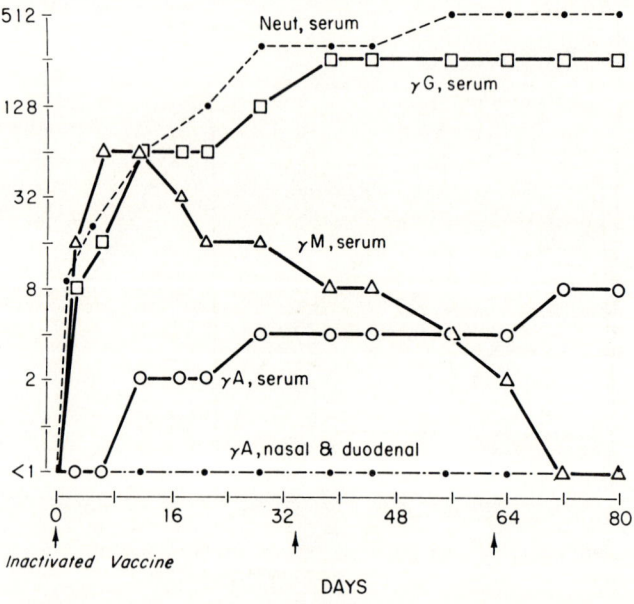

Fig. 11. Production of IgM, IgG, and IgA antibody against poliovirus type 1 in serum and secretions after immunization with three doses of trivalent inactivated virus at monthly intervals, beginning at 2 months of age. From Ogra et al. (1968).

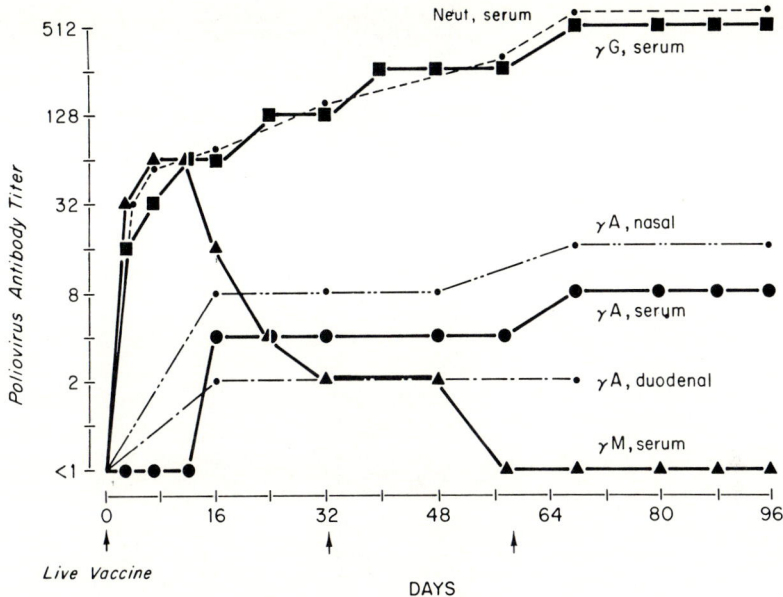

Fig. 12. Production of IgM, IgG, and IgA antibody against poliovirus type 1 in serum and secretions after immunization with live attenuated poliovirus types 1, 2, and 3, given sequentially at monthly intervals, beginning at 2 months of age. From Ogra *et al.* (1968).

tibody was detected in low titers in one-fourth of the infants aged 2 months; no sera contained IgM. IgM and IgG were detected 3 days after the first vaccine dose. The IgM titers rose more rapidly than those of IgG and became maximal during the second week before declining to undetectable levels by 8–10 weeks. IgM declined more slowly in recipients of inactivated virus as they had repeated antigenic stimulation (3 doses). IgG titers in both groups continued to rise for 7–10 weeks before leveling off. Serum IgA titers were not detected until 2 weeks after initial immunization; they rose slowly over a 3-month period. After the booster at 12 months, IgM titers showed a transient rise to previous levels, thus duplicating the findings in rabbits (Fig. 13). Recipients of live virus had neutralizing IgA in their nasal and duodenal secretions after 16–21 days, which persisted for at least 90 days (duodenal) and 300 days (nasal); recipients of inactivated virus had no secreted IgA antibody to poliovirus.

Studies of guinea pigs infected with arboviruses (Bellanti *et al.*, 1965) and of humans infected with mumps virus (Brown *et al.*, 1970; Daugharty *et al.*, 1973), Coxsackie virus (Schmidt *et al.*, 1968), influ-

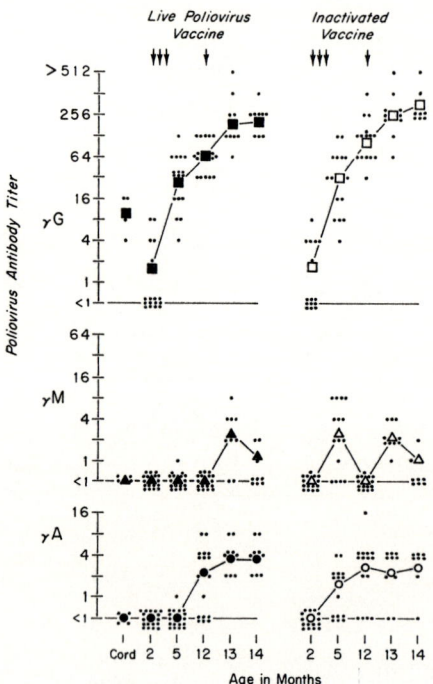

Fig. 13. Serum poliovirus type 1 immunoglobulin responses after immunization with live attenuated or inactivated virus; individual and geometric mean titers are shown. Note the IgM responses after booster immunization. From Ogra *et al.* (1968).

enza virus (Brown and O'Leary, 1971), or inoculated with soluble adenovirus antigens (Lehrich *et al.*, 1966) have demonstrated IgM and IgG patterns similar to those following poliovirus infection and suggest that this pattern of antibody response is a general phenomenon. The IgM response following natural influenza infection or immunization appears to be unique in one study in that the IgM was exclusively of a 7 S form (Brown and O'Leary, 1973).

B. *Elicitation of Specific Immunoglobulin Classes*

Particular antigens of a virus appear to be capable of eliciting a response of a specific class of immunoglobulin, as do nonviral antigens (Schirrmacher and Rajewsky, 1970). Cowan (1970) and Brown and Smale (1970) have shown that IgM and IgG produced in guinea pigs infected with foot-and-mouth disease virus are specific for distinctive antigenic determinants on the virus particle, and Miyamoto *et al.* (1971) have described differential reactions of 7 S and 19 S antibodies with HSV antigens in infected cells. Most patients with warts produce only IgM antibodies to the human wart virus (Goffe et al., 1966; Pyrhonen and Penttinen, 1972). Recently, Lee et al. (1974) reported that normal $B6C3F_1$ mouse sera contains 19 S antibodies that react with antigenic determinants on 3 structural proteins of MuLV while antibodies in the 7 S fraction react with only one of these proteins, p15.

Several explanations can be offered for the preferential elicitation of particular immunoglobulin classes by these viral antigens. A trivial explanation for not finding IgM against a particular antigen is that the IgM response is transient unless there is continued antigenic stimulation. An exclusively IgM response may occur with small immunogenic stimuli, as discussed above. Thus, wart virus, growing only in the epidermis, does not have ready access to the bloodstream or lymphatics to immunize the host. This has led to the suggestion that susceptibility to recurrent attacks of warts may be related to failure of very small doses of antigen to promote an IgG response, the presence of the latter being a good indicator of healing (Pyrhonen and Penttinen, 1972).

C. Genetic Control of Antiviral Antibody Responses

The genetic control of immune responses to certain antigens has been demonstrated in guinea pigs and mice and appears to be under the control of the Ir genes in the H-2 complex (see Benacerraf and McDevitt, 1972; McDevitt and Landy, 1973). Nonresponders produce only IgM antibody to the specific antigen (Grumet, 1972) unless certain conditions such as an allogeneic stimulus are imposed (Ordal and Grumet, 1972). Similar situations with viral antigens may also occur, but have not yet been described. However, an increased humoral response to measles virus has been associated with HL-A3 in man (Arnason et al., 1974). An increased incidence of multiple sclerosis is associated with HL-A3 but there is no such association with optic neuritis, which often evolves clinically into multiple sclerosis. Also, patients with optic neuritis have normal levels of antibody to measles virus. The association of high titers of antibody to measles virus with multiple sclerosis may thus reflect the prevalence of high titers to the virus in people with the HL-A3 genotype.

D. Genetic Control of Virus-Induced Diseases

Many examples of genetically controlled resistance to infection within a species are known (Allison, 1965). Thus, several major genes confer resistance to chickens and chick cells against infection by particular strains of avian leukemogenic viruses or Rous viruses coated by them. The control of murine leukemogenesis is multigenic, with different genes controlling viral expression (Akv-1 and Akv-2 genes), viral replication (Fv-1 gene), and resistance to Gross virus and virus-transformed cells (the Rgv-1 gene) (Lilly and Pincus, 1973; Rowe, 1973). The Rgv-1 gene is linked to H-2 and influences late disease patterns. It is only by inference, however, that its mechanism is thought to involve immune responses. The immunopathological disease caused by LCM virus infection of adult mice has been reported associated with H-2 (Oldstone et al., 1973). This finding is not universally found in all laboratories (possibly because of virus strain differences), and awaits detailed immunologic analysis.

IV. Secretory Antibody Responses

Viruses infecting seromucous surfaces such as the respiratory or alimentary tracts must pass a first line of defense consisting of secretory antibody and inhibitory mucoprotein secretions. Francis (1942) first noted the presence of anti-influenzal antibody in human nasal secretions and for years it has been thought that virus infections of the mucous membranes could confer specific local immunity. It is now clear that the main antibody in seromucous secretions is IgA, although a compensatory increase in the levels of other immunoglobulins, especially IgM, occurs in the secretions of people with IgA deficiency (see Tomasi and Bienenstock, 1969). Thus, antibody in nasal secretions against rhinoviruses (Rossen et al., 1966), parainfluenza 1 virus (Smith et al., 1966), and influenza virus (Rossen et al., 1966; Alford et al., 1967) is predominantly IgA. However, the role of IgA antibodies in recovery from virus infections and prevention of reinfection is less clear.

Fazekas de St. Groth and Graham (1954) reported that the immunity of mice to reinfection with influenza virus is more closely correlated with the presence of antibody in nasal secretions than with antibody in serum. Several groups of investigators have reported that parenteral administration of inactivated viruses increases levels of serum IgG and IgM antibodies, but not levels of IgA antibodies in nasal secretions, whereas natural infection results in the formation of IgA secretory antibodies and better resistance to reinfection (Rossen et al., 1966; Smith et al., 1966; Alford et al., 1967). This does not necessarily imply that IgA is responsible for the resistance to reinfection because the natural infection could have other effects, including local stimulation of T lymphocytes. Claims that local IgA production and protection follow aerosol administration of inactivated influenza virus (Waldman et al., 1970) have not been confirmed in other laboratories (Shore et al., 1973) and further work on the subject is required.

One of the arguments of Sabin (1959) in support of live poliovirus immunization is that it would stimulate local secretory antibody production, thereby limiting excretion of the virus and transmission in the population. Ogra (1973) has presented evidence that production of IgA antibody is a local reaction. Immunization of selected segments of the large intestine in subjects with double-barreled colostomies induced an IgA antibody response against poliovirus in the immunized segment with little or no response elsewhere. However, subcutaneous immunization with killed poliovirus has not only eliminated paralytic disease but also the transmission of the virus in the Swedish population, as shown by large scale examinations of feces of persons admitted to hospital for any reason (Perkins, 1974).

Deficiency of secretory IgA is not rare, occurring in about 1 in 500 persons in Western Europe and North America. Most such individuals remain healthy, although some have recurrent sinopulmonary and gastrointestinal infections (Schwartz and Buckley, 1971). Thus, in some individuals IgG and IgM antibodies appear able to substitute for IgA antibodies in secretions.

V. Thymus Dependence of Viral Antigens

After the exposure of animals to most antigens the formation of antibodies by cells of the B lymphocyte lineage requires helper effects of T lymphocytes (Miller et al., 1971). This has given rise to the concept of the "thymus dependence" of antigens, some antigens being more dependent than others on T lymphocytes for a normal humoral response. Originally, thymus dependence was defined in terms of the amount of serum antibody formed to an antigen in a T lymphocyte-deprived animal. Later, it was found that IgM responses are less dependent on T lymphocytes than those of other immunoglobulin classes and that humoral responses to certain "thymus independent" antigens (pneumococcal polysaccharide type III) are regulated by T lymphocytes. "Thymus dependence" is thus a relative term and depends on animal species and strain as well as mode of antigen presentation. Generally, "thymus-independent" antigens are large, slowly metabolized molecules with repeating antigenic determinants (epitopes). It might be expected that some viruses, many of which possess antigenic polyvalency inherent in their structures, could have some epitopes in the proper repeating spatial relationship to be immunogenically thymus-independent.

Until the recent availability of the athymic nude mouse, neonatal thymectomy or treatment with ALS was used to deplete animals of T lymphocytes and ascertain the thymus dependence of virus antigens. Although these methods of T lymphocyte depletion are not effective by present standards, the results obtained will be reviewed. Thus, neonatal thymectomy did not abolish the production of HI antibodies to polyoma virus in mice (Miller et al., 1964; Mori et al., 1966) or rats (Allison and Taylor, 1967), or to influenza virus (Svet-Moldavsky et al., 1964) or Coxsackie B5 virus (cited in Mori et al., 1967) in mice. Titers of complement-dependent neutralizing antibodies (probably IgM) to HSV in CF-1 mice neonatally thymectomized were similar to those of control mice (Mori et al., 1970). The other method of T lymphocyte depletion, pretreatment of mice with ALS, did not diminish the production of HI antibodies to vaccinia virus (Hirsch et al., 1968b), CF antibodies to LCM virus (Hirsch et al., 1968a), or HI antibodies to influenza virus (Hirsch and Murphy, 1968).

In addition to the ineffective methods of T lymphocyte deprivation in these studies, the continuing antigen presentation that occurs in virus infections must be considered. Svet-Moldavsky et al. (1964) have demonstrated that the abrogation of antibody response to sheep erythrocytes observed in neonatally thymectomized mice can be overcome by repeated immunizations. Mori et al. (1970) reported that neonatally thymectomized mice inoculated with Japanese encephalitis virus had diminished HI titers which, however, rose to normal levels after repeated inoculations.

A few studies have suggested thymus dependence for some virus antigens. Thind and Price (1971) reported markedly depressed levels of neutralizing antibodies to Langat virus (a togavirus) in mice neonatally thymectomized and infected 6 weeks later. Virelizier et al. (1974b) have recently analyzed the role of T cell helper effects in the formation of antibodies against influenza virus hemagglutinin. Two hemagglutinins, each containing a cross-reactive determinant(s) and a strain-specific determinant, were used and antibody formation against each of these could be quantitated independently by immunodiffusion. Immunization of thymectomized, irradiated, and bone-marrow reconstituted (TXBM) mice showed a strong thymus

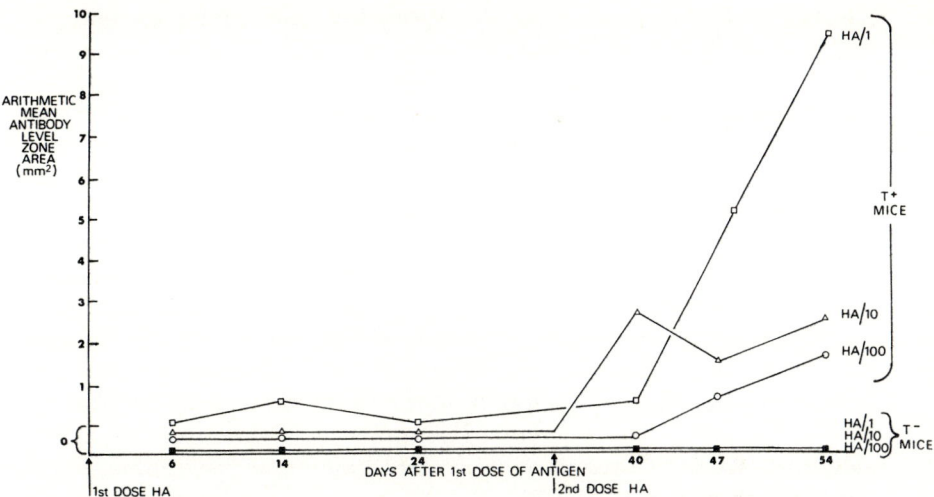

Fig. 14. Thymus dependence of influenza virus hemagglutinin (HA). Levels of antibody to HA were determined by radial immunodiffusion after immunization with various dilutions of HA of normal (T+) or TXBM (T−) mice. From Virelizier et al. (1974b).

dependence of antibody formation against both determinants (Fig. 14). Haller and Lindenmann (1974) and W. H. Burns (unpublished observations) have confirmed the thymus dependence of HI antibody formation to influenza virus in nude mice. B. Rager-Zisman and A. C. Allison (unpublished observations, 1974) observed that, in neonatally thymectomized mice infected as adults with HSV, levels of serum neutralizing antibodies were much lower than in intact animals; A. C. Allison and W. H. Burns have confirmed this finding in TXBM mice and nude mice (unpublished observations). Discrepancies between these findings and previous reports concerning HSV and influenza virus probably stem from the use of mice inadequately depleted of T lymphocytes in the earlier reports.

Since mice sham thymectomized, irradiated, and bone-marrow reconstituted make poor responses to some antigens months after reconstitution (Howard *et al.*, 1971; Mitchell and Humphrey, 1973), lesions in addition to T lymphocyte depletion must be present in TXBM mice. Although nude mice may possess abnormalities in addition to those presently recognized, they are probably the best animals for studying thymus dependence. W. H. Burns (unpublished observations) has compared the humoral responses of nude mice and their normal (nu/+, +/+) littermates to infections with a number of viruses. Insignificant or very low (probably IgM) levels of neutralizing antibodies were found in nude mice infected with Coxsackie B1 virus, encephalomyocarditis virus, West Nile virus, VSV, or HSV. No HI antibodies were detected after infections with influenza or Sendai viruses and no CF antibodies were detected after infection with mouse adenovirus. However, infection with Sindbis virus resulted in high titers (1:1000) of neutralizing antibody, solely of the IgM class; this titer was comparable to that in control littermates and was sustained for 2 weeks. The antigens of Sindbis virus that react with neutralizing antibody are two membrane glycoproteins. Using rabbit antisera, Kennedy (1974) has demonstrated that the antigenic determinants of Semliki Forest virus (an alphavirus similar to Sindbis virus) are in the polypeptide portions rather than the carbohydrate moieties of the envelope glycoproteins. It will be of interest to determine if the "thymus-independent" antigenic determinants of Sindbis virus similarly reside in the protein part of the molecules. Recently, "natural" antibody in sera of nude mice has been detected that neutralizes a xenotropic virus isolated from these mice (S. Cross, H. M. Morse, and J. Hartley, personal communication, 1974). Presumably the antibody (predominantly IgM) is directed against viral envelope proteins and/or glycoproteins.

VI. B Lymphocyte Memory and "Original Antigenic Sin"

On theoretical grounds it might be supposed that vaccination with a series of antigenically related viral vaccines would produce a broad immunity against all the viruses of a group, e.g., type A influenza viruses or flaviviruses. However, this aim is difficult to achieve because of a property of immunologic memory that Francis (1955) has called "original antigenic sin." The response of various age groups of the human population to vaccinations with different strains of influenza A virus showed that the serologic response of an individual is dominated throughout his life by the type of antibody produced as a result of his first exposure to an influenza A virus (Francis, 1953, 1955; Davenport and Hennessy, 1956). This type of response is characteristic of infections of long-lived animals with any virus of which there are several cross-reacting antigenic types, e.g., flaviviruses—group B arthropod-bone viruses (Hearn and Rainey, 1963), paramyxoviruses (van der Veen and Sonderkamp, 1965), and enteroviruses (Mietens et al., 1964). It can be reproduced in laboratory animals either by successive infections with cross-reacting viruses or successive vaccination with inactive vaccines made from such cross-reacting viruses. The phenomenon is also observed when mice are immunized with purified cross-reactive influenza virus hemagglutinins (Virelizer et al., 1974a). Analogous responses have been reported in animals immunized with cross-reactive serum albumins, HL-A antigens, and haptens. Westaway et al. (1974) recently reported that, after sequential infections of rabbits with related togaviruses, the cross-reactive antibodies produced after rechallenge were of the IgG class while IgM antibodies were specific for the most recent immunizing virus. In geographic areas where flavivirus infections are common and serologic diagnosis difficult because of cross-reacting antibodies and the recall phenomenon, determination of IgM specificity can permit diagnosis (Edelman et al., 1973; Edelman and Pariyanonda, 1973).

Thus, the original antigenic sin phenomenon is not only of general interest from the theoretical point of view but of practical importance in immunization programs and in serologic epidemiology. It is paradoxical, since it implies a qualitative failure in the specificity of immunologic memory. The cellular basis of the phenomenon is unknown, and investigations in detail have begun using two purified influenza hemagglutinins, H_0 and H_1, possessing specific as well as cross-reactive determinants (Virelizier et al., 1974a,b). As mentioned above, formation of antibody against both these determinants is thymus-dependent. However, the thymus dependence of antibody formation against the cross-reactive determinant could be overcome by repeated inoculations of hemagglutinin in TXBM mice, indicating the presence of memory in these animals. Strong, secondary type responses were observed in primed, thymus-deprived mice after reconstitution with syngeneic virgin thymus cells, showing that specific immunologic memory is elicited by both determinants despite the absence of detectable antibody secretion. These observations are interpreted as examples of immunologic recognition and memory mediated by B lymphocytes. They suggest that the helper effect of T lymphocytes is exerted at a late stage in the differentiation of specific populations of B cells into antibody-secreting cells.

These findings are similar to those of Roelants and Askonas (1972) and I. M. Zitron (personal communication) for nonviral antigens. A similar interpretation might explain the results of Yamanouchi et al. (1974b) who reported that acute infection with rinderpest virus depressed the primary response of rabbits to sheep erythrocytes, but left intact the secondary response after reimmunization 3 weeks later. Rinderpest virus, like measles virus which it closely resembles, may transiently impair T cell helper effects yet allow B lymphocyte proliferation.

Several experiments have shown that B lymphocyte memory is responsible for original antigenic sin. Thus, when spleen cells from mice primed with H_0 are transferred to normal or irradiated recipients and the latter are challenged with H_1, secondary responses to specific H_0 determinants, as well as cross-reactive determinants, are obtained. Treatment of the spleen cells with anti-θ sera and complement does not affect this type of recall. However, similar experiments using irradiated recipients show that, in addition to the memory which is responsible for the special type of recall, there is a T lymphocyte memory that increases specifically the response to the determinant on the first hemagglutinin (H_0) which is not cross-reactive.

VII. Neutralization

A. Mechanisms of Neutralization

The decrease in infectious titer after mixing antibody and virus is termed neutralization and has been reviewed by Svehag (1968). Most studies have been carried out in the fluid phase *in vitro* and each system of virus–cell–antibody–complement components presents unique features. The influence of the host cell was shown by Kjellen and Schlesinger (1959), who found different levels of residual infectivity of VSV when the same virus–antibody complexes were assayed on chick and human cells. Complexes of virus and mammalian antibody were more efficiently neutralized when propagated on mammalian cells than chicken cells, whereas chicken antibody was more effective with chicken cells. Philipson (1966) reported analogous findings with poliovirus when assayed on monkey and human cells, and others have made similar observations with various virus–host cell systems (Lafferty, 1963a; Hawkes, 1964). Thus neutralization is a complex process involving three components: virus, antibody, and host cell. Neutralization *in vivo* where leukocytes and accessory factors are present may differ in important respects from that observed in cell cultures.

The initial interaction between virus and antibody has been extensively studied. Some workers found the interaction to be reversible, e.g., with influenza virus (Burnet *et al.*, 1937; Fazekas de St. Groth, 1962; Lafferty, 1963a), while others felt it was essentially irreversible, e.g., with poliovirus (Dulbecco *et al.*, 1956; Mandel, 1961; Philipson, 1966), adenovirus (Kjellen, 1962), NDV (Granoff, 1965), and HSV (Yoshino and Taniguchi, 1965b). Philipson (1966), using a two-phase aqueous polymer system that distributes free and antibody-bound virus in different phases, examined the interaction of poliovirus with various immunoglobulins. After a short lag, IgM antibody bound virus irreversibly while IgG antibody, following first-order kinetics, bound virus rapidly and irreversibly. Using a countercurrent distribution procedure with a total dilution factor of 10^{18}, only a small fraction of poliovirus–antibody complexes could be dissociated. Mandel (1961) showed that such complexes were stable for 50 days when resuspended in media without antibody. However, dissociation can occur and infectious poliovirus recovered after exposure of the complexes to acid or alkali (Mandel, 1961), treatment with fluorocarbon (Ketler et al., 1961), sonication (Keller, 1965), or exposure to proteolytic enzymes (Keller, 1968).

The Fc part of the immunoglobulin molecule determines many of its biologic properties (complement fixation, placental transfer, binding to certain cells) and its influence on virus neutralization has been examined indirectly by observing neutralization with Fab fragments. The purity of Fab fragments varied in different experiments, but generally Fab was found to neutralize influenza virus (Lafferty, 1963b), poliovirus (Vogt et al., 1964), HSV (Ashe et al., 1968, and LDV (Notkins et al., 1968), but not adenovirus type 5 (Kjellen, 1964, 1965).

Antibody in proper amounts can agglutinate or coat virions and prevent their adsorption, as has been shown for NDV (Rubin and Franklin, 1957) and poliovirus (Mandel, 1962; Keller, 1966). However, virus–antibody complexes can sometimes adsorb to host cells, although complexes containing the larger IgM do so more slowly than those containing IgG perhaps because of greater steric hindrance (Mandel, 1967). Adsorbed complexes may penetrate more slowly and be more susceptible to further neutralization by added antisera than nonadsorbed free virus (Rubin and Franklin, 1957; Rubin, 1957; Mandel, 1962).

Correlations between antigenic structure and neutralization have been made for several viruses, and a few examples will now be considered. The neutralization of adenovirus takes place in two steps, with firm initial antibody–virus binding followed by increasing inactivation (Kjellen, 1962). Although either univalent or bivalent Fab fragments bind to adenovirus and block whole antibody HI activity, neither fragment blocks the neutralizing activity of whole antibody. Since HA is mediated by the fiber γ antigen while neutralization requires interaction with the hexon ϵ antigen, this could be explained if Fab fragments bind to γ but not to ϵ. Binding of Fab fragments of antisera prepared against capsid subunits would clarify this. Since antisera against the hexon ϵ antigens neutralize (Wilcox and Ginsberg, 1963; Kjellen and Pereira, 1968; Philipson, 1969) while those against fibers usually do not (Kjellen and Pereira, 1968; Pettersson et al., 1968), neutralizing antibody may not prevent adsorption to host cells but may alter a later step such as uncoating. Intrasubgroup heterotypic antisera neutralize adenovirus type 5 at low pH, and addition of these heterotypic sera to homotypic sera at normal pH enhances neutralization (Kjellen and Pereira, 1968). It was suggested that low pH or the interaction of homotypic antibody with the outer aspect of hexons might expose inner sites with subgroup specificity which then could react with heterotypic antibody and enhance neutralization. According to this view, conformational changes of the hexons are important in adenovirus neutralization, possibly leading to faulty uncoating and degradation in heterophagic vacuoles, as has been described for antibody-complexed NDV and vaccinia (Dales and Kajioka, 1964; Silverstein and Marcus, 1964; Dales, 1969).

Foot-and-mouth disease virus (FMDV) is an icosohedral particle which has been shown to have three classes of antibody-binding sites (Brown and Smale, 1970). One is a 12 S protein subunit on the faces of the particles which can be separated from the virus by heat or acid treatment and reacts only with IgG. Both sites at the vertices bind IgG and one, which is trypsin sensitive, is the only site of attachment of IgM antibody. Neutralization studies with antisera against whole virus and adsorbed with trypsin-treated virus or 12 S subunits indicate that both vertex sites are involved in neutralization while the face site is not (Rowlands et al., 1971).

Virion glycoproteins appear to be important antigens involved in the neutralization of many viruses. The G protein of VSV is a glycoprotein forming the spikes that protrude from the virus coat and can be solubilized by detergents and purified. Antisera produced against this protein have good neutralizing activity (Kelley et al., 1972). The envelope glycoprotein of another rhabdovirus, rabies, can also be extracted and purified; it can induce neutralizing antibody and protects animals against later challenge with rabies virus (Wiktor et al., 1973) and offers a new form of vaccine. Cohen et al. (1972) have reported purification from HSV-infected cell of a virion glycoprotein that is capable of stimulating in rabbits monoprecipitin antisera that neutralize HSV. Other workers have isolated envelope glycoproteins from HSV types 1 and 2 which react with type-specific neutralizing antibodies (Powell et al., 1974).

Neutralization of influenza virus results primariily from the interaction of antibody with hemagglutinin although high concentrations of antibody to neuraminidase can neutralize some virus strains (Kilbourne et al., 1968). Antibodies to hemagglutinin can prevent virion attachment to cells while antibodies to neuraminidase do not. Both antibodies prevent viropexis and in their presence virions remain at the cell surface (Dourmashkin and Tyrrell, 1974). Antineuraminidase may also interfere with egress of virus from infected cells.

B. Complement-Dependent Neutralization

The capacity of "natural antibody" (thought to be IgM) and early immune IgM antibody to neutralize viruses is increased by reaction with the complement system. Normal human sera and rabbit early immune sera require complement to neutralize T coliphages whereas late immune sera of humans and rabbits do not (Muschel and Toussaint, 1962). After inoculation of rabbits with HSV, early (8-day) sera contained both IgM and IgG antibodies which required complement for neutralization (Yoshino and Taniguchi, 1964, 1965a). Late sera contained both IgM and IgG which could neutralize HSV without complement, but complement increased the IgM neutralizing capacity and raised the neutralization rate constant but not titer of late IgG (Hampar et al., 1968). Neutralizing antibody against rubella virus, especially IgM and early IgG, also requires complement (Rawls et al., 1967; Leerhoy, 1968). The inefficiency of early and late IgM and early IgG antibody against equine arteritis virus in neutralization was not affected by complement, but an exception to the above findings is the observation that late IgG antibody to this virus is strongly dependent on complement for neutralization (Hyllseth and Pettersson, 1970; Radwan and Burger, 1973). This finding was noted in sera from five species and is therefore probably characteristic of the virus rather than the source of antibody.

It is not clear how complement increases neutralization. Since the antibody in early immune sera often has low avidity for virus, it is possible that the reaction with complement stabilizes the virus–antibody complex. In the HSV system, however, the complex of virus and early sera is stable and some other mechanism must be operative (Yoshino and Taniguchi, 1965b). These complexes can be neutralized by late sera, so that the binding of early serum antibodies must leave crucial sites for infection exposed. The accumulation of complement proteins on the virion surface may cover these important sites and interfere with adsorption, penetration, or uncoating; aggregation of virus particles can also occur (Oldstone et al., 1974).

Virus–antibody complexes of HSV and equine arteritis virus adsorbed to cell surfaces were found to be susceptible to complement during the early period of cell–complex interaction, suggesting that complement can influence a step later than adsorption (Yoshino and Taniguchi, 1967; Radwan and Burger, 1973). Since penetration of virus–antibody complexes into cells is known to be prolonged compared to virus alone, reaction with complement at this stage may be important.

The sequence of complement component reactions with the virus–antibody complex is the same as for other antigen–antibody systems. Studies using purified components of complement and HSV or NDV complexed with early IgM have shown that C1 and C4 are required for neutralization and that the effects of suboptimal amounts of C4 can be supplemented by the addition of C2 and C3 (Daniels et al., 1969, 1970; Linscott and Levinson, 1969). Similar findings for complement enhancement of HI activity of early IgM antibody bound to influenza virus have been reported (Reno and Hoffman, 1972). Oldstone et al. (1974) found that complement-enhanced neutralization of polyoma virus requires C3 as well as C1, C2, and C4. Enhanced neutralization occurred primarily by agglutination of virus–antibody complexes.

Electron microscopic studies have demonstrated that avian infectious bronchitis virus, a coronavirus with a host-derived lipid coat containing 200 Å projections, can undergo complement-dependent virolysis similar to complement-dependent erythrocyte lysis (Berry and Almeida, 1968; Almeida and Waterson, 1969). Antibody from infected chickens reacted only with the virus-specified projections, recognizing the virion membrane as self (host-derived). However, antibody from rabbits immunized with virus grown in chickens reacted with the virion membrane and projections, whereas rabbit antibody to uninfected chicken cells reacted only with the membrane. The neutralizing capacity of all three antisera was enhanced by complement, and electron microscopy showed complement attached to projections when antibody was bound there and 100 Å holes in the membrane after complement reacted with antibody at that site. Complement-mediated virolysis has also been described for rubella virus (Almeida and Laurence, 1969), influenza virus (Almeida and Waterson, 1969), Gross leukemogenic (AKR) virus (Oroszlan and Gilden, 1970), and equine arteritis virus (Radwan et al., 1973).

The preceding discussion has considered only the classical complement activation pathway, which initially requires the conversion of C1 to C1 and subsequent interaction of C1 with C4 and C2 before activation of C3 and the remaining components. Interest has recently turned toward an alternate pathway in which C3 is activated without interaction of the preceding three components (Osler and Sandberg, 1973). Certain immunoglobulins or immunoglobulin fragments, after binding antigen, can activate complement by the alternate pathway. Guinea pig $\gamma 2$ antibodies efficiently activate complement by the classic pathway in which interaction of the Fc portion of the antibody molecule with C1 is essential. However, the $F(ab')_2$ fragments of $\gamma 2$ immunoglobulins activate complement via the alternate pathway. A. L. Sandberg (personal communication) has used $F(ab')_2$ fragments of anti-HSV $\gamma 2$ to determine whether complement-dependent enhancement of HSV neutralization can occur by the alternate pathway. She found that the $F(ab')_2$ fragments bound to the virus but were not as efficient in enhancing neutralization as were the parent undigested antibodies. Furthermore, there was only minimal lysis of HSV-infected rabbit kidney cells by the alternate pathway after binding of the $F(ab')_2$ fragments to the cell membrane. More viruses must be examined before conclusions can be drawn concerning the importance of the alternate pathway in virus neutralization, but there may be a specific requirement for the first complement components in the enhancement of neutralization of some viruses.

The *in vivo* consequences of complement reactions with virus-antibody complexes are often detrimental to the host, producing arteritis, glomerulonephritis, and choroiditis (Oldstone and Dixon, 1971; Oldstone, 1974). In addition, C3 bound to complexes may facilitate their attachment to macrophages, neutrophils, and B lymphocytes, which have C3 receptors. This could enhance their clearance by such cells if viral growth is restricted in them or, conversely, facilitate virus growth and spread if the cells are susceptible.

C. Infectious Complexes and Antiglobulin Neutralization

The residual infectivity of virus after exposure to excess antibody is called the persistent fraction, the presence and nature of which has been reviewed by Notkins (1971) and Majer (1972). Burnet *et al.* (1937) first noted the existence of a nonneutralizable fraction of an animal virus, and studies of many viruses *in vitro* (picornaviruses, togaviruses, myxoviruses, herpesviruses, poxviruses, and reoviruses) and *in vivo* (lactate dehydrogenase virus, H-1 virus, Visna virus, and Aleutian mink disease virus) demonstrate the generality of the phenomenon. That the virus in the persistent fraction is not a genetic variant was shown in studies demonstrating similar behavior of non-neutralized virus progeny and the parent population in neutralization tests (Dulbecco et al., 1956; Notkins et al., 1966b; Hahon, 1970b; Majer and Link, 1970).

The persistent fraction has been shown to consist of virus–antibody complexes by physiochemical methods—density-gradient centrifugation (Kjellen, 1965), countercurrent distribution (Philipson, 1966), and ratezonal centrifugation (Notkins et al., 1971). However, most studies have been based on the use of antiglobulins (Ashe and Notkins, 1966), when antibody directed against the antiviral immunoglobulin is reacted with the virus–antibody complexes and any increase in neutralization noted. Notkins et al. (1966b) found the persisting infectious virus in the plasma of mice infected with LDV to be in virus–antibody complexes which could be neutralized by treatment with antisera against mouse immunoglobulins. With rabbit antibody against HSV, Ashe and Notkins (1967) found that the persistent fraction could be markedly reduced with antisera against rabbit immunoglobulins, although such antisera had no effect on virus not "sensitized."

Using antiglobulins against various immunoglobulin classes, it has been shown that IgM, IgG, and IgA can sensitize virus. Studies of unfractionated antisera demonstrate that the sensitizing antibodies in mice infected with LDV are IgG and IgA; anti-mouse IgM did not neutralize the persistent fraction (Notkins et al., 1968). Human antisera to Venezuelan equine encephalitis (VEE) virus, likewise, had sensitizing IgG and IgA but not IgM antibodies (Hahon, 1970b). Hampar et al. (1968) could sensitize HSV with IgM antibody from rabbit late immune sera but not from early sera.

The sites of antiglobulin interaction have been examined. Univalent antiviral Fab fragments were found to sensitize HSV (Ashe et al., 1968, 1969) and poliovirus (Keller, 1968) and anti-Fab could neutralize sensitized VEE virus (Hahon, 1970b), indicating that the Fab portion of the sensitizing antibody can bind to the antiglobulin and result in neutralization. The persistent fraction of VEE virus could also be neutralized with anti-allotype antiglobulin for an Fc allotype and with anti-Fc antiglobulin, demonstrating that the Fc portion can also bind the antiglobulin.

Virus sensitization is generally thought to occur when antibodies are attached to noncritical sites on the virion, exposure of which is not required to initiate infection. This may hinder attachment of other antibodies to critical sites. If suboptimal amounts of antisera are reacted with virus, it is found after subsequent addition of antiglobulin that a large fraction of virus has been sensitized but not

7. Virus Infections and Immune Responses

neutralized by the antiviral antibody (Ashe and Notkins, 1967; Notkins et al., 1968). Thus, it was found that for LDV sensitization occurs sooner than neutralization and for both LDV and HSV that as sensitization increases the neutralization constant diminishes. Presumably, antiglobulin binding to antiviral antibody at noncritical sites sterically hinders interaction of virus with cells. Accordingly, univalent antiglobulin Fab fragments neutralize sensitized virus less well than larger whole antiglobulin (Ashe et al., 1968; Notkins et al., 1968).

Rheumatoid factor (RF), a human IgM with specificity for the Fc portion of aggregated or complexed IgG antibodies, has also been found to react with virus–IgG antibody complexes (Ashe et al., 1971). Rabbit or human anti-HSV IgG antibody was reacted with HSV and then with human RF. No reduction in the persistent fraction of these HSV–IgG–RF complexes occurred unless the preparations were allowed to react further with complement or anti-human IgM antiglobulin. Apparently the attachment of RF provides new sites for complement reaction and attachment on the complex. If Fab fragments of anti-HSV were used to sensitize the virus, no enhancement of neutralization was observed after reaction with complement or anti-IgM, presumably because of the inability of RF to attach to the Fab fragment. Hayashi et al. (1973) have shown that RF can bind to infected cells after they have been exposed to antiviral antibody. Whether RF plays a protective role *in vivo* by enhancing neutralization of infectious virus–antibody complexes is unknown. Alternatively, by enhancing the complement-fixing capacity of complexes it may lead to increased pathology in immune complex diseases.

VIII. Capacity of Macrophages to Support Virus Replication

Mims (1964) has summarized evidence that viruses introduced into the lungs or other sites are taken up by macrophages in the local tissues and in lymph nodes, where they are demonstrable by immunofluorescence. Likewise, viruses entering the blood from the primary site of multiplication or introduced into the bloodstream (e.g., by arthropod vectors) are removed by Kupffer cells and other macrophages lining blood sinuses. Usually, the viruses cannot multiply sufficiently well in the macrophages of adult hosts to spread to other cells which are highly susceptible, such as hepatic parenchymal cells. However, if the macrophage barrier is bypassed by exposing liver parenchymal cells directly to infection (e.g., by injecting virus into the bile duct) a lethal infection with widespread multiplication of virus in parenchymal cells results. Similarly, the brain is a highly susceptible organ, and intracerebral injection of many viruses in adult animals will result in lethal infections.

If macrophages represent an important barrier to the spread of infection there should be a relationship between the capacity of a virus to multiply in macrophages and virulence in adult animals. Such a relationship exists, and is most strikingly demonstrated where major genetic factors determine the susceptibility to infection. Bang and Warwick (1960) found that adult mice of the Princeton (PRI) strain are susceptible to lethal infection with the Nelson strain of mouse hepatitis virus (MHV-2), whereas the C3H strain of mice is resistant. Mating experiments show that the susceptibility to infection segregates as a single Mendelian dominant genetic factor. It was found, moreover, that cultures of hepatic or peritoneal macrophages taken from susceptible hosts support multiplication of MHV with cytopathic effects, whereas macrophages from resistant mice do not. This interesting observation showed that inherited resistance is a property of individual macrophages, manifested *in vitro* in the absence of an acquired immune response. Observations on other MHV strains also emphasize the relationship between virulence and the capacity of viruses to multiply in macrophages. Thus, the avirulent strain MHV-1 does not multiply in macrophages, whereas the virulent strain MHV-3, which after intraperitoneal injection into adult mice of most strains produces a lethal hepatitis, multiplies readily in mouse peritoneal macrophages with giant cell formation (Fig. 15) (Allison and Mallucci, 1965). Only the A strain of mice resists infection with MHV-3 as adults, and cultures of peritoneal macrophages from this strain again show no cytopathic effects after exposure to MHV-3 (J. L. Virelizier and A. C. Allison, unpublished observations, 1974).

Parallelism between inherited resistance of mice to viruses and the capacity of their mononuclear phagocytes to support virus multiplication is not confined to the murine hepatitis viruses. Another system that has been analyzed in detail is the inherited resistance against arthropod-borne viruses of the B group. Sabin (1954) found that the striking difference in susceptibility of HSVS and PRI mice to yellow fever virus is determined by a single pair of genes, with resistance dominant. The PRI mice also show marked resistance to other flaviviruses. This resistance is not a general one to all types of virus; in fact, the PRI mice which are resistant to flaviviruses are highly susceptible to MHV-2, and the two resistance factors segregate in-

7. Virus Infections and Immune Responses 521

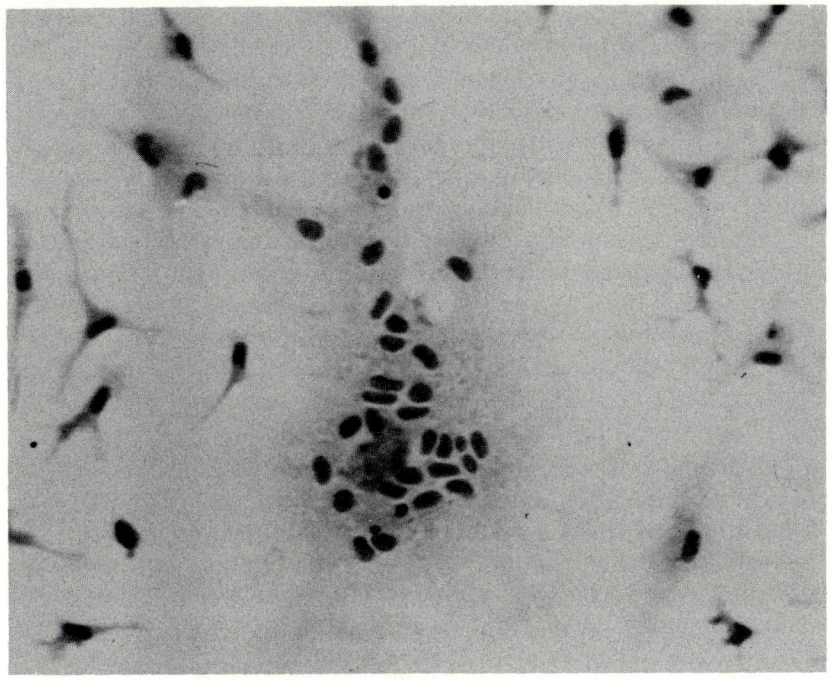

Fig. 15. Mouse peritoneal macrophages infected with mouse hepatitis virus (MHV-3), showing giant cell formation. ×200.

dependently among the offspring of hybrids (Kantoch *et al.*, 1963). It was shown by Goodman and Koprowski (1962) that macrophages from susceptible mice support multiplication of flaviviruses very efficiently, whereas macrophages from resistant mice do not. Similar observations have subsequently been made in Koprowski's laboratory on mice congenic for the resistance gene. B. Rager-Zisman and A. C. Allison (unpublished observations, 1974) have found that encephalomyocarditis virus, which is virulent in adult mice, can replicate in macrophages. Hence, there is little doubt that the capacity of a virus to multiply in macrophages is an important aspect of virulence, but not of course the only one.

It was also found (Zisman *et al.*, 1969) that the resistance of weanling mice to intraperitoneal injection of herpes simplex virus could be broken down by injections of silica particles or of rabbit anti-mouse macrophage serum. Both these treatments lead to rapid mortality beginning 5 days after infection, with high titers of virus in the liver and virus-induced hepatic necrosis. This is the result expected if the Kupffer cell barrier to the spread of virus had been broken down. In contrast, anti-lymphocytic serum resulted in a later mortality with lower concentrations of virus in the liver and no hepatitis, but a higher viremia and encephalitis. This might be expected if there was a slow buildup of virus in the blood, owing to failure of an acquired immune response, with secondary spread across the blood–brain barrier.

From all these observations we conclude that macrophages are important in preventing spread of viruses from primary sites of infection to highly susceptible cells, such as those of the liver parenchyma or brain. As will be discussed next, macrophages of newborn animals carry out this function very inefficiently, but the capacity to contain virus infections and prevent spread to susceptible cells matures rapidly during the first few weeks of postnatal life in mice.

IX. Ontogeny of Macrophage Resistance to Viral Infections

Allison and his colleagues have analyzed the role of the macrophage barrier to the spread of viruses and its development in newborn animals. Experiments with herpes simplex virus in mice can be used to illustrate the point, which probably applies also to many viruses as well as to other intracellular infections. Intraperitoneal inoculation of newborn mice with herpes simplex virus is followed by rapid spread of virus to the viscera, encephalitis, and death, whereas similar injections into weanling or adult mice result in no viral spread to the liver or brain and no morbidity or mortality. The resistance to intraperitoneal infection develops rapidly during the first few weeks of life. Transfers of peritoneal macrophages from adult CBA to syngeneic suckling mice were able to confer a large measure of protection against intraperitoneal infection with herpesvirus; similar transfers of peritoneal lymphocytes from adult animals were without any protective effect (Hirsch et al., 1970). Further studies showed that the adult macrophages, particularly when stimulated by prior injections of proteose-peptone, were much more efficient at taking up and preventing the spread of virus than macrophages from suckling animals, whether stimulated or not. This was reflected in the diminished capacity of infected adult macrophages to establish infectious centers when cultured together with susceptible cells, and similar findings were reported by Johnson (1964).

In addition to this diminished capacity of adult macrophages to transfer virus to contiguous cells, which for various reasons was thought not to be due to release of interferon and the basis of which is still not well defined, adult macrophages may replicate the virus less well than macrophages from neonates. This view is reinforced by studies of Stevens and Cook (1971a) showing that herpes simplex virus in adult mouse macrophages undergoes an abortive cycle of replication, with synthesis of virus nucleic acids and antigens, and the formation of nascent capsids lacking dense cores, in the nucleus. Hence, a late stage of herpesvirus synthesis, perhaps involving DNA metabolism or nucleocapsid formation, appears to be blocked in adult mouse macrophages.

The human counterpart to these experiments is the severe, generalized infection which herpes simplex virus produces in newborn children (Wheeler and Huffines, 1965; Nahmias et al., 1969). Usually this is herpesvirus type 2 acquired during childbirth from a maternal genital infection; occasionally it is type 1 infection. The virus disseminates widely, to the central nervous system, liver and other organs, and administration of antibody has not provided any demonstrable protection. The great majority of children die. Immaturity of macrophages in the human newborn may well be an important contributory factor allowing the dissemination of the infection. That the Kupffer cell barrier is poorly developed in human fetuses and newborns is suggested by involvement of hepatic parenchymal cells in congenital rubella infections; this is not seen in adult cases of rubella (Stern and Williams, 1966). Rager-Zisman and Allison (1973b) also found that newborn mice could be protected from intraperitoneal inoculation of Coxsackie B virus by syngeneic adult peritoneal exudate cells; the presence of very small amounts of antibody increased the protective effects.

Maturation of macrophage virucidal capacity during the first few weeks of life may be linked to cell-mediated immunity and stimulation with bacterial or other antigens. The work of Mackaness (1970) and others suggests that a lymphocyte-mediated immune response increases the capacity of macrophages to kill organisms unrelated to those providing the antigenic stimulus. Allison (1965) reported that macrophages taken later from neonatally thymectomized animals support the multiplication of the avirulent virus MHV-1, whereas the virus multiplies to a very limited extent in macrophages from intact adult animals. This work has been continued using the more virulent MHV-3 strain of virus in genetically resistant A strain mice; they succumb to MHV-3 if infected soon after birth or if they are neonatally thymectomized and infected as adults (Dupuy et al., 1973; Levy-Leblond and Dupuy, 1974).

The latter investigators and J. L. Virelizier and A. C. Allison (unpublished observations, 1974) have found that peritoneal macrophages taken from neonatally thymectomized mice support the multiplication of the virus, with giant cell formation, whereas those from normal mice of the same age do not. Also, TXBM mice of the resistant A strain when tested 2 weeks after thymus deprivation are resistant to MHV-3 and no virus replication was observed in cultures of peritoneal macrophages from such animals. However, when similar mice were tested 3 months after thymus deprivation, at a time when most macrophages present probably have developed in an environment deficient in T lymphocytes and putative thymic hormones, they were found to be susceptible to MHV-3 infection and peritoneal macrophages replicated the virus *in vitro*.

Macrophages from thymus-deprived mice have generally been thought to be normal. However, the above observations demonstrate that at least one property of "mature" macrophages, virucidal capacity, depends on the presence of the thymus and/or T lymphocytes during at least some of their development. Other macrophage functions, such as participation in granuloma formation, are deficient in newborn and neonatally thymectomized mice (Yang and Skinsnes, 1973). However, transfer experiments with macrophages from these animals are necessary before conclusions can be made concerning the role of T lymphocytes (which is established) and the developmental dependence of these macrophages on the thymus and T cells. Experiments demonstrating the inability of macrophages from newborn animals to participate in immune responses *in vivo* (see Hardy *et al.*, 1973) should be reexamined with this possibility in mind.

X. Surface Changes of Virus-Infected Cells

A. *Virus-Coded Antigens*

1. VIRION ANTIGENS

Many viruses have envelopes derived from host cell membranes and all viruses are intimately related to host cell membranes during adsorption, penetration, and replication. This can lead to profound changes in the cell membrane as well as the basic physiology and behavior of the cell and its relationship to its environment (see review by Allison, 1971). Infection with most viruses results in cell membrane alterations that can be detected by the appearance of new antigens and sometimes as a change in the ability to bind particular lectins or other materials. Table III lists viruses now known to produce antigenic changes in host membranes as detected biologically in transplantation studies or directly by immunofluorescence, immunoradiolabeling, immunoelectron microscopy, and assays employing cytotoxic antibody or lymphoid cells. It should be noted that the antisera used in many assays were produced by active infection with the virus, and antigenic changes may represent virus-induced host cell alterations and not antigens the structures of which are encoded in the virus genome.

Most of the surface antigens appear early in infection. Thus, cells infected with influenza virus produce viral protein in 1 hour (Noll, 1962) and virus-specific cell surface antigens are detectable 4 hours after infection (Hahon and Eckert, 1972). New surface antigens appear on cells infected by NDV at 3 hours, VEE and Sindbis viruses at 4 hours, vaccinia virus at 4 hours, HSV at 6 hours, and measles, rinderpest, and canine distemper viruses at 20 to 24 hours. Studies with protein and nucleic acid synthesis inhibitors have demonstrated that new protein must be synthesized before the antigens are detectable (i.e., the antigens are not adsorbed virions) but that nucleic acid synthesis is not usually required. Thus the antigenic changes probably represent early functions of the virus genome. An apparent exception is the transplantation rejection antigen (TRA) produced by SV40 infection, which does not appear in lytic infection but appears late in the transformation of nonpermissive cells (Smith and Mora, 1972).

Infection by some viruses produces no detectable surface antigens. Picornaviruses, although associated with cytoplasmic membranes during development, do not bud through membranes and lack membrane envelopes. Perhaps significantly in this regard, they also lack carbohydrates which, in those viruses containing carbohydrates, are attached to virus proteins while the latter are embedded in host membranes. Cells infected by Coxsackie B5 virus (a picornavirus) have no surface antigens detectable by immunofluorescence or radiolabeling (Hayashi et al., 1973). A strain of vaccinia virus has been reported which does not produce a major surface antigen normally found early during infection (Ito and Barron, 1972b).

Most cells transformed by the Moloney variant of murine sarcoma virus (MSC) also produce helper murine leukemogenic virus and possess surface antigens specified by the latter virus. A few MSV-transformed cell lines not producing helper virus are available and Strouk et al. (1972) could not detect virus-specific surface antigens

TABLE III

Demonstration of Virus-Specific Surface Antigens on Infected Cells

Virus	Assay[a]	Reference
Murine leukemogenic	CT	Slettenmark-Wahren and Klein, 1962
	CT	Geering et al., 1966
	IEM	Aoki et al., 1970, 1972
	CT	Shirai et al., 1971
	CT	Stockert et al., 1971
	LC	Proffitt et al., 1973
Murine mammary tumor	IA	Nishioka et al., 1969
Feline leukemia	IEM	Oshiro et al., 1971
	RI	Boone et al., 1973
Avian tumor	IEM	Gelderblom et al., 1972
	LC	Kurth and Bauer, 1972
	IEM	Gelderblom and Bauer, 1973
	IEM	Phillips and Perdue, 1974
Orthomyxoviruses		
Influenza	IEM	Duc-Nguyen et al., 1966
	CT	Brier et al., 1971
	IF	Hahon and Eckert, 1972
Paramyxoviruses		
Mumps	IEM	Duc-Nguyen and Rosenblum, 1967
	LC	Speel et al., 1968
Sendai	CT	Eaton and Scala, 1969
SV5	CT	Holmes et al., 1969
Measles, rinderpest,	IF	Yamanouchi et al., 1970
canine distemper	LC	Rustigian et al., 1971
	LC	Labowskie et al., 1974
Respiratory syncitial	LA	Epsmark, 1965
Togaviruses		
Chikungunya	IF	Mantani and Igarashi, 1971
VEE	IF	Hahon, 1970a
EEE	CT	Catanzaro et al., 1974
Sindbis	HA	Burge and Pfefferkorn, 1967
	IF, LC	McFarland, 1974
Dengue	CT, IEM	Catanzaro et al., 1974
Rhabdoviruses		
Rabies	CT	Fernandes et al., 1964
	CT	Wiktor et al., 1968
Arenaviruses		
LCM	LC	Lundstedt, 1969
	CT, LC	Oldstone et al., 1969
	LC	Wright et al., 1972
	IF, LC	Cole et al., 1973
	LC	Marker and Volkert, 1973
	LC	Zinkernagel and Doherty, 1974

7. Virus Infections and Immune Responses

TABLE III (Cont.)

Virus	Assay[a]	Reference
Adenoviruses		
Adenovirus type 12	CT	Berman, 1967
	IF	Hollinshead and Alford, 1969
	IF	Vasconcelos-Costa, 1970
	IF	Vasconcelos-Costa et al., 1973
Herpesviruses		
Herpes simplex	IF	O'Dea and Dineen, 1957
	CT	Roane and Roizman, 1964
	IA	Epsmark, 1965
	IEM	Nii et al., 1968
	CT	Brier et al., 1971
	IF	Lowry et al., 1971
	IEM	Miyamoto et al., 1971
	IF	Nahmias et al., 1971
	IA	Ito and Barron, 1972a
	CT	Smith et al., 1972
Varicalla-zoster	IF	Gershon et al., 1974
Cytomegaloviruses	IF	Thé and Langenhuysen, 1972
Epstein–Barr	IF	Klein et al., 1968
	IF	Dunkel and Zeigel, 1970
Marek's disease	IF	Chen and Purchase, 1970
Poxviruses		
Vaccinia, cowpox, monkeypox	IA, IF	Miyamoto and Kato, 1968, 1971
	IF	Ueda et al., 1969
	CT	Brier et al., 1971
	RI	Hayashi et al., 1972
	IA	Ito and Barron, 1972b
Shope fibroma	IF, CT	Ishimoto and Ito, 1969, 1971
	IF	Tompkins et al., 1970b
Papova		
SV40	CT	Smith et al., 1970
	RI	Ting and Herberman, 1970
	CT	Wright and Law, 1971
	RI	Kedar et al., 1972
Polyoma	IF	Irlin, 1967
	IF	Malmgren et al., 1968
	RI	Ting and Herberman, 1970

[a] Key: CT, antibody + complement cytotoxicity; IA, immune adherence; IEM, immunoelectron microscopy; IF, immunofluorescence; LC, lymphocyte-mediated cytotoxicity; RI, radioimmunoassay.

on such cells using hemadsorption and lymphocyte cytotoxicity assays. Stephenson and Aaronson (1972) failed to detect transplantation antigens on similar cell lines, but Law and Ting (1970) did find transplantation antigens and the issue is not settled.

2. NONVIRION ANTIGENS

Some virus-induced surface antigens are thought to be virus coded but are not found in the virion. Gross leukemogenic virus produces a variety of antigens in infected cells (Aoki et al., 1972), among which are nonvirion surface antigens (GCSAa and GCSAb). Similarly, the transplantation antigens of adenoviruses, SV40, and polyoma virus have not been identified in virions.

B. Alteration of Host Antigens or Receptors

1. APPEARANCE OF "NEW" HOST ANTIGENS

Some recognizable new surface antigens probably result from unmasking of antigenic substructure already present or derepression of host genes. Cells of a hamster kidney line (BHK) which normally have no demonstrable Forssman antigen acquired it after transformation with SV40, polyoma virus, or Rous sarcoma virus (Fogel and Sachs, 1962; O'Neill, 1968; Robertson and Black, 1969).

2. CHANGES IN LECTIN RECEPTORS

The appearance on transformed cells of accessible receptors for lectins, glycoproteins from plants and invertebrates capable of agglutinating certain cells by binding with particular carbohydrates, may also represent an unmasking phenomenon or rearranging of membrane components. Burger (1973) has reviewed the subject and it appears that lectin receptors on normal and transformed cells may be present in equal amounts. Virus transformation or mild treatment of normal cells with proteases does not lead directly to clustering of lectin-binding receptors, but does increase the mobility of lectin-binding sites which can cluster in the presence of multivalent lectins (Rosenblith et al., 1973).

Even so, there are demonstrable changes in the concentrations of membrane components and related enzymes during the transformation process (Brady et al., 1973). Sialic acid levels were found to be reduced in SV40 (Wu et al., 1968) and polyoma virus (Ohta et al., 1968) transformed cells when compared to parental cells; there is

7. Virus Infections and Immune Responses

usually a reduction in higher ganglioside homologues as well (Brady and Mora, 1970). The higher gangliosides are formed by the sequential addition of various hexose moieties and sialic acid and is mediated by transferase enzymes. An examination of one transferase involved has revealed it to be markedly reduced in most SV40 and polyoma virus transformed cells (Brady et al., 1973). Viral alterations in enzymes concerned with membrane biosynthesis and structure (such as ganglioside transferases) might alter phenotypic expression in much the same way as the lysogenic conversion of *Salmonella* by ϵ phage (Robbins and Uchida, 1965).

3. Appearance of an Fc Receptor

The appearance on cells infected with HSV of a receptor that binds the Fc portion of rabbit or human IgG molecules has been reported (Watkins, 1965; Yasuda and Milgrom, 1968; Shimizu, 1971; Westmoreland and Watkins, 1974). The Fc receptor appeared on the surfaces of all infected cells tested, including fibroblasts and epithelial cells from mice, hamsters, monkeys, and humans. Receptors appeared on HeLa cells within 4 hours after infection and at 11 hours after infection an estimated 5×10^4 molecules of IgG per cell bound to the cell membrane during 30 minutes at 37°C. Experiments with actinomycin D and puromycin suggested an early need for RNA synthesis after infection and for continuing synthesis of receptors. No evidence was obtained to suggest unmasking of Fc receptors already present in a cryptic form. Antisera against uninfected host cells or HSV blocked the subsequent attachment of immunoglobulin to the infected cells. This could be due to steric hindrance or the Fc receptor might contain host and viral antigenic determinants; a viral protein glycosylated by host enzymes and functioning as an Fc receptor could have this characteristic. It is not known whether the virus codes for a protein which is the receptor itself or which can be glycosylated by cellular enzymes and resemble the Fc receptor known to be present on macrophages, neutrophils, B lymphocytes, and possibly some T lymphocytes. Alternatively, infection could result in derepression of the appropriate host gene(s) controlling synthesis of the receptor. This latter possibility is intriguing in view of recent suggestions that the Fc receptor is a product of the Ir gene complex. Since these genes control some immune responses, infection of lymphocytes by viruses that activate genes in this complex might affect immune responses or perhaps permit autoimmune responses.

4. Loss of Host Antigens

Virus infections can result not only in the appearance of "new" host antigens, but also in the diminution of normal membrane antigens. Hecht and Summers (1972) found a 70% reduction in the capacity of VSV-infected mouse cells to adsorb cytolytic antibodies directed against H-2 antigen. This was not due to inhibition of protein synthesis as treatment of cells with cycloheximide for a similar time period did not reduce the H-2 concentration, nor did infection with encephalomyocarditis virus which inhibits host protein synthesis. Whether other cell antigens, particularly tumor antigens, will behave similarly during infection merits examination. At least one tumor antigen is known to cocap and thus to be linked with H-2 antigen and conceivably may be altered by those factors influencing H-2 density (Gooding and Edidin, 1974). Recently, Hecht and Summers (1974) reported that NDV-infected L (mouse) cells lose 50% of their H-2 antigen.

C. Capping of Viral Antigens

The polar redistribution (capping) of surface immunoglobulins (Taylor et al., 1971) and receptors for immune complexes (Miller et al., 1973) on lymphocytes and of transplantation antigens on a variety of cell types (Kourilsky et al., 1972) has been reported by many laboratories and much speculation concerning its physiological importance has arisen. Joseph and Oldstone (1974) have described capping of measles virus antigen on infected HeLa cells; it required active cell metabolism and multivalent antibody. Capping has also been observed for mumps antigen on infected cells (K. Hayashi, personal communication) and for gs-1 and gs-3 antigens on Gross virus-induced leukemic cells (Yoshiki et al., 1974a) and may be a general phenomenon for virus-specific cell surface antigens.

Capping of viral antigens on the surface of infected cells could have a number of consequences. If viral nucleocapsids must align themselves beneath membrane containing viral proteins before budding (e.g., myxoviruses), capping could interfere with viral morphogenesis and release. Alteration of the density of viral antigens on the cell surface might result in ineffective interaction of the cell with lymphocytes (Cole et al., 1973) or of the attached antibody with complement (Brier et al., 1971). Some nonlytic infections thus protected from effective immune responses might persist.

D. Antigenic Modulation

A phenomenon similar to capping that results in reversible losses of surface antigens, termed antigenic modulation, can also occur. A host antigen, the TL (thymus-leukemia) antigen in mice, is an organ-specific allotypic determinant on thymocytes of certain mouse strains with its genetic locus near the D end of the H-2 locus (Boyse et al., 1965; Boyse and Old, 1969). Leukemias induced by leukemogenic viruses in the TL-positive mouse strains result in the appearance of the TL antigen on leukemic cells. If such leukemic cells are transplanted to TL-negative animals previously immunized with TL antigen and producing antibody to it, the antigen is quickly lost from the cell surface but can reappear if the leukemic cells are transplanted back to a TL-positive host (lacking antibody to TL). Phenotypic expression of TL was found to markedly reduce the demonstrable quantity of H-2 antigens, especially those specified by the D region. With loss of TL by antigen modulation, an increase in the H-2 antigens was observed (Boyse et al., 1968; Old et al., 1968). Antigenic modulation for the GCSAa antigen of leukemic cells, which appears to be coded by the Gross leukemia virus rather than the host, has also been reported (Aoki et al., 1972).

E. Possible Combinations of Host and Viral Antigenic Determinants

Recent experiments by Zinkernagel and Doherty (1974) raise the interesting possibility that some virus-induced surface antigens may be combinations of virus and host material. These investigators reported that lymphocytes from LCM-infected mice are capable of mediating a cytotoxic reaction only with infected target cells which share similarity at either the K or D region of the H-2 locus. The reactive lymphocytes were sensitive to anti-θ and complement and thus are T lymphocytes. (It should be mentioned that Cole et al. (1973) found no such H-2 requirement in a similar system.) R. V. Blanden (personal communication) has obtained similar results using ectromelia virus. One explanation for this phenomenon is that the interaction of cytotoxic T lymphocytes with somatic cells requires an intimate contact that is strongly dependent on some degree of histocompatibility, as is suggested for the interaction of helper T lymphocytes and B lymphocytes (Katz et al., 1973a,b). An alternative explanation is that the immune lymphocytes recognize a composite antigen consisting of virus protein and H-2 material, or that the virus infection results in altered H-2 antigens that are no longer recognized by the lymphocytes as "self."

XI. Evidence for Cell-Mediated Immunity to Viral Antigens

A. Introduction

Over the past couple of decades knowledge of the structure of antibodies and their protective and pathological roles in immunity have been well defined. Currently, much interest is centered on understanding lymphoid cells and cell-mediated immunity. Various methods have been used to illustrate the presence of cell-mediated immunity against virus-specific antigens. Each has its own advantages and limitations. Although delayed hypersensitivity to many viruses or viral antigens has been demonstrated, it must be interpreted with caution. For example, some reactions are elicited by antigens from the heterologous cells in which viruses are grown. Antibody-mediated reactions to replicating antigens may be maximal between 24 and 72 hours after intradermal inoculation; even the histology may be ambiguous. Of the *in vitro* tests for cell-mediated immunity, MIF production correlates better with delayed hypersensitivity than does blast transformation (David and Schlossman, 1968; Rocklin *et al.*, 1970). With peptides of tobacco mosaic virus and glucagon, delayed skin reactions correlated with the production of MIF by lymphoid cells *in vitro*, but not always with the stimulation of DNA synthesis on the exposure of host lymphocytes to the antigens (Spitler *et al.*, 1970; Senyk *et al.*, 1971). It seems that MIF production is a particularly good *in vitro* correlate of delayed hypersensitivity in guinea pigs, but attempts to obtain MIF production with cells from other species, including man, have not been easily reproducible in all laboratories.

Many studies of lymphocyte stimulation by viruses have been performed, but for the most part they have been inadequately controlled to exclude the possible involvement of host cell antigens and to characterize the participating cells. The manner of antigen presentation—whether infected cells or virus, infectious or inactivated—can determine the type and extent of response obtained. The blastogenic response primarily represents antigenic recognition by lymphocytes, and Gershon *et al.* (1973) have found that for T lymphocytes this may not correlate with the development of recognized T lymphocyte

7. Virus Infections and Immune Responses

functions. The lymphocyte cytotoxicity assays represent effector functions as well as antigen recognition (Bach et al., 1973) and may be complicated by factors (such as immune complexes) that influence either of these functions.

What is considered cell-mediated immunity in the animal is a complex multicomponent phenomenon involving functionally different lymphocyte populations as well as macrophages, K cells and antibodies, soluble mediators, and other factors. Obviously, to assay one component of this process *in vitro* is rather artificial, and all *in vitro* assays must be interpreted with caution. Even so, from these investigations some useful generalizations are beginning to emerge. Sensitization of T lymphocytes in virus infections is an early event, being demonstrable 3 to 7 days after infection, reaching a peak of cytotoxic reactivity at 7 to 14 days and then falling to near background levels. A population of memory cells, not themselves cytotoxic but able to generate cytotoxic effector cells, then persists for weeks or months. The finding of stimulated DNA synthesis by lymphocytes in the presence of virus antigen does not necessarily imply T lymphocyte sensitization, especially in secondary responses where B lymphocyte proliferation may predominate.

This section can consider this large subject only in outline form. Evidence for delayed hypersensitivity (DH) to virus antigens will be briefly mentioned and the *in vitro* correlates summarized.

B. Poxviruses

1. Vaccinia Virus

In 1907, von Pirquet suggested that hypersensitivity contributes to the local inflammatory lesion of primary vaccinia, and vaccinia virus has continued to be used in studies of DH. Broom (1947) demonstrated in humans that prevaccination lesions can occur in the absence of specific antibody and Turk et al. (1962), by injecting virus-antiserum mixtures, produced typical DH reactions in guinea pigs without demonstrable humoral antibody. Allison (1967) could passively transfer DH against vaccinia in inbred guinea pigs with peritoneal exudate cells but not with serum. Pincus and Flick (1963) used anti-mononuclear cell antisera to inhibit local vaccinia skin lesions in guinea pigs.

In vitro studies have shown that lymphoid cells from humans immunized with vaccinia can respond specifically to antigenic challenge by generating MIF (Tompkins *et al.*, 1970a). Spleen and peripheral blood lymphocytes from vaccinia-infected rabbits, when exposed to UV-inactivated vaccinia, were found to incorporate up to thirty times as much thymidine into their DNA as appropriate controls (Rosenberg *et al.*, 1972a). This stimulation was observed from 3 to at least 120 days after infection and was at its peak during the second week of infection. Elfenbein and Rosenberg (1973) have subsequently shown that both T and B lymphocytes participate in this proliferation. Using heat-inactivated vaccinia virus, Epstein *et al.* (1972) have demonstrated transformation and interferon production by human lymphocytes from immune donors.

2. Ectromelia Virus

This poxvirus of mice, which cross-reacts with vaccinia virus, produces a severe and often fatal disease. Fenner (1949) showed that there is an allergic component as measured by swelling of the foot on challenge with live virus at various times after primary infection. The allergy was first seen on the seventh day and increased in magnitude thereafter. Since generalized infection of the skin occurs on the sixth day, Fenner considered it unlikely that allergy played an important part in localizing virus in the skin. However, more recent studies by Blanden (1970, 1971) have further defind the role of cell-mediated immunity to this virus *in vivo*.

Gardner *et al.* (1974) have used a chromium-release cell-mediated cytotoxicity assay with infected L cells as target cells to study the generation of immune lymphocytes after infection. Mouse spleen cells showed cytotoxic activity 2 days after immunization and this activity peaked at 6 days before declining to low levels by day 10. This activity was not diminished by the removal of macrophages or the addition of antisera to ectromelia or by exogenous interferon, but was abrogated by prior treatment of the lymphocytes with anti-θ antibody and complement and thus is mediated by T lymphocytes.

3. Fibroma Virus

When inoculated into the skin of adult domestic rabbits, this poxvirus induces a rapidly growing tumor that subsequently regresses. Intradermal challenge with virus on the fifth day produced DH reactions (Allison, 1966; Allison and Friedman, 1966). *In vitro* production of MIF can also be elicited from lymphocytes obtained 5 days after virus inoculation (Tompkins *et al.*, 1970a).

C. Herpesviruses

1. Herpes Simplex Virus

HSV can elicit DH reactions in a large proportion of adults and a lower proportion of children (Nagler, 1944; Rose and Molloy, 1947; Anderson and Kilbourne, 1961). DH to HSV in guinea pigs was demonstrated by Brown (1953) and later Lausch et al. (1966) showed that DH could be induced by a single injection of infective HSV. The skin reaction can be elicited by a soluble antigen (Anderson and Kilbourne, 1961; Jawetz et al., 1951, 1955), and recently Rogers et al. (1972) demonstrated that DH can be induced in guinea pigs with a soluble antigen. It will be interesting to determine if DH can be induced and/or elicited with the glycoprotein recently shown to be a neutralizing antigen for HSV (Cohen et al., 1972; Powell et al., 1974).

In vitro studies demonstrated that inactivated HSV can stimulate DNA synthesis in sensitized lymphocytes (Rosenberg et al., 1972a) and differentiate type 1 and type 2 virus (Rosenberg et al., 1972b).

2. Epstein–Barr Virus

Gerber and Lucas (1972) have shown that peripheral blood lymphocytes from previously infected subjects are stimulated to incorporate thymidine by UV-inactivated EB virus whereas lymphocytes from seronegative subjects are not stimulated.

3. Cytomegaloviruses

It has already been noted that the various in vitro tests purporting to demonstrate cell-mediated immunity may depend crucially on the manner of antigen presentation and may reflect different functions of lymphocytes. The former point is well demonstrated in the report of Thurman et al. (1973) concerning MIF production and transformation of lymphocytes from CMV-infected patients after exposure of the lymphocytes to virus or to virus-infected cells. The lymphocytes from CMV-infected patients responded by production of MIF when cultured with purified virus but were transformed only by culture with CMV-infected cell lines. Virus-specific antigens on the virion surface and the membranes of infected cells probably differ quantitatively and qualitatively, and may elicit different lymphocyte responses or stimulate different lymphocyte populations.

D. Myxoviruses

Beveridge and Burnet (1944) found skin hypersensitivity of the DH type with influenza virus. Interestingly, they stated that live attenuated virus administered intranasally was more effective in inducing skin hypersensitivity than killed virus vaccine injected subcutaneously. Mice inoculated with inactivated influenza virus developed cell-mediated immunity as shown by *in vitro* tests (Feinstone *et al.*, 1969). Hellman *et al.* (1972) reported the stimulation by PR8 influenza virus of thymidine incorporation into spleen cells of sensitized mice, beginning 7 days after infection and peaking at 14 days before declining. MIF assays have been employed by Wetherbee (1973) to demonstrate systemic cell-mediated responses in guinea pigs infected intranasally with influenza virus. Gadol *et al.* (1974) compared MIF production by lymphocytes from bronchial washes or spleens of guinea pigs infected intranasally or by the footpad route. Intranasal infection led to MIF production predominantly by lung lymphocytes whereas parenteral inoculation resulted mainly in systemic immunity.

E. Paramyxoviruses

1. Mumps Virus

Enders *et al.* (1945) demonstrated dermal hypersensitivity to mumps virus and positive reactions were related to immunity. DH has been produced in guinea pigs with mumps virus (Glasgow and Morgan, 1957) and Speel *et al.* (1968) showed that spleen cells from mice immunized with mumps virus are toxic to Chang cells persistently infected with mumps. Lymphocytes from mice infected with mumps virus have been shown to produce MIF *in vitro* (Feinstone *et al.*, 1969). Using inactivated mumps virus, Smith *et al.* (1972) have demonstrated stimulation of DNA synthesis in human lymphocytes after primary exposure and for up to 40 years after primary exposure and correlated this with delayed skin sensitivity.

2. Measles Virus and SSPE Agent

Skin testing with measles virus has been complicated by contaminating antigens derived from cells used to culture the virus (Isacson, 1968). A number of *in vitro* assays have been employed to assess cell-mediated immunity to measles virus and the closely related agent of subacute sclerosing panencephalitis (SSPE). A colony-

7. Virus Infections and Immune Responses

inhibition assay used lymphocytes from monkeys infected with measles virus and BSC-1 cells persistently infected with the virus (Rustigian et al., 1971). Labowskie et al. (1974) reported that lymphocytes from seropositive individuals were capable of morphological destruction and lysis of cell lines persistently infected with measles. This reaction could be blocked by pretreatment of the target cells with antisera to measles. Thurman et al. (1973) and Ahmed et al. (1974) reported that lymphocytes from seropositive individuals produced MIF and lymphotoxin on exposure to purified measles virus, but interestingly, blastogenic responses did not occur on exposure of the lymphocytes to virus preparations but, as with CMV, were elicited when the lymphocytes were cultured with virus-infected cells.

There has been much controversy concerning the nature of cell-mediated immunity in general and to measles antigens or virus in particular in patients with subacute sclerosing panencephalitis. There are reports of diminished lymphocyte responses to PHA (Kolar, 1968) and lack of normal dermal hypersensitivity reactions to common test antigens as well as delayed rejection of skin allografts (Gerson and Haslam, 1971). However, Jabbour et al. (1969) found all of eight patients tested to have normal skin responses to *Candida* and two of three patients could be sensitized to dichloronitrobenzene. J. F. Soothill (private communication) has found normal lymphocyte responses to PHA in eight cases. Normal *in vitro* cell-mediated immunity to antigens other than measles was reported for twenty cases (Moulias et al., 1971). A generalized defect in cell-mediated immunity is therefore not established.

Two reports on five patients with SSPE confirm normal reactivity of lymphocytes from SSPE patients in MIF and lymphotoxin-release assays using virus preparations of measles or the SSPE agent as the antigen, or in transformation assays using SSPE-infected cells as the stimulant (Thurman et al., 1973; Ahmed et al., 1974). A blocking factor found in high concentration in the cerebrospinal fluids of SSPE patients and in lesser concentration in their sera was found to block the reactions of lymphocytes from SSPE patients and normal seropositive individuals in the MIF, lymphotoxin-release, and transformation assays specifically for the SSPE agent and not against other antigens (Sell et al., 1973; Ahmed et al., 1974). This factor is heat-labile, larger than MW 150,000, sensitive to the actions of trypsin and neuraminidase, neutralized by rheumatoid factor, and may be an antigen–antibody complex.

Using the lymphocyte-mediated cytotoxicity assay of Labowskie *et al.* (1974), J. A. Bellanti and his colleagues (personal communication) have confirmed the normal reactivity of lymphocytes from seven SSPE patients against measles-infected cells. These workers also found specific blocking factors in the sera of these patients. In conclusion it appears that SSPE patients have the capacity to mount cell-mediated immune responses in general and to measles-SSPE virus antigens in particular, but reaction to the latter are thwarted by blocking factors, possibly immune complexes, that are found predominantly in the CSF.

F. Murine Leukemogenic Viruses

Cell-mediated responses to murine leukemias have been recognized for years. However, congenital infections by the murine leukemia viruses formerly were thought to result in tolerance to the virus antigens and only recently has circulating antibody to these viruses been demonstrated. The concept of "split tolerance" in which humoral responses are not accompanied by cell-mediated responses was then suggested. Recently, Proffitt *et al.* (1973) presented evidence for cell-mediated immunity in carrier C3H mice for Moloney leukemia virus. Lymphocytes from such animals mediated cytotoxic reactions against syngeneic cells infected with Moloney leukemia virus but not against uninfected cells. Wahren and Metcalf (1970) had reported similar results using C3H carrier mice (for Moloney MuLV) and embryo cell cultures from these mice as target cells; lymphocytes from normal C3H mice were not cytotoxic for these target cells. The latter investigators also reported cytotoxic reactions of lymphocytes from preleukemic AKR mice for cell monolayers of AKR embryos or of AKR thymic epithelial cells. Many tissues of AKR mice are known to possess Gross MuLV antigens and these target cells probably possessed viral antigens since the cytotoxic reaction was prevented by pretreatment of the target cells with antisera to Gross cell surface antigens. At variance with the above studies, Chieco-Bianchi *et al.* (1974) have reported no cytotoxic reactions between spleen lymphocytes from adult C57BL/6 mice infected neonatally with Moloney MuLV and syngeneic Moloney MuLV-infected target cells. Differences in the production of the virus carrier state and in the cytotoxic assays employed may account for this discrepancy. In this last study a chromium-release assay was used while in the previous studies a microcytotoxicity assay (similar to colony inhibition assays) was used and important differences in these assays are known (Biesecker *et al.*, 1973; Bloom *et al.*, 1973).

G. Togaviruses

1. Sindbis Virus

Beginning a few days after footpad inoculation of mice with Sindbis virus, lymphocytes from draining nodes and spleen underwent blastogenesis after exposure to the virus (Griffin and Johnson, 1973). This sensitivity peaked 6 days after infection and returned to control levels by 16 days. Lysis of infected syngeneic mouse embryo cells by immune lymphocytes followed a similar but slightly shorter time course (McFarland, 1974). This latter function was sensitive to treatment with anti-θ antisera and complement and thus probably represents a T lymphocyte activity.

2. Venezuelan Equine Encephalitis Virus

Stimulation of spleen lymphocytes from immune mice by Venezuelan equine encephalitis virus (VEE) was reported by Adler and Rabinowitz (1973). The reactivity of lymphocytes from mice receiving one immunizing dose of virus was abolished by treatment with anti-θ sera and complement, while that of lymphocytes from mice receiving two immunizing doses was not. Reactivity of the latter lymphocytes was sensitive to treatment with antisera against mouse immunoglobulin plus complement. These results suggest that after primary immunization antigen recognition and proliferation in the immune spleen cell population are due to T lymphocytes while after secondary immunization the reactive cells are predominantly B lymphocytes. These findings are in agreement with those of Elfenbein and Rosenberg (1973) for vaccinia virus.

3. Rubella Virus

A chromium-release assay using persistently infected BHK cells has been described and only peripheral blood lymphocytes from seropositive subjects were cytotoxic in this assay (Steele et al., 1973). Smith et al. (1973) have described an assay to measure the blastogenic responses of human lymphocytes after exposure to rubella antigen. Using a similar assay Lee and Sigel (1974) examined the influence of immune complexes on the blastogenic responses of blood lymphocytes from immune rabbits after exposure to inactivated rubella virus. The response was not altered by the presence of complexes of virus and anti-rubella IgG but virus complexes with anti-rubella IgM were markedly inhibitory. Normal IgM mixed with rubella virus or anti-rubella IgM mixed with poliovirus or influenza virus had no effect. In a study with HSV (Rosenberg et al., 1972a) hyperimmune sera mixed with HSV did not inhibit blastogenesis; anti-HSV antibodies in this sera probably were of the IgG class. Examination of the effects on immune responses of virus–antibody complexes with attention to antibody class will be of especial interest with measles virus and the SSPE agent.

H. Arenaviruses

There is considerable evidence for *in vivo* cell-mediated responses after infection of adult rodents with LCM virus (Lehmann-Grube, 1971; Cole, 1974). For example, Tosolini and Mims (1971) described the time course of the development of DH reactions in acutely infected mice by using the footpad test. *In vitro* assays have employed persistently infected L cells as target cells for immune lymphocytes. Benson (1962) first showed that immune spleen lymphocytes inhibited the adherence and growth of infected L cells, and this phenomenon was studied in more detail by Lundstedt (1969). Similar studies demonstrating cytotoxic effects of immune lymphocytes have employed the Hellstrom method (Wright et al., 1972) and chromium-release assays (Oldstone et al., 1969; Cole et al., 1973; Marker and Volkert, 1973; Zinkernagel and Doherty, 1974). Cole et al. (1973) have demonstrated that the immune lymphocytes responsible for this specific cytotoxicity are sensitive to anti-θ antisera and complement. Effector activity appears a few days after infection, peaks at 10 days, and then falls sharply off—a pattern similar to that after infection with ectromelia virus or Sindbis virus.

Recent reports from three laboratories indicate that the immune spleen cells obtained early during infection differ from late immune spleen cells (Mims and Blanden, 1972; Johnson et al., 1974; Volkert et al., 1974). The former cells, in addition to being cytotoxic in *in vitro* assays, possessed antiviral activities and protected mice during acute lethal infections. Late immune cells lacked these properties *in re* acutely infected mice, but had strong antiviral activity when transplanted to chronically infected mice—a situation in which early immune cells had little effect. Also, the cytotoxic and antiviral activities of the early immune cells were relatively resistant to X-irradiation, while the antiviral activity (on transfer to chronically infected mice) of late immune cells was radiation sensitive. Functions of both populations of cells were sensitive to treatment with anti-θ antisera and complement, and thus T lymphocytes are involved in both populations. Perhaps the late immune cells comprise relatively few actively cytotoxic T lymphocytes but many "memory" T lymphocytes capable, over a period of time longer than that involved in acute infection, of producing a large population of cytotoxic cells.

XII. Persistence of Immunity to Viruses

A lifelong immunity against reinfection is produced by many viruses, including smallpox, poliomyelitis, yellow fever, and the acute childhood exanthemas. In 1847 Panum showed that in the Faroe islands, where successive measles epidemics were separated by intervals of 65 and 31 years, each epidemic infected all those who had not been previously exposed but spared those who had been exposed. Reports of antibodies persisting in the absence of reinfection include those against yellow fever virus for 75 years (Sawyer, 1931), poliomyelitis among the Eskimos for 40 years (Paul et al., 1951), and Rift Valley fever for 12 years (Sabin and Blumberg, 1947). Reexposure to virus may increase the duration of immunity. Thus, Krugman et al. (1966) found rises in neutralizing antibody titers in immune subjects exposed to measles, and similar observations have been made on vaccinated subjects exposed to smallpox (Downie and McCarthy, 1958).

Two explanations have been put forward for prolonged anti-viral immunity in the absence of reinfection; according to one there is persistence of specific clones of immunocompetent cells (Burnet, 1959) and according to the other persistence of virus (Olitsky and Long, 1929a,b). Observations of antibody in rabbits 2 years after inoculation with inactivated poliovirus (Svehag, 1964b) and similar data in man after administration of killed virus vaccines show that immunologic memory exists, but whether it can explain a lifetime of antibody production in the absence of further antigenic stimulation is uncertain.

Many viruses are known to persist after infection, and in 1929 Olitsky and Long (1929a) suggested "that the immunity in virus diseases may be linked with the persistence in the body of the living virus." De Koch (1924) found the blood of a horse recovered from an attack of equine pernicious anemia to be infectious 7 years later. The salivary gland virus of guinea pigs could be recovered any time after infection and in the presence of antibody (Cole and Kuttner, 1926). Vaccinia virus was isolated from rabbits 4 months after inoculation (Olitsky and Long, 1929a,b). Measles virus has been isolated from brain and lymph nodes of patients with subacute sclerosing panencephalitis (Horta-Barbosa et al., 1969; Payne et al., 1969) and from the lymph nodes and spleens of normal subjects some years after infection (Enders-Ruckle, 1965). Adenoviruses are commonly isolated from human tonsillar and adenoidal tissues (Israel, 1962; Strohl and Schlesinger, 1965), and in rabbits they persist for long periods in splenic and lymph node cells (Pereira and Kelly, 1957; Reddick and Lefkowitz, 1969; Allison, 1970; Faucon et al., 1974). Mouse cytomegaloviruses can be isolated from the spleen and lymph nodes of chronically infected mice (Henson et al., 1972). Some viruses such as lymphocytic choriomeningitis virus and lactate dehydrogenase virus often persist for the lifetime of host animals even in the presence of antibody.

The human herpesviruses are well known for their latency and tendency to establish recurring infections. Human CMV is often isolated from leukocytes of normal persons (Diosi et al., 1969; Perham et al., 1971; Lang, 1972). EB virus may be induced in lymphocytes years after recovery from infectious mononucleosis (Diehl et al., 1968). Varicella-zoster virus remains dormant for years after chicken pox and reappears clinically as zoster. Initial HSV infection presents as a childhood stomatitis with subsequent positive titers for CF and neutralizing antibody (Yoshino et al., 1962). HSV can later be isolated from asymptomatic subjects as well as those with herpetic lesions (Buddingh et al., 1953; Kaufman et al., 1967). Over 40 years ago Goodpasture (1929) suggested that the virus remains in a dormant state between recurrences in the sensory ganglia. Direct proof for this concept was lacking until recently, when Stevens and Cook (1971b) isolated HSV from the spinal ganglia of mice weeks after recovery from posterior paralysis following virus inoculation of hind footpads, and from rabbit trigeminal ganglia months after recovery from corneal infection (Nesburn et al., 1972; Stevens et al., 1972). Virus was recovered only from the ganglia and not from proximal or distal nerve structures except during acute infection. Virus could not be detected in the ganglia by electron microscopy or by infectious virus assay, and only after the ganglia were explanted and cultured for a period of time *in vitro* could virus be recovered. Recovery of HSV from *in vitro* cultures of human trigeminal ganglia obtained at autopsy from patients without active herpes infection has now been reported (Bastian et al., 1972; Baringer and Swoveland, 1973). J. R. Baringer (1974) has recently isolated type 2 (genital) herpes from the sacral ganglia of humans. It appears that the virus is activated by the explantation and culture, probably due to metabolic changes in the neurons subsequent to injury rather than to the removal of the tissue to an environment free of immune responses. This interpretation is consistent with the finding that HSV can be activated in dorsal ganglia after sciatic nerve injury (Walz et al., 1974) and with the well-known observation that proximal rhizotomy of the human trigeminal ganglion results in activation of HSV (Cushing, 1905; Carton and Kilbourne, 1952).

XIII. Tolerance to Viral Antigens

The work of Traube in the 1930's showed that in mouse colonies vertical transmission from mothers to offspring of lymphocytic choriomeningitis (LCM) virus establishes a symptomless lifelong infection in which no antiviral antibody is demonstrable in the circulating blood. Infection of adult mice with LCM leads to an immunopathological disease and antibody formation. The lack of antibody after congenital LCM virus infection was one of the observations that led Burnet and Fenner (1949) to postulate the existence of immunologic tolerance. More recently, Oldstone and Dixon (1967) and Benson and Hotchin (1969) have demonstrated in mice congenitally infected with LCM virus the presence of antiviral antibody and the accumulation in the kidneys of immune complexes containing viral antigen and antibody (Oldstone and Dixon, 1971). Hence, the congenitally infected mice are able to make some antibody against viral antigens. Volkert and Hannover-Larsen (1965) found that, if spleen cells from LCM-immune mice (infected as adults) are transferred to syngeneic congenitally infected carrier animals, very high levels of antibody are formed, but no immunopathological disease results.

The simplest interpretation of these findings appears to be that LCM viral antigens produce a tolerance resembling that occurring with autoantigens in low dose, namely that T lymphocytes specific for viral antigens become unresponsive while specific B lymphocytes remain able to respond to antigen (Allison, 1973). In the absence of specific helper cells, only a small amount of antibody is produced, and this combines with antigen liberated into the circulation to form immune complexes which accumulate in the kidney, leading eventually to immunopathological glomerulonephritis. However, when virus-specific T cells are supplied by adoptive immunization, a helper effect greatly increases antibody formation in the recipients. A helper role of T cells in antibody formation against LCM viral antigens is demonstrated by the experiments of Cole et al. (1972).

Adoptive immunization of congenitally infected LCM virus carrier mice with spleen cells from syngeneic immune donors resulted in high antibody levels, as already described, but treatment of the spleen cells with anti-θ serum before transfer virtually abolished this effect. Thus, even in the presence of B cells from immune donors, little antibody is formed unless sensitized T cells are also present. The interpretation of these experiments is complicated by the fact that in the recipients the level of virus is reduced, so that the antigenic load is less and the chances of finding free antibody are increased. However, the levels of antibody in recipients are so high that this is unlikely to be the whole explanation.

For a long time it was thought that mice congenitally infected with leukemogenic viruses would likewise be tolerant to virus-specific antigens. However, Aoki et al. (1966) detected antibody to Gross leukemogenic virus cell surface antigens (GCSA's) in the sera of old C57BL/6 mice. Mellors et al. (1969) found that Gross soluble antigens, a mixture of virus-specific antigens (Aoki et al., 1972), increased in the sera of NZB mice until 9 months of age, after which increasing titers of antibody to these antigens could be detected and immune elimination of the viral antigen occurred while glomerulonephritis progressed; renal eluates contained 7 S antibody to Gross soluble antigen (Mellors et al., 1971). Previously preparation in mice of antisera to Gross virus had resulted in the production of antibodies against GCSAs but not of neutralizing antibodies directed against virion envelope antigens (GVEA's). This led to the hypothesis that, due to occult infections early in life, mice might be tolerant to VEA's. However, old NZB mice were found to make "natural antibody" to GVEA's (Aoki et al., 1970). Recently, Yoshiki et al. (1974b) reported that NZB, NZW, and their F_1 hybrid mice contain remarkably high concentrations of the viral envelope glycoprotein gp69/71, and that this protein is deposited as immune complexes in the glomeruli of these mice in much greater concentration than the major structural protein of the virion, p30.

Studies of the high-leukemic AKR mouse strain have also provided evidence for antibody responses to endogenous infections of Gross leukemogenic virus. Oldstone et al. (1972) reported glomerulonephritis developed spontaneously in AKR mice and renal eluates contained antibodies to GCSA's and complement-fixing antibodies to internal viral components. Using immunofluorescence, Markham et al. (1972) found IgG antibody and complement along with the viral antigens gs-1 and gs-3 in the kidneys of 8- to 10-month-old AKR mice. Hollis et al. (1974) eluted from AKR mouse kidneys IgM and IgG antibodies directed against the virion reverse transcriptase; as expected, these antibodies reacted with mouse and feline but not avian reverse transcriptase. Much of the antibody against AKR virus antigen found in the glomeruli may be directed to viral antigens produced *in situ* by infected cells, especially mesangial cells (Pascal *et al.*, 1973; Yoshiki *et al.*, 1974b).

Other strains of mice also produce natural antibody to Gross viral antigens. Thus low-leukemic RF mice (Hanna *et al.*, 1972) and C57BL/6 mice (Porter *et al.*, 1973) produce antiviral antibody and develop chronic glomerulonephritis; over half of the antibody eluted from kidneys of the latter mice at 1 year of age reacted with GCSA's. Predominantly IgM antibodies to GVEA's were also deteced in sera and glomeruli of C57BL/6 mice as well as in B6C3F$_1$, BALB/c, and AKR mice (Ihle *et al.*, 1973; Batzing *et al.*, 1974). Using a sensitive radioimmune precipitation assay in which serum is reacted with isotopically labeled virus and the complexes formed then precipitated with appropiate antiglobulins, antibodies to GVEA's (mainly IgG) have been detected in the sera of most inbred mouse strains studied (Nowinski and Kaehler, 1974), and some of these antigens have been characterized as virion envelope glycoproteins (Ihle *et al.*, 1974). Recently, Lee *et al.* (1974) examined the sera of normal B6C3F$_1$ mice and found 19 S antibody which reacted with 3 antigenic components of Gross MuLV—gp69/71, a second viral envelope glycoprotein with MW 43,000 daltons, and the small virus core protein p15. Antibody in the 7 S fraction reacted only with the nonenvelope protein, p15. Only 19 S antibody neutralized the xenotropic BALB:virus-2, which cross-reacts with Gross virus (*vide infra*).

Humoral responses are also made to other vertically transmitted murine oncornaviruses. Hirsch *et al.* (1969) and Branca *et al.* (1972) found that mice congenitally infected with Moloney leukemogenic and sarcoma viruses have complexes of viral antigen and antibody in their glomeruli. Recently, endogenous murine oncornaviruses, released spontaneously from cells of BALB/c and NZB mice and unable to grow in mouse cells but able to grow in cells of other species and thus called xenotropic viruses, have been isolated and designated BALB:virus-2 and NZB-MuLV, respectively. Neutralizing antibodies to these two viruses are cross-reactive and widespread, being present in high titers in 2-month-old mice of all strains tested except the NIH strain (Aaronson and Stephenson, 1974). These investigators suggest that previous studies detecting "natural" antibody to the Gross viral antigens may have been primarily directed against the BALB:virus-2 class of endogenous viruses but cross-reactive at a lower level with Gross-type virus. Some cross-reactivity between BALB:virus-2 and Gross leukemogenic virus does exist since antisera against the latter virus neutralized the former, but normal BALB/c sera which neutralized BALB:virus-2 did not neutralize viruses of the Gross or FMR subgroups and the antigenic relationships of these viruses awaits clarification. Another xenotropic virus has been isolated from athymic nude mice and neutralizing antibody to this virus, mainly IgM, has been detected in high titers in the nude mice from which the virus was isolated; this sera also neutralized BALB:virus-2 and NZB-MuLV (S. Cross, H. M. Morse, and J. Hartley, personal communication, 1974).

Mice infected *in utero* or neonatally or inheriting viral genomes in a Mendelian, chromosomal fashion can make antibody responses to the viral antigens and thus are not tolerant to these antigens in the classic sense. Whether they can also mount cell-mediated immune responses to these viral antigens is less clear. Recently, Proffitt *et al.* (1973) have found that lymphocytes from C3H carrier mice (carrying Moloney leukemogenic virus) are cytotoxic to cells bearing virus-specific antigens. If these reactions are mediated by T lymphocytes, a lack of tolerance is suggested. Similar observations for Gross leukemogenic virus (MuLV-G) have been published by Wahren and Metcalf (1970). Absence of tolerance in mice neonatally infected with polyoma virus has been found by Allison (1970): lymphocytes from such animals were able to protect immunosuppressed recipients from polyoma tumor formation. Many investigators have described T lymphocyte-mediated cytotoxicity of cell cultures in which LCM virus is replicating (*vide supra*). It is observed in mice infected with LCM virus as adults but not in carrier mice infected as newborns. This supports the view that the carrier mice do not have T lymphocytes reactive against virus-specific antigens, not necessarily the same antigens that enter the circulating blood. These studies suggest that it is more difficult to induce tolerance to virus-specific antigens than was formerly supposed, although some examples of selective tolerance (e.g., specifically induced unresponsiveness of T lymphocytes after congenital LCM infection) appear to exist. It is not yet known whether this is due to deletion or inactivation of T lymphocytes or temporary inhibition of their responses by antigen or immune complexes.

XIV. Cooperative Effects of Viral Antigens on Immunogenicity

Examples of a response to a strong immunogen increasing the response to a second, weaker immunogen coupled to it have been extensively studied, especially carrier effects in which a hapten has been coupled to different carrier proteins (Katz and Benacerraf, 1972; Leskowitz, 1972). In an analogous way the presence of the highly immunogenic chicken isoantigen B along with the weaker isoantigen A on the same cells will elicit a stronger than normal immune response to the latter (Schierman and McBride, 1967). Conceivably, highly immunogenic viral coat proteins may increase the response to less immunogenic components. Tumor transplantation antigens are often weakly immunogenic, and the immunogenicity of various tumors has been improved by association of the tumor antigens with stronger immunogens by forming somatic hybrids with more antigenic cells (Watkins and Chen, 1969), or by virus infection (reviewed by Lindenmann, 1974). Thus, Lindenmann and Klein (1967) prepared viral oncolysates by infecting Ehrlich ascites tumor cells with influenza virus and showed that immunization of mice with such preparations would protect them against 100 lethal doses of the uninfected tumor cells eleven days later. Even if inactivated, partially purified virus from oncolysates was protective, indicating direct viral lysis of the tumor *in vivo* was not involved. Antisera to the virus (prepared against influenza virus grown in eggs) eliminated the protective effect and simple mixtures of virus and tumor cells were not effective, indicating that close coupling of viral and tumor antigens was required. These findings have been confirmed (Hakkinen and Halonen, 1971). Since the virions were not rigorously purified after oncolysis, it cannot be decided from these experiments whether the immunogen was fragments of cell membrane containing virus antigens or virions containing host material. The latter interpretation is favored in similar experiments with VSV and fowl-plague virus in which the viral oncolysates were immunogenic only when prepared following the appearance of progeny virus, long after the incorporation of virus proteins into cell membranes (Lindenmann, 1970).

Immunizing hamsters with highly purified and inactivated VSV grown in SV40-transformed hamster cells, Ansel (1974) induced transplantation immunity to the same and another SV40-transformed cell line. Although similar immunization with VSV grown in a spontaneously transformed hamster cell line conferred no such immunity, more cell lines transformed by SV40 and other viruses must be studied before specificity for the SV40 transplantation rejection antigen (TRA) is established in this system. Also, it is unclear whether the SV40 TRA was incorporated into the virion structure or adsorbed onto its surface as a contaminant; some host material is incorporated into VSV virions (*vide supra*), but cell surface antigens can be adsorbed onto the virions (Hecht and Summers, 1972).

In other studies virus was not purified from tumor lysates and tumor cell membranes containing virus antigens may be the immunogen. Thus, Eaton *et al.* (1973) reported increased immunogenicity of a Gross virus lymphoma when syngeneic mice were immunized with lysates of tumor cells infected with NDV or Sendai virus, and membrane fractions were more effective than concentrated virus. Kobayashi *et al.* (1970) have shown that infection of rat tumors with Friend virus increases their immunogenicity and similar findings in the hamster for SV40-transformed human cells have been reported using oncolysates prepared by infection with NDV (Axler and Girardi, 1970). A syngeneic system using SV40-transformed 3T3 cells transplanted to BALB/c mice and oncolysates produced by influenza virus or VSV yielded similar results (Boone *et al.*, 1971, 1974; Boone and Blackman, 1972). Boone *et al.* (1974) found that tumor immunity cannot be induced by viral oncolysates if mice are first made tolerant to the virus by cyclophosphamide treatment. This was considered evidence for a carrier–hapten relationship between the virus and tumor antigens, but interpretation is difficult because of the complexities of cyclophosphamide treatment (Aisenberg, 1973; Lagrange *et al.*, 1974).

The use of viral oncolysates from human tumors to improve the immunizing efficiency of patients to their own tumors following surgery, radiotherapy, or chemotherapy is potentially important, especially if inactivation of the virus does not diminish tumor immunogenicity. Infection of cancer patients with various viruses has sometimes been thought to have beneficial effects (Webb and Smith, 1970). However, critical evaluation of this approach is required. The cooperative effect in virus infections may also prove useful in the preparation of antisera to cellular isoantigens in allogeneic systems (Lindenmann and Klein, 1964) and of potent antilymphocyte sera in xenogeneic systems (Bandlow *et al.*, 1972, 1973).

Cooperative phenomena may also help explain the broadening reactivity of late viral antisera, since the immune response to minor viral determinants may be stimulated by response to stronger ones. Certain types of autoimmunity may involve cooperative effects if self-antigens are coupled to strongly immunogenic viral antigens during infection. It has been shown that immunization of chickens with egg-grown influenza virus results in antibody production against an autologous mucopolysaccharide antigen (*vide supra*) present embryologically in endodermal cells lining the allantoic cavity and in the liver and bile of adults (Harboe and Haukenes, 1966; Harboe *et al.*, 1966; Schoyen *et al.*, 1966); no pathological lesions were reported. Virus particles have been found in NZB mice, which manifest many autoimmune phenomena (Mellors et al., 1969), in dogs with a lupus syndrome (Lewis, 1974), and possibly in patients with systemic lupus erythematosus (reviewed by Andres et al., 1972), but the role of viruses in these autoimmune phenomena has yet to be clearly defined.

XV. Influence of Virus Infections on Immune Responses

Several viruses are known to influence the activity of the immune system (see review by Notkins et al., 1970). Many virus infections result in nonspecific immunoglobulin elevation (LDV, VEE, Rauscher leukemia, Aleutian mink disease, equine infectious anemia) or depression (most leukomogenic viruses). Some infections, as with Aleutian mink disease virus, result in elevated immunoglobulins but a diminished humoral response to unrelated antigens (Porter et al., 1965; Kenyon, 1966; Lodmell et al., 1970). Mice infected with murine leukomogenic viruses have diminished circulating antibody to sheep erythrocytes and bovine serum albumin. The Jerne plaque technique has been used to demonstrate at a cellular level a diminished response to sheep erythrocytes in mice infected with mouse CMV (Osborn et al., 1968), Rowson–Parr virus (Bendinelli and Nardini, 1973), Friend virus (Salaman and Wedderburn, 1966; Chan et al., 1968), Rauscher leukomogenic virus (Siegel et al., 1969; Bennett and Steeves, 1970), and Moloney leukomogenic virus (Salaman and Wedderburn, 1966).

Cell-mediated immunity may also be affected, as shown by prolonged skin-graft rejection in mice following infections with LDV (Dent et al., 1965; Howard et al., 1969), Marek's disease virus (Purchase et al., 1968), and NDV (Woodruff and Woodruff, 1974). Von Pirquet (1908) noted that measles infection resulted in a decreased dermal hypersensitivity to tuberculin, and this phenomenon has been observed during natural measles infection (Nablant, 1937; Beck, 1962) and shortly after vaccination with attenuated virus (Mellman and Wetton, 1963; Brody and McAlister, 1964; Starr and Berkovich, 1964). Transient diminished skin test responses to antigens of *Candida* and vaccinia virus, dinitrochlorobenzene, and poison ivy have also been observed following attenuated measles virus vaccination (Blumhardt et al., 1968; Fireman et al., 1969). Lymphocytes from subjects recently vaccinated with the attenuated virus showed transient diminished blastogenesis and DNA synthesis *in vitro* when exposed to measles antigen, tuberculin, and *Candida* antigens, but not to appropriate concentrations of PHA (Smithwick and Berkovich, 1966; Fireman et al., 1969; Finkel and Dent, 1973). Yamanouchi et al. (1974b) reported marked suppression of dermal hypersensitivity to PPD in sensitized rabbits for 2 weeks following infection with rinderpest virus.

Transient suppression of tuberculin sensitivity has also been reported during a few other viral infections. Suppression was observed during the acute phase of paralytic poliomyelitis (Carnevale and Iovino, 1959) and after immunization of tuberculous children with Sabin 1 vaccine (Berkovich and Starr, 1966). The latter authors reported one-third of the tuberculous children studied became tuberculin negative 4 to 6 weeks after Sabin immunization, and this state persisted for as long as 2 months. The long delay between vaccination and suppression was unexplained. The same authors (Starr and Berkovich, 1964) reported that 8 of 17 tuberculous children with varicella infection became tuberculin negative near the end of the 14-day incubation period and during the exanthem; reactivity returned to normal in a few days.

Nonspecific functions such as clearance by the reticuloendothelial system (RES) may be depressed (LDV, ectromelia, LCM, dengue, Sandfly fever) or elevated (VEE, murine leukemia viruses) by virus infections. Infection by LDV presents a special example of impaired clearance. Following infection, phagocytic activity of the RES as reflected by carbon particle clearance is only transiently impaired (Mahy, 1964) while there is permanent impairment of the clearance of certain enzymes (LDH, isocitrate dehydrogenase, malate dehydrogenase, aspartate transaminase) but not others (alkaline phosphatase, alanine transaminase). Little consideration has been given to the clearance of endogenous enzymes (those enzymes that are useful intracellularly but which, after becoming extracellular due to cell leakage or cell death, have no known extracellular functions). It has long been held that the RES plays a role in clearing proteins generally (Hyman and Paldino, 1960) and, based on their studies showing decreased clearance of endogenous enzymes after RES blockade, Wakim and Fleisher (1963) suggested a similar role for the RES in clearing endogenous proteins. Infection by LDV, which replicates almost exclusively in macrophages *in vitro*, appears specifically to eliminate or impair the function of a subpopulation of macrophages or cells of the RES responsible for clearance of certain endogenous enzymes. The specificity of the clearance cells for certain enzymes is presumably on a nonimmunological basis since there is no evidence to suggest that the extracellular enzymes are structurally (an-

7. Virus Infections and Immune Responses

tigenically) altered and therefore the animal should be tolerant to them. One can postulate that specific membrane receptors for the enzymes cleared exist on a particular population of cells infected by LDV. Because of its selective tropism, LDV may prove to be a useful tool to define and explore the functions of subpopulations of macrophages, especially in regard to their clearance functions.

There are many ways in which virus infections influence the immune system. Lytic infections may affect the thymus. Rowe and Capps (1961) described a virus, recently characterized as a herpesvirus (Parker *et al.*, 1973) which causes transient massive destruction of thymus cortex and medulla in newborn mice. Studies by S. Cross and H. M. Morse (personal communication) demonstrate that this virus (called the thymic agent) replicates in thymocytes of newborn mice and later can be found only in the salivary glands. Several weeks after infection, lymphocytes from thymus, lymph node, and spleen have minimal reactivity in the graft-versus-host reaction; lymph node cells show normal reactivity at 8 weeks postinfection. Mitogenic responses to T lymphocyte mitogens but not to lipopolysaccharide are also depressed for weeks (G. H. Cohen, personal communication). A human herpesvirus, varicella-zoster, can also grow in the thymus. Cheathem *et al.* (1956) observed evidence of virus growth in thymuses of children dying of fatal varicella infections. Many intranuclear inclusion bodies were seen in thymus reticular cells and Hassall's corpuscles were necrotic.

Measles infection of humans can result in thymus changes. White and Boyd (1973) studied autopsy material from eight children less than 3 years of age who died during or shortly after measles infection. Beginning 4 days after the onset of illness, there was severe aggregation and syncytial formation of thymocytes in the thymus cortex and subsequent total loss of cortex in some cases. No recovery of cortex was discernible until 3 or 4 months after infection. Examination of other lymphoid tissues, including spleen and mesenteric lymph nodes, did not reveal similar changes. In tissue cultures a prominent cytopathic effect of measles infection is syncytial formation (Enders and Peebles, 1954). White and Boyd felt the syncytial cell formation in the thymus differed from the Warthin–Finkeldey "giant cells" (Warthin, 1931) found in peripheral lymphoid tissue during the prodromal stage of measles. It is difficult to relate these thymus observations to the previously noted suppression of delayed hypersensitivity reactions by measles infection since, in mice at least, the effects of thymectomy on cell-mediated immunity are not seen for weeks. More likely, immunosuppression occurs because of

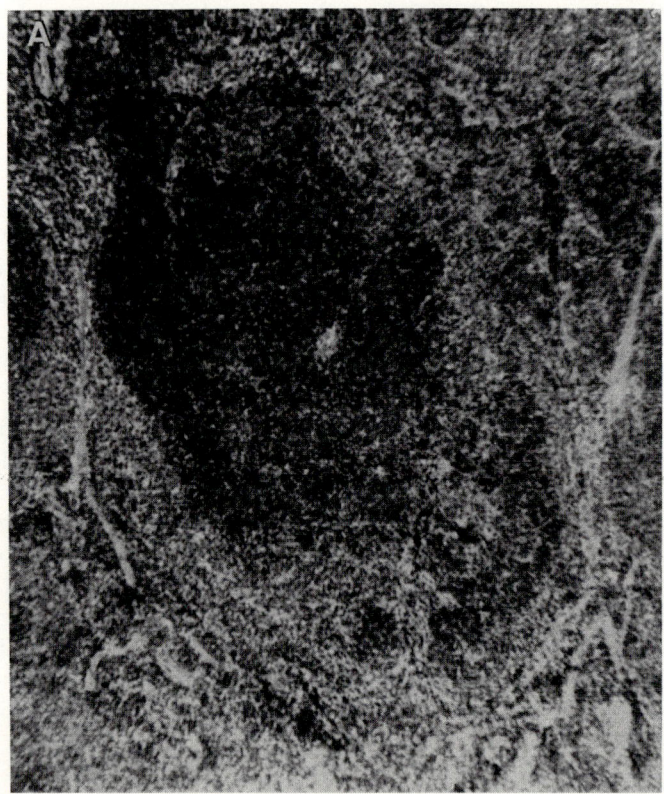

Fig. 16. Effect of infection with lactate dehydrogenase virus (LDV) on thymus-dependent area of mouse spleen. (A) Section of normal BALB/c mouse spleen showing white pulp. (B) Section of BALB/c mouse spleen 48 hours after infection with LDV. Note depletion of lymphocytes in periarteriolar (thymus-dependent) area of white pulp.

direct effects of measles virus on lymphocytes as demonstrated *in vitro*. Infections by other viruses of the medipest subgroup of paramyoviruses also produce lesions in the thymus as well as in other lymphoid tissues. Canine distemper virus infections of dogs produced thymus necrosis (McCullough *et al.*, 1973), as did rinderpest virus infections of rabbits (Yamanouchi *et al.*, 1974a).

Infection of mice with LDV causes transient depletion of thymus-dependent areas of lymph nodes and spleen (Fig. 16) (Proffitt *et al.*, 1972; Snodgrass *et al.*, 1972). Although LDV can grow in macrophage cultures, it does not replicate in lymphocyte cultures and cannot be demonstrated by electron microscopy within the lympho-

7. Virus Infections and Immune Responses

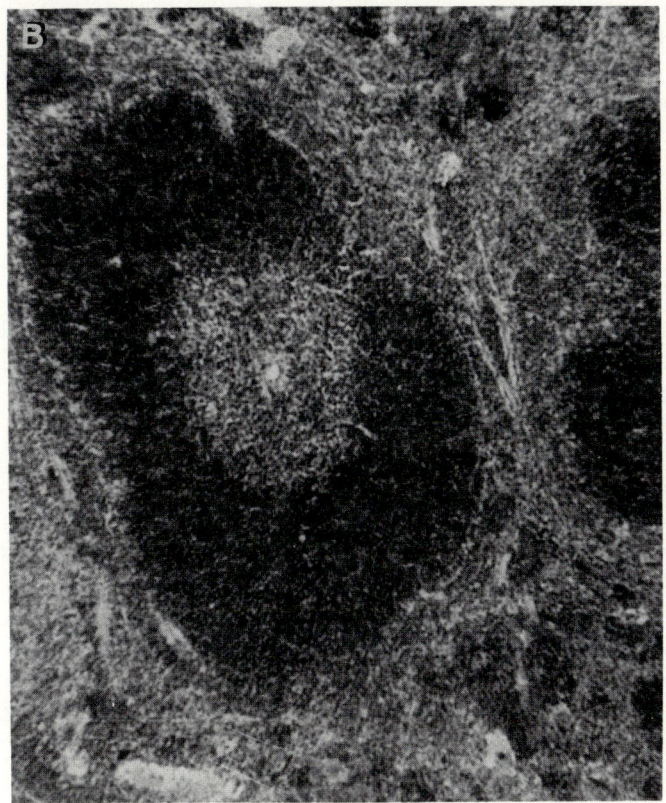

Fig. 16B.

cytes of infected spleens (Snodgrass *et al.*, 1972). It is postulated that its toxic effect on lymphocytes is mediated by viral growth in dendritic macrophages near the lymphocytes with disruption of tropic influences or the release of toxic materials. Alterations in T lymphocyte migrations could also result. Peripheral lymphoid necrosis is a common feature of infections by mouse hepatitis virus (Hirano and Ruebner, 1965; Biggart and Ruebner, 1970) as well as the medipest viruses already mentioned. The bursal infectious agent, an avian virus that causes lymphoid necrosis in young chickens resulting in a syndrome termed Gumboro disease, replicates in thymus, lymph nodes, spleen, and the bursa of Fabricius (Cheville, 1967). A severe inflammatory reaction occurs in the bursa, which is the only lymphoid organ that does not repopulate with lymphocytes after infection. During infection, viral antigen and virus particles can be detected in macrophages in the bursa but not in the affected lymphocytes. Damage to the lymphocytes may therefore be indirect and possibly of an autoimmune nature.

Many viruses are known to replicate in lymphocytes (Mims, 1964; Gresser and Lang, 1966; Edelman and Wheelock, 1967; Wheelock and Toy, 1973) and infections may result in chromosomal abnormalities (Nichols, 1966) and cell death. Persistent infections may result in more subtle disturbances of cell function. It has been hypothesized that infected lymphocytes may have alterations in protein synthesis, responses to hormones, interactions with other lymphoid cells, macrophages, or antigens, and in migration characteristics. Migration of lymphocytes *in vivo* is partly determined by cell membrane characteristics such as sialic acid content (Woodruff and Gesner, 1969; Berney and Gesner, 1970). The surfaces of infected cells are often altered (*vide supra*) and the appearance on cell membranes of viral neuraminidase after infection with SV5 can result in release of cell membrane sialic acid (Klenk and Choppin, 1970, 1971; Klenk *et al.*, 1970). Woodruff and Woodruff (1974) have reported that inoculation of NDV into rats causes a transient diversion of homing thoracic duct lymphocytes from lymph nodes and spleen to liver with resulting depletion of lymphocytes in thymus-dependent areas of nodes and spleen. This appeared to be due to viral neuraminidase acting on the lymphocyte surface. The importance of this phenomenon in natural infections is not clear.

Theoretically, latent infections in lymphocytes might convert to productive or lytic infections when the lymphocytes are stimulated to divide. Virus activation occurs in graft-versus-host reactions and in mixed lymphocyte reactions (Hirsch *et al.*, 1970, 1972), and the induced viruses (endogenous leukemogenic viruses) were found primarily in blastogenic lymphocytes (André-Schwartz *et al.*, 1973). Presumably, the viral genome is present in the phenotypically normal cells as postulated by the oncogene theory (Todaro and Huebner, 1972) and is activated by processes triggered by an allogeneic stimulus.

The importance of immunologic activation of viruses to human disease is suggested by the high incidence of malignancies of the RES found in renal allograft patients (Penn and Starzl, 1972). Relevant to this, Hirsch *et al.* (1973) reported that mice receiving ALS treatment as well as allografts had an increased incidence of activated viruses in their spleens compared to those receiving allografts without ALS treatment; no animals receiving ALS alone produced virus. Thus, host-versus-graft reactions can activate oncogenic viruses, especially if the host is receiving ALS therapy. Human lymphocytes stimulated with ALS replicate VSV (Edelman and Wheelock, 1968b) and HSV (Kleinman et al., 1972) to higher titers than untreated cells.

The activation of nononcogenic viruses from lymphocytes by allogeneic stimulation is suggested by the cytomegalovirus posttransfusion syndrome. Isolation of CMV from donors or recipients prior to blood transfusion is rare (Mirkovic et al., 1971) and lymphocyte–lymphocyte interactions may be required. A similar situation may exist for EB virus activation after transfusion (Henle et al., 1970). Whether severe or chronic infections may also activate viruses is not known.

Some viruses, such as VSV (Edelman and Wheelock, 1967, 1968a), yellow fever (Wheelock and Edelman, 1969), mumps (Duc-Nguyen and Henle, 1966), and HSV (Nahmias et al., 1964), grow little—if at all—in lymphocytes unless they are stimulated with PHA or antilymphocyte sera (Edelman and Wheelock, 1968b). VSV appears to grow predominantly in blastogenic T lymphocytes and perhaps preferentially in those with cytotoxic potential (Kano et al., 1973). Concanavalin A and pokeweed mitogen stimulation of spleen lymphocytes resulted in 33-fold and 17-fold increases in virus plaque-forming cells, respectively, while lipopolysaccharide stimulation resulted in only a two-fold increase above background. Prior treatment of cells with anti-θ sera and complement or the use of athymic nude mouse spleen cells resulted in no virus plaque-forming cells. Mixed cultures of DBA/2 and CBA lymphocytes produced many cytotoxic lymphocytes and large numbers of virus plaque-forming cells were observed while cultures of BALB/c and DBA/2 lymphocytes resulted in even more blastogenesis but less cytotoxicity, and few virus plaque-forming cells were observed.

Infections by viruses requiring lymphocyte proliferation for their own replication, occurring fortuitously or activated from a latent state at a time of antigenic stimulation, might eliminate a rapidly dividing clone of immunocompetent cells specific for the stimulating antigen. Conceivably, a virus lytically infecting lymphoid cells at a time when they are responding to the antigenic stimulus provided by the virus itself might eliminate clones of immune cells specific for those virus antigens. Thus, specific states of tolerance similar to those produced by cyclophosphamide treatment of animals after antigenic exposure or virus infection (Nathanson and Cole, 1970) might arise.

Several approaches have been taken to establish which population of lymphocytes is primarily affected by virus infections. The ability of infected cells to participate in graft-versus-host reactions (Purchase et al., 1968; Howard et al., 1969; Bennett and Steeves, 1970), reject skin grafts (Howard et al., 1969), and be stimulated by PHA or an in vitro allogeneic exposure (Hagry et al., 1970) has been used to determine the immunocompetence of infected T lymphocytes, and transfer-reconstitution experiments with infected bone marrow cells have been used to ascertain B lymphocyte competence (Bennett and Steeves, 1970; Shearer et al., 1973). Interpretation of these experiments is difficult since transfers of infected cells often result in transfer of infectious virus as well. Experiments with Friend virus are particularly complicated by contamination with Rowson–Parr virus, lymphatic leukemia virus, and LDV (Bennett and Steeves, 1970). In a recent transfer-reconstitution experiment, Shearer et al. (1973) demonstrated that the antibody response to a D-amino acid polypeptide (a thymus-independent antigen) was significantly reduced after infection of bone marrow cells with the SJL/J leukemogenic virus, regardless of whether thymocytes were infected or not. Hence, infection with this virus may result in a decrease in the response of B lymphocytes, but the experiments provide no information on possible effects on T lymphocytes. Peled and Haran-Ghera (1974) found that infection of mice with the radiation leukemia (Gross) virus resulted in depressed responses of spleen cells to sheep erythrocytes but normal responses to the thymus-independent antigens polyvinylpyrrolidine and pneumococcal polysaccharide SIII. They concluded that the immunosuppressive effect of this virus is on T lymphocytes.

The direct effect of measles virus infection on lymphocytes has been investigated by H. McFarland (personal communication). A mouse-adapted strain of virus was used to infect mice and measles antigen was present in spleen for 6 to 12 days after inoculation, but T lymphocytes were not killed as demonstrated by normal numbers of lymphocytes sensitive to anti-θ and complement. Mice were primed with ovalbumin-DNP (OA-DNP), a carrier–hapten conjugate, or with chicken γ-globulin (CGG), a secondary carrier, and their spleen cells used in combination to adoptively immunize irradiated recipient mice; secondary anti-hapten responses were measured after challenge with the appropriate conjugate. The effect of measles virus infection was ascertained by infecting either the CGG primed donor or the OA-DNP primed donors, and it was found that infection of CGG primed donors resulted in diminished anti-hapten responses while infection of OA-DNP donors had no effect on the response. Sindbis virus infection of the carrier donor did not affect the response. Although these studies demonstrate an effect of measles virus infection on the helper cell population of T lymphocytes, impairment of other T lymphocyte activity may be responsible for the observed impairment of delayed hypersensitivity.

Finally, virus infections can abrogate tolerance. Inoculation of BALB/c mice with subimmunogenic amounts of pneumococcal polysaccharide (SIII), a relatively thymus-independent antigen, results in unresponsiveness to subsequent immunogenic amounts of antigen; this state lasts for months and is specific for SIII (Baker et al., 1974). Tolerance in this system appears to be mediated by suppressor T cells since it is broken by the administration of ALS along with SIII; also, tolerance to SIII cannot be induced in athymic nude mice. P. J. Baker and W. H. Burns (unpublished observations) have found that infection with LDV will abrogate tolerance, although to a lesser extent than ALS administration. This is not due to an adjuvant effect since well-known adjuvants like complete Freund's adjuvant, poly I-C, and lipopolysaccharide do not abrogate tolerance in this system. Figure 16 shows that 48 hours after infection the thymus-dependent areas of the spleen (and lymph nodes) are depleted of lymphocytes and have the appearance of lymphoid tissue following administration of ALS. Whether LDV alters T cell migration or is directly or indirectly toxic to T cells is not clear. It is doubtful that the virus selectively impairs the functions of suppressor T cells, but rather impairs the functions of all or most T cells. In this system with SIII as antigen, the predominant influence of T cells on specific B cells is a suppressive one and destruction or impairment of T cell functions results in a diminution of their suppressive effect. Thus, as demonstrated here, virus infections can unbalance the normal regulatory mechanisms of the immune system. The frequency of virus infections in all animals, the presence of "endogenous viruses" in most or all cells, and the persistent and latent infections by "exogenous viruses" in many cells require an awareness by immunologists of the influences of these viruses on immune responses.

XVI. Concluding Remarks

During the past two decades the science of immunology has advanced rapidly. The various classes and subclasses of immunoglobulins have been recognized and their structures and properties elucidated. Interactions of T and B lymphocytes and macrophages in the induction of immune responses have been extensively documented. Reactions of receptor immunoglobulins on B lymphocytes and the mechanism of synthesis of immunoglobulins in their progeny have been analyzed. Products of T lymphocytes activated by antigens and mitogens have been defined, and their effects on macrophages and other cells studied. Components of the complement system have been isolated and characterized, and the alternate path of activation of the complement system has been recognized.

At the same time considerable advances have been made in molecular virology and genetics. The structures of viruses, their nucleic acids, the specific polymerases involved in their replication, and the mechanisms of synthesis of the protein and glycoprotein components of their capsids and envelopes have all been studied in detail. The genetics of animal viruses and the genetic control of immune responses have received increasing attention. Temperature-sensitive mutants of viruses have been used to study their mode of replication and the mechanisms of malignant transformation. Human patients and experimental animals with inherited deficiencies of immunoglobulin or complement component formation and thymus deficiencies have already provided valuable information about differential susceptibility to infections.

For the most part the developments in immunology, virology, and genetics have been parallel but independent. In the future, the accumulated information and powerful analytical methods developed in these disciplines should be pooled for a combined approach to problems that have so far seemed intractable.

Some benefits of this sort of approach are already apparent. Many remarkable features of humoral immune responses came to light during the course of studies of antibodies against viruses. These include some of the earliest analyses of secretory antibodies, later shown to be mainly of IgA specificity, and features of immunologic memory such as "original antigenic sin" and IgM memory following repeated exposure to small doses of antigen. The cellular basis of these responses is still imperfectly understood, and with the high sensitivity of the plaque neutralization system, viral antigens offer interesting material for further study. Current studies analyzing at the cellular level the formation of B lymphocyte memory, the response of such B cells to the same or cross-reactive antigens and the influence of T lymphocytes on that recall should provide basic knowledge concerning T and B lymphocyte interactions.

Studies have just begun on the thymus dependence of viral

antigens, most of which resemble other proteins in being thymus-dependent. However, one (Sindbis envelope glycoprotein) is relatively thymus-independent and biochemical analysis of this molecule may provide insights concerning this interesting property.

The science of immunology began with observations of Jenner and later von Pirquet on the body's responses, beneficial and pathological, to virus infections. The devastating effects on patients with thymus deficiencies of virus infections usually mild in normal humans was the first indication of the biologic importance of cell-mediated immunity. Virus infections (as with ectromelia virus) of experimental animals have provided model systems for analyzing *in vivo* the roles of various lymphoid cells. The recent development of *in vitro* assays for various lymphocyte functions make feasible correlative studies with *in vivo* activities of different lymphocyte populations. Interesting information from such studies, particularly those using LCM virus, has already been discussed.

Mechanisms of immunity mediated by T lymphocytes and the part they play in protection against some virus infections are still imperfectly understood, but still less is known about the biologic importance of the cytotoxic system in which antibody sensitizes virus-infected target cells for destruction by nonspecific effector (K) lymphoid cells. This has recently been shown to occur *in vitro* with herpesvirus-infected cells and could play a role in immunity and immunopathology (Rager-Zisman and Bloom, 1974; Shore *et al.*, 1974). Model systems of viral infections should be useful in defining the importance of this phenomenon.

Finally, although first noted by von Pirquet almost 70 years ago, the effects of virus infections on immune responses has only recently received much attention. As already discussed, the presence of viral antigens with less immunogenic antigens may enhance responses to the latter. Viruses that infect or affect particular populations of lymphoid cells, e.g., the thymic agent and LDV, have been reported and the latter can abrogate tolerance to certain antigens. The tropism of viruses may prove to be a useful property for selectively depleting animals of certain lymphocyte populations. The causative role of such viruses in diseases and autoimmune phenomena is still relatively unexplored.

References

Aaronson, S. A., and Stephenson, J. R. (1974). *Proc. Nat. Acad. Sci. U. S.* **71**, 1957.
Adler, W. H., and Rabinowitz, S. (1973). *J. Immunol.* **110**, 1354.

Ahmed, A., Strong, D. M., Sell, K. W., Thurman, G. B., Knudsen, R. C., Wistar, R., and Grace, W. R. (1974). *J. Exp. Med.* **139**, 902.
Aisenberg, A. (1973). *Transplant. Proc.* **5**, 1221.
Alford, R. H., Rossen, R. D., Butler, W. T., and Kasel, J. A. (1967). *J. Immunol.* **98**, 724.
Allison, A. C. (1965). *Arch. Gesamte Virusforsch.* **17**, 280.
Allison, A. C. (1966). *J. Nat. Cancer Inst.* **36**, 869.
Allison, A. C. (1967). *Brit. Med. J.* **23**, 60.
Allison, A. C. (1970). *In* "Immunity and Tolerance in Oncogenesis" (L. Severi, ed.), p. 563.
Allison, A. C. (1971). *Int. Rev. Exp. Pathol.* **10**, 181.
Allison, A. C. (1973). *Ann. Rheum. Dis.* **32**, 283.
Allison, A. C. (1974). *Transplant. Rev.* **19**, 3.
Allison, A. C., and Burns, W. H. (1972). *In* "Immunogenicity" (F. Borek, ed.), pp. 155–203. North-Holland Publ., Amsterdam.
Allison, A. C., and Friedman, R. M. (1966). *J. Nat. Cancer Inst.* **36**, 859.
Allison, A. C., and Mallucci, L. (1965). *J. Exp. Med.* **121**, 463.
Allison, A. C., and Taylor, R. B. (1967). *Cancer Res.* **27**, 703.
Almeida, J. D., and Laurence, G. D. (1969). *Amer. J. Dis. Child.* **118**, 101.
Almeida, J. D., and Waterson, A. P. (1969). *Advan. Virus Res.* **15**, 307.
Anderson, W. A., and Kilbourne, E. D. (1961). *J. Invest. Dermatol.* **37**, 25.
Andres, G. A., Spiele, H., and McCluskey, R. T. (1972). *Progr. Clin. Immunol.* **1**, 23.
André-Schwartz, J., Schwartz, R. S., Hirsch, M. S., Phillips, S. M., and Black, P. H. (1973). *J. Nat. Cancer Inst.* **51**, 507.
Ansel, S. (1974). *Int. J. Cancer* **13**, 773.
Aoki, T., and Johnson, P. A. (1972). *J. Nat. Cancer Inst.* **49**, 183.
Aoki, T., and Todaro, G. (1973). *Proc. Nat. Acad. Sci. U. S.* **70**, 1598.
Aoki, T., Boyse, E. A., and Old, L. J. (1966). *Cancer Res.* **26**, 1415.
Aoki, T., Boyse, E. A., Old, L. J., de Harven, E., Hammerling, U., and Wood, H. A. (1970). *Proc. Nat. Acad. Sci. U. S.* **65**, 569.
Aoki, T., Herberman, R. B., Johnson, P. A., Liu, M. and Sturm, M. M. (1972). *J. Virol.* **10**, 1208.
Appleyard, G., Oram, J. D., and Stanley, J. L. (1970). *J. Gen. Virol.* **9**, 179.
Arnason, B. G., Fuller, T. C., Lehrich, J. R., and Wray, S. W. (1974). *J. Neurol. Sci.* **22**, 419.
Ashe, W. K., and Notkins, A. L. (1966). *Proc. Nat. Acad. Sci. U. S.* **46**, 447.
Ashe, W. K., and Notkins, A. L. (1967). *Virology* **33**, 613.
Ashe, W. K., Mage, M., Mage, R., and Notkins, A. L. (1968). *J. Immunol.* **101**, 500.
Ashe, W. K., Mage, M., and Notkins, A. L. (1969). *Virology* **37**, 290.
Ashe, W. K., Daniels, C. A., Scott, G. S., and Notkins, A. L. (1971). *Science* **172**, 176.
Axler, D. A., and Girardi, A. J. (1970). *Proc. Amer. Ass. Cancer Res.* **11**, 4.
Bach, F. H., Segall, M., Zier, K. S., Sondel, P. M., and Atler, B. J. (1973). *Science* **180**, 403.
Baker, P. J., Stashak, P. W., Amsbaugh, D. F., and Prescott, B. (1974). *J. Immunol.* **112**, 2020.
Bandlow, G., Kieling, F., and Thomssen, R. (1972). *Med. Microbiol. Immunol.* **157**, 335.
Bandlow, G., Koszinowski, U., and Thomssen, R. (1973). *Arch. Gesamte Virusforsch.* **40**, 63.
Bang, F. B., and Warwick, A. (1960). *Proc. Nat. Acad. Sci. U. S.* **46**, 1065.
Baringer, J. R. (1974). *N. Engl. J. Med.* **291**, 828.

7. Virus Infections and Immune Responses

Baringer, J. R., and Swoveland, P. (1973). *N. Engl. J. Med.* **288**, 648.
Bastian, F. O., Rabson, A. S., Yee, C. L., and Tralka, T. S. (1972). *Science* **178**, 306.
Batzing, B. L., Yurconic, M., and Hanna, M. G. (1974). *J. Nat. Cancer Inst.* **52**, 117.
Beck, V. (1962). *Amer. J. Dis. Child.* **103**, 242.
Bellanti, J. A., Russ, S. B., Holmes, G. E., and Buescher, E. L. (1965). *J. Immunol.* **94**, 1.
Benacerraf, B., and McDevitt, H. O. (1972). *Science* **175**, 273.
Bendinelli, M., and Nardini, L. (1973). *Infec. Immunity* **7**, 160.
Bennett, M., and Steeves, R. A. (1970). *J. Nat. Cancer Inst.* **44**, 1107.
Benson, L. (1962). *N. Y. State Dep. Health Annu. Rep. Div. Lab. Res.*, pp. 41–42.
Benson, L., and Hotchin, J. (1969). *Nature (London)* **222**, 1045.
Berkovich, S., and Starr, S. (1966). *N. Engl. J. Med.* **274**, 67.
Berman, L. (1967). *J. Exp. Med.* **125**, 983.
Berney, I. N., and Gesner, B. M. (1970). *Immunology* **18**, 681.
Berry, D. M., and Almeida, J. D. (1968). *J. Gen. Virol.* **3**, 97.
Beveridge, W. I., and Burnet, F. M. (1944). *Med. J. Aust.* **1**, 85.
Biesecker, L. J., Fitch, F. W., Rowley, D. A., Scollard, D., and Stuart, F. (1973). *Transplantation* **16**, 421.
Biggart, J. D., and Ruebner, B. H. (1970). *J. Med. Microbiol.* **3**, 627.
Blacklow, N. R., Hoggan, M. D., Austin, J. B., and Rowe, W. P. (1969). *Amer. J. Epidemiol.* **90**, 501.
Blanden, R. V. (1970). *J. Exp. Med.* **132**, 1035.
Blanden, R. V. (1971). *J. Exp. Med.* **133**, 1074 and 1090.
Bloom, B. R., Landy, M., and Lawrence, H. S. (1973). *Cell Immunol.* **6**, 331.
Blumhardt, R., Pappano, J. E., and Moyes, D. C. (1968). *J. Amer. Med. Ass.* **206**, 2739.
Boone, C. W., Blackman, K., and Brandchaft, P. (1971). *Nature (London)* **231**, 265.
Boone, C. W., and Blackman, K. (1972). *Cancer Res.* **32**, 1018.
Boone, C. W., Brandchaft, P., Irving, D., and Gilden, R. (1972). *Int. J. Cancer* **9**, 685.
Boone, C. W., Gordin, F., and Kawakami, T. G. (1973). *J. Virol.* **11**, 515.
Boone, C. W., Paranjpe, M., Orme, T., and Gillette, R. (1974). *Int. J. Cancer* **13**, 543.
Bose, H. R., and Sagik, B. P. (1970). *J. Virol.* **5**, 410.
Boyse, E. A., and Old, L. J. (1969). *Annu. Rev. Genet.* **3**, 269.
Boyse, E. A., Old, L. J., and Stockert, E. (1965). *In* "Immunopathology" (P. Grabar and P. Miescher, eds.), vol. 4, pp. 23–40. Schwabe, Basel.
Boyse, E. A., Stockert, E., and Old, L. J. (1968). *J. Exp. Med.* **128**, 85.
Brady, R. O., and Mora, P. T. (1970). *Biochim. Biophys. Acta* **218**, 308.
Brady, R. O., Fishman, P. H., and Mora, P. T. (1973). *Fed. Proc., Fed. Amer. Soc. Exp. Biol.* **32**, 102.
Branca, M., de Petris, S., Allison, A. C., Harvey, J., and Hirsch, M. S. (1972). *Clin. Exp. Immunol.* **9**, 853.
Brier, A. M., Wohlenberg, C., Rosenthal, J., Mage, M., and Notkins, A. L. (1971). *Proc. Nat. Acad. Sci. U. S.* **68**, 3073.
Brody, J. A., and McAlister, R. (1964). *Amer. Rev. Resp. Dis.* **90**, 607.
Broom, J. C. (1947). *Lancet* **1**, 364.
Brown, F., and Smale, C. J. (1970). *J. Gen. Virol.* **7**, 115.
Brown, G. C., and O'Leary, T. P. (1971). *J. Immunol.* **107**, 1486.
Brown, G. C., and O'Leary, T. P. (1973). *J. Immunol.* **110**, 889.
Brown, G. C., Baublis, J. V., and O'Leary, T. P. (1970). *Immunol.* **104**, 861.
Brown, J. A. H. (1953). *Brit. J. Exp. Pathol.* **34**, 290.
Buddingh, G. J., Schrum, D. I., Lanier, J. C., and Guidry, D. J. (1953). *Pediatrics* **11**, 595.

Burge, B. W., and Huang, A. S. (1970). *J. Virol.* **6**, 176.
Burge, B. W., and Pfefferkorn, E. (1967). *J. Virol.* **1**, 956.
Burge, B. W., and Strauss, J. H. (1970). *J. Mol. Biol.* **47**, 449.
Burger, M. M. (1973). *Fed. Proc., Fed. Amer. Soc. Exp. Biol.* **32**, 91.
Burnet, F. M. (1959). "A Clonal Selection Theory of Acquired Immunity," Cambridge Univ. Press, London and New York.
Burnet, F. M., and Fenner, F. (1949). "The Production of Antibodies," 2nd ed. Macmillan, New York.
Burnet, F. M., Keogh, E. V., and Lush, D. (1937). *Aust. J. Exp. Biol. Med. Sci.* **15**, 226.
Carnevale, A., and Iovino, A. (1959). *Gi. Mal. Infet. Parassit.* **11**, 919.
Carton, C. A., and Kilbourne, E. D. (1952). *N. Engl. J. Med.* **246**, 172.
Cartwright, B., and Brown, F. (1972). *J. Gen. Virol.* **15**, 243.
Cartwright, B., Smale, C. J., and Brown, F. (1970). *J. Gen. Virol.* **7**, 19.
Casals, J. (1957). *Trans. N. Y. Acad. Sci.* [2] **19**, 219.
Catanzaro, P. J., Brandt, W. E., Hogrefe, W. R., and Russell, P. K. (1974). *Infec. Immunity* **10**, 381.
Chan, G., Rancourt, M. W., Ceglowski, W. S., and Friedman, H. (1968). *Science* **159**, 437.
Cheathem, W. J., Weller, T. H., Dolan, T. F., and Dower, J. C. (1956). *Amer. J. Pathol.* **32**, 1015.
Cheville, N. F. (1967). *Amer. J. Pathol.* **51**, 527.
Chen, J. H., and Purchase, H. G. (1970). *Virology* **40**, 410.
Chieco-Bianchi, L., Sendo, F., Aoki, T., and Barrera, O. L. (1974). *J. Nat. Cancer Inst.* **52**, 1345.
Choppin, P. W., Compans, R. W., Scheid, A., McSharry, J. J., and Lazarowitz, S. G. (1972). *In* "Membrane Research" (C. F. Fox, ed.), pp. 163–185. Academic Press, New York.
Cohen, G. H., Ponce de Leon, M., and Nichols, C. (1972). *J. Virol.* **10**, 1021.
Cole, G. A. (1974). *Progr. Med. Virol.* **18**, 94.
Cole, G. A., Nathanson, N., and Prendergast, R. A. (1972). *Nature (London)* **238**, 335.
Cole, G. A., Prendergast, R. A., and Henney, C. S. (1973). *In* "Lymphocytic Choriomeningitis and Other Arenaviruses" (F. Lehmann-Grube, ed.) p. 61. Springer-Verlag, Berlin and New York.
Cole, R., and Kuttner, A. G. (1926). *J. Exp. Med.* **44**, 855.
Collins, J., and Black, P. H. (1973). *J. Nat. Cancer Inst.* **51**, 95 and 115.
Compans, R. W. (1971). *Nature (London), New Biol.* **229**, 114.
Compans, R. W. (1973). *Virology* **51**, 56.
Compans, R. W., Klenk, H., Caliguiri, L. A., and Choppin, P. W. (1970). *Virology* **42**, 880.
Cowan, K. M. (1970). *J. Immunol.* **104**, 423.
Cushing, H. (1905). *J. Amer. Med. Ass.* **44**, 1002.
Dales, S. (1969). *In* "Lysosomes in Biology and Pathology" (J. T. Dingle and H. B. Fell, eds.), vol. 2, pp. 69–86. North-Holland Publ., Amsterdam.
Dales, S., and Kajioka, R. (1964). *Virology* **24**, 278.
Daniels, C. A., Borsos, T., Rapp, H. J., Snyderman, R., and Notkins, A. L. (1969). *Science* **165**, 508.
Daniels, C. A., Borsos, T., Rapp, H. J., Snyderman, R., and Notkins, A. L. (1970). *Proc. Nat. Acad. Sci. U. S.* **65**, 528.
Daugharty, H., Warfield, D. T., Hemingway, W. D., and Casey, H. L. (1973). *Infec. Immunity* **77**, 380.

7. Virus Infections and Immune Responses

Davenport, F. M., and Hennessy, A. V. (1956). *J. Exp. Med.* **104**, 85.
David, J. R., and Schlossman, S. F. (1968). *J. Exp. Med.* **128**, 1451.
de Koch, G. (1924). *Trop. Vet. Bull.* **12**, 136.
Dent, P. B., Peterson, R., and Good, R. A. (1965). *Proc. Soc. Exp. Biol. Med.* **119**, 869.
Diehl, V., Henle, G., Henle, W., and Kohn, G. (1968). *J. Virol.* **2**, 663.
Diosi, P., Moldovan, E., and Tomescu, N. (1969). *Brit. Med J.* **4**, 660.
Dourmashkin, R. R., and Tyrrell, D. A. J. (1974). *J. Gen. Virol.* **24**, 129.
Downie, A. W., and McCarthy, K. (1958). *J. Hyg.* **56**, 479.
Duc-Nguyen, H., and Henle, W. (1966). *J. Bacteriol.* **42**, 258.
Duc-Nguyen, H., and Rosenblum, E. N. (1967). *J. Virol.* **1**, 415.
Duc-Nguyen, H., Rose, H. M., and Morgan, C. (1966). *Virology* **28**, 404.
Dulbecco, R., Vogt, M., and Strickland, A. (1956). *Virology* **2**, 162.
Dunkel, V. C., and Zeigel, R. F. (1970). *J. Nat. Cancer Inst.* **44**, 133.
Dupuy, J. M., Levy-Leblond, E., and Le Prévost, C. (1973). *Abstr., 10th Annu. Meet., Reticuloendothel. Soc.* p. 1.
Eaton, M. D., and Scala, A. R. (1969). *Proc. Soc. Exp. Biol. Med.* **132**, 20.
Eaton, M. D., Heller, J. A., and Scala, A. R. (1973). *Cancer Res.* **33**, 3293.
Edelman, R., and Pariyononda, A. (1973). *Amer. J. Epidemiol.* **98**, 29.
Edelman, R., and Wheelock, E. F. (1967). *J. Virol.* **1**, 1139.
Edelman, R., and Wheelock, E. F. (1968a). *J. Virol.* **2**, 440.
Edelman, R., and Wheelock, E. F. (1968b). *Lancet* **1**, 771.
Edelman, R., Nisalak, A., Pariyanonda, A., Udomsakdi, S., and Johnsen, D. (1973). *Amer. J. Epidemiol.* **97**, 208.
Elfenbein, G. J., and Rosenberg, G. L. (1973). *Cell. Immunol.* **7**, 516.
Enders, J. F., and Peebles, T. C. (1954). *Proc. Soc. Exp. Biol. Med.* **86**, 277.
Enders, J. F., Cohen, S., and Kane, L. W. (1945). *J. Exp. Med.* **81**, 119.
Enders-Ruckle, G. (1965). *Arch. Gesamte Virusforsch.* **16**, 182.
Epsmark, J. A. (1965). *Arch. Gesamte Virusforsch.* **17**, 89.
Epstein, L. B., Stevens, D. A., and Merigan, T. C. (1972). *Proc. Nat. Acad. Sci. U. S.* **69**, 2632.
Faucon, N., Chardonnet, Y., and Sohier, R. (1974). *Infec. Immunity* **10**, 11.
Faulkner, P., and Dobos, P. (1968). *Can. J. Microbiol.* **14**, 45.
Fazekas de St. Groth, S. (1962). *Advan. Virus Res.* **9**, 1.
Fazekas de St. Groth, S., and Graham, D. M. (1954). *Aust. J. Exp. Biol. Med. Sci.* **32**, 369.
Feinstone, S. M., Beachey, E. H., and Rytel, M. W. (1969). *J. Immunol.* **103**, 844.
Fenner, F. (1949). *J. Immunol.* **63**, 341.
Fernandes, M. V., Wiktor, T. J., and Koprowski, H. (1964). *J. Exp. Med.* **120**, 1099.
Finkel, A., and Dent, P. B. (1973). *Cell. Immunol.* **6**, 41.
Fireman, P., Friday, G., and Kumate, J. (1969). *Pediatrics* **43**, 264.
Fogel, M., and Sachs, L. (1962). *J. Nat. Cancer Inst.* **29**, 239.
Francis, T., Jr. (1942). *Harvey Lect.* p. 69.
Francis, T., Jr. (1953). *Ann. Intern. Med.* **39**, 203.
Francis, T., Jr. (1955). *Ann. Intern. Med.* **43**, 454.
Friedman, M., Lilly, F., and Nathenson, S. G. (1974). *J. Virol.* **14**, 1126.
Gadol, N., Johnson, J. E., and Waldman, R. H. (1974). *Infec. Immunity* **9**, 858.
Gardner, I., Bowern, N. A., and Blanden, R. V. (1974). *Eur. J. Immunol.* **4**, 63 and 68.
Geering, G. L., Old, L. J., and Boyse, E. A. (1966). *J. Exp. Med.* **124**, 753.
Gelderblom, H., and Bauer, H. (1973). *Int. J. Cancer* **11**, 466.
Gelderblom, H., Bauer, H., and Graf, T. (1972). *Virology* **47**, 416.

Gerber, P., and Lucas, S. J. (1972). *Cell. Immunol.* **5,** 318.
Gershon, A. A., Steinberg, S., and Brunell, P. A. (1974). *N. Engl. J. Med.* **290,** 243.
Gershon, R. K., Maurer, P. H., and Merryman, C. F. (1973). *Proc. Nat. Acad. Sci. U. S.* **70,** 250.
Gerson, K. L., and Haslam, R. (1971). *N. Engl. J. Med.* **285,** 78.
Glasgow, L. A., and Morgan, H. R. (1957). *J. Exp. Med.* **106,** 45.
Goffe, A. P., Almeida, J., and Brown, F. (1966). *Lancet* **2,** 607.
Gooding, L. R., and Edidin, M. (1974). *J. Exp. Med.* **140,** 61.
Goodman, T., and Koprowski, H. (1962). *J. Cell. Comp. Physiol.* **59,** 333.
Goodpasture, E. W. (1929). *Medicine (Baltimore)* **8,** 223.
Granoff, A. (1965). *Virology* **25,** 38.
Gresser, I., and Lang, D. J. (1966). *Progr. Med. Virol.* **8,** 62.
Griffin, D. E., and Johnson, R. T. (1973). *Cell. Immunol.* **9,** 426.
Grimes, W. J., and Burge, B. W. (1971). *J. Virol.* **7,** 309.
Grumet, F. C. (1972). *J. Exp. Med.* **135,** 110.
Haase, A. T., and Pereira, H. G. (1972). *J. Immunol.* **108,** 633.
Hagry, P., Rago, D., and Defendi, V. (1970). *J. Nat. Cancer Inst.* **44,** 1311.
Haheim, L. R., and Haukenes, G. (1973a). *Acta Pathol. Microbiol. Scand.* **81,** 440.
Haheim, L. R., and Haukenes, G. (1973b). *Acta Pathol. Microbiol. Scand.* **81,** 657.
Hahon, N. (1970a). *Infec. Immunity* **2,** 713.
Hahon, N. (1970b). *J. Gen. Virol.* **6,** 361.
Hahon, N., and Eckert, H. L. (1972). *Infec. Immunity* **6,** 730.
Hakkinen, L., and Halonen, P. (1971). *J. Nat. Cancer Inst.* **46,** 1161.
Hall, W. W., and Martin, S. J. (1973). *J. Gen. Virol.* **19,** 175.
Hall, W. W., and Martin, S. J. (1974). *J. Gen. Virol.* **22,** 363.
Haller, O., and Lindenmann, J. (1974). *Nature (London)* **250,** 679.
Hampar, B., Notkins, A. L., Mage, M., and Keehn, M. A. (1968). *J. Immunol.* **100,** 586.
Hanna, M. G., Tennant, R. W., Yuhas, J. M., Clapp, N. K., Batzing, B. L., and Snodgrass, M. J. (1972). *Cancer Res.* **32,** 2226.
Harboe, A., and Haukenes, G. (1966). *Acta Pathol. Microbiol. Scand.* **68,** 98.
Harboe, A., Schoyen, R., and Bye-Hansen, A. (1966). *Acta Pathol. Microbiol. Scand.* **67,** 573.
Hardy, B. Globerson, A., and Danon, D. (1973). *Cell. Immunol.* **9,** 282.
Harrison, S. C., David, A., Jumblatt, J., and Darnell, J. E. (1971). *J. Mol. Biol.* **60,** 521.
Hartley, J. W., Rowe, W. P., Capps, W. I., and Huebner, R. J. (1969). *J. Virol.* **1,** 152.
Haukenes, G., Harboe, A., and Mortensson-Egnund, K. (1966). *Acta Pathol. Microbiol. Scand.* **66,** 510.
Hawkes, R. (1964). *Aust. J. Exp. Biol. Med. Sci.* **42,** 465.
Hayashi, K., Rosenthal, J., and Notkins, A. L. (1972). *Science* **176,** 516.
Hayashi, K., Niwa, A., Rosenthal, J., and Notkins, A. L. (1973). *Intervirology* **2,** 48.
Hearn, H. J., and Rainey, T. C. (1963). *J. Immunol.* **90,** 720.
Hecht, T. T., and Summers, D. F. (1972). *J. Virol.* **10,** 578.
Hecht, T. T., and Summers, D. F. (1974). *J. Virol.* **14,** 162.
Hellman, A., Fowler, A. K., Steinman, H. G., and Buzzard, P. M. (1972). *Proc. Soc. Exp. Biol. Med.* **141,** 106.
Henle, W. G., Henle, G., Scriba, M., Joyner, C. R., Harrison, F. S., Essen, R., Paloheimo, J., and Klemola, E. (1970). *N. Engl. J. Med.* **282,** 1068.
Henson, D., Strano, A. J., Slotnik, M., and Goodheart, C. (1972). *Proc. Soc. Exp. Biol. Med.* **140,** 802.
Higginbotham, J. D., Schoyen, R., Mortensson-Eghund, K., How, M. J., and Harboe, A. (1971). *Acta Pathol. Microbiol. Scand.* **79,** 349.

Hirano, T., and Ruebner, B. H. (1965). *Lab. Invest.* **14**, 488.
Hirsch, M. S., and Murphy, F. A. (1968). *Lancet* **2**, 37.
Hirsch, M. S., Murphy, F. A., and Hicklin, M. D. (1968a). *J. Exp. Med.* **127**, 757.
Hirsch, M. S., Nahmias, A. J., Murphy, F. A., and Kramer, J. H. (1968b). *J. Exp. Med.* **128**, 121.
Hirsch, M. S., Allison, A. C., and Harvey, J. J. (1969). *Nature (London)* **223**, 739.
Hirsch, M. S., Zisman, B., and Allison, A. C. (1970). *J. Immunol.* **104**, 1160.
Hirsch, M. S., Phillips, S. M., Solnik, C., Black, P. H., and Schwartz, R. S. (1972). *Proc. Nat. Acad. Sci. U. S.* **69**, 1069.
Hirsch, M. S., Ellis, D. A., Black, P. H., Monaco, A. P., and Wood, M. L. (1973). *Science* **180**, 500.
Holland, J. J., and Kiehn, E. D. (1970). *Science* **167**, 202.
Hollinshead, A., and Alford, T. C. (1969). *J. Gen. Virol.* **5**, 411.
Hollis, V. W., Aoki, T., Barrera, O., Oldstone, M. B. A., and Dixon, F. J. (1974). *J. Virol.* **13**, 448.
Holmes, K. V., Klenk, H., and Choppin, P. W. (1969). *Proc. Soc. Exp. Biol. Med.* **131**, 651.
Horta-Barbosa, L., Fuccillo, D. A., Sever, J., and Zeman, W. (1969). *Nature (London)* **221**, 974.
Hosaka, Y., and Shimiza, Y. K. (1972). *Virology* **49**, 627.
Howard, J. G., Christie, G. H., Courtenay, B. M., Leuchars, E., and Davies, A. J. S. (1971). *Cell. Immunol.* **2**, 614.
Howard, R. J., Notkins, A. L., and Mergenhagen, S. E. (1969). *Nature (London)* **221**, 873.
Howe, C., Lee, L. T., Harboe, A., and Haukenes, G. (1967). *J. Immunol.* **98**, 543.
Hummeler, K., Anderson, T. F., and Brown, R. A. (1962). *Virology* **16**, 84.
Hummeler, K., Koprowski, H., and Wiktor, T. (1967). *J. Virol.* **1**, 152.
Hyllseth, B., and Pettersson, U. (1970). *Arch. Gesamte Virusforsch.* **32**, 337.
Hyman, C., and Paldino, R. L. (1960). *Ann. N. Y. Acad. Sci.* **88**, 232.
Igarashi, A., Nithiuthai, P., and Rojanasuphot, S. (1970). *Biken J.* **13**, 229.
Igarashi, A., Fukuoka, T., and Fukai, K. (1971). *Biken J.* **14**, 353.
Ihle, J. N., Yurconic, M., and Hanna, M. G. (1973). *J. Exp. Med.* **138**, 194.
Ihle, J. N., Hanna, M. G., Roberson, L. E., and Kenney, F. T. (1974). *J. Exp. Med.* **139**, 1568.
Ikeda, H., Pincus, T., Yoshiki, T., Strand, M., August, J., Boyse, E., and Mellors, R. (1974). *J. Virol.* **14**, 1274.
Irlin, I. S. (1967). *Virology* **32**, 725.
Isacson, P. (1968). *Perspect. Virol.* **6**, 141.
Isacson, P., and Koch, A. E. (1965). *Virology* **27**, 129.
Ishimoto, A., and Ito, Y. (1969). *Virology* **39**, 595.
Ishimoto, A., and Ito, Y. (1971). *J. Nat. Cancer Inst.* **46**, 353.
Israel, M. S. (1962). *J. Pathol. Bacteriol.* **84**, 169.
Ito, M., and Barron, A. L. (1972a). *J. Immunol.* **108**, 711.
Ito, M., and Barron, A. L. (1972b). *Proc. Soc. Exp. Biol. Med.* **140**, 374.
Jabbour, J. T., Roane, J. A., and Sever, J. (1969). *Neurology* **19**, 929.
Jawetz, E., Coleman, V., and Allende, M. F. (1951). *J. Immunol.* **67**, 197.
Jawetz, E., Coleman, V., and Merrill, E. (1955). *J. Immunol.* **75**, 28.
Jenner, E. (1798). "An Inquiry into the Causes and Effects of the Variolae Vacciniae" p. 13. Sampson-Low, London.
Johnson, E. D., Nathanson, N., and Cole, G. A. (1974). *Fed. Proc., Fed. Amer. Soc. Exp. Biol.* **33**, 729.

Johnson, R. (1964). *J. Exp. Med.* **120**, 359.
Joseph, B. S., and Oldstone, M. B. A. (1974). *J. Immunol.* **113**, 1205.
Kano, S., Bloom, B. R., and Howe, M. L. (1973). *Proc. Nat. Acad. Sci. U. S.* **70**, 2299.
Kantoch, M., Warwick, A., and Bang, F. B. (1963). *J. Exp. Med.* **117**, 781.
Kates, M., Allison, A. C., Tyrrell, D. A. J., and James, A. T. (1961). *Biochim. Biophys. Acta* **52**, 455.
Katz, D., and Benacerraf, B. (1972). *Advan. Immunol.* **15**, 1.
Katz, D., Hamaoka, T., and Benacerraf, B. (1973a). *J. Exp. Med.* **137**, 1405.
Katz, D., Hamaoka, T., Dorf, M. E., and Benacerraf, B. (1973b). *Proc. Nat. Acad. Sci. U. S.* **70**, 2624.
Kaufman, N. E., Brown, D. C., and Ellison, E. M. (1967). *Science* **156**, 1628.
Kedar, E., Aaronov, A., Goldblum, N., and Sulitzeanu, D. (1972). *Int. J. Cancer* **9**, 536.
Keller, R. (1965). *J. Immunol.* **94**, 143.
Keller, R. (1966). *J. Immunol.* **96**, 96.
Keller, R. (1968). *J. Immunol.* **100**, 1071.
Kelley, J. M., Emerson, S. U., and Wagner, R. (1972). *J. Virol.* **10**, 1231.
Kennedy, S. I. T. (1974). *J. Gen. Virol.* **23**, 129.
Kenyon, A. J. (1966). *Amer. J. Vet. Res.* **27**, 1780.
Ketler, A., Hinuma, Y., and Hummeler, K. (1961). *J. Immunol.* **86**, 22.
Kilbourne, E. D., Laver, W. G., Schulman, J., and Webster, R. G. (1968). *J. Virol.* **2**, 281.
Kjellen, L. (1962). *Virology* **14**, 484.
Kjellen, L. (1964). *Arch. Gesamte Virusforsch.* **14**, 189.
Kjellen, L. (1965). *Immunology* **8**, 557.
Kjellen, L., and Pereira, H. G. (1968). *J. Gen. Virol.* **2**, 177.
Kjellen, L., and Schlesinger, R. W. (1959). *Virology* **7**, 236.
Klein, G., Pearson, G., Nadkarni, J. S., Nadkarni, J. J., Klein, E., Henle, G., Henle, W., and Clifford, P. (1968). *J. Exp. Med.* **128**, 1011.
Kleinman, L. F., Kibrick, S., Ennis, F., and Polgar, P. (1972). *Proc. Soc. Exp. Biol. Med.* **141**, 1095.
Klenk, H., and Choppin, P. W. (1970). *Proc. Nat. Acad. Sci. U. S.* **66**, 57.
Klenk, H., and Choppin, P. W. (1971). *J. Virol.* **7**, 416.
Klenk, H., Compans, R. W., and Choppin, P. W. (1970). *Virology* **42**, 1158.
Klenk, H., Rott, R., and Becht, H. (1972a). *Virology* **47**, 579.
Klenk, H., Scholtissek, C. and Rott, R. (1972b). *Virology* **49**, 723.
Kobayashi, H., Sendo, F., Kaji, H., Shirai, T., Saito, H., Takeichi, N., Hosokawa, M., and Kodama, T. (1970). *J. Nat. Cancer Inst.* **44**, 11.
Kolar, O. (1968). *Neurology* **18**, 107.
Kourilsky, F. M., Silvestre, D., Neauport-Sautres, C., Loosfelt, Y., and Dausset, J. (1972). *Eur. J. Immunol.* **2**, 249.
Krugman, S., Giles, J. P., Friedman, H., and Stone, S. (1966). *Pediatrics* **66**, 471.
Kurth, R., and Bauer, H. (1972). *Virology* **47**, 426.
Labowskie, R. J., Edelman, R., Rustigian, R., and Bellanti, J. A. (1974). *J. Infec. Dis.* **129**, 233.
Lafferty, K. J. (1963a). *Virology* **21**, 61.
Lafferty, K. J. (1963b). *Virology* **21**, 76.
Lagrange, P. H., Mackaness, G. B., and Miller, T. E. (1974). *J. Exp. Med.* **139**, 1529.
Lang, D. (1972). *Arch. Gesamte Virusforsch.* **37**, 365.
Lausch, R., Swyers, J., and Kaufman, H. (1966). *J. Immunol.* **96**, 981.
Laver, W. G. (1973). *Advan. Virus Res.* **18**, 57.

Laver, W. G., and Webster, R. G. (1973). *Virology* **51**, 383.
Laver, W. G., Suriano, J. R., and Green, M. (1967). *J. Virol.* **1**, 723.
Law, L., and Ting, R. (1970). *J. Nat. Cancer Inst.* **44**, 615.
Lazarowitz, S. G., Compans, R. W., and Choppin, P. W. (1971). *Virology* **46**, 830.
Lazarowtiz, S. G., Compans, R. W., and Choppin, P. W. (1973). *Virology* **52**, 199.
Lee, J. C., and Sigel, M. M. (1974). *Cell. Immunol.* **13**, 22.
Lee, J. C., Hanna, M. G., Ihle, J. N., and Aaronson, S. A. (1974). *J. Virol.* **14**, 773.
Lee, L. T., Howe, C., Meyer, K., and Choi, H. (1969). *J. Immunol.* **102**, 1144.
Leerhoy, J. (1968). *Acta Pathol. Microbiol. Scand.* **73**, 275.
Lehmann-Grube, F. (1971). *Virol. Monogr.* **10**, 1.
Lehrich, J. R., Kasel, J. A., and Rossen, R. D. (1966). *J. Immunol.* **97**, 654.
Leskowitz, S. (1972). *In* "Immunogenicity" (F. Borek, ed.), pp. 131–151. North-Holland Publ., Amsterdam.
Levy-Leblond, E., and Dupuy, J. M. (1974). *Fed. Proc., Fed. Amer. Soc. Exp. Biol.* **33**, 743.
Lewis, R. (1974). *Int. Rev. Exp. Pathol.* **13**, 55.
Lilly, F., and Pincus, T. (1973). *Advan. Cancer Res.* **17**, 231.
Lilly, F., and Steeves, R. (1974). *Biochim. Biophys. Acta* **355**, 105.
Lindenmann, J. (1970). *Arch. Gesamte Virusforsch.* **31**, 61.
Lindenmann, J. (1974). *Biochim. Biophys. Acta* **355**, 49.
Lindenmann, J., and Klein, P. A. (1964). *Proc. Soc. Exp. Biol. Med.* **117**, 446.
Lindenmann, J., and Klein, P. A. (1967). *J. Exp. Med.* **126**, 93.
Link, H., Panelius, M., and Salmi, A. A. (1973). *Arch. Neurol. (Chicago)* **28**, 23.
Linscott, W., and Levinson, W. (1969). *Proc. Nat. Acad. Sci. U. S.* **64**, 520.
Lodmell, D. L., Haddow, W. J., Munoz, J. J., and Whitford, H. W. (1970). *J. Immunol.* **104**, 878.
Lowry, S. P., Bronson, D. L., and Rawls, W. E. (1971). *J. Gen. Virol.* **11**, 47.
Lundstedt, C. (1969). *Acta Pathol. Microbiol. Scand.* **75**, 139.
McCullough, B., Krakowka, S., and Koestner, A. (1973). *Amer. J. Pathol.* **74**, 155.
McDevitt, H. O., and Landy, M., eds. (1973). "Genetic Control of Immune Responsiveness: Relationship to Disease Susceptibility." Academic Press, New York.
McFarland, H. (1974). *J. Immunol.* **113**, 173.
Mackaness, G. (1970). *In* "Mononuclear Phagocytes" (R. van Furth, ed.), pp. 461–484. Blackwell, Oxford.
McSharry, J. J., Compans, R. W., and Choppin, P. W. (1971). *J. Virol.* **8**, 722.
Mahy, B. W. J. (1964). *Virology* **24**, 481.
Majer, M. (1972). *Curr. Top. Microbiol. Immunol.* **58**, 69.
Majer, M., and Link, F. (1970). *Clin. Exp. Immunol.* **7**, 283.
Malmgren, R., Takemoto, K., and Carney, P. (1968). *J. Nat. Cancer Inst.* **40**, 263.
Mandel, B. (1961). *Virology* **14**, 316.
Mandel, B. (1962). *Cold Spring Harbor Symp. Quant. Biol.* **27**, 123.
Mandel, B. (1967). *Virology* **31**, 238.
Mantani, M., and Igarashi, A. (1971). *Biken J.* **14**, 131.
Marker, O., and Volkert, M. (1973). *J. Exp. Med.* **137**, 1511.
Markham, R. V., Sutherland, J. C., Cimino, E. F., Drake, W. P., and Mardiney, M. R. (1972). *Rev. Eur. Etud. Clin. Biol.* **17**, 690.
Mellman, W., and Wetton, R. (1963). *J. Lab. Clin. Med.* **61**, 453.
Mellors, R., Aoki, T., and Huebner, R. J. (1969). *J. Exp. Med.* **129**, 1045.
Mellors, R. C., Shirai, T., Aoki, T., and Huebner, R. J. (1971). *J. Exp. Med.* **133**, 113.
Mietens, C., Hummeler, K., and Henle, W. (1964). *J. Immunol.* **92**, 17.

Miller, G. W., Saluk, P. H., and Nussenzweig, V. (1973). *J. Exp. Med.* **138**, 495.
Miller, J. F. A. P., Ting, R. C., and Law, L. W. (1964). *Proc. Soc. Exp. Biol. Med.* **116**, 323.
Miller, J. F. A. P., Basten, A., Sprent, J., and Cheers, C. (1971). *Cell. Immunol.* **2**, 469.
Mims, C. A. (1964). *Bacteriol. Rev.* **28**, 30.
Mims, C. A., and Blanden, R. V. (1972). *Infec. Immunity* **6**, 695.
Mirkovic, R., Werch, J., South, M. A., and Benyesh-Melnick, M. (1971). *Infec. Immunity* **3**, 45.
Mitchell, G., and Humphrey, J. (1973). In "Germinal Centers of Lymphoid Tissue" (B. Janovic, ed.), p. 125. Plenum, New York.
Miyamoto, H., and Kato, S. (1968). *Biken J.* **11**, 343.
Miyamoto, H., and Kato, S. (1971). *Biken J.* **14**, 311.
Miyamoto, H., Morgan, C., Hsu, K., and Hampar, B. (1971). *J. Nat. Cancer Inst.* **46**, 629.
Mori, R., Nomoto, K., Kimura, G., and Takeya, K. (1966). *Arch. Gesamte Virusforsch.* **18**, 186.
Mori, R., Tasaki, T., Kimura, G., and Takeya, K. (1967). *Arch. Gesamte Virusforsch.* **21**, 459.
Mori, R., Kimoto, K., and Takeya, K. (1970). *Arch. Gesamte Virusforsch.* **29**, 32 and 38.
Moulias, R. L., Reinert, P. H., and Goust, J. M. (1971). *N. Engl. J. Med.* **285**, 1090.
Moyer, S., and Summers, D. F. (1974). *Cell* **1**, 63.
Muschel, L. H., and Toussaint, A. J. (1962). *J. Immunol.* **89**, 35.
Nablant, J. (1937). *Amer. Rev. Tuberc.* **36**, 773.
Nagler, F. P. O. (1944). *J. Immunol.* **48**, 213.
Nahmias, A. J., Kibrick, S., and Rosan, R. (1964). *J. Immunol.* **93**, 69.
Nahmias, A. J., Dowdle, W. R., Josey, W. E., Naib, Z. M., Painter, L. M., and Luce, C. (1969). *J. Pediat.* **75**, 1194.
Nahmias, A. J., del Buono, I., Schneweis, K. E., Gordon, D. S., and Thies, D. (1971). *Proc. Soc. Exp. Biol. Med.* **138**, 21.
Nathanson, N., and Cole, G. A. (1970). *Advan. Virus Res.* **16**, 397.
Nesburn, A. B., Cook, M. L., and Stevens, J. G. (1972). *Arch. Ophthalmol.* **88**, 412.
Nichols, W. W. (1966). *Amer. J. Hum. Genet.* **18**, 81.
Nii, S. C., Morgan, C., Rose, H. M., and Hsu, K. C. (1968). *J. Virol.* **2**, 1172.
Nishioka, K., Irie, R. F., Kawana, T., and Takeuchi, S. (1969). *Int. J. Cancer* **4**, 139.
Noll, H. (1962). *Cold Spring Harbor Symp. Quant. Biol.* **27**, 256.
Norrby, E. (1969a). *J. Gen. Virol.* **5**, 221.
Norrby, E. (1969b). *J. Virol.* **4**, 657.
Norrby, E., and Gollmar, Y. (1972). *Infec. Immunity* **6**, 240.
Norrby, E., and Hammarskjold, B. (1972). *Microbios* **5**, 17.
Norrby, E., and Wadell, G. (1969). *J. Virol.* **4**, 663.
Norrby, E., and Wadell, G. (1972). *Virology* **48**, 757.
Norrby, E., Marusyk, H., and Hammarskjold, B. (1969). *Virology* **38**, 477.
Norrby, E., Link, H., and Olsson, J. (1974). *Arch. Neurol. (Chicago)* **30**, 285.
Notkins, A. L. (1971). *J. Exp. Med.* **134**, 41s.
Notkins, A. L., Mergenhagen, S., Rizzo, A., Scheele, C., and Waldmann, T. (1966a). *J. Exp. Med.* **123**, 347.
Notkins, A. L., Mahar, S., Scheele, C., and Goffman, J. (1966b). *J. Exp. Med.* **124**, 81.
Notkins, A. L., Mage, M., Ashe, W. K., and Mahar, S. (1968). *J. Immunol.* **100**, 314.
Notkins, A. L., Mergenhagen, S. E., and Howard, R. J. (1970). *Annu. Rev. Microbiol.* **24**, 525.

Notkins, A. L., Rosenthal, J., and Johnson, B. (1971). *Virology* **43**, 321.
Nowinski, R. C., and Kaehler, S. L. (1974). *Science* **185**, 869.
O'Dea, J. F., and Dineen, J. K. (1957). *J. Gen. Microbiol.* **17**, 19.
Ogra, P. (1973). *In* "Airborne Transmission and Airborne Infection" (J. Hers and K. Winkler, eds.), pp. 280–282. Oosthoek Publ. Co., Utrecht.
Ogra, P., Karzon, D. T., Righthand, F., and MacGillivray, M. (1968). *N. Engl J. Med.* **279**, 893.
Ohta, N., Pardee, A. B., McAuslan, B. R., and Burger, M. M. (1968). *Biochim. Biophys. Acta* **158**, 98.
Old, L. J., Stockert, E., Boyse, E. A., and Kim, J. H. (1968). *J. Exp. Med.* **127**, 523.
Oldstone, M. B. A. (1974). *Progr. Med. Virol.* **19**, 123.
Oldstone, M. B. A., and Dixon, F. J. (1967). *Science* **158**, 1193.
Oldstone, M. B. A., and Dixon, F. J. (1971). *J. Exp. Med.* **134**, 32s.
Oldstone, M. B. A., Habel, K., and Dixon, F. J. (1969). *Fed. Proc., Fed. Amer. Soc. Exp. Biol.* **28**, 429.
Oldstone, M. B. A., Aoki, T., and Dixon, F. J. (1972). *Proc. Nat. Acad. Sci. U. S.* **69**, 134.
Oldstone, M. B. A., Dixon, F. J., Mitchell, G. F., and McDevitt, H. O. (1973). *J. Exp. Med.* **137**, 1201.
Oldstone, M. B. A., Cooper, N. R., and Larson, D. L. (1974). *J. Exp. Med.* **140**, 549.
Olitsky, P. K., and Long, P. H. (1929a). *J. Exp. Med.* **50**, 263.
Olitsky, P. K., and Long, P. H. (1929b). *Science* **69**, 170.
Olshevsky, U., and Becker, Y. (1972). *Virology* **50**, 277.
O'Neill, C. H. (1968). *J. Cell Sci.* **3**, 405.
Ordal, J. C., and Grumet, F. C. (1972). *J. Exp. Med.* **136**, 1195.
Oroszlan, S., and Gilden, R. V. (1970). *Science* **168**, 1478.
Osborn, J. E., Blazkovec, A. A., and Walker, D. L. (1968). *J. Immmunol.* **100**, 835.
Oshiro, L. S., Riggs, J. L., Taylor, D., Lennette, E. H., and Huebner, R. J. (1971). *Cancer Res.* **31**, 1100.
Osler, A., and Sandberg, A. (1973). *Progr. Allergy* **17**, 51.
Parker, J. C., Vernon, M. L., and Cross, S. S. (1973). *Infec. Immunity* **7**, 305.
Parks, W. P., Scolnick, E. M., Ross, J., Todaro, G. J., and Aaronson, S. A. (1972). *J. Virol.* **9**, 110.
Pascal, R. R., Koss, M. N., and Kassel, R. L. (1973). *Lab. Invest.* **29**, 150.
Pasternak, G. (1967). *Nature (London)* **214**, 1364.
Paul, J. R., Riordan, J. T., and Melnick, J. L. (1951). *Amer. J. Hyg.* **54**, 275.
Payne, F. E., Baublis, J. V., and Itabashi, H. H. (1969). *N. Engl. J. Med.* **281**, 585.
Pedersen, C. E., Slocum, D. R., and Eddy, G. A. (1973). *Infec. Immunity* **8**, 901.
Peled, A.. and Haran-Ghera, N. (1974). *Immunology* **26**, 323.
Penn, I., and Starzl, T. E. (1972). *Transplantation*, **14**, 407.
Pereira, H. G., and Kelly, B. (1957). *Nature (London)* **180**, 615.
Perham, T. G., Caul, E. O., Coneway, P. J., and Mott, M. G. (1971). *Brit. J. Heematol.* **20**, 307.
Perkins, F. T. (1974). *In* "Prophylaxis of Infectious and other Diseases" (T. Inderbitzin, ed.). Karger, Basel (in press).
Pettersson, U., Philipson, L., and Hoglund, S. (1968). *Virology* **35**, 204.
Pfefferkorn, E., and Hunter, H. S. (1963). *Virology* **20**, 433.
Philipson, L. (1966). *Virology* **28**, 35.
Philipson, L. (1969). *Int. Virol.* **1**, 90.
Phillips, E. R., and Perdue, J. F. (1974). *J. Cell Biol.* **61**, 743.

Pincus, W. B., and Flick, J. A. (1963). *J. Infec. Dis.* **113**, 15.
Plummer, G., Goodheart, C. R., Henson, D., and Bowling, C. (1969). *Virology* **39**, 134.
Porter, D. D., Dixon, F. J., and Larson, A. E. (1965). *Blood* **25**, 736.
Porter, D. D., Porter, H. G., and Cox, N. A. (1973). *J. Immunol.* **111**, 1626.
Powell, K. L., Buchan, A., Sim, C., and Watson, D. H. (1974). *Nature (London)* **249**, 360.
Proffitt, M. R., Congdon, C. C., and Tyndall, R. L. (1972). *Int. J. Cancer* **9**, 193.
Proffitt, M. R., Hirsch, M. S., and Black, P. H. (1973). *J. Immunol.* **110**, 1183.
Purchase, H. G., Chubband, R. C., and Biggs, P. M. (1968). *J. Nat. Cancer Inst.* **40**, 583.
Pyrhonen, S., and Penttinen, K. (1972). *Lancet* **2**, 1330.
Radwan, A. I., and Burger, D. (1973). *Virology* **51**, 71.
Radwan, A. I., Burger, D., and Davis, W. C. (1973). *Virology* **53**, 372.
Rager-Zisman, B., and Allison, A. C. (1973a). *J. Gen. Virol.* **19**, 329.
Rager-Zisman, B., and Allison, A. C. (1973b). *J. Gen. Virol.* **19**, 339.
Rager-Zisman, B., and Bloom, B. R. (1974). *Nature (London)* **251**, 542.
Rawls, W. E., Desmayter, J., and Melnick, J. L. (1967). *Proc. Soc. Exp. Biol. Med.* **124**, 167.
Reddick, R. A., and Lefkowitz, S. S. (1969). *J. Immunol.* **103**, 687.
Renkonen, O., Kaarainen, L., Simons, K., and Gahmberb, C. G. (1971). *Virology* **46**, 318.
Reno, P. W., and Hoffman, E. M. (1972). *Infec. Immunity* **6**, 945.
Roane, P. R., and Roizman, B. (1964). *Virology* **22**, 1.
Robbins, P., and Uchida, T. (1965). *J. Biol. Chem.* **240**, 375.
Robertson, H. T., and Black, P. H. (1969). *Proc. Soc. Exp. Biol. Med.* **130**, 363.
Rocklin, R. E., Meyers, O. L., and David, J. R. (1970). *J. Immunol.* **104**, 95.
Roelants, G. E., and Askonas, B. A. (1972). *Nature (London), New Biol.* **239**, 63.
Rogers, H. W., Scott, L. V., and Patnode, R. A. (1972). *J. Immunol.* **109**, 801.
Roizman, B., and Heine, J. W. (1972). *In* "Membrane Research" (C. F. Fox, ed.), pp. 203-207. Academic Press, New York.
Rose, H. M., and Molloy, E. (1947). *Fed. Proc., Fed. Amer. Soc. Exp. Biol.* **6**, 432.
Rosen, L. (1960). *Amer. J. Hyg.* **71**, 120.
Rosenberg, G. L., Farber, P. A., and Notkins, A. L. (1972a). *Proc. Nat. Acad. Sci. U. S.* **69**, 756.
Rosenberg, G. L., Wohlenberg, C., Nahmias, A. J., and Notkins, A. L. (1972b). *J. Immunol.* **109**, 413.
Rosenblith, J. Z., Ukena, T. E., Yin, H. H., Berlin, R. D., and Karnovsky, M. J. (1973). *Proc. Nat. Acad. Sci. U. S.* **70**, 1625.
Rossen, R. D., Douglas, R. G., Cate, T. R., Couch, R. B., and Butler, W. T. (1966). *J. Immunol.* **97**, 532.
Rowe, W. P. (1973). *Cancer Res.* **33**, 3061.
Rowe, W. P., and Capps, W. I. (1961). *J. Exp. Med.* **113**, 831.
Rowlands, D. J., Sanger, D. V., and Brown, F. (1971). *J. Gen. Virol.* **13**, 85.
Rubin, H. (1957). *Virology* **4**, 533.
Rubin, H., and Franklin, R. (1957). *Virology* **3**, 84.
Rustigian, R., Randall, E., and Winston, S. H. (1971). *Bacteriol. Proc.* p. 183.
Sabin, A. (1954). *Res. Publ., Ass. Res. Nerv. Ment. Dis.* **33**, 57.
Sabin, A. (1957). *Spec. Publ. N. Y. Acad. Sci.* **5**, 113.
Sabin, A. (1959). *In* "Immunity and Virus Infection" (V. Najjer, ed.), p. 211. Wiley, New York.

Sabin, A., and Blumberg, R. W. (1947). *Proc. Soc. Exp. Biol. Med.* **64**, 385.
Salaman, M. H., and Wedderburn, N. (1966). *Immunology* **10**, 445.
Salmi, A., Gollmar, Y., Norrby, E., and Panelius, M. (1973). *Acta Pathol. Microbiol. Scand.* **81**, 621.
Sawyer, W. A. (1931). *J. Prev. Med.* **5**, 413.
Scharff, M. D., and Lewinton, L. (1963). *Virology* **19**, 491.
Scheid, A., and Choppin, P. W. (1973). *J. Virol.* **11**, 263.
Scheid, A., and Choppin, P. W. (1974). *Virology* **57**, 475.
Scheid, A., Cliguiri, L. A., Compans, R. W., and Choppin, P. W. (1972). *Virology* **50**, 640.
Schierman, L. W., and McBride, R. A. (1967). *Science* **156**, 658.
Schirrmacher, V., and Rajewsky, K. (1970). *J. Exp. Med.* **132**, 1019.
Schlesinger, R. W. (1969). *Advan. Virus Res.* **14**, 2.
Schmidt, N. J., Lennette, E. H., and Dennis, J. (1968). *J. Immunol.* **100**, 99.
Schoyen, R., Harboe, A., and Wang, L. (1966). *Acta Pathol. Microbiol. Scand.* **68**, 103.
Schulze, I. (1973). *Advan. Virus Res.* **18**, 1.
Schwartz, D. P., and Buckley, R. H. (1971). *N. Engl. J. Med.* **284**, 513.
Sell, K. W., Thurman, G. B., Ahmed, A., and Strong, D. M. (1973). *N. Engl. J. Med.* **288**, 215.
Senyk, G., Williams, E. B., Nitecki, D. E., and Goodman, J. W. (1971). *J. Exp. Med.* **133**, 1294.
Shearer, G. M., Mozes, E., Haran-Ghera, N., and Bentwich, Z. (1973). *J. Immunol.* **110**, 736.
Shimizu, Y. (1971). *Arch. Gesamte Virusforsch.* **33**, 338.
Shirai, T., Hiroshi, K., Takeichi, N., Sendo, F., Saito, H., Hosokawa, M., and Kobayashi, H. (1971). *J. Nat. Cancer Inst.* **46**, 449.
Shore, S., Potter, C. W., and Stuart-Harris, G. H. (1973). In "Airborne Transmission and Airborne Infection" (J. Hers and K. Winkler, eds.), pp. 290–294. Oosthoek Publ. Co., Utrecht.
Shore, S. L., Nahmias, A. J., Starr, S. E., Wood, P. A., and McFarlin, D. E. (1974). *Nature (London)* **251**, 350.
Siegel, B. V., Neher, G. H., and Morton, J. I. (1969). *Lab. Invest.* **20**, 347.
Silverstein, S., and Marcus, P. (1964). *Virology* **23**, 370.
Skehel, J. J. (1972). *Virology* **49**, 23.
Slettenmark-Wahren, B., and Klein, E. (1962). *Cancer Res.* **22**, 947.
Smith, C. B., Purcell, R. H., Bellanti, J. A., and Chanock, R. M. (1966). *N. Engl. J. Med.* **275**, 1145.
Smith, K. A., Chess, L., and Mardiney, M. R. (1972). *Cell. Immunol.* **5**, 597.
Smith, K. A., Chess, L., and Mardiney, M. R. (1973). *Cell. Immunol.* **8**, 321.
Smith, K. O. (1965). *J. Immunol.* **94**, 976.
Smith, R. W., and Mora, P. T. (1972). *Virology* **50**, 233.
Smith, R. W., Morganroth, J., and Mora, P. T. (1970). *Nature (London)* **227**, 141.
Smithwick, E. M., and Berkovich, S. (1966). *Proc. Soc. Exp. Biol. Med.* **123**, 276.
Snodgrass, M. J., Lowrey, D. S., and Hanna, M. (1972). *J. Immunol.* **108**, 877.
Speel, L. F., Osborn, J. E., and Walker, D. L. (1968). *J. Immunol.* **101**, 409.
Spitler, L., Benjamin, E., Young, J. D., Kaplan, H., and Fudenberg, H. H. (1970). *J. Exp. Med.* **131**, 133.
Springer, G. F., and Schuster, R. (1964). *Klin. Wochenschr.* **42**, 221.
Stanley, P. M., and Haslam, E. A. (1971). *Virology* **46**, 764.
Stanley, P. M., Gandhi, S. S., and White, D. O. (1973). *Virology* **53**, 92.
Starr, S., and Berkovich, S. (1964). *Pediatrics* **33**, 769.

Steele, R. W., Honsan, S. A., Vincent, M. M., Fuccillo, D. A., and Bellanti, J. A. (1973). *J. Immunol.* **110**, 1502.
Steeves, R. A. (1968). *Cancer Res.* **28**, 338.
Stephenson, J. R., and Aaronson, S. (1972). *J. Exp. Med.* **135**, 503.
Stern, H., and Williams, B. M. (1966). *Lancet* **1**, 293.
Stevens, J. G., and Cook, M. L. (1971a). *J. Exp. Med.* **133**, 19.
Stevens, J. G., and Cook, M. L. (1971b). *Science* **173**, 843.
Stevens, J. G., Nesburn, A. B., and Cook, M. L. (1972): *Nature (London), New Biol.* **235**, 216.
Stockert, E., Old, L. J., and Boyse, E. A. (1971). *J. Exp. Med.* **133**, 1334.
Strand, M., Lilly, F., and August, J. T. (1974). *Proc. Nat. Acad. Sci. U. S.* **71**, 3682.
Strauss, J. H., Burge, B. W., Pfefferkorn, E. R., and Darnell, J. E. (1968). *Proc. Nat. Acad. Sci. U. S.* **59**, 533.
Strauss, J. H., Burge, B. W., and Darnell, J. E. (1970). *J. Mol. Biol.* **47**, 437.
Strohl, W. A., and Schlesinger, R. W. (1965). *Virology* **26**, 208.
Strouk, V., Grundner, G., Fenyo, E., Lamon, E., Skurzak, H., and Klein, G. (1972). *J. Exp. Med.* **136**, 344.
Svehag, S. (1964a). *J. Exp. Med.* **119**, 225.
Svehag, S. (1964b). *J. Exp. Med.* **119**, 517.
Svehag, S. (1968). *Progr. Med. Virol.* **10**, 1.
Svehag, S., and Mandel, B. (1964a). *J. Exp. Med.* **119**, 1.
Svehag, S., and Mandel, B. (1964b). *J. Exp. Med.* **119**, 21.
Svet-Moldavsky, G. T., Zinbar, S. N., and Spector, N. M. (1964). *Nature (London)* **202**, 353.
Taylor, J. M., Hampson, A. W., and White, D. (1969). *Virology* **39**, 419.
Taylor, R. B., Duffus, P. H., Raff, M. C., and dePetris, S. (1971). *Nature (London), New Biol.* **233**, 225.
Thé, T. H., and Langenhuysen, M. M. C. (1972). *Clin. Exp. Immunol.* **11**, 475.
Thind, I. S., and Price, W. H. (1971). *Bacteriol. Proc.* p. 183.
Thurman, G. B., Ahmed, A., Strong, D. M., Knudsen, R. C., Grace, W. R., and Sell, K. W. (1973). *J. Exp. Med.* **138**, 839.
Ting, C. C., and Herberman, R. B. (1970). *J. Nat. Cancer Inst.* **44**, 729.
Todaro, G., and Huebner, R. J. (1972). *Proc. Nat. Acad. Sci. U. S.* **69**, 1033.
Tomasi, T. B., and Bienenstock, J. (1969). *Advan. Immunol.* **9**, 1.
Tompkins, W. A. F., Adams, C., and Rawls, W. E. (1970a). *J. Immunol.* **104**, 502.
Tompkins, W. A. F., Crouch, N. A., Tevethia, S. S., and Rawls, W. E. (1970b). *J. Immunol.* **105**, 1181.
Tosolini, F. A., and Mims, C. A. (1971). *J. Infec. Dis.* **123**, 134.
Tozawa, H., Watanabe, M., and Ishida, N. (1973). *Virology* **55**, 242.
Turk, J. G., Allison, A. C., and Oxman, M. (1962). *Lancet* **1**, 405.
Ueda, Y., Ito, M., and Tagaya, I. (1969). *Virology* **38**, 180.
Uhr, J. W., and Finkelstein, M. S. (1963). *J. Exp. Med.* **117**, 457.
van der Veen, J., and Sonderkamp, H. J. A. (1965). *Arch. Gesamte Virusforsch.* **15**, 721.
Vandvik, B., and Norrby, E. (1973). *Proc. Nat. Acad. Sci. U. S.* **70**, 1060.
Vasconcelos-Costa, J. (1970). *J. Gen. Virol.* **8**, 69.
Vasconcelos-Costa, J., Geralden, A., and Carvalho, Z. (1973). *Virology* **52**, 337.
Virelizier, J. L., Postlewaite, R., Schild, G., and Allison, A. C. (1974a). *J. Exp. Med.* **140**, 1559.
Virelizier, J. L., Allison, A. C., and Schild, G. (1974b). *J. Exp. Med.* **140**, 1571.
Vogt, A., Kopp, R., Maass, G., and Reich, L. (1964). *Science* **145**, 1447.

Volkert, M., and Hannover-Larsen, J. (1965). *Progr. Med. Virol.* **7**, 160.
Volkert, M., Marker, O., and Bro-Jorgensen, K. (1974). *J. Exp. Med.* **139**, 1329.
von Pirquet, C. (1907). *In* "Klinische Studien uber Vakzination und Medizinale Allergie," Deuticke, Leipzig.
von Pirquet, C. (1908). *Deut. Med. Wochenschr.* **34**, 1297.
Wadell, G. (1972). *J. Immunol.* **108**, 622.
Wadell, G., and Norrby, E. (1969). *J. Virol.* **4**, 671.
Wahren, B., and Metcalf, D. (1970). *Clin. Exp. Immunol.* **7**, 373.
Wakim, K. G., and Fleisher, G. A. (1963). *J. Lab. Clin. Med.* **61**, 86.
Waldman, R. H., Wood, S. H., Torres, E. J., and Small, P. A. (1970). *Amer. J. Epidemiol.* **91**, 575.
Waldman, R. H., Spencer, C. S., and Johnson, J. E. (1972). *Cell. Immunol.* **3**, 294.
Walz, M. A., Price, R. W., and Notkins, A. L. (1974). *Science* **184**, 1185.
Warthin, A. S. (1931). *Arch. Pathol.* **11**, 864.
Watkins, J. F. (1965). *Virology* **26**, 746.
Watkins, J. F., and Chen, L. (1969). *Nature (London)* **223**, 1018.
Watson, D. H., and Wildy, P. (1963). *Virology* **21**, 100.
Webb, H. E., and Smith, C. E. (1970). *Lancet* **1**, 1206.
Webster, R. G. (1965). *Immunology* **9**, 501.
Webster, R. G. (1968a). *Immunology* **14**, 29.
Webster, R. G. (1968b). *Immunology* **14**, 39.
Westaway, E. G., Della-Porta, A. J., and Reedman, B. M. (1974). *J. Immunol.* **112**, 656.
Westmoreland, D., and Watkins, J. F. (1974). *J. Gen. Virol.* **24**, 167.
Wetherbee, R. G. (1973). *J. Immunol.* **111**, 157.
Wheeler, C. J., and Huffines, W. (1965). *J. Amer. Med. Ass.* **191**, 455.
Wheelock, E. F., and Edelman, R. (1969). *J. Immunol.* **103**, 429.
Wheelock, E. F., and Toy, S. T. (1973). *Advan. Immunol.* **16**, 123.
White, R. G., and Boyd, J. F. (1973). *Clin. Exp. Immunol.* **13**, 343.
Wigand, R., and Fliedner, D. (1968). *Arch. Gesamte Virusforsch.* **24**, 25.
Wiktor, T. J., Kuwert, E., and Koprowski, H. (1968). *J. Immunol.* **101**, 1271.
Wiktor, T. J., György, E., Schlumberger, H., Sokol, F., and Koprowski, H. (1973). *J. Immunol.* **110**, 269.
Wilcox, W. C., and Ginsberg, H. S. (1963). *Proc. Soc. Exp. Biol. Med.* **114**, 37.
Woodruff, J., and Gesner, B. (1969). *J. Exp. Med.* **129**, 551.
Woodruff, J. F., and Woodruff, J. J. (1974). *Infec. Immunity* **9**, 969.
Wright, P. W., and Law, L. W. (1971). *Proc. Nat. Acad. Sci. U. S.* **68**, 973.
Wright, P. W., Brodine, S., Lowy, D. R., and Rowe, W. P. (1972). *Fed. Proc., Fed. Amer. Soc. Exp. Biol.* **30**, 760.
Wrigley, N. G., Skehel, J. J., Charlwood, P. A., and Brand, C. M. (1973). *Virology* **51**, 525.
Wu, H., Meezan, E., Black, P. H., and Robbins, P. W. (1968). *Fed. Proc., Fed. Amer. Soc. Exp. Biol.* **27**, 814.
Yamanouchi, K., Kobune, F., Fukada, A., Hayami, M., and Shishido, A. (1970). *Arch. Gesamte Virusforsch.* **29**, 90.
Yamanouchi, K., Chino, F., Kobune, F., Fukuda, A., and Yoshikawa, Y. (1974a). *Infec. Immunity* **9**, 199.
Yamanouchi, K., Fukuda, A., Kobune, F., Yoshikawa, Y., and Chino, F. (1974b). *Infec. Immunity* **9**, 206.
Yang, H. Y., and Skinsnes, O. K. (1973). *RES, J. Reticulendothel. Soc.* **14**, 181.
Yasuda, J., and Milgrom, F. (1968). *Int. Arch. Allergy Appl. Immunol.* **33**, 151.

Yoshiki, T., Mellors, R. C., Hardy, W. D., and Fleissner, E. (1974a). *J. Exp. Med.* **139,** 925.
Yoshiki, T., Mellors, R. C., Strand, M., and August, J. T. (1974b). *J. Exp. Med.* **140,** 1011.
Yoshino, K., and Taniguchi, S. (1964). *Virology* **22,** 193.
Yoshino, K., and Taniguchi, S. (1965a). *Virology* **26,** 44.
Yoshino, K., and Taniguchi, S. (1965b). *Virology* **26,** 61.
Yoshino, K., and Taniguchi, S. (1967). *Virology* **31,** 260.
Yoshino, K., Taniguchi, S., Furuse, R., Najima, T., Fujii, R., Minanitani, M., Tada, R., and Kubota, H. (1962). *Jap. J. Med. Sci. Biol.* **15,** 235.
Zinkernagel, R. M., and Doherty, P. C. (1974). *Nature (London)* **248,** 701.
Zisman, B., Hirsch, M. S., and Allison, A. C. (1969). *J. Immunol.* **104,** 1155.

Author Index

Numbers in italics refer to the pages on which the complete references are listed.

A

Aaronov, A., 527, *566*
Aaronson, S. A., 388, *440*, 499, 505, 528, 545, *559*, *567*, *569*, *572*
Aas, K., 293, 295, 297, 306, 307, 346, *350*, *352*
Abbot, A., 238, *261*
Abdel-Akher, M., 4, *110*
Abdou, N. I., 248, *260*
Abeyounis, C. J., 400, *435*
Abramson, H. A., 276, 277, *350*, *353*
Acher, R., 308, *352*
Ackermann, B., 375, *446*
Ada, G. L., 89, 91, *121*, 165, *184*, 207, 214, 215, 220, 221, 223, 224, 225, 226, 231, 232, 235, 236, 237, 238, 239, 243, 249, 254, *260*, *261*, *262*, *265*, *266*, *269*
Adams, C., 534, *572*
Adams, M. H., 27, 28, *110*
Adkinson, N. F., Jr., 308, *358*
Adler, W. H., 200, *266*, 539, *559*
Ahmed, A., 535, 537, *560*, *571*, *572*
Ahrons, S., 372, 373, *437*
Aird, J., 104, *125*
Aisenberg, A., 548, *560*
Albert, E. A., 362, 373, 400, *435*, *442*
Albert, E. D., 363, 399, *435*, *441*
Alberto, R., 274, 288, *355*
Alexander, H. E., 39, 40, 76, *125*
Alford, R. H., 506, *560*
Alford, T. C., 527, *565*
Alkan, S. S., 129, 169, 171, 172, 173, 175, 78, 182, *183*, *187*, 243, *261*
Allan, D., 194, 208, *261*
Allan, P. Z., 52, 84, *110*, *114*
Allen, F. H., Jr., 372, *440*
Allen, J. L., 92, *110*
Allende, M. F., 535, *565*

Allison, A. C., 482, 491, 505, 508, 509, 511, 520, 521, 523, 533, 534, 542, 543, 545, 546, *560*, *561*, *565*, *566*, *570*, *572*, *574*
Alm, G. V., 219, 231, *264*
Almeida, J. D., 505, 516, *560*, *561*, *564*
Alspaugh, M. A., 391, *437*
Aluotto, B. B., 465, *476*
Amante, L., 211, 248, *266*
Ambler, J., 292, 307, *350*
Amiel, J. L., 364, 432, *435*
Amos, D. B., 337, *351*, 363, 370, 376, 380, 382, 383, 386, 387, 390, *435*, *438*, *439*, *444*, *447*
Amsbaugh, D. F., 87, 88, 90, 92, 93, 94, *110*, *111*, 557, *560*
Amspacher, W. H., 279, *357*
Anacker, R. L., 7, *122*
Anderson, C. L., 194, *261*
Anderson, E. S., 40, 41, *110*, *111*
Anderson, H. R., 214, *261*
Anderson, P. R., 42, *125*
Anderson, T. F., 484, *565*
Anderson, W. A., 535, *560*
Andersson, B., 92, 93, *111*, 233, *269*
Andersson, J., 93, *111*, *120*, 201, 207, 208, 209, 210, 211, 245, 253, 257, 258, *261*, *265*
Andersson, K., 255, *266*
Andersson, L. G., 194, *266*
André, J., 293, *350*
Andres, G. A., 549, *560*
André-Schwartz, J., 554, *560*
Andrews, P., 287, *350*
Anfinsen, C. B., 151, *186*
Ansel, S., 498, 547, *560*
Anthony, B. F., 49, *120*
Antonini, E., 150, *186*
Aoki, T., 385, 388, 391, *435*, *439*, 499,

575

526, 528, 531, 538, 544, 549, *560*, *562*, *565*, *567*, *569*
Appella, E., 418, 421, *441*, *445*
Appleyard, G., 496, *560*
Arakatsu, Y., 52, 68, 69, 93, *111*, 140, *183*
Araujo, P., 43, 44, 81, *111*
Arbesman, C. E., 308, *352*
Archibald, A. R., 46, *111*
Archibald, W. J., 4, *111*
Armstrong, A. S., 400, 433, *439*
Arnason, B. G., 505, *560*
Arnon, R., 137, 139, 149, 151, 164, *183*, *185*
Arquilla, E. R., 144, *183*
Artenstein, M. S., 84, *114*
Ashe, W. K., 513, 518, 519, *560*, *568*
Ashford, A. E., 327, *354*
Ashman, R. F., 240, 241, 249, *261*
Ashwell, G., 2, 52, 68, 69, 77, 93, *111*, 140, *183*
Ashwell, M. A., 398, *435*
Askonas, B. A., 102, 103, *121*, 221, 235, 236, 237, 238, *261*, 265, 267, 511, *570*
Asofsky, R., 94, *110*, 173, *183*
Aster, R. H., 383, *435*
Atassi, M., Z., 135, 141, *183*
Atler, B. J., 533, *560*
Attallah, N. A., 316, *350*
Atwell, J. L., 179, *185*, 194, 207, 216, *261*, *265*
August, J. T., 499, 544, 545, *565*, *572*, *574*
Augustin, R., 275, 276, 277, 283, 291, 293, 298, *350*
Austen, K. F., 152, *187*, 202, 260, *264*, 268, 273, 274, *356*
Austin, C. M., 235, 243, *261*, *266*
Austin, J. B., 485, *561*
Austrian, R., 103, 104, *118*
Averbeck, A. K., 273, *352*
Avery, O. T., 2, 73, 77, 89, 93, *111*, *113*, *114*, *115*, 133, 147, *183*, *184*
Avrameas, S., 213, *261*
Axelson, N. H., 292, *350*
Axler, D. A., 548, *560*

B

Babers, F. H., 2, 73, 93, *114*, *147*, *184*
Bach, F. H., 533, *560*
Bach, J. F., 218, 219, *261*, 364, *435*

Bach, M. L., 429, *435*
Bacon, J. S. D., 101, *111*
Baddiley, J., 27, 28, 31, 45, 46, 83, *111*, *112*, *113*, *118*, *123*, *125*
Baecher, L., 316, *355*
Baer, H., 168, *184*, 285, 300, 327, 346, *350*, *352*
Bagdian, G., 17, 60, 66, 71, 72, *111*, *124*
Bagian, G., 58, *120*
Baker, E. E., 106, *111*
Baker, H. J., 279, *357*
Baker, P. J., 49, 87, 88, 90, 92, 93, *111*, 218, *261*, 557, *560*
Baldwin, R. L., 287, *359*
Balfour, T. C., 387, *443*
Ballou, C. E., 4, 47, 48, 53, 90, *111*, *117*, *118*, *121*, *124*
Balner, H., 333, *350*, 363, 367, 374, *435*, *446*
Bamburg, J. R., 35, *112*
Bandlow, G., 548, *560*
Bang, F. B., 520, 521, *560*, *566*
Bankhurst, A. D., 215, 248, *261*, *264*
Baringer, J. R., 542, *560*, *561*
Barker, L. F., 466, *476*
Barker, S. A., 27, 32, 33, *111*, 134, *183*, 292, *350*
Baron, B., 279, *352*
Barrera, O. L., 538, 544, *562*, *565*
Barron, A. L., 525, 527, *565*
Barth, R. F., 385, 388, *435*
Barthold, D. R., 94, *110*
Basten, A., 171, *185*, 194, 195, 197, 205, 237, 238, 240, 247, 249, *261*, *263*, 266, 507, *568*
Bastian, F. O., 542, *561*
Batchelor, F. R., 293, *350*
Batchelor, J. R., 362, 364, 374, 381, *435*, *444*
Battisto, J. R., 107, *111*
Batzing, B. L., 545, *561*, *564*
Baublis, J. V., 503, 542, *561*, *569*
Bauer, H., 526, *563*, *566*
Bauer, J. A., 367, *435*
Bauminger, S., 200, 201, 255, 257, *263*, *264*, *267*
Baur, S., 207, *261*, *269*
Bayona, I. G., 278, *352*
Bayse, G. S., 216, *261*, *266*
Bazaral, M., 339, *350*, *353*

Author Index

Beachey, E. H., 536, *563*
Bearn, A. G., 420, 427, *435*
Becht, H., 491, *566*
Bechtol, K. B., 249, *263*
Beck, V., 549, *561*
Becker, M. J., 169, 172, 174, *183*
Becker, Y., 455, *476*, 485, *569*
Beckman, B. L., 469, *471*
Beiser, S. M., 136, *183*
Belin, L., 281, 282, 287, 288, 292, 293, 305, 306, 324, 325, 326, 327, *350*, *355*
Bell, E., 396, *444*
Bellanti, J. A., 345, *357*, 503, 506, 526, 537, *561*, *566*, *571*, *572*
Belzer, F. O., 364, *437*
Benacerraf, B., 19, 26, 89, 94, *111*, *123*, 144, 145, 163, 164, 166, 178, *183*, *184*, *185*, *186*, 197, 205, 226, 231, 239, 243, 244, 247, 250, 255, *261*, *264*, 265, 269, 333, *350*, *354*, 368, *435*, *441*, 505, 531, 547, *561*, *566*
Benaim, C., 278, *358*
Benajam, A., 383, *437*
Benderli, H., 148, 180, *183*
Bendinelli, M., 549, *561*
Ben Efraim, S., 175, *187*
Benjamin, E., 532, *571*
Benjamini, E., 140, 141, 146, 165, 168, *183*, *187*, 243, *267*, *268*, 313, 348, *350*
Bennett, D., 385, *439*
Bennett, M., 549, 556, *561*
Bennich, H., 273, 287, 288, 307, 346, *351*, *352*, *353*, *359*
Benson, A. A., 470, *476*
Benson, L., 540, 543, *561*
Bent, V. D., 364, *436*
Benton, A. W., 308, *358*
Bentwich, Z., 221, *266*, 556, *571*
Benyesh-Melnick, M., 555, *568*
Berah, M., 385, *435*
Berg, D., 47, 84, *117*, 137, *185*
Berg, T., 346, *352*
Berger, A., 148, 180, *183*
Berggård, I., 251, *266*, 420, 421, 427, 429, *435*, *437*, *443*
Berke, R. A., 323, *359*
Berken, A., 205, *261*
Berkovich, S., 549, 550, *561*, *571*
Berlin, R. D., 528, *570*
Berman, L., 527, *561*

Bernard, G. E., 372, *440*
Berney, I. N., 554, *561*
Bernhard, W. G., 2, 73, 83, 106, *115*
Bernier, G. M., 420, *435*
Bernoco, D., 200, *261*, 373, 389, 390, 391, 392, 397, 431, *436*
Bernstein, I. L., 292, 328, 329, *351*, *353*
Bernstein, M., 218, *261*
Bernstein, R. L., 64, 68, 74, *122*
Bernton, H. S., 275, 278, *351*, *358*
Berrens, L., 278, 281, 290, 292, 295, 311, 312, *350*, *356*
Berry, D. M., 516, *561*
Berst, M., *111*
Bert, G., 207, *261*
Bertrams, J., 387, *436*
Beutel, H., 383, 390, *438*
Beveridge, W. I., 536, *561*
Bezer, A. E., 3, 84, 85, 91, 93, *117*, *124*
Bhatnagar, S. S., 104, *111*
Bianco, C., 194, 205, 253, *261*, *263*
Bias, W. B., 280, 283, 287, 288, 295, 304, 305, 321, 322, 330, 334, 335, 337, 338, 339, 340, 342, 343, 345, *351*, *355*
Biberfeld, G., 452, 460, 471, *476*
Biberfeld, P., 452, 460, *476*
Bick, S. M., 27, *111*
Bienenstock, J., 506, *572*
Biesecker, L. J., 538, *561*
Biggart, J. D., 553, *561*
Biggs, P. M., 549, 556
Billing, R., 376, 406, 427, 429, *436*, *438*
Billingham, R. E., 364, 366, *436*, *445*
Binns, R. M., 366, *447*
Biozzi, G., 26, 87, 89, *116*, 217, 218, *261*, 266, 434, *436*
Biro, C. E., 375, *442*
Bister, F., 9, *125*
Bitter-Saermann, D., 253, *263*
Björndal, H., 5, 18, 19, 35, 74, *111*, *112*
Black, J. H., 330, *359*
Black, P. H., 526, 528, 538, 546, 554, *560*, *562*, 565, *570*, *573*
Black, P. L., 330, 338, 339, *350*
Blackley, C. H., 275, *351*
Blacklow, N. R., 485, *561*
Blackman, K., 548, *561*
Blanden, R. V., 107, *112*, *119*, 207, 244, *263*, 534, 540, *561*, *563*, *568*

Blaurock, A. E., 198, 269
Blazkovec, A. A., 549, 569
Bleiweis, A. S., 43, 112
Bleumink, E., 295, 311, 351
Bloch, K. J., 97, 98, 121, 273, 293, 351, 356
Blomberg, B., 94, 112
Blomgren, H., 93, 111
Bloom, B. R., 538, 555, 559, 561, 566, 570
Bloth, B., 204, 268
Bluestone, R., 344, 356, 357, 373, 447
Blumberg, R. W., 541, 571
Blumenthal, M. N., 337, 351
Blumhardt, R., 549, 561
Boatman, E. S., 452, 460, 461, 476
Bockman, D. E., 214, 265
Bodey, G. P. S., 408, 439
Bodmer, J. G., 363, 381, 431, 436, 443
Bodmer, W. F., 343, 344, 351, 363, 370, 381, 383, 390, 431, 436, 439, 442, 443
Böhlck, I., 105, 106, 122
Boiarski, K. W., 475, 477
Boivin, A., 9, 112
Bonilla-Soto, O., 292, 351
Bonner, S. V., 459, 478
Bonynge, C. W., 25, 112
Boone, C. W., 526, 548, 561
Borberg, H., 406, 436
Borek, F., 54, 123, 146, 151, 163, 183, 187, 313, 351
Borel, Y., 254, 261
Boring, J. R., III, 26, 105, 123
Borsos, R., 372, 436
Borsos, T., 206, 262, 516, 562
Borzynski, E. A., 49, 120
Bos, E., 366, 446
Bose, H. R., 496, 548, 561
Bostock, J., 275, 351
Bott, E. M., 25, 112
Bourne, H. R., 260, 264
Bouthiller, Y., 218, 261
Bowen, R., 331, 351
Bowern, N. A., 207, 244, 263, 534, 563
Boyd, J. F., 551, 573
Boyd, W. C., 170, 184
Boyse, E. A., 194, 195, 207, 211, 214, 215, 219, 246, 249, 262, 268, 269, 369, 385, 387, 388, 391, 392, 432, 435, 436, 439, 441, 442, 499, 526, 531, 544, 560, 561, 563, 565, 569, 572

Boyum, A., 369, 373, 436
Bradbury, S. M., 307, 308, 351, 358
Bradley, B., 366, 447
Brady, R. O., 528, 529, 561
Bramson, S., 395, 436, 440
Branca, M., 545, 561
Brand, C. M., 490, 573
Brandchaft, P., 548, 561
Brandt, R., 293, 351
Brandt, W. E., 526, 562
Branton, D., 198, 199, 267, 268
Bratlie, A., 364, 366, 370, 398, 399, 430, 445, 446
Braun, D., 97, 112
Braun, D. G., 96, 98, 112, 113
Braun, O. H., 49, 119
Braun, W., 259, 269
Braun, W. E., 399, 436
Brautbar, C., 382, 395, 431, 436
Brdicka, R., 366, 445
Bredt, W., 452, 467, 476
Breese, S. S., 42, 125
Brent, L., 362, 364, 435, 436
Bretscher, M. S., 199, 262
Bretscher, P., 93, 112, 172, 183, 252, 262
Brewerton, D. A., 344, 351
Bridger, G. P., 322, 351
Brier, A. M., 526, 527, 530, 561
Brimacombe, J. S., 27, 30, 32, 53, 78, 111, 116
Britton, C. J. C., 277, 283, 351
Britton, S., 92, 112
Brock, T. D., 153, 184
Broder, S., 373, 436
Brodine, S., 526, 540, 573
Brody, J. A., 549, 561
Brody, T., 234, 262
Bro-Jorgensen, K., 540, 573
Bromer, W., 144, 183
Bron, C., 436
Bronson, D. L., 527, 567
Brooke, M. S., 89, 112
Broom, J. C., 533, 561
Brown, D. C., 542, 566
Brown, D. G., 96, 113
Brown, F., 497, 498, 504, 505, 514, 561, 562, 564, 570
Brown, G. C., 503, 504, 561
Brown, J., 77, 96, 121
Brown, J. A. H., 535, 561
Brown, R., 7, 122

Brown, R. A., 484, 565
Brown, R. K., 150, 183
Brownstone, A., 153, 183
Brubaker, R. R., 11, 13, 116, 122
Bruce, C. A., 218, 305, 323, 325, 326, 327, 351, 355
Bruley, M., 387, 442
Brundish, D. E., 31, 83, 112
Brunet, R., 295, 304, 353
Bruning, J. W., 364, 383, 389, 436, 438
Brunnell, P. A., 527, 564
Brunner, H., 467, 476
Brunner, K. T., 249, 262, 388, 391, 436
Brunner, M., 279, 351
Bryant, R. E., 373, 439
Bube, F. W., 408, 446
Bucci, E., 150, 186
Buchan, A., 485, 514, 535, 570
Buchanan, J. G., 27, 28, 46, 111, 112, 113, 118, 123, 125
Buckley, C. E., 337, 351
Buckley, R. H., 507, 571
Buddingh, G. J., 542, 561
Buell, D. N., 395, 436
Buescher, E. L., 503, 561
Bullock, W. W., 225, 266
Bulman, H. N., 163, 184
Bulman, N., 137, 183
Bunting, J. R., 203, 269
Burg, C., 194, 269
Burge, B. W., 495, 496, 497, 498, 526, 562, 564, 572
Burger, D., 316, 355, 515, 516, 570
Burger, M. M., 528, 562, 569
Burka, E. R., 396, 441
Burke, G. C., 136, 183
Burnet, F. M., 170, 187, 192, 262, 433, 436, 483, 512, 517, 536, 541, 543, 561, 562
Burns, W. H., 482, 560
Burris, C., 454, 478
Burtin, P., 287, 353
Bush, M. E., 182, 183, 243, 261
Busse, W. W., 323, 351
Bustin, M., 194, 208, 262, 263
Butler, K., 134, 183
Butler, W. T., 390, 440, 506, 560, 570
Buttery, S. H., 468, 477, 478
Buzzard, P. M., 536, 564
Bye-Hansen, A., 492, 548, 564
Byrt, P., 207, 220, 224, 225, 226, 232, 235, 236, 237, 238, 239, 249, 260, 261, 262, 269

C

Caffrey, M., 344, 351
Caldes, G., 471, 474, 478
Caliguiri, L. A., 491, 562
Callaghan, O. H., 301, 351
Callahan, G. N., 366, 436
Callewart, G. L., 295, 299, 308, 328, 358
Calne, R. Y., 366, 447
Campbell, D. H., 137, 163, 183, 186, 280, 282, 285, 286, 287, 288, 289, 291, 293, 295, 296, 297, 300, 316, 318, 319, 346, 351, 352, 353, 354, 355, 359
Campbell, J. H., 89, 96, 112
Campbell, P., 213, 264, 268
Cannon F. D., 363, 444
Cantor, H., 173, 183
Canty, T. G., 249, 262
Capková, J., 368, 438
Capps, W. I., 498, 551, 564, 570
Capra, J. D., 160, 183, 185, 299, 304, 356
Carbonara, A. O., 285, 355
Carnevale, A., 550, 562
Carney, P., 527, 567
Carpenter, C. B., 260, 268
Carroll, W. R., 27, 122
Carswell, E. A., 385, 439
Carton, C. A., 543, 562
Cartwright, B., 497, 562
Carvalho, Z., 527, 572
Casals, J., 495, 562
Casey, H. L., 503, 562
Cashman, T., 142, 185
Caspari, E. L., 77, 124
Casper, W., 86, 122
Castro, E., 468, 477
Castro-Murillo, E., 357
Catanzaro, P. J., 526, 562
Cate, T. R., 506, 570
Cathou, R. E., 97, 102, 116, 154, 183, 203, 262, 269
Caul, E. O., 542, 569
Caulfield, A. H. W., 277, 351
Cavalli-Sforza, L. L., 370, 436
Cavanaugh, J. J. A., 331, 357
Cebra, J. J., 134, 136, 160, 184, 186, 211, 264
Ceglowski, W. S., 549, 562
Celada, F., 381, 436

Centis, D., 381, 384, 406, *438*
Ceppellini, C., 200, *261*
Ceppellini, R., 26, 105, *112*, 362, 364, 368, 373, 381, 389, 390, 391, 392, 397, 402, 408, 418, 431, *436*, *440*, *446*
Cerottini, J. C., 208, 216, 248, 249, *262*, *264*, 388, 391, *436*
Cesari, I. M., 160, *187*
Ceska, M., 282, *352*
Chaicumpa, W., 107, *112*
Chambers, D. C., 278, *358*
Chan, E. L., 246, *264*
Chan, G., 549, *562*
Chang, E. B., 313, 333, *352*
Changeux, J.-P., 259, *266*
Chanock, R. M., 460, 465, 466, 467, 471, 474, *476*, *478*, 506, *571*
Chaouat, M., 391, *444*
Chaparas, S. D., 168, *184*
Chapel, H. M., 397, *436*
Chapuis, B., 249, *262*
Chardonnet, Y., 542, *563*
Chargaff, E., 39, 40, 76, *125*
Charlton, R. K., 406, *436*
Charlwood, P. A., 490, *573*
Chase, G. A., 305, 342, *355*
Chase, R. M., Jr., 400, *444*
Cheathem, W. J., 551, *562*
Cheers, C., 171, *185*
Chen, F. W., 97, *112*
Chen, J. H., 527, *562*
Chen, L., 547, *573*
Cheng, J., 274, 288, *355*
Cherry, M., 368, 371, *445*
Chesebro, B., 204, *268*
Chess, L., 527, 536, 539, *571*
Chessin, L. N., 395, *436*
Cheville, N. F., 553, *562*
Chiapetta, G., 107, *111*
Chieco-Bianchi, L., 538, *562*
Chiller, J. M., 94, *112*, 231, 253, *262*, *265*
Chinitz, A., 333, *355*
Chino, F., 511, 550, 552, *573*
Chionglo, T. D., 43, *112*
Chipman, D. M., 180, *184*
Chittenden, G. J. F., 28, *112*
Chobot, R., 276, *358*
Choi, H., 492, *567*
Choi, T. K., 96, *122*
Choppin, P. W., 489, 491, 494, 497, 498, 526, 554, *562*, *565*, *566*, *567*, *571*

Choy, Y. M., 32, 34, *112*, *113*
Chrambach, A., 415, *444*
Christensen, T., 293, 295, 297, 306, *352*
Christie, G. H., 3, 26, 83, 85, 86, 87, 89, 90, 91, 92, 93, 94, 103, *116*, 509, *565*
Chubband, R. C., 549, 556, *570*
Cikes, M., 387, 393, 395, *437*
Cimino, E. F., 544, *567*
Cividalli, G., 221, *266*
Claesson, M. H., 372, 373, *437*
Claman, H. N., 177, *186*
Clapp, N. K., 545, *564*
Clark, W. R., 42, *112*
Clarke, J., 230, 231, *262*
Clarke, M., 278, *358*
Claudemans, C. P. J., 29, *115*
Claus, D., 11, *112*
Clayburgh, J., 249, *264*
Clerici, E., 147, *187*
Cleve, H., 201, *264*
Clifford, H. T., 291, *359*
Clifford, P., 206, 212, *265*, 527, *566*
Cliguiri, L. A., 494, *471*
Cline, W. L., 460, *478*
Clyde, W. A., 465, 466, *476*
Coca, A. F., 274, 276, 311, *352*, *353*
Cochrum, K. C., 364, *437*
Cohen, G. H., 485, 514, 535, *562*
Cohen, I., 390, *435*
Cohen, S., 3, 99, *112*, 536, *563*
Cohn, M., 3, 99, 100, 101, 102, *112*, *114*, *119*, *125*, 160, 172, *183*, *187*, 252, *262*
Cole, B. C., 467, *476*
Cole, G. A., 249, *264*, 526, 530, 531, 540, 543, 555, *562*, *565*, *568*
Cole, R., 541, *562*
Coleman, L. H., 467, *476*
Coleman, V., 535, *565*
Colldahl, H., 306, *353*
Collier, A. M., 454, *476*
Collier, E. M., 383, *445*
Collins, F. M., 107, *112*, *119*
Collins, J., *562*
Collins, R. D., 373, *439*
Colombani, J., 383, 390, 398, 399, *437*
Colombani, M., 383, 390, 398, 399, *437*
Colon, S. M., 213, 248, *264*, *267*, 420, 422, 423, 424, *439*
Compans, R. W., 489, 490, 491, 494, 496, 497, 498, 554, *562*, *566*, *567*, *571*
Cone, R. E., 179, *185*, 194, 201, 207, 208,

214, 215, 216, 217, 248, *261, 262, 265,*
267
Coneway, P. J., 542, 569
Congdon, C. C., 552, 570
Connell, J. T., 283, 295, 299, 301, 322,
323, 327, 336, 347, *352, 354*
Conrad, H. E., 5, 32, 34, 35, *112, 114, 122*
Conway-Jacobs, A., 152, *186*
Cook, M. L., 523, 542, 546, *568, 572*
Cooke, R. A., 274, 276, 311, 318, 330, 331,
352, 358
Cooley, D. G., 378, *438*
Coombs, R. R. A., 207, *262,* 277, 283, *351*
Coons, A. H., 89, *117*
Cooper, H. E., 383, *435*
Cooper, M. D., 214, 215, 216, 217, 219,
229, 249, *262, 265, 269*
Cooper, M. G., 165, *184,* 226, 231, 232,
237, 238, 239, 243, 249, 252, 254, *261,*
262
Cooper, N. R., 376, 377, 378, 380, 382,
394, 395, 412, *438, 441,* 516, *569*
Corley, R. B., 337, *351*
Corneil, I., 134, *184*
Cotten, I., 382, *442*
Cottew, G. S., 468, *476, 478*
Cottrell, R. C., 295, 299, 308, 328, *358*
Couch, R. B., 506, *570*
Coulson, E. J., 278, 295, *358*
Courtenay, B. M., 3, 26, 83, 85, 86, 87, 89,
90, 91, 92, 93, 94, 103, *116,* 509, *565*
Coutinho, A., 26, 93, *112,* 241, 254, *262*
Cowan, K. M., 504, *562*
Cox, N. A., 545, *570*
Coynault, C., 72, 74, *124*
Craig, L. C., 283, *352*
Craig, S. W., 211, *264*
Cramer, M., 112
Crandall, M. A., 153, *184*
Cresswell, P., 250, 262, 392, 419, 420,
422, 423, 424, 425, 431, *437, 439, 444*
Crifó, S., 301, *352*
Cromwell, H. W., 276, *356, 358*
Crone, M., 219, 231, 249, 250, *262*
Crosnier, J., 364, *435, 439*
Cross, A. M., 171, *185*
Cross, S. S., 551, *569*
Crossley, G., 316, *355*
Crouch, N. A., 527, *572*
Crowle, A. J., 107, *112*
Cruickshank, C. N. D., 292, *350*

Crumpton, M. J., 135, 140, 141, *184,* 194,
208, 223, *261, 262*
Cuatrecasas, P., 286, *352*
Cullen, S., 200, *261,* 389, 390, 391, 392,
397, 431, *435, 436*
Cunningham, A. J., *262*
Cunningham, B. A., 251, *266,* 421, 429,
437, 443
Cunnington, A. M., 309, 310, *355*
Curtis, S. N., 43, *112*
Curtoni, E. S., 364, 402, 408, 418, *440*
Curvall, M., 18, *112*
Cushing, H., 543, *562*

D

Dagorn, M. B., 60, *113*
Dales, S., 514, *562*
D'Amaro, J., 367, 383, *435, 437*
Dambrosio, F., 374, *438*
Danielli, J. F., 430, *437*
Daniels, C. A., 516, 519, *560, 562*
Danon, D., 524, *564*
Dardenne, M., 218, *261*
Darnell, J. E., 398, *439,* 495, 496, *564,*
572
Das, A., 29, *113*
Daugharty, H., 503, *562*
Dausset, J., 200, *265,* 341, *352,* 362, 363,
383, 385, 386, 388, 389, 390, 391, 392,
398, 399, 401, 431, 432, *435, 437, 438,*
440, 441, 442, 443, 530, *566*
Davenport, F. M., 510, *563*
David, A., 496, *564*
David, C. S., 250, *262, 269,* 399, *437*
David, J. J., 156, *185*
David, J. R., 532, *563, 570*
Davidson, A. G., 279, *352*
Davie, J. M., 98, *113, 120,* 173, 174, *184,*
220, 224, 226, 231, 234, *262, 265, 266*
Davies, A. J. S., 3, 83, 91, 93, 94, 103, *116,*
171, *184,* 509, *565*
Davies, D. A. L., 364, 400, 402, *437, 442*
Davies, D. R., 154, *186,* 203, *267*
Davis, B. D., 382, *437*
Davis, B. J., 287, *352*
Davis, W. C., 374, 388, 389, 391, *437,* 516,
570
Davson, H., 430, *437*
Deane, H. W., 89, *117*
Debray-Sachs, M., 364, *435*

Decker, J., 223, 230, 231, *262*, *265*
Decreusefond, C., 218, *261*
Deeb, B. J., 468, 475, *476*
Defendi, V., 556, *564*
de Groot, M. L., 333, *350*
de Harven, E., 388, 391, *435*, *439*, 499, 526, 544, *560*
Deisseroth, A., 260, *268*
de Koch, G., 541, *563*
de la Chapelle, A., 396, *438*
Delamore, I. W., 432, *447*
del Buono, I., 527, *568*
Delespesse, G. J., 338, 339, *351*
Della Corte, E., 209, 210, *263*
Della-Porta, A. J., 511, *573*
De Luca, C., 233, *263*
Deluca, D., 223, *265*
Del Villano, B. C., 395, 396, 397, 398, *438*, *443*
Delvin, H. B., 40, *113*
Démant, P., 364, 368, 371, *438*, *439*, *445*
Dennis, J., 503, *571*
Denny, F. W., 465, 466, *476*
Dent, P. B., 549, 550, *563*
de Petris, S., 200, 240, 242, 249, *263*, *267*, *268*, 389, 392, *445*, 530, 545, *561*, *572*
Dersjant, H., 363, 367, *435*
Desai, P. R., 108, *120*, *123*, 400, 433, *442*
Descamps, B., 364, *439*
Desmayter, J., 515, *570*
Des Prez, R. M., 378, *438*
Deutsch, G. F., 137, 139, 149, *186*
Deutsch, H. F., 202, *267*, 295, *352*
Dewdney, J. M., 293, *350*
de Weck, A. L., 293, 315, 316, 317, *352*, 367, *438*
de Witt, C., 106, *125*
DeWitt, C. W., 366, *436*, *445*
Dhir, S. P., 53, *113*, 468, 469, *476*
DiCossano, D. L., 207, *261*
Diehl, V., 403, *447*, 542, *563*
Diener, E., 200, 201, 222, 223, 232, 240, 255, 256, *263*
Dierich, M. P., 395, 397, *438*
Dietrich, F. M., 315, *352*
DiGenio, T., 106, 107, *119*
DiLapi, M. M., 2, 73, 83, 106, *115*
Dineen, J. K., 527, *569*
Diosi, P., 542, *563*
Dische, Z., 287, *352*

Dixon, F. J., 87, *113*, 213, *265*, 395, 432, *411*, *442*, 506, 517, 526, 540, 543, 544, 549, *565*, *569*, *570*
Dixon, R. J., 27, 28, *113*
Dobos, P., 496, *563*
Dobson, R. L., 295, 296, *355*
Doherty, P. C., 244, *269*, 526, 531, 540, *574*
Dolan, T. F., 551, *562*
Domer, J., 292, *357*
Domermuth, C. H., 467, *476*
Donch, J. J., 157, *184*
Doonan, S., 295, 308, 328, *358*
Dorf, M. E., 250, *265*, *269*, 333, *350*, 531, *566*
Dormont, J., 364, *435*
Dorrington, K. J., 259, *263*
Dorsey, F. C., 337, *351*
Dos Reis, A. P., 383, 390, *438*
Douglas, R., 383, *436*
Douglas, R. G., 506, *570*
Dourmashkin, R. R., 206, *264*, 372, *436*, 515, *563*
Dowdle, W. R., 523, *568*
Dower, J. C., 551, *562*
Downie, A. W., 541, *563*
Drach, G. W., 107, 108, *113*
Drake, W. P., 544, *567*
Dresser, D. W., 89, 91, *113*, 214, *261*
Dubos, R. J., 89, *113*
Duc-Nguyen, H., 526, 555, *563*
Dudin, J., 98, *113*
Dudman, W. F., 27, 33, 82, 83, *113*, *115*
Duffus, P. H., 200, *268*, 389, 392, *445*
Duffus, W. P. H., 530, *572*
Dukor, P., 171, *185*, 205, 253, *263*
Dulbecco, R., 512, 518, *563*
Dunkel, V. C., 527, *563*
Dupuy, J. M., 523, *563*, *567*
Dutton, D., 46, *111*
Dutton, G. G. S., 32, 34, *112*, *113*
Dutton, R. W., 163, *184*, 197, 235, 249, *263*, *265*
Dwyer, J. M., 221, 230, 231, 249, *263*

E

East, J., 171, *184*
Eastlake, A., 151, *186*
Eaton, M. D., 460, 477, 526, 548, *563*

Author Index

Eckert, H. L., 525, 526, *564*
Eddy, G. A., 496, *569*
Edelman, G. M., 201, 203, 223, 234, 251, 258, *261, 263, 266, 267, 269,* 421, 429, *443*
Edelman, R., 511, 526, 537, 554, 555, *563, 566, 573*
Edidin, M., 200, *263,* 385, 386, 389, 430, *438, 439, 440,* 530, *564*
Edstrom, R. D., 19, 58, *113*
Edward, D. G., 450, 451, 464, *476*
Edwards, P. R., 64, *113*
Eernisse, J. G., 363, *446*
Eggersten, G., 26, *116*
Ehrlich, P., 191, *263*
Eichenberger, E., 6, 49, *113, 120, 125*
Eichmann, K., 96, 98, *112, 113, 118*
Einstein, A. B., Jr., 374, 401, *438*
Eisel, R. J., 406, *439*
Eisen, H. N., 131, 137, 163, 170, *184, 185, 187*
Elfenbein, G. J., 534, 539, *563*
Elliot, S., 80, *115*
Elliott, E. V., 171, *184*
Elliott, W. B., 308, *352*
Ellis, D. A., 554, *565*
Ellison, E. M., 542, *566*
Ellman, L., 378, *439*
Elsayed, S. M., 293, 295, 297, 306, 307, *350, 353*
Elson, C. J., 201, *263*
Elson, J., 26, 87, 89, 90, 91, *116*
Emerson, S. U., 497, 514, *566*
Ende, H. A., 292, *356*
Enders, J. F., 536, 551, *563*
Enders-Ruckle, G., 542, *563*
Engel, L. D., 465, *476*
Engelman, D. M., 197, 198, *263, 269*
Engers, H. D., 201, 221, *263*
Engleberger, F. M., 157, *185*
Ennis, F., 555, *566*
Epley, J. D., 35, *112*
Epsmark, J. A., 526, 527, *563*
Epstein, L. B., 534, *563*
Eriksen, J. L., 32, 33, *113, 116*
Eriksson, R., 282, *352*
Erlandson, A. L., 40, *113*
Escobar, M. R., 64, *113*
Eshhar, Z., 194, 208, *262, 263*
Eskeland, T., 213, *265*

Essen, R., 555, *564*
Estrada-Parra, S., 27, 28, 53, 55, 76, 81, *113*
Etheredge, E. E., 384, 404, *438*
Etiévant, M., 17, 60, 64, *111, 113*
Evans, C. A., 387, *443*
Evans, W. H., 389, *438*
Evering, S., 322, *357*
Ey, P. L., 201, 211, 212, 213, 248, *263*
Ezzell, R., 223, *265*

F

Faber, J. E., 465, *476*
Fahey, J. L., 362, 364, 374, 395, 401, 403, 406, 412, *436, 438, 441*
Falsen, E., 293, *350*
Fanger, M. W., 259, *263,* 420, *435*
Fantoni, A., 396, *438*
Farber, P. A., 534, 535, 540, *570*
Farina, C., 374, *438*
Farmer, V. C., 101, *111*
Farnham, S. B., 409, *440*
Farr, S. R., 49, *120*
Fasman, G., 137, 139, 149, *186,* 202, 267
Faucon, N., 542, *563*
Fauconnet, M., 363, *441*
Faulkner, P., 496, *563*
Faur, Y., 395, *440*
Faux, J., 292, 293, *356*
Fazekas de St. Groth, S., 506, 512, *563*
Feeley, J. C., 106, *125*
Fehmel, F., 37, *113*
Feigen, G. A., 316, *352*
Feinberg, A. R., 278, *358*
Feinberg, J. G., 277, 287, 291, *352*
Feinberg, S. M., 278, 292, *352, 358*
Feingold, N., 398, *437*
Feinstein, A., 202, 204, 207, *262, 263*
Feinstone, S. M., 536, *563*
Feldmann, M., 93, *113,* 197, 200, 205, 240, 242, 247, 249, 256, *262, 263, 267*
Felix, A., 42, 104, 106, *113*
Fellous, M., 385, 386, *438*
Felton, L. D., 26, 87, 89, 90, *113*
Fenner, F., 192, *262,* 534, 543, *562, 563*
Fenyo, E., 525, *572*
Ferber, E., 194, *263*
Fernald, G. W., 465, 466, *476*
Fernandes, M. V., 526, *563*
Ferraresi, R. W., 107, *114*

Ferrebee, J. W., 363, *444*
Ferrone, S., 372, 373, 374, 375, 376, 377, 378, 380, 381, 382, 383, 384, 386, 388, 391, 393, 394, 395, 396, 397, 398, 399, 400, 401, 403, 404, 406, 407, 408, 412, 414, 416, 425, 426, 427, 428, 429, 431, *436*, *438*, *439*, *441*, *442*, *445*, *446*
Fialkow, P. J., 212, *267*
Fine, D. P., 378, *438*
Fink, J., 292, *357*
Finkel, A., 550, *563*
Finkelstein, M. S., 500, *572*
Finkelstein, S., 364, 432, *447*
Finn, J., 144, *183*
Fireman, P., 549, 550, *563*
Fischetti, T., 418, *441*
Fisher, M. W., 40, *113*
Fishman, P. H., 528, 529, *561*
Fitch, R. W., 538, *561*
Fitzgerald, P. L., 39, 40, 76, *125*
Fitzgerald, W. A., 464, *476*
Fjeldborg, O., 382, *440*
Flaherty, L., *436*
Flanagan, J. F., 364, *441*
Fleischmann, J. G., 98, *113*
Fleisher, G. A., 550, *573*
Fleissner, E., 499, 530, *574*
Fleming, W. L., 77, *124*
Flick, J. A., 533, *570*
Fliedner, D., 488, *573*
Flodin, P., 282, 287, *357*
Florent, G., 206, *267*
Fogel, M., 528, *563*
Fong, R., 381, *439*
Fong, S., 243, *267*
Forbes, J. F., 432, *439*
Forest, N., 66, *124*
Forni, L., 179, *186*, 200, 201, 206, 211, 221, 241, 242, 247, 248, 249, *265*, *266*, *267*, 390, 392, *441*
Foster, A. B., 33, *111*
Fotino, M., 336, *354*
Foucard, T., 346, *352*
Fournier, C., 218, *261*
Fowler, A. K., 536, *564*
Fox, H. H., 474, *476*
Fox, I., 278, *352*
Fraefel, W., 308, *352*
Framberg, K., 11, *120*
Francis, T., 311, *352*

Francis, T., Jr., 506, 510, *563*
Franecki, B. H., 384, *438*
Franek, F., 160, *184*
Frank, M. M., 378, *439*
Franklin, H. A., 403, *442*
Franklin, R., 308, *358*, 513, *570*
Frederiks, E., 364, 406, *446*
Freed, J. H., 249, *263*
Freedman, S. O., 292, 308, *352*
Freeman, G. G., 9, *113*
Freeman, M. E., 42, *125*
Freeman, T., 287, 288, 307, *356*
Freiereich, E. J., 408, *439*
Frelinger, J. A., 250, *262*
Frenzl, B., 366, *445*
Freundt, E. A., 450, 451, *476*
Frey, J. R., 367, *438*
Friberg, S., Jr., 387, 393, *437*
Friday, G., 549, 550, *563*
Friedhoff, F., 395, *440*
Friedman, H., 92, *110*, *113*, 541, 549, *562*, *566*
Friedman, M., 499, *563*
Friedman, R. M., 534, *560*
Fries, J. H., 279, 322, 330, *352*, *359*
Frick, O. L., 306, *357*
Fricsay, M., 6, *113*
Fröhland, S., 249, *263*
Fromme, I., 11, 20, *118*, *122*
Fronticelli, C., 150, *186*
Frye, L. D., 200, *263*, 389, 430, *439*
Fuccillo, D. A., 542, 565, *572*
Fuchs, S., 141, 142, 143, 164, *184*, *185*, *187*
Fudenberg, H. H., 156, 168, *187*, 532, *571*
Fujii, R., 542, *574*
Fujita, N. J., 156, *185*
Fukada, A., 511, 526, 550, 552, *573*
Fukai, K., 496, *565*
Fukazawa, Y., 64, *125*
Fukuoka, T., 496, *565*
Fuller, N. A., 60, 64, *113*
Fuller, T. C., 505, *560*
Furcaig, I., 382, *442*
Furuse, R., 542, *574*

G

Gabb, B. W., 363, 383, *435*, *439*
Gadol, N., 536, *563*
Gafni, M., 194, 208, *263*

Author Index

Gahan, L. C., 32, 34, *114*
Gahmberb, C. G., 495, *570*
Gaither, T., 378, *439*
Gajewski, M., 373, *439*
Galanos, C., 4, 6, 9, 13, 20, 21, 22, 23, 24, 56, *114, 119, 122*
Gale, J. L., 466, 474, *476*
Gall, W. E., 203, *267*
Gallagher, R., 363, 375, 380, *446*
Gallmeier, W. M., 387, *436*
Galper, J. B., 398, *439*
Gandhi, S. S., 490, *571*
Gardner, I., 207, *263*, 534, *563*
Garegg, P. J., 41, *114*
Garovoy, M. R., 260, *268*
Garvin, J. E., 373, *440*
Gay, L. N., 276, *352*
Geckeler, W. R., 94, *112*
Geering, G. L., 526, *563*
Geiduschek, E. P., 409, *439*
Gelanos, C., 253, 257, *261*
Gelderblom, H., 526, *563*
Gell, P. G. H., 163, 164, 166, 178, *183, 184*, 206, 207, *268*
Gelzer, J., 50, 51, *114*
Geralden, A., 527, *572*
Gerber, P., 373, 375, 381, 386, 395, *444*, 535, *564*
Gerety, R. J., 107, *114*
Gerloff, R. K., 459, *476*
Gerner, R. F., 403, *442*
Gershon, A. A., 527, *564*
Gershon, R. K., 532, *564*
Gerson, K. L., 537, *564*
Gerulat, B. F., 142, *185*
Gervais, A. G., 388, *439*
Gerwing, J., 165, *184*
Gesner, B. M., 554, *561, 573*
Gettner, H. H., 276, 277, *350, 353*
Ghalambor, M. A., 26, *125*
Ghanta, V. K., 100, 103, *114*
Gibofsky, A., 382, *439*
Gilden, R. V., 516, *561, 569*
Giles, J. P., 541, *566*
Gill, P., 475, *476*
Gill, T. J., III, 141, 142, 149, *184*, 304, 313, *352*
Gillette, R., *561*
Ginsberg, H. S., 487, 514, *573*
Girard, A., 4, 7, *122*

Girard, R., 17, 55, 60, *114, 124*
Girardi, A. J., 548, *560*
Givol, D., 154, 157, 160, *184*, 194, 204, 208, *263*
Glade, P. R., 373, *436*
Glasgow, L. A., 536, *564*
Glaudemans, C. P. J., 27, *122*
Glazer, A. N., 99, *114*
Gleich, G. J., 52, *110, 114*, 273, 290, 301, 346, *352, 359*
Glick, A. D., 373, *439*
Glick, M. C., 412, *447*
Globerson, A., 524, *564*
Glynn, A. A., 26, 103, 104, 105, *114, 116*
Glynn, L. E., 108, *120*
Gmeiner, J., 23, *114, 119*
Godfrey, H., 327, 346, *350*
Godfrey, H. P., 168, *184*
Goebel, W. F., 2, 27, 28, 41, 68, 71, 73, 93, *110, 114, 122*, 133, 147, *183, 184*
Götze, D., 374, 393, 401, 408, 412, 414, 418, *438, 439, 443, 444*
Götze, O., 378, *439*
Goetzl, E. J., 160, *184*
Goffe, A. P., 505, *564*
Goffman, J., 518, *568*
Gold, W. M., 323, *353*
Goldberg, E. H., 385, *439*
Goldberg, L. S., 373, *447*
Goldberg, M., 278, *353*
Goldberg, N. D., 260, *264*
Goldblum, N., 527, *566*
Goldfarb, A. R., 276, 292, 300, 301, 305, 327, *351, 353*
Goldschneider, I., 84, *114*
Goldstein, I. J., 4, 5, *114*
Gollmar, Y., 495, *568, 571*
Gomez, I., 53, 55, *113*
Good, R. A., 219, 231, *263*, 387, *446*, 549, *563*
Goodfriend, L., 280, 283, 285, 287, 288, 295, 299, 303, 304, 305, 321, 322, 334, 335, 339, 343, 345, *353, 354, 355, 356, 357, 358*
Goodheart, C. R., 484, 542, *564, 570*
Gooding, L. R., 530, *564*
Goodman, J. W., 129, 134, 135, 137, 139, 141, 157, 162, 163, 166, 167, 169, 171, 172, 173, 174, 175, 178, 182, *183, 184*, 186, 187, 243, *261*, 532, *571*

Goodman, T., 521, *564*
Goodpasture, E. W., 542, *564*
Gorczynski, R. M., 234, *263*
Gordin, F., 526, *561*
Gordon, D. S., 527, *568*
Gordon, H. G., 374, 401, *438*
Gordon, J., 329, *357*
Gordon, W. G., 293, *358*
Gorer, P. A., 362, 365, *439*
Gormus, B. J., 31, 32, 33, *114*
Gotschlich, E. C., 83, 84, *114, 115*
Gottschalk, A., 287, *353*
Gould, H. J., 142, *184*
Gourlay, R. N., 467, 468, *476, 477*
Goust, J. M., 537, *568*
Grabar, P., 287, *353*
Graber, C. D., 388, 391, *447*
Grace, W. R., 535, 537, *560, 572*
Graf, T., 526, *563*
Graham, D. M., 506, *563*
Graham, T. C., 366, *445*
Granoff, A., 512, *564*
Graw, R. G., Jr., 406, *439*
Grayston, J. T., 53, *113*, 451, 468, 469, *476, 477, 478*
Greaves, M. F., 200, 201, 206, 207, 210, 211, 216, 218, 219, 249, 257, 259, *263, 264, 266*
Grecek, D. R., 399, *436*
Greely, A., 106, 107, *119*
Green, I., 163, *184*
Green, M., 485, *567*
Green, N. M., 202, 203, *264, 269*
Greenert, S., 328, 329, *353*
Greenwalt, T. J., 373, *439*
Grégoire, C., 329, *357*
Gresser, I., 554, *565*
Grey, H. M., 100, 101, *114, 124*, 194, 208, 211, 213, 216, 248, *261, 264, 265, 267, 268*, 420, 422, 423, 424, 425, *437, 439*
Griffin, D. E., 539, *564*
Griffiths, B. W., 295, 301, 304, 312, *353*
Grimes, W. J., 497, *564*
Grollmann, A. P., 53, *124*
Gronwall, A., 84, *114*
Grossberg, A. L., 129, 132, 136, 149, *186*
Grothaus, E. A., 382, *439*
Grove, E. F., 276, *353*
Grumet, F. C., 247, *264*, 505, *564, 569*
Grundbacher, F. J., 95, *114*
Grundner, G., 525, *572*

Guidry, D. J., 542, *561*
Guilbert, B., 213, *261*
Guild, W. R., 468, *477*
Gussoni, C., 301, *353*
Gutterman, J. U., 408, *439*
Guy, R. C. E., 27, 30, *114*
Guyer, R. B., 199, *267*
György, E., 514, *573*

H

Haager, O., 203, *267*
Haase, A. T., 488, *564*
Habel, K., 526, 540, *569*
Haber, E., 3, 95, 96, 97, 98, 102, *112, 114, 116, 117, 121*, 134, 152, 154, 175, *183, 184, 187*, 202, *264*
Habermann, E., 278, 293, 308, *353, 356*
Habicht, G. S., 94, *112*
Hackman, R. H., 278, *353*
Haddad, Z. H., 282, 285, 287, 288, 291, 295, 297, 300, 318, *353, 355*
Hadden, E. M., 260, *264*
Hadden, J. W., 260, *264*
Haddow, W. J., 549, *567*
Haddox, M. K., 260, *264*
Hägg, L. B., 223, 241, 246, 249, *267*
Hämmerling, G. J., 20, 21, 94, *114, 115*, 222, 224, 227, 228, *264, 268*
Hämmerling, U., 49, *115, 123*, 215, *264*, 388, 391, *435, 439*, 499, 526, 544, *560*
Hagiwara, S., 66, *124*
Hagry, P., 556, *564*
Haheim, L. R., 491, 492, *564*
Hahn, R. G., 475, *477*
Hahn, Y., 246, 266
Hahon, N., 467, 478, 518, 525, 526, *564*
Haimovich, J., 140, 160, *184*
Hakkinen, L., 547, *564*
Hakomori, S., 5, 53, *113, 114*
Hakomori, S. I., 469, *476*
Hall, L. A. R., 132, *186*
Hall, W. W., 494, *564*
Haller, G. J., 475, *477*
Haller, O., 509, *564*
Halliday, W. J., 87, 93, *114, 118*
Halliwell, R. E., 339, *357*
Halonen, P., 547, *564*
Hamaguchi, K., 409, *439*
Hamaoka, T., 226, 239, 244, 255, 265, 531, *566*
Hamburger, J., 364, 401, *439, 444*

Hamburger, R. N., 339, *350*, *353*
Hamilton, J. A., 255, *264*
Hamilton, J. K., 4, *110*
Hamlin, J., 144, *183*
Hamlin, N. M., 100, 103, *114*
Hammarskjold, B., 487, 488, 495, *568*
Hammer, D., 106, *114*
Hampar, B., 504, 515, 518, 527, *564*, *568*
Hampson, A. W., 489, *572*
Hampton, S. F., 318, *358*
Hanaoka, T., 363, *444*
Hanessian, S., 4, 40, *115*
Hanna, M. G., 505, 545, 552, 553, *561*, *564*, *565*, *567*, *571*
Hanna, M. J., 545, *565*
Hannig, K., 194, *269*
Hannover-Larsen, J., 543, *573*
Hansen, C. T., 94, *110*
Hanson, L. Å., 26, 49, 108, *115*, *116*
Haran-Ghera, N., 556, *569*, *571*
Harboe, A., 491, 548, *564*, *565*, *571*
Hardy, B., 524, *564*
Hardy, W. D., 499, 530, *574*
Hargreaves, F. E., 292, 293, *356*
Harris, A., 382, *437*
Harris, A. W., 94, *120*, 215, *264*
Harris, M., 146, 165, *187*, 243, *268*
Harris, R., 386, 387, *439*
Harris, R. L., 295, 296, 316, *355*
Harrisdangkul, V., 51, 93, 102, *115*
Harrison, F. S., 555, *564*
Harrison, S. C., 496, *564*
Harrold, A. J., 307, 320, *357*
Hart, D. A., 259, *263*
Hart, F. D., 344, *351*
Hartley, B. S., 181, *184*
Hartley, J. W., 498, *564*
Hartmann, P. E., 64, *125*
Harvey, J., 545, *561*
Hasegawa, T., 382, *446*
Hasenclever, H. F., 53, *115*, *120*, *124*
Haskell, T., 4, 40, *115*
Haskins, W. T., 7, *122*
Haslam, E. A., 489, *571*
Haslam, R., 537, *564*
Hauber, T. H., 382, *446*
Haughton, G., 388, *439*
Haukenes, G., 491, 492, 548, *564*, *565*
Hauptfeld, V., 250, *264*
Hauschka, T. S., 386, *439*
Havas, H. F., 255, *264*

Hawkes, R., 512, *564*
Hay, G. W., 4, 5, *114*, *115*
Hayami, M., 526, *573*
Hayashi, J. A., 43, *112*
Hayashi, K., 519, 525, 527, *564*
Hayflick, L., 382, 395, 431, *436*, 467, 474, *476*, *478*
Hayry, P., 194, *266*
Hayward, B. J., 291, *350*
Hayward, J. A., 207, 234, *266*
Hearn, H. J., 510, *564*
Heath, E. C., 19, 26, 58, *113*, *125*
Hebald, S., 318, *358*
Hecht, T. T., 387, *439*, 530, 547, *564*
Hedin, P. J., 366, 370, 430, *445*
Hedrick, S. R., 168, *184*
Heidelberger, M., 2, 27, 28, 29, 30, 33, 49, 53, 61, 72, 73, 76, 77, 78, 79, 80, 81, 82, 83, 84, 88, 106, *113*, *114*, *115*, *116*, *119*, *121*, *124*, 128, 133, 147, *184*
Heimlich, E. M., 296, 316, *355*
Heine, J. W., 484, *570*
Heller, J. A., 548, *563*
Hellerqvist, C. G., 5, 11, 17, 60, 74, *111*, *115*, *116*
Hellman, A., 536, *564*
Hellström, K. E., 386, *439*
Hemingway, W. D., 503, *562*
Hemmingson, E. J., 219, 231, *264*
Henle, G., 527, 542, 555, *563*, *564*, *566*
Henle, W., 510, 527, 542, 555, *563*, *566*, *567*
Henle, W. G., 555, *564*
Hennessy, A. V., 510, *563*
Henney, C. S., 163, *184*, 249, 260, *264*, 526, 530, 531, 540, *562*
Henriksen, S. D., 32, 33, *113*, *116*
Henry, C., 176, *184*, 233, *264*
Henson, D., 484, 542, *564*, *570*
Herberman, R. B., 382, 386, *439*, *446*, 526, 527, 528, 531, 544, *560*, *572*
Herbertson, S., 306, *353*
Herbst, M., 203, *267*
Heremans, J. F., 285, *355*
Herman, J., 169, *187*
Hersh, E. M., 408, *439*
Herzenberg, L. A., 211, 246, 249, *263*, *264*
Herzig, G. P., 406, *439*
Heslop-Harrison, J., 327, *354*
Heumann, H., 406, *436*

Heyns, K., 42, *116*
Hickey, C. A., 388, *441*
Hicklin, M. D., 508, *565*
Hickman, J., 2, 77, *111*
Higashi, N., 453, *477, 478*
Higginbotham, J. D., 27, 29, 30, 82, 83, *113, 115, 116*, 492, *564*
Hijmans, W., 206, *269*
Hildemann, W. H., 366, *442*
Hill, B. M., 288, *354*
Hiller, M. C., 383, *445*
Himmelspach, K., 4, 9, 61, 68, 69, 70, 71, 73, 93, *114, 116, 118*
Hinuma, Y., 513, *566*
Hinzová, E., 368, *438, 439*
Hiramoto, R. N., 100, 103, *114*
Hirano, T., 553, *565*
Hirase, S., 26, *116*
Hirata, A. A., 108, *116, 120, 123*, 390, 391, 400, 406, 433, *439, 442, 443*
Hiroshi, K., 526, *571*
Hirsch, M. S., 508, 521, 522, 526, 538, 545, 546, 554, *560, 561, 565, 570, 574*
Hirschfeld, J., 371, *439*
Hirschhorn, K., 373, 395, *436*
Hirst, J. W., 100, *114, 119*
Hitchcock, A. S., 291, *353*
Hixon, R., 107, *111*
Hjorth, N., 347, *353*
Hoborn, J., 293, *350*
Hochman, J., 157, *184*
Hochwald, G. M., 214, *268*
Hodge, L. D., 395, *441*
Hodges, R. G., 2, 73, 83, 84, 106, *115, 119*
Hoecker, G., 385, 386, *439, 443*
Hoehne, J. H., 323, *351*
Hoffman, E. M., 516, *570*
Hofmann, S., 16, *123*
Hofmeister, F., 409, *439*
Hogarth-Scott, R. S., 292, 307, *353*
Hogg, N. M., 160, *186*, 206, 219, 249, *263, 264*
Hoggan, M. D., 485, *561*
Hoglund, S., 514, *569*
Hogman, C., 366, 370, 395, 430, *440, 445*
Hogrefe, W. R., 526, *562*
Holland, J. J., 491, *565*
Hollers, J. C., 200, 201, *268*
Hollingdale, M. R., 463, 464, 468, 473, 474, 475, *477*

Hollinshead, A., 527, *565*
Hollis, V. W., 544, *565*
Holm, S. E., 108, *116*
Holme, T., 5, 17, 41, 60, 74, *114, 115, 116*
Holmes, G. E., 503, *561*
Holmes, K. V., 526, *565*
Holmgren, J., 26, 108, *116*
Holowka, D. A., 97, 102, *116*
Hong, R., 429, *435*
Honsan, S. A., *572*
Hooker, S. B., 170, *184*
Hood, L., 96, *113*
Hopkins, S. J., 278, *359*
Hopper, J. E., 156, *187*
Hopton, J. W., 134, *183*
Horn, R. G., 373, *439*
Hornbrook, M. M., 273, 333, *353*
Horne, R. W., 47, *121*
Hornick, C. L., 205, *264*
Hors, J., 341, *352*, 385, 399, *435, 437*
Horta-Barbosa, L., 542, *565*
Horton, R. E., 107, *123*
Hosaka, Y., 494, *565*
Hosokawa, M., 526, 548, *566, 571*
Hotchin, J., 543, *561*
How, M. J., 27, 30, 53, 78, *111, 114, 116*, 492, *564*
Howard, C. J., 103, 104, 105, *114, 116*
Howard, J. G., 3, 26, 83, 85, 86, 87, 89, 90, 91, 92, 93, 94, 103, *116*, 195, 232, 252, *261, 264*, 509, *565*
Howard, R. J., 549, 556, *565, 568*
Howe, C., 491, 492, *565, 567*
Howe, M. L., 555, *566*
Hsieh, B., 301, *357*
Hsu, K. C., 504, 527, *568*
Hsu, S. H., 280, 287, 288, 295, 304, 305, 321, 322, 334, 339, 343, 345, *355*
Hu, C. C., 107, *112*
Huang, A. S., 497, *562*
Huang, S. W., 429, *435*
Hudson, L., 234, *267*
Huebner, R. J., 498, 526, 544, 549, 554, *564, 567, 569, 572*
Hütteroth, T. H., 201, *264*
Huffines, W., 523, *573*
Hug, K., 211, *267*
Huijmans-Evers, A. G. M., 465, *477*
Hume, D. M., 401, *444*

Hummeler, K., 484, 497, 510, 513, 565, 566, 567
Humphrey, J., 509, 568
Humphrey, J. H., 91, 120, 171, 184, 221, 232, 235, 236, 237, 238, 239, 261, 264, 265, 372, 436
Hungerer, D., 37, 53, 55, 74, 116
Hunter, A., 374, 399, 416, 438
Hunter, B. M., 122
Hunter, H. S., 495, 569
Hurni, H., 6, 113
Hurwitz, E., 78, 88, 121, 160, 184
Hussain, R., 292, 295, 299, 307, 308, 353, 358
Hyllseth, B., 515, 565
Hyman, C., 550, 565

I

Iannetti, G., 301, 352
Igarashi, A., 496, 526, 565, 567
Ihle, J. N., 505, 545, 565, 567
Ikeda, H., 499, 565
Imm, W., 194, 263
Inbar, D., 154, 157, 184
Ingelman, B., 84, 114
Inuoe, M., 213, 265
Ioppolo, C., 150, 186
Iovino, A., 550, 562
Irie, R. F., 526, 568
Irlin, I. S., 527, 565
Irving, D., 561
Isacson, P., 494, 536, 565
Isbell, H. S., 4, 116, 120
Iscaki, S., 158, 185
Iseki, S., 64, 117
Ishida, N., 494, 572
Ishimoto, A., 527, 565
Ishizaka, K., 273, 283, 288, 314, 315, 318, 319, 320, 322, 327, 333, 335, 337, 338, 339, 347, 351, 353, 354, 355, 356, 358, 382, 440
Ishizaka, T., 273, 315, 333, 353, 382, 440
Ishizaki, T., 309, 356
Ishizuka, M., 259, 269
Israel, M. S., 542, 565
Israels, L. G., 194, 266
Israels, M. C. O., 432, 447
Itabashi, H. H., 542, 569
Ito, M., 525, 527, 565, 572
Ito, Y., 527, 565

Ivanyi, P., 368, 401, 439, 440
Ivasková, E., 401, 440
Iverson, G. M., 177, 187
Iwazaki, Y., 401, 440

J

Jabbour, J. T., 537, 565
Jackson, R. L., 199, 267
Jackson, S. A., 160, 186
Jacob, M. J., 26, 89, 90, 91, 116
Jacobbi, L., 375, 441
Jacobson, E. B., 246, 264
Jaffee, I., 39, 122
James, A. T., 491, 566
James, D. C. O., 344, 351
James, W. D., 460, 471, 474, 476, 478
Janeway, C. A., Jr., 91, 117, 176, 184
Jann, B., 4, 5, 9, 12, 13, 16, 20, 21, 23, 26, 37, 38, 53, 54, 55, 63, 74, 76, 80, 115, 116, 117, 118, 120, 121, 122, 123, 124
Jann, K., 3, 4, 5, 6, 7, 9, 12, 13, 16, 19, 20, 21, 25, 26, 36, 37, 38, 52, 53, 54, 55, 56, 74, 80, 104, 115, 116, 117, 118, 119, 120, 121, 122, 123, 124, 125
Janossy, G., 200, 201, 210, 264, 266
Jansen, I., 213, 265, 395, 441
Jarrett, E., 338, 339, 351
Jaton, J. C., 96, 97, 98, 112, 117, 118, 121
Jawetz, E., 535, 565
Jeanes, A., 4, 26, 121, 122
Jeffries, W., 150, 186
Jenkin, C. R., 107, 108, 117, 122
Jenkin, H. M., 453, 467, 469, 477
Jenner, E., 480, 565
Jensen, K. E., 465, 478
Jensenius, J. C., 208, 213, 215, 248, 264
Jerne, N. K., 85, 117, 162, 171, 173, 176, 184, 186, 192, 193, 264
Jersild, C., 366, 370, 430, 445
Jocius, I. B., 100, 103, 125
Jørgensen, O., 372, 373, 437
Johansson, B., 213, 265
Johansson, S. G. O., 273, 286, 287, 288, 307, 346, 351, 352, 353, 359
Johns, M. A., 106, 107, 119
Johnsen, D., 511, 563
Johnson, A. H., 390, 440
Johnson, B., 518, 569
Johnson, B. W., 362, 365, 441
Johnson, C. N., 99, 117

Johnson, E. D., 540, 565
Johnson, G. S., 260, 266
Johnson, J. E., 536, 563, 573
Johnson, M. H., 385, 386, 440
Johnson, P., 277, 280, 281, 282, 283, 284, 285, 295, 297, 298, 299, 300, 351, 353, 355
Johnson, P. A., 526, 528, 531, 544, 560
Johnson, R. T., 522, 539, 564, 566
Johnson, T. M., 373, 440
Johnston, I. R., 101, 117
Johnston, J. H., 21, 117
Johnston, R. J., 21, 117
Jones, D., 101, 111
Jones, G., 201, 213, 264
Jones, G. H., 47, 117
Jones, J. K. N., 28, 30, 117, 120
Jones, P. P., 211, 264
Jones, R. T., 346, 352
Jones, V., 169, 172, 174, 185
Joseph, B. S., 530, 566
Josey, W. E., 523, 568
Joyce, R. L., 25, 112
Joyner, C. R., 555, 564
Jumblatt, J., 496, 564
Jureziz, R., 154, 186
Jutila, J. W., 93, 120
Jyo, T., 293, 354

K

Kaarainen, L., 495, 570
Kabat, E. A., 4, 29, 30, 46, 47, 49, 50, 51, 52, 55, 68, 69, 70, 84, 85, 91, 93, 100, 102, 110, 111, 114, 115, 117, 118, 119, 122, 124, 125, 134, 135, 136, 137, 138, 140, 141, 148, 149, 159, 160, 183, 184, 185, 187, 202, 264, 279, 311, 354, 382, 437, 440
Kaehler, S. L., 545, 569
Kärkäinen, J., 4, 5, 117
Kahan, B. D., 362, 364, 367, 368, 373, 385, 402, 403, 404, 407, 408, 410, 412, 414, 415, 418, 419, 420, 425, 440, 442, 443, 444
Kahane, I., 199, 265, 472, 473, 475, 477, 478
Kaijser, B., 103, 107, 108, 116, 117
Kailin, E. W., 279, 354
Kaiser, S. J., 2, 73, 83, 106, 115
Kaji, H., 548, 566
Kajioka, R., 514, 562
Kalica, A. R., 467, 476
Kaliner, M., 260, 268
Kammann, O., 275, 354
Kandutsch, A. A., 364, 440
Kane, L. W., 536, 563
Kang, S., 41, 117
Kano, K., 400, 401, 435, 444
Kano, S., 555, 566
Kantoch, M., 521, 566
Kantor, F. S., 163, 186
Kaplan, H., 168, 187, 532, 571
Kaplan, J., 137, 139, 187
Kaplan, M. H., 89, 117
Karakawa, W. W., 42, 82, 98, 117, 121
Karnovsky, M. J., 89, 112, 200, 201, 215, 264, 269, 374, 377, 389, 440, 446, 528, 570
Karush, F., 132, 133, 185, 205, 264
Karzon, D. T., 502, 504, 569
Kasel, J. A., 504, 506, 560, 567
Kashiwagi, K., 64, 117
Kass, E. H., 467, 477
Kassel, R. L., 545, 569
Katagiri, J., 157, 185
Katagiri, M., 250, 268
Kates, M., 491, 566
Kathan, R. H., 199, 264
Kato, S., 527, 568
Katsutani, T., 293, 354
Katz, D., 531, 547, 566
Katz, D. H., 197, 215, 226, 231, 239, 244, 247, 250, 255, 264, 265, 266
Katz, M., 96, 117, 121
Kauffmann, F., 2, 5, 12, 16, 26, 35, 41, 42, 56, 58, 61, 62, 63, 64, 72, 76, 117, 118, 125
Kauffmann, G., 87, 89, 90, 113
Kaufman, H., 535, 566
Kaufman, N. E., 542, 566
Kaufman, W., 279, 322, 354
Kauzman, W., 409, 440
Kawai, T., 292, 293, 309, 310, 354, 357
Kawakami, T. G., 526, 561
Kawana, T., 526, 568
Kay, J. W. D., 400, 433, 439
Kayman, H., 357
Kearney, R., 87, 93, 118
Kedar, E., 527, 566
Keehn, M. A., 515, 518, 564

Kehoe, J. M., 160, *185*, 299, 304, *356*
Keiderling, W., 6, *125*
Keith, A., 198, *268*
Keleti, J., 11, *118*
Keller, H. U., 236, *264*
Keller, J. M., 64, 68, 74, *122*
Keller, R., 513, 518, *566*
Kelley, J. M., 497, 514, *566*
Kelly, B., 542, *569*
Kemp, J. P., 306, *357*
Kendall, F. G., 2, 49, 72, 78, *115*
Kennedy, D. A., 27, 28, *118*
Kennedy, S. I. T., 496, 510, *566*
Kennedy, F. T., 545, *565*
Kenny, G. E., 53, *113*, 452, 454, 455, 456, 457, 459, 460, 461, 462, 463, 464, 465, 466, 468, 469, 470, 471, 472, 474, 475, *476*, *477*, *478*
Kenyon, A. J., 549, *566*
Keogh, E. V., 512, 517, *562*
Kersey, J., 387, *446*
Kersey, J. H., 388, *440*
Ketler, A., 513, *566*
Kettman, J. R., 249, *265*
Kibrick, S., 555, *566*, *568*
Kickhöfen, B., *119*
Kiehn, E. D., 491, *565*
Kieling, F., 548, *560*
Kiessling, G., 42, *116*
Kilbourne, E. D., 515, 535, 543, *560*, *562*, *566*
Kim, J. H., 387, 391, *442*, 531, *569*
Kimball, J. W., 97, 102, *116*, *118*
Kimoto, K., 508, *568*
Kimura, G., 508, *568*
Kimura, J., 233, *264*, *269*
Kincade, P. W., 214, 229, *265*
Kindred, B., 244, *265*
Kindt, T. J., 35, 96, *112*, *118*
King, T. P., 281, 283, 285, 295, 299, 301, 302, 303, 305, 312, 322, 327, 336, 347, *352*, *354*
Kinski, R. G., 87, *116*
Kirk, D. L., 396, *442*
Kirov, S. M., 214, 215, *265*
Kissmeyer-Nielsen, F., 345, *354*, 366, 368, 370, 381, 382, 383, 398, 399, 430, *439*, *440*, *445*, *446*
Kjellen, L., 487, 512, 513, 514, 518, *566*
Kjerbye, K. E., 383, 398, 399, *445*, *446*

Klein, D., 250, *264*, 395, *440*
Klein, E., 206, 212, 213, *265*, *267*, 526, 527, *566*, *571*
Klein, G., 206, 212, *265*, *267*, 387, 393, 395, *437*, 525, 527, *566*, *572*
Klein, J., 250, *264*, 363, 365, 368, 369, 371, 395, 399, 430, *437*, *440*
Klein, P. A., 547, 548, *567*
Klein, W. J., Jr., 390, *435*
Kleinhammer, G., 61, 70, 71, *118*
Kleinman, L. F., 555, *566*
Klemola, E., 555, *564*
Klenk, H., 491, 526, 554, *562*, *565*, *566*
Klinman, N. R., 163, *185*
Klotz, I. M., 409, *440*
Knapp, S., 144, *183*
Knecht, J. C., 103, 104, *118*
Knight, W. B., 278, *352*
Knox, R. B., 327, *354*
Knudsen, R. C., 535, 537, *560*, *572*
Kobayashi, H., 526, 548, *566*, *571*
Kobune, F., 511, 526, 550, 552, *573*
Koch, A. E., 494, *565*
Koch, C., 219, 231, 249, 250, *262*
Koch, C. T., 364, 406, *446*
Kocourek, J., 4, *118*
Kodama, T., 548, *566*
Koessler, K. K., 275, *354*
Koestner, A., 552, *567*
Kohn, G., 542, *563*
Kojis, F. E., 278, *354*
Kolar, O., 537, *566*
Komoto, K., 293, *354*
Konrad, P., 364, 432, *447*
Kontainen, S., 163, *185*
Kontou-Karakitsos, K., 331, *354*
Kopacka, B., 60, 64, *124*
Kopp, R., 513, *572*
Koprowski, H., 497, 514, 521, 526, *563*, *564*, *565*, *573*
Koren, H. S., 178, *187*
Koshland, D., 259, *265*
Koshland, M. E., 156, 157, *185*
Koss, M. N., 545, *569*
Koszinowski, U., 548, *560*
Kotelko, K., 73, 74, *118*
Kountz, S. L., 364, *427*
Kourilsky, F. M., 200, *265*, *266*, *267*, 386, 388, 389, 390, 391, 392, 431, *440*, *442*, *443*, *445*, 530, *566*

Kovartovsky, J., 472, 473, 475, *477*, *478*
Krakowka, S., 552, *567*
Kramer, J. H., 508, *565*
Kramer, K., 47, *122*
Kratky, O., 203, *267*
Krause, M. D., 43, *112*
Krause, R. M., 3, 43, 44, 81, 95, 96, 98, *111*, *112*, *113*, *118*, *120*, *121*, 154, *185*
Kreis, H., 364, *435*
Kreisler, M., 363, 364, 432, 433, *411*, *446*
Kreiter, V. P., 250, *268*, 406, *442*
Kremer, W. B., 387, *444*
Kren, V., 366, *445*
Krenova, D., 366, *445*
Kristofová, H., 392, *440*
Kröger, E., 49, *119*
Krüger, L., 12, 16, 63, *118*
Krueger, R. G., 396, *445*
Krugman, S., 541, *566*
Krupey, J., 292, 308, *352*
Kruyff, J. J., 68, *120*
Kubo, R. T., 208, 211, 216, 248, *264*, *265*, 420, 422, 423, 424, 425, *431*, *439*
Kubota, H., 542, *574*
Küstner, H., 274, 279, 311, *357*
Kuhns, W. J., 395, *436*, *440*
Kulczycki, A., 154, *183*
Kumate, J., 549, 550, *563*
Kundur, V., *357*
Kunkel, H. G., 3, 95, *118*
Kunz, H. W., 141, 142, 149, *184*
Kuo, C. C., 459, 464, *477*
Kurahashi, K., 60, *124*
Kurn, N., 148, 180, *183*
Kurth, R., 526, *566*
Kuttner, A. G., 541, *562*
Kuwert, E., 387, *436*, 526, *573*

L

Labowskie, R. J., 526, 537, *566*
Lackland, H., 96, *113*
Lafferty, K. J., 512, 513, *566*
Lafleur, L. A., 208, 255, *261*, *266*
Lagrange, P. H., 548, *566*
Lalezari, P., 372, *440*, *446*
Lambertenghi-Deliliers, G., 372, *441*
Lamelin, J.-P., 207, *265*
Lamm, M., 204, *265*
Lamon, E., 525, *572*
Lancefield, R. C., 42, 44, *118*, *119*

Landsteiner, K., 128, 129, 132, 136, 141, 147, 149, *185*, 191, *265*
Landy, M., 26, 42, 105, *112*, *125*, 218, 219, 231, *261*, *263*, 538, *561*
Lang, D. J., 542, 554, *564*, *566*
Langenhuysen, M. M. C., 527, *572*
Langman, R. E., 226, 232, 238, *262*, *265*
Lanier, J. C., 542, *561*
Lapkoff, C. B., 283, 299, 304, *353*, *356*
Lapresle, C., 135, *185*
Larm, O., 17, 29, 30, *116*, *118*
Larson, A. E., 549, *570*
Larson, D. L., 516, *569*
Larson, J. B., 346, *352*
Laskov, R., 218, *265*
Latta, H., 373, *446*
Laurell, C. B., 464, *477*
Laurence, G. D., 516, *560*
Lausch, R., 535, *566*
Laver, W. G., 485, 489, 493, 515, *566*, *567*
Law, L. W., 418, *441*, 508, 527, 528, *567*, *568*, *573*
Lawrence, D. A., 178, 179, *185*, 225, *265*
Lawrence, H. S., 538, *561*
Lawson, C. J., 41, *118*
Lawton, A. R., 214, *265*
Lazarowitz, S. G., 489, *562*, *567*
Lazary, S., *352*
Le-Ba Nhan, 37, 53, 55, *118*
Lee, J. C., 505, 539, 545, *567*
Lee, L. T., 491, 492, *565*, *567*
Lee, S., 401, *439*
Lee, S.-T., 194, *266*
Lee, Y. C., 47, *118*
Leerhoy, J., 515, *567*
Lefkowitz, S. S., 542, *570*
Legrand, L., 392, 398, 399, *437*, *441*
Lehmann, V., 6, 20, 23, 56, *119*
Lehmann-Grube, F., 540, *567*
Lehrer, H. I., 137, 139, *187*
Lehrich, J. R., 504, 505, *560*, *567*
Leidy, G., 39, 40, 76, *122*, *125*
LeLuc, B., 17, 71, 72, 74, *124*
Lemcke, R. M., 451, 456, 463, 464, 467, 468, 469, 470, 471, 473, 474, 475, *477*, *478*
Le Minor, L., 58, 64, 66, 71, 72, 74, *118*, *119*, *124*
Lengerová, A., 392, *440*

Author Index

Lennartz, *122*
Lennette, E. H., 503, 526, *569*, *571*
Leon, M. A., 100, 101, 102, 103, *118*, *121*, *125*
Leonard, E. J., 200, *265*
Le Prévost, C., 523, *563*
Lerman, L. S., 286, *351*
Lerner, R., 213, *265*
Lerner, R. A., 382, 395, 396, 397, 398, *438*, *441*
Leskowitz, S., 169, 172, 174, *185*, 331, 357, 547, *567*
Lesley, J. F., 249, *265*
Leuchars, E., 3, 83, 91, 93, 94, 103, *116*, 171, *184*, *185*, 509, *565*
Leung, C. Y., 140, 141, 165, *183*, *187*
Leupen, M. J., 309, 310, *359*
Leventhal, M., 210, *264*, 374, 377, 389, *440*
Levin, H. A., 145, 169, 172, 174, *183*, *185*
Levine, B. B., 137, *185*, 243, *261*, 293, 314, 315, 329, 333, 335, 336, *354*, *358*, *359*
Levine, H., 137, 138, 145, *185*, *187*
Levine, L., 49, *125*, 137, 139, 149, *186*, *187*, 202, *267*
Levine, S., 373, *441*
Levinson, W., 516, *567*
Levy, D. A., 273, 274, 286, 287, *354*, *356*
Levy, J. P., 386, 388, 391, *440*, *442*, *445*
Levy-Leblond, E., 523, *563*, *567*
Lewinton, L., 484, *571*
Lewis, B. A., 4, 5, *114*, *115*
Lewis, H., 201, 213, 248, *266*, *269*
Lewis, R., *567*
Liacopoulos-Briot, M., 217, 218, *261*, *266*
Lichenberg, L., 92, *118*
Lichtenstein, L. M., 260, *264*, 273, 274, 280, 281, 286, 287, 288, 289, 293, 299, 300, 303, 304, 305, 308, 309, 310, 312, 316, 317, 318, 319, 322, 323, 325, 326, 327, 328, 336, 337, 345, 346, 347, *350*, *351*, *354*, *355*, *356*, *357*, *358*
Lie, S. O., 364, *446*
Liebermann, R., 99, *121*
Liebich, H. G., 194, *269*
Liebig, R., 68, *121*
Lietze, A., 296, 347, *355*
Liew, F. Y., 205, *265*
Lightstone, A. C., 279, 322, *352*

Lilly, F., 200, *266*, 389, 431, 432, *441*, *442*, 499, 506, *563*, *567*, *572*
Lin, J. S., 467, *477*
Lincoln, K., 26, *116*
Lindberg, A. A., 5, 17, 60, 74, *115*, *116*, *118*
Lindberg, B., 5, 11, 13, 17, 18, 19, 29, 30, 32, 34, 35, 41, 53, 60, 74, *111*, *112*, *114*, *115*, *116*, *118*, *122*
Lindblom, B., 366, 370, 430, *445*
Lindblom, J. B., 250, *266*, 420, 421, 422, 426, *443*
Lindenmann, J., 509, 547, 548, *564*, *567*
Link, F., 518, *567*
Link, H., 495, *567*, *568*
Linscott, W. D., 377, *441*, 516, *567*
Lipke, P. N., 48, 90, *111*, *118*
Lisowska-Bernstein, B., 207, 215, 216, 217, 246, 248, *265*
Little, C. C., 362, 365, *441*
Little, J. R., 131, *185*
Litwin, S. D., 201, *264*
Lodmell, D. L., 549, *567*
Loeb, L., 362, 365, *441*
Lönngren, J., 5, 17, 18, 19, 32, 34, 35, *112*, *116*, *118*
LoGrippo, G. A., 463, *478*
Long, P. H., 483, 541, *569*
Longbottom, J. L., 292, 293, *356*
Loor, F., 199, 200, 201, 223, 241, 246, 249, *265*, *267*, 390, 392, *441*
Loosfelt, Y., 200, *265*, 389, 390, 391, 392, *440*, 530, *566*
Losick, R., 7, *118*
Louis, J., 231, *265*
Low, B., 366, 370, 430, *445*
Low, I. E., 460, *477*
Lowell, F. C., 293, 331, *356*, *357*
Lowrey, D. S., 552, 553, *571*
Lowry, S. P., 527, *567*
Lowy, D. R., 526, 540, *573*
Lucas, D. R., 373, *441*
Lucas, S. J., 535, *564*
Luce, C., 523, *568*
Lüderitz, O., 3, 4, 6, 7, 9, 11, 12, 13, 16, 17, 18, 19, 20, 21, 22, 23, 24, 25, 36, 38, 48, 49, 51, 52, 53, 56, 57, 58, 59, 61, 62, 63, 64, 66, 71, 72, 74, 79, 86, 104, *111*, *113*, *114*, *115*, *118*, *119*, *120*,

122, 123, 124, 125, 134, 146, 185, 253, 257, 261
Luescher, E., 286, 351
Lundblad, A., 100, 119
Lundstedt, C., 526, 540, 567
Luria, S. E., 60, 61, 74, 124, 141, 187
Lush, D., 512, 517, 562
Lutsky, I. I., 454, 477
Lyklema, A. W., 309, 310, 359
Lyman, M., 274, 288, 355
Lynn, R. J., 467, 476

M

Maass, G., 513, 572
McAlister, R., 549, 561
McAuslan, B. R., 528, 569
McBride, R. A., 547, 571
McCabe, W. R., 106, 107, 119
McCarthy, K., 541, 563
McCarty, M. C., 43, 44, 72, 118, 119
McCleary, C. W., 41, 118
McClelland, J. D., 363, 380, 445
McCluskey, R. T., 549, 560
McConahey, P. J., 213, 265, 395, 441
McCredie, K. B., 408, 439
McCullough, B., 552, 567
McDevitt, H. O., 94, 111, 114, 144, 145, 185, 221, 222, 235, 236, 247, 249, 261, 263, 264, 265, 333, 350, 354, 355, 368, 432, 435, 441, 442, 505, 506, 561, 569
McDonald, J. C., 375, 401, 441
McDonough, D. J., 102, 115
McEwan, M., 150, 183
McFarland, H., 526, 539, 567
McFarlin, D. E., 559, 571
MacGillivray, M., 502, 504, 569
McIntire, F. C., 108, 120, 123, 319, 356, 400, 433, 439, 442
MacIntire, K. R., 100, 101, 103, 118, 119, 194, 204, 207, 219, 249, 268
Mackaness, G. B., 107, 112, 119, 523, 548, 566, 567
Mackay, I. R., 221, 230, 231, 249, 263
McKenna, J. L., 373, 439
McLaughlin, J., 42, 112
MacLeod, C. M., 2, 73, 83, 84, 106, 115, 119
MacPherson, C. F. C., 2, 84, 115
MacPherson, L., 230, 231, 262

McSharry, J. J., 489, 497, 498, 562, 567
Mäkelä, O., 64, 104, 119, 125, 163, 185, 225, 266
Mäkelä, P. H., 6, 7, 8, 13, 20, 21, 63, 64, 104, 115, 119, 120, 121, 124, 125
Mage, M., 513, 518, 519, 526, 527, 530, 560, 561, 564, 568
Mage, R., 50, 77, 119, 137, 149, 185, 513, 518, 519, 560
Mahar, S., 513, 518, 519, 568
Mahy, B. W. J., 550, 567
Maini, V., 32, 116
Maizel, J. V., 287, 357
Maja, M., 207, 261
Majer, M., 517, 518, 567
Makino, T., 60, 124
Malley, A., 295, 296, 316, 347, 355
Mallucci, L., 520, 523, 560
Malmgren, B., 7, 122
Malmgren, R., 527, 567
Maloney, C. J., 285, 300, 327, 346, 350
Manchee, R. J., 478
Mancini, G., 285, 355
Mandel, B., 500, 501, 502, 512, 513, 567, 572
Mandel, T. E., 194, 199, 226, 232, 261, 265
Mangalo, R., 158, 185
Maniloff, J., 452, 453, 455, 477
Manire, G. P., 453, 455, 467, 477, 478
Mann, D. L., 362, 364, 374, 401, 403, 406, 407, 412, 438, 441
Mannik, M., 3, 95, 118
Manning, J. K., 86, 93, 120, 121
Manson, L. A., 364, 388, 441
Mantani, M., 526, 567
Maoz, A., 164, 185
Marcelli-Barge, A., 399, 437
Marchalonis, J. J., 94, 120, 179, 185, 194, 201, 207, 208, 214, 215, 216, 217, 223, 246, 248, 261, 262, 265, 267
Marchant, R., 171, 184
Marchesi, V. T., 199, 265, 267, 268
Marchioro, T. L., 363, 445
Marcus, P., 514, 571
Marcuson, E. C., 213, 264
Marder, V. J., 383, 445
Mardiney, M. R., 527, 536, 539, 544, 567, 571
Marfey, P. S., 141, 184
Margolies, M. N., 96, 97, 98, 117

Author Index

Marker, O., 526, 540, 550, 567, 573
Markham, R. V., 544, 567
Markley, S., 107, *120*
Markovitz, A., 41, *117*, *120*
Marks, P. A., 396, *438*, *441*
Marmion, B. P., 469, 470, 471, *477*, *478*
Marney, S. R., Jr., 378, *438*
Maron, E., 164, *185*
Marsh, D. G., 280, 281, 282, 283, 284, 285, 287, 288, 289, 291, 293, 295, 296, 297, 298, 299, 300, 304, 305, 309, 310, 313, 314, 316, 318, 319, 321, 322, 323, 324, 325, 326, 327, 328, 330, 333, 334, 335, 336, 337, 338, 339, 340, 341, 342, 343, 345, 346, *351*, *352*, *353*, *354*, *355*, *356*, *357*
Martin, R. O., 46, *111*
Martin, S. J., 494, *564*
Marusyk, H., 487, 488, *568*
Mason, S., 215, 221, 249, *263*, *264*, *265*
Massaro, A. L., 207, *261*
Masuda, T., 222, 224, 227, 228, *264*
Masurel, M., 364, *436*
Mathé, G., 364, 432, *435*
Matsuhashi, S., 63, *120*
Matsumoto, A., 453, 467, *477*, *478*
Matsumozo, T., *124*
Matter, A., 207, *265*
Mattiuz, P. L., 364, 382, 399, 402, 408, 418, *440*, *441*
Maunsell, K., 309, 310, *355*
Maurer, P. H., 84, 87, *113*, *120*, 135, 137, 142, *185*, 202, *265*, 279, 311, *354*, 532, *564*
Mavligit, G., 408, *439*
May, C. D., 274, 288, *355*
May, J., 378, *439*
Mayer, H., 7, 11, 17, 20, 71, 72, *118*, *119*, *120*, *122*, *124*, *125*
Mayer, M. M., 4, 49, *117*, 382, *440*
Medawar, P. B., 362, 363, 364, 402, *436*, *441*
Medlin, J., 91, *120*
Meezan, E., 528, *573*
Melchers, F., 201, 207, 208, 209, 210, 211, 245, 257, *261*, *265*
Melkonian, G. A., 68, *121*
Mellman, W., 549, *567*
Mellors, R. C., 499, 530, 544, 545, 549, 565, 567, *574*
Melnick, J. L., 515, 541, *569*, *570*

Mendell, N. R., 337, *351*
Mendershausen, P. B., 47, *124*
Mendes, N. F., 364, *441*
Merchant, D. J., 395, *440*
Mercuriali, F., 382, 399, *441*
Mergenhagen, S. E., 549, 556, *565*, *568*
Merigan, T. C., 534, *563*
Merrill, E., 535, *565*
Merrill, J. P., 260, *268*
Merryman, C. F., 532, *564*
Mery, A. M., 364, 432, *435*
Mesrobeanu, L., 9, *112*
Messeter, L., 366, 370, 430, *445*
Metcalf, D., 538, 546, *573*
Metzgar, R. S., 364, 374, 385, 386, 387, 401, 407, *441*, *444*
Metzger, A. L., 344, *356*
Metzger, H., 160, *184*, 204, 205, *265*, *355*
Meyer, K., 492, *567*
Meyers, O. L., 532, *570*
Meyers, R. L., 316, *352*
Michael, J. G., 328, 329, *353*
Michaeli, D., 164, *185*
Michel, M. F., 43, 44, 98, *113*, *120*, *125*
Michelson, M. M., 373, *443*
Mickey, M. R., 363, 364, 376, 380, 381, 382, 390, 398, 399, 432, 433, *435*, *441*, *442*, *443*, *446*
Middleton, V. L., 387, *443*
Miescher, P., 363, *441*
Mietens, C., 510, *567*
Miggiano, V. C., 373, 389, 390, 391, *436*, *442*
Mihaesco, C., 150, *187*
Miles, P., 144, *183*
Milford, E. L., 276, *355*
Milgrom, F., 400, 401, *435*, *444*, 462, *477* 529, *573*
Mill, P., 47, *120*
Miller, A., 223, 233, *263*, *265*
Miller, E. C., 98, *120*
Miller, E. J., 98, *113*, *121*
Miller, F., 204, *265*
Miller, G., 176, *186*
Miller, G. W., 530, *568*
Miller, J. F. A. P., 171, *185*, 194, 205, 206, 218, 223, 224, 225, 237, 238, 239, 242, 247, 248, 249, 255, *261*, *264*, *266*, *268*, 269, 507, 508, *568*
Miller, J. L., 374, 407, *441*
Miller, R. G., 234, *263*

Miller, T. E., 548, 566
Millette, C. F., 223, 234, 263, 267
Mills, G. T., 27, 120
Milner, F. H., 280, 284, 295, 297, 298, 300, 355
Milner, K. C., 7, 122
Milstein, C., 3, 99, 112, 158, 159, 185
Mims, C. A., 519, 540, 568, 572
Minanitani, M., 542, 574
Minchin Clarke, H. G., 287, 288, 307, 356
Minden, P., 49, 120
Mirkovic, R., 555, 568
Mishell, R. I., 178, 187, 197, 235, 263
Mitchell, G., 146, 165, 187, 509, 568
Mitchell, G. F., 243, 255, 266, 268, 432, 442, 506, 569
Mitchell, W. D., 53, 115, 120
Mitchison, N. A., 89, 91, 93, 94, 113, 120, 153, 172, 176, 177, 183, 185, 194, 267
Mittal, K. K., 108, 120, 123, 374, 376, 381, 382, 390, 398, 399, 400, 401, 406, 412, 418, 433, 436, 438, 440, 442
Miyajima, T., 390, 391, 406, 442
Miyakawa, Y., 406, 421, 442
Miyamoto, H., 504, 527, 568
Miyamoto, T., 293, 309, 310, 356
Miyuzaki, T., 27, 30, 120
Möller, E., 218, 225, 232, 266, 366, 370, 386, 430, 439, 445
Möller, G., 26, 92, 93, 111, 112, 120, 241, 254, 258, 261, 262, 388, 442
Moldovan, E., 542, 563
Mole, L. E., 160, 186, 299, 304, 356
Mollison, P. L., 382, 443
Molloy, E., 535, 570
Molulsky, A. G., 330, 358
Monaco, A. P., 554, 565
Monod, J., 259, 266
Montgomery, R., 5, 123
Monto, A. S., 106, 107, 125
Moore, D. H., 276, 277, 350, 353, 382, 437
Moore, E. E., 276, 356
Moore, G. E., 373, 395, 403, 406, 442, 443
Moore, M. A. S., 214, 266
Moore, M. B., 276, 356, 358
Moorhead, J. W., 177, 186
Mora, P. T., 525, 527, 528, 529, 561, 571
Morgan, C., 504, 526, 527, 563, 568
Morgan, H. R., 536, 564

Morgan, W. T. J., 4, 73, 120, 121
Morganroth, J., 260, 268, 527, 571
Mori, R., 508, 568
Morowitz, H. J., 452, 453, 455, 468, 477
Moroz, C., 246, 266
Morris, J. H., 281, 292, 295, 350, 356
Morris, P. J., 94, 120, 432, 439
Morris, R., 344, 356
Morrison, D. C., 253, 262
Morrison, M., 216, 261, 266
Mortensson-Egnund, K., 492, 564
Morton, J. I., 549, 571
Morton, J. J., 295, 352
Moscona, A. A., 396, 442
Mott, M. G., 542, 569
Motta, R., 387, 442
Moulder, J. W., 455, 467, 469, 477
Moulias, R. L., 537, 568
Mouton, D., 218, 261, 434, 436
Moyer, J. D., 4, 120
Moyer, S., 498, 568
Moyes, D. G., 549, 561
Mozes, E., 92, 118, 120, 123, 249, 266, 268, 556, 571
Mozes, S., 143, 187
Müller-Eberhard, H. J., 378, 439
Müller-Seitz, E., 9, 12, 16, 120, 121
Mufson, M. A., 474, 476
Mukherjee, G. N., 401, 441
Mullen, Y., 366, 442
Muller, J. Y., 218, 261
Munn, E., 204, 263
Munoz, J. J., 549, 567
Munro, A. J., 247, 251, 268
Muramatsu, T., 419, 442
Murphy, F. A., 508, 565
Murphy, G. B., 372, 399, 437, 440
Murphy, J. J., 399, 436
Muschel, L. H., 104, 120, 515, 568
Myers, W. G., 236, 266

N

Nabholtz, M., 390, 442
Nablant, J., 549, 568
Nadel, J. A., 323, 356
Nadkarni, J. J., 206, 212, 265, 527, 566
Nadkarni, J. S., 527, 566
Nadkarni, J. W., 206, 212, 265
Nagler, F. P. O., 535, 568

Author Index

Nahmias, A. J., 508, 523, 527, 535, 555, 559, 565, 568, 570, 571
Naib, Z. M., 523, 568
Naide, Y., 7, 8, 13, 120, 121
Najarian, J. S., 384, 404, 438
Najima, T., 542, 574
Nakada, H. I., 41, 118
Nakamuro, K., 250, 268, 420, 421, 442, 445
Nakla, L. S., 108, 120
Naor, D., 219, 220, 221, 226, 232, 266
Nardini, L., 549, 561
Nase, S., 162, 171, 173, 186, 194, 267
Nass, M. K., 412, 447
Natali, P. G., 374, 388, 391, 394, 399, 412, 416, 438, 443
Naterman, H. L., 318, 356
Nathanson, N., 540, 543, 555, 562, 565, 568
Nathenson, S. G., 362, 364, 397, 402, 403, 407, 412, 414, 419, 431, 437, 441, 444, 445, 499, 563
Natvig, J. B., 249, 263
Nauciel, C., 172, 186
Neauport-Sautes, C., 200, 265, 266, 267, 389, 390, 391, 392, 431, 440, 442, 443, 530, 566
Ne'eman, Z., 472, 477
Neerbout, R., 364, 432, 447
Neher, G. H., 549, 571
Neill, J. M., 77, 124
Neimark, H. C., 455, 457, 459, 477
Nelken, D., 382, 442
Nelson, R. A., Jr., 375, 442
Nesburn, A. B., 542, 546, 568, 572
Neter, E., 7, 26, 49, 119, 120, 125
Neufeld, F., 25, 86, 120
Neumann, W., 278, 356
Neumüller, G., 93, 120
Newberry, W. M., 260, 268
Newell, J. M., 275, 276, 282, 332, 356
Newton, R. M., 470, 471, 477
Nghiem, H. O., 58, 120
Nicholls, A., 344, 351
Nichols, C., 485, 514, 535, 562
Nichols, W. W., 554, 568
Nickoryak, C. A., 150, 183
Nicolai, M. G., 386, 388, 391, 440, 442, 445
Nicolson, G. L., 198, 268, 389, 430, 445

Nii, S. C., 527, 568
Nikaido, H., 3, 6, 7, 8, 11, 12, 13, 21, 52, 53, 56, 57, 58, 59, 61, 62, 64, 66, 119, 120, 121
Nilsson, K., 18, 112
Nimmich, W., 11, 18, 19, 27, 31, 32, 33, 34, 35, 53, 82, 83, 112, 115, 118, 121
Nisalak, A., 511, 563
Nishioka, K., 526, 568
Nisonoff, A., 96, 122, 154, 156, 186, 187, 259, 263
Nitecki, D. E., 129, 137, 139, 149, 162, 166, 167, 169, 171, 172, 173, 174, 175, 178, 182, 183, 184, 187, 243, 261, 532, 571
Nithiuthai, P., 496, 565
Niwa, A., 519, 525, 564
Noble, M., 146, 165, 187, 243, 268
Noll, H., 525, 568
Nomoto, K., 508, 568
Noon, L., 345, 356
Norcross, N. L., 43, 122
Nordin, A. A., 85, 117, 249, 262
Nordin, P., 68, 121
Nordling, S., 194, 266
Noreen, H., 337, 351
Norman, P. S., 281, 283, 285, 287, 288, 292, 293, 295, 299, 300, 301, 303, 305, 309, 310, 312, 317, 318, 319, 322, 323, 327, 328, 336, 337, 346, 347, 350, 351, 354, 355, 356
Norrby, E., 485, 487, 488, 489, 494, 495, 568, 571, 572, 573
Northcote, D. H., 47, 121
Nossal, E. T. V., 93, 113
Nossal, G. J. V., 89, 123, 201, 213, 214, 215, 221, 229, 231, 235, 236, 238, 243, 248, 261, 266, 269, 434, 442
Nota, N. R., 217, 266
Notani, G., 100, 101, 112
Notkins, A. L., 513, 515, 516, 517, 518, 519, 525, 526, 527, 530, 534, 535, 540, 543, 549, 556, 560, 561, 562, 564, 565, 568, 569, 570, 573
Novey, H. S., 323, 359
Nowinski, R. C., 545, 569
Nurminen, M., 6, 20, 22, 23, 56, 119
Nussenzweig, V., 176, 186, 194, 205, 253, 261, 263, 530, 568

O

Ochoa, P., 157, *185*
O'Dea, J. F., 527, *569*
Ørskov, F., 4, 12, 16, 26, 37, 38, 53, 54, 55, 74, 76, 80, *115, 116, 117, 118, 121*
Ørskov, I., 4, 12, 16, 26, 37, 38, 53, 54, 55, 74, 76, 80, *115, 116, 117, 121*
Ogilvie, B. M., 292, 307, *353*
Ogra, P., 502, 504, 507, *569*
Oh, S. K., 393, 398, 404, 406, 407, 408, 409, 410, 412, 425, 426, 427, 428, 429, *442, 443, 444*
Ohanian, S. H., 214, *268*
Ohle, H., 68, *120*
Ohman, J. L., Jr., 293, *356*
Ohta, N., 528, *569*
O'Konski, C. T., 203, *262*
Okumura, K., 344, *378*
Old, L. J., 194, 207, 219, 249, *268*, 369, 387, 388, 391, 392, 432, *435, 436, 439, 441, 442*, 499, 526, 531, 544, *560, 561, 563, 569, 572*
Oldstone, M. B. A., 382, 395, 432, *441, 442*, 506, 516, 517, 526, 530, 540, 543, 544, 565, 566, *569*
O'Leary, T. P., 503, 504, *561*
Olhagen, B., 382, *442*
Olitsky, P. K., 483, 541, *569*
Oliveira, B., 378, *444*
Olling, S., 103, 107, *117*
Olsen, S., 382, *440*
Olshevsky, U., 485, *569*
Olsson, J., 495, *568*
O'Neill, C. H., 528, *569*
Onn, T., 41, *114*
Onozaki, K., 258, *266*
Oram, J. D., 496, *560*
Orange, R. P., 273, 274, *356*
Ordal, J. C., 505, *569*
Orentas, D. G., 26, *121, 123*
Organick, A. B., 454, *477*
Orgel, H. A., 339, *350, 353*
Orme, T., *561*
Ornstein, L., 286, 287, *356*
Oroszlan, S., 516, *569*
Orr, K. B., 194, *266*
Orr, T. S. C., 292, 307, *350*
Osborn, J. E., 526, 536, 549, *569, 571*
Osborn, M. J., 6, 7, *121*
Osborne, T. B., 128, *187*
Oshima, S., 309, *356*
Oshiro, L. S., 526, *569*
Osler, A. G., 273, 274, 286, 287, 288, 317, *354, 356*, 378, *444*, 517, *569*
Osmond, D., 229, 238, *266*
Osoba, D., 234, *266*
Osterland, C. K., 98, 101, *113, 120, 121*
Ostertag, M., 331, *358*
O'Sullivan, S., 293, 295, *356*
Osunkoya, B. O., 200, *266*
Otsuka, T., 293, *354*
Otten, J., 260, *266*
Ottinger, B., 87, 89, 90, *113*
Ouchterlony, Ö., 49, *121*
Ovary, Z., 163, *186*, 315, *356*
Owen, J. J. T., 214, *266*
Oxman, M., 533, *572*

P

Padlan, E. A., 154, *186*
Padley, P. J., 277, 283, *353*
Paetkau, V. H., 200, 201, 222, 223, 232, 240, 255, *263*
Page, L. A., 451, *477*
Page, L. B., 202, *264*
Painter, L. M., 523, *568*
Painter, T. J., 4, *121*
Paldino, R. L., 550, *565*
Palm, J., 363, 364, 366, 388, *441, 442*
Palmstierna, H., 292, *356*
Paloheimo, J., 555, *564*
Pan, J., 475, *476*
Panelius, M., 495, 567, *571*
Papaconstantinou, J., 396, *445*
Papermaster, B. W., 373, 384, 395, 419, *440, 442, 443, 444*
Papermaster, D. S., 141, 149, *184*
Papermaster, V. M., 373, 395, *442, 443*
Pappano, J. E., 549, *561*
Pappenheimer, A. M., Jr., 77, 89, 96, 97, *112, 117, 118, 121*
Paranjpe, M., *561*
Paraskevas, F., 194, *266*
Pardee, A. B., 528, *569*
Parish, C. R., 89, 91, *121*, 165, *186*, 207, 234, 238, *266*
Parish, W. E., 273, *356*
Pariyanonda, A., 511, *563*

Author Index

Parker, C. W., 101, *121*, 260, *268*
Parker, J. C., 551, *569*
Parker, M. I., 49, *122*
Parkhouse, R. M. E., 102, 103, *121*, 207, 208, 209, 210, 211, 245, *263*, *266*
Parks, W. P., 499, *569*
Parrott, D. M. V., 171, *184*
Parsell, Z., 104, *123*
Partridge, S. M., 73, *120*
Pasanen, V., 218, *261*
Pascal, R. R., 545, *569*
Passmore, H. C., 368, *443*
Pasten, I., 260, *266*
Pasternak, C. A., 393, *443*, *447*
Pasternak, G., 499, *569*
Patel, R., 364, 382, 432, 433, *443*
Path, F. C., 104, *123*
Patnode, R. A., 535, *570*
Patrick, R., 194, 253, *261*
Patrucco, R., 314, 333, *356*
Patt, J. K., 466, *476*
Patterson, R., 319, *356*
Paul, C., 206, *267*
Paul, J. R., 541, *569*
Paul, W. E., 19, 26, 89, *123*, 163, 173, 174, *184*, *186*, 200, 201, 207, 220, 224, 226, 231, 234, 243, *262*, *265*, *266*, *268*
Pavlovskis, O. R., 49, *121*
Payne, F. E., 542, *569*
Payne, R. O., 363, 364, 382, 395, 431, *436*, *437*, *443*
Pazur, J. H., 42, 82, *117*
Peakman, E. M., 373, *441*
Pearson, C. M., 344, *357*
Pearson, G., 527, *566*
Pedersen, C. E., 496, *569*
Pedersen, K. O., 4, *124*
Peebles, T. C., 551, *563*
Pegrum, G. D., 387, *443*
Peled, A., 556, *569*
Pellegrino, A., 373, 381, 383, 384, 385, 386, 388, 391, 394, 398, 403, 404, 406, 408, 412, *443*
Pellegrino, M. A., 364, 373, 374, 375, 376, 377, 378, 380, 381, 382, 383, 384, 385, 386, 388, 391, 393, 394, 395, 396, 397, 398, 400, 401, 402, 403, 404, 406, 407, 408, 409, 410, 412, 414, 415, 416, 418, 419, 425, 426, 427, 428, 429, 431, *436*, *438*, *439*, *440*, *442*, *443*, *444*, *446*
Penn, I., 554, *569*
Penttinen, K., 505, *570*
Pepys, J., 290, 292, 293, *356*
Pepys, M. G., 253, *266*
Percy, D. H., 307, 308, *351*
Perdue, J. F., 526, *569*
Pereira, H. G., 487, 488, 514, 542, *564*, *566*, *569*
Perham, T. G., 542, *569*
Perkins, F. T., 507, *569*
Perkins, H. A., 364, *437*
Perkins, W. D., 200, 215, *269*, 389, *446*
Perlin, A. D., *110*
Perlman, F., 278, 316, *355*, *356*
Perlzweig, W. A., 86, *121*
Pernis, B., 179, *186*, 200, 201, 206, 211, 221, 241, 242, 247, 248, 249, *265*, *266*, *267*, 390, 392, *441*
Perper, R. J., 373, *443*
Perry, M. B., 28, *117*
Perry, S., 406, *439*
Peterson, E. A., 282, *356*
Peterson, P. A., 250, 251, *266*, 420, 421, 422, 426, 429, *437*, *443*
Peterson, R., 549, *563*
Pettersson, U., 514, 515, *565*, *569*
Pfefferkorn, E. R., 495, 496, 526, *562*, *569*, *572*
Phair, J. P., 163, *186*
Philips, D. C., 99, *117*, 154, *186*
Philipson, L., 512, 513, 514, 518, *569*
Phillips, E. R., 526, *569*
Phillips, E. W., 320, *357*
Phillips, R. A., 234, *263*
Phillips, S. M., 554, *560*, *565*
Phills, J. A., 307, 320, *357*
Piat, S., 200, *267*, 392, *443*
Pike, B. L., 214, 215, 229, 231, *266*
Pilotti, A., 17, *116*
Pilz, I., 203, *267*
Pinchuck, P., 142, *185*
Pinckard, R. N., 49, *121*
Pincus, C., 176, *186*
Pincus, J. H., 96, 97, 98, *121*
Pincus, T., 499, *560*, *565*, *567*
Pincus, W. B., 533, *570*
Pink, J. R. L., 158, 159, *185*
Pinto da Silva, P., 199, *267*
Pirie, N. W., 450, *477*
Pirofsky, B., 211, *265*

Pitt, R. M., 42, 104, 106, *113*
Pittman, M., 106, *125*
Pitt-Rivers, R., 153, *183*
Pizarro, O., 385, *443*
Plackett, P., 468, 469, 470, 471, 472, *477*, *478*
Plummer, G., 484, *570*
Pohlit, H., 165, *186*
Pokorno, Z., 385, 386, *446*
Polackova, M., 385, 386, *446*
Polak, L., 367, *438*
Polgar, P., 555, *566*
Poljak, R. J., 202, 203, *267*
Polkowski, J., 150, *183*
Pollack, J. D., 461, 474, *478*
Polley, M. J., 382, *443*
Pollock, M. E., 459, 460, *478*
Ponce de Leon, M., 485, 514, 535, *562*
Ponterius, G., 293, *351*
Porath, J., 282, 287, 306, *353*, *357*
Porter, D. D., 545, 549, *570*
Porter, H. G., 545, *570*
Porter, J. F., 32, 33, *114*
Porter, R. R., 135, 136, 160, 180, *186*, 204, *267*
Posborg Petersen, V., 382, *440*
Postlewaite, R., 511, *572*
Potter, C. W., 507, *571*
Potter, M., 3, 99, 100, 101, *121*, *122*, 154, 179, *186*
Poulik, M. D., 420, 421, 422, 423, 424, 425, 426, 427, 428, 429, *435*, *436*, *439*, *443*, *445*
Povlsen, C. O., 212, *267*
Powell, K. L., 485, 514, 535, *570*
Prausnitz, C., 274, 279, 311, *357*
Prehm, P., 21, *121*
Prendergast, R. A., 249, *264*, 526, 530, 531, 540, 543, *562*
Prescott, B., 49, 87, 88, 89, 90, 92, 93, 94, *110*, *111*, *113*, 471, 474, *478*, 557, *560*
Press, E. M., 135, 136, 160, *186*
Pressman, D., 129, 132, 136, 149, 158, *186*, *187*, 250, *268*, 406, 420, 421, *442*, *445*
Pretlow, T. G., 100, 103, *114*
Preud'homme, J. L., 200, 211, *267*, 392, *443*
Price, R. W., 543, *573*

Price, W. H., 508, *572*
Princler, G., 101, *119*
Probst, H., 253, *263*
Proctor, D. F., 322, *351*, *357*
Proffitt, M. R., 526, 538, 546, 552, *570*
Pruzansky, J. J., 319, *356*
Puchwein, G., 203, *267*
Pulaski, E. J., 279, *357*
Purcell, R. H., 460, 465, 466, *478*, 506, *571*
Purchase, H. G., 527, 549, 556, *562*, *570*
Putnam, F. W., 206, *267*
Pye, J., 194, 205, 237, 238, 239, *261*
Pyrhonen, S., 505, *570*

Q

Quinlan, M., 322, *357*

R

Rabellino, E., 213, 248, *264*, *267*, *268*
Rabinowitz, S., 539, *559*
Rabson, A. S., 542, *561*
Rack, L., 250, *266*
Rackemann, F. M., 277, 279, 306, 331, *357*
Radola, B. J., 286, 287, *357*
Radwan, A. I., 515, 516, *570*
Raff, M. C., 171, *186*, 194, 200, 207, 211, 219, 240, 241, 242, 248, 249, *261*, *263*, *267*, *268*, 389, 392, *445*, 530, *572*
Raff, R., 16, *119*
Raffel, S., 107, *114*, 315, *357*
Rager-Zisman, B., 523, 559, *570*
Rago, D., 556, *564*
Rainey, T. C., 510, *564*
Rajbhandary, U. L., 46, *111*
Rajewsky, K., 162, 165, 171, 173, 176, 177, *185*, *186*, 215, *264*, 504, *571*
Ralph, W. B., 337, *351*
Ramos, A., 385, *443*
Rancourt, M. W., 549, *562*
Randall, E., 526, 537, *570*
Rantz, A. L., 106, 107, *125*
Ranzi, T., 372, *441*
Rao, C. V. N., 27, *121*
Rapaport, F. T., 363, 399, 400, 401, *437*, *441*, *444*
Rapp, H. J., 206, 262, 516, *562*
Rappaport, H. G., 276, *353*
Raschke, W. C., 48, 53, 90, *111*, *118*, *121*

Author Index

Rask, L., 420, 421, 422, 426, *443*
Ratner, B., 330, *357*
Ravitch, M. M., 246, *264*
Rawls, W. E., 515, 527, 534, 567, 570, 572
Ray, A., 160, *186*
Raynaud, M., 158, 172, *185, 186*
Razin, S., 467, 471, 472, 473, 474, 475, 476, 577, 478
Rebers, P. A., 27, 28, 76, 78, 88, *113, 115, 121*
Reddick, R. A., 542, *570*
Reed, C. E., 296, 323, 347, *351, 355*
Reed, N. D., 86, 93, *120, 121*
Reed, W. D., 77, 96, *121*
Reed, W. P., 107, 108, *113*
Reedman, B. M., 511, *573*
Rees, D. A., 41, 55, *118, 121*
Reeves, R. E., 27, 28, *110, 122*
Reich, L., 513, *572*
Reichlin, M., 150, *186*
Reinert, P. H., 537, *568*
Reis, H. E., 387, *436*
Reisfeld, R. A., 96, *122*, 362, 364, 367, 368, 373, 374, 375, 376, 377, 378, 380, 381, 382, 383, 384, 388, 391, 393, 394, 395, 396, 397, 398, 399, 400, 401, 402, 403, 404, 406, 407, 408, 409, 410, 412, 414, 415, 418, 419, 420, 425, 426, 427, 428, 429, 431, *436, 438, 439, 440, 442, 443, 444, 446*
Reisner, E. G., 383, 390, *438*
Reizkoyá, J., 392, *440*
Renkonen, O., 495, *570*
Reno, P. W., 516, *570*
Resch, K., 194, *263*
Reske, K., 13, 19, *122*
Reyes, F., 218, *261*
Ribi, E., 7, *122*
Riblet, R. J., 246, *264*
Ricci, M., 293, 310, *357*
Rice, S. A., 100, 101, *112*
Richards, F. F., 202, *264*
Richiardi, P., 382, 399, *441*
Richter, M., 329, *357*
Rieber, E.-P., 249, *267*
Riethmüller, G., 249, *267*
Rietschel, E. T., 6, 20, 22, 23, 24, 56, *114, 119, 122*
Rifkind, R. A., 396, *438*
Riggs, J. L., 526, *569*

Righthand, F., 502, 504, *569*
Rinny, A., 207, 215, 216, 217, 246, 248, *265*
Riordan, J. T., 541, *569*
Ripe, E., 292, *356*
Risse, H. J., 13, *119*
Rittenberg, M. B., 163, *186*
Ritter, D. B., 459, *476*
Rizzo, A., *568*
Roane, J. A., 537, *565*
Roane, P. R., 527, *570*
Roantree, R. J., 104, *122*
Robbins, K. C., 301, *357*
Robbins, P. W., 7, 17, 60, 61, 64, 66, 68, 74, *118, 122, 124*, 141, *187*, 528, 529, *570, 573*
Roberson, L. E., 545, *565*
Roberts, W. K., 28, *112*
Robertson, H. T., 528, *570*
Robinson, B., 2, 73, 83, 84, 106, *115, 119*
Robolt, O. A., 158, *187*
Rockey, J. H., 339, *357*
Rocklin, R. E., 532, *570*
Rodbard, D., 415, *444*
Rodkey, L. S., 96, *122*
Rodwell, A., 451, *478*
Roebber, M., 280, 283, 285, 295, 303, 304, *354, 357*
Roelants, G. E., 163, 171, 175, 179, *186*, 220, 221, 223, 225, 227, 232, 236, 237, 238, 239, 241, 246, 249, *264, 267*, 511, *570*
Rogentine, G. N., Jr., 364, 373, 375, 381, 386, 395, 403, 412, *441, 444*
Rogers, A. H., 41, *111*
Rogers, A. W., 220, *267*
Rogers, H. W., 535, *570*
Roitt, I. M., 213, 249, *263, 264*
Roizman, B., 484, 527, *570*
Rojanasuphot, S., 496, *565*
Rolfs, M. R., 363, *443*
Rolley, R. T., 201, 223, 246, *262, 267*
Romeo, D., 5, 7, *122*, 253, *267*
Rosan, R., 555, *568*
Rose, B., 329, *357*
Rose, H. M., 526, 527, 535, *563, 568, 570*
Rose, N. R., 432, *446*
Rosell, K. G., 35, *112*
Rosen, L., 484, *570*
Rosenbaum, N., 41, *120*

Rosenberg, E., 39, 122
Rosenberg, G. L., 534, 535, 539, 540, 563, 570
Rosenberg, L. T., 467, 478
Rosenblith, J. Z., 528, 570
Rosenblum, E. N., 526, 563
Rosenfelder, G., 6, 20, 23, 56, 119
Rosenthal, A. S., 200, 201, 207, 224, 234, 262, 267, 268
Rosenthal, J., 518, 519, 525, 526, 527, 530, 561, 564, 569
Rosenthal, R. R., 323, 351
Ross, J., 499, 569
Ross, M. R., 467, 469, 477
Rossbach, E. A., 279, 354
Rossen, R. D., 390, 440, 504, 506, 560, 567, 570
Rossi-Fanelli, A., 150, 186
Roth, I. L., 25, 123
Rothengatter, G., 366, 446
Rothfield, L., 5, 7, 122, 253, 267
Rothschild, K. J., 197, 267
Rothwell, T. L. W., 292, 307, 353
Rotman, B., 381, 436
Rotman, M., 154, 184
Rott, R., 491, 566
Rovis, L., 100, 122
Rowe, A. J., 202, 263
Rowe, D. S., 211, 267
Rowe, W. P., 485, 498, 499, 506, 526, 540, 551, 561, 564, 570, 573
Rowinska, D., 364, 439
Rowlands, D. J., 514, 570
Rowley, D., 107, 108, 112, 117, 122
Rowley, D. A., 538, 561
Rowley, J. R., 306, 324, 350
Roy, N., 27, 29, 115, 122
Rubin, B., 177, 186
Rubin, H., 513, 570
Rubinstein, P., 385, 443
Rudbach, J. A., 7, 86, 121, 122
Ruden, U., 5, 18, 112, 118
Rudikoff, S., 154, 186
Ruebner, B. H., 553, 561, 565
Rüde, E., 73, 74, 123
Ruschmann, E., 13, 16, 23, 24, 119, 122
Russ, S. B., 503, 561
Russell, H., 43, 122
Russell, P. K., 526, 562
Russell, P. S., 385, 388, 400, 435, 444
Rustigian, R., 526, 537, 566, 570
Rutishauser, U., 223, 234, 263, 267
Ruys, A. C., 465, 477
Rydén, A., 223, 225, 241, 246, 249, 267
Rygaard, J., 212, 267
Rysen, J. E., 207, 265
Rytel, M. W., 536, 563

S

Sabin, A., 502, 507, 520, 541, 570, 571
Sablovic, D., 194, 269
Sachs, D. H., 151, 186, 400, 444
Sachs, L., 528, 563
Safferman, R. S., 292, 351
Safford, J. W., Jr., 400, 443
Sage, H. J., 137, 139, 149, 186, 202, 267
Sagik, B. P., 496, 548, 561
Sagin, F. J., 42, 125
Saha, A., 316, 355
Saito, H., 526, 548, 566, 571
Saito, T., 47, 53, 124
Sakai, T., 117
Sakurai, Y., 258, 266
Salaman, M. H., 549, 571
Salfner, B., 406, 408, 436, 446
Salman, S., 322, 357
Salmi, A. A., 495, 567, 571
Saluk, P. H., 530, 568
Salvaggio, J., 292, 331, 354, 357
Salvin, S. B., 166, 186
Samuelson, K., 11, 13, 17, 34, 53, 116, 118, 122
Sandberg, A., 517, 569
Sandberg, A. L., 378, 444
Sandberg, L., 366, 370, 430, 445
Sanderson, A. R., 364, 381, 384, 392, 397, 402, 407, 419, 429, 437, 444, 446
Sandford, P. A., 5, 32, 34, 114, 122
Sanford, J. P., 122
Sanger, D. V., 514, 570
Santer, V., 194, 267
Santilli, J., 345, 357
Sanz, E., 316, 352
Saplin, B. J., 135, 141, 183
Sarma, V. R., 203, 267
Sarvas, M., 104, 119, 125
Sasaki, T., 63, 122, 124
Sato, S., 309, 356
Sato, W., 367, 438
Sawardeker, J. S., 4, 122

Author Index

Sawyer, W. A., 541, *571*
Scala, A. R., 526, 548, *563*
Schachman, H. K., 4, *122*, 287, *357*
Schalch, D. S., 49, *122*
Scharff, M. D., 484, *571*
Schechter, A. N., 151, *186*
Schechter, B., 54, *123*, 136, 137, 139, 140, 146, 147, 151, 152, *186*, *187*
Schechter, I., 136, 137, 139, 140, 146, 147, 148, 149, 151, 180, *183*, *184*, *186*, *187*, 235, 255, *265*, *267*
Schechter, T., 54, *123*
Scheele, C., 518, *568*
Scheid, A., 489, 494, *562*, *571*
Scheid, M., 385, *439*
Schenkein, I., 207, *261*, 293, *358*
Scher, M., 47, *122*
Scherp, H. W., *115*
Schiemann, O., 86, *122*
Schierman, L. W., 547, *571*
Schiffman, G., 103, 104, *118*
Schild, G., 508, 509, 511, *572*
Schimpl, A., 172, *187*
Schippers, H. M. A., 364, *446*
Schirrmacher, V., 162, 171, 173, *186*, 504, *571*
Schlecht, S., 13, 21, 105, 106, *119*, *122*
Schlesinger, M., 194, *267*, 387, 391, *444*
Schlesinger, R. W., 485, 512, 542, 566, *571*, *572*
Schlessinger, D., 396, *441*
Schlosshardt, J., 13, *119*, *122*
Schlossman, S. F., 50, *122*, 137, 138, 145, 169, 175, *185*, *187*, 234, 243, *267*, 532, *563*
Schlosstein, L., 344, *357*
Schlumberger, H., 514, *573*
Schmidhauser-Kopp, M., 6, *113*
Schmidt, C. G., 387, *436*
Schmidt, G., 9, 13, 20, 21, 38, 76, *117*, *119*, *122*, *123*
Schmidt, N. J., 503, *571*
Schmidt, W. C., 39, 43, *123*
Schneeberger, E. E., 320, *357*
Schneider, C. H., 352
Schneider, K. F., 4, 37, 53, 54, 55, *117*
Schneider, U., 403, *447*
Schneweis, K. E., 527, *568*
Scholtissek, C., *566*
Scholtus, M., 383, *436*

Schoyen, R., 492, 548, *564*, *571*
Schrader, J. W., 253, *267*
Schramm, G., 86, *123*
Schroeder, E., 152, *187*
Schrum, D. I., 542, *561*
Schuit, H. R. E., 206, *269*
Schulman, J., 515, *566*
Schulte-Holthausen, H., 13, *119*, 403, *447*
Schultz, J. S., 406, *444*
Schulze, I., 489, 491, 493, *571*
Schuster, R., 491, *571*
Schwartz, B. D., 397, 431, *437*, *444*
Schwartz, D. P., 507, *571*
Schwartz, H. J., 331, *354*
Schwartz, M., 292, 320, 330, *357*
Schwartz, R. S., 554, *560*, *565*
Schwartzman, R. M., 339, *357*
Schwarzman, S., 26, 105, *123*
Schwarzmüller, E., 58, *123*
Scibienski, R., 243, *267*, 313, 348, *350*
Scollard, D., 538, *561*
Scolnick, E. M., 499, *569*
Scott, G. S., 519, *560*
Scott, J. E., 26, *123*
Scott, L. V., 535, *570*
Scott, R. B., 396, *444*
Scott, R. E., 199, *267*, 268
Scriba, M., 555, *564*
Scudeller, G., 200, *261*, 381, 389, 390, 391, 392, 397, 431, *436*, *446*
Seabury, J., 292, *357*
Segal, A. T., 306, *357*
Segal, D. M., 154, *186*
Segall, M., 533, *560*
Segrest, J. P., 199, *265*, *267*
Sehon, A. H., 292, 308, 316, 329, *350*, *352*, *357*
Seibel, E., 408, *446*
Seigler, H. F., 385, 386, 387, 401, 407, *441*, *444*
Sela, M., 54, 73, 91, 92, 110, *117*, *118*, *120*, *123*, 129, 136, 137, 139, 140, 141, 142, 143, 144, 146, 147, 149, 151, 152, 169, 172, 174, *183*, *184*, *186*, *187*, 194, 208, 235, 249, 251, 255, *262*, *263*, *265*, *266*, *267*, 268, 304, 313, 333, *357*
Seligmann, M., 150, *187*, 211, *267*
Sell, K. W., 535, 537, *560*, *571*, *572*
Sell, S., 206, 207, *268*
Seltmann, G., 16, *123*

Sendo, F., 526, 538, 548, *562*, *566*, *571*
Senik, A., 388, 391, *440*
Senterfit, L. B., 461, 465, 474, *478*
Senyk, G., 163, 164, 166, 167, *185*, *186*, *187*, 532, *571*
Sercarz, E., 223, 230, 231, *262*, 265
Sergent, J. S., 378, *438*
Sever, J., 537, 542, *565*
Sevier, E. D., 425, 426, 427, 428, 429, *443*
Shabarova, Z. A., 27, *123*
Shanbrom, E., 364, 375, 432, *446*, *447*
Shapiro, A. L., 287, *357*
Sharon, N., 99, *124*, 180, *184*
Sharpless, N. S., 463, *478*
Shaw, E. J., 469, 470, 471, 472, *478*
Shaw, N., 46, *123*, 472, *478*
Shearer, G. M., 92, *118*, *120*, *123*, 245, 249, *266*, *268*, 556, *571*
Shellam, G. R., 89, *123*
Shelton, E., 204, *268*
Shepherd, G. W., 308, *352*
Sheppard, J. R., 260, *268*
Sher, A., 100, 102, *125*
Sherman, W. B., 275, 287, 292, 300, 318, 320, 321, 330, *357*, *358*
Sherr, C. J., 207, *261*
Shevach, E. M., *267*
Shimada, A., 402, 414, *445*
Shimada, T., 363, *444*
Shimiza, Y. K., 494, *565*
Shimizu, A., 206, *267*
Shimizu, M., 140, 141, *183*
Shimizu, Y., 529, *571*
Shin, H. S., 378, *444*
Shinoda, T., 206, *267*
Shipolini, R. A., 295, 299, 308, 328, *358*
Shirai, T., 526, 544, 548, *566*, *567*, *571*
Shishido, A., 526, *573*
Shiurba, R., 366, *445*
Shons, A. R., 404, *438*
Shore, S., 507, *571*
Shreffler, D. C., 242, 250, *262*, *265*, 363, 365, 368, 371, 395, 399, 406, 430, *437*, *440*, *442*, *444*, *445*
Shulman, N. R., 383, *445*
Shulman, S., 278, 293, 315, *358*
Shutt, R. H., 396, *445*
Siddiqui, I. R., 33, *111*
Siebel, E., 406, *436*
Siegel, B. V., 549, *571*

Siegel, M., 132, *186*
Siegesmund, K. A., 454, *477*
Sievers, K., 49, *119*
Sigel, M. M., 102, *115*, 539, 545, *567*
Silberman, D. E., 330, *357*
Silverman, L., 374, 388, 389, *437*
Silvers, W. K., 366, *445*
Silverstein, A. M., 163, *183*
Silverstein, S., 514, *571*
Silverton, E. W., 203, *267*
Silvestre, D., 200, *265*, *266*, *267*, 386, 388, 389, 390, 391, 392, 431, *440*, *442*, *443*, *445*, 530, *566*
Sim, C., 485, 514, 535, *570*
Simmons, D. A. R., 5, 16, 18, 19, 21, *117*, *118*, *123*
Simmons, N. S., 99, *114*
Simon, M., 6, 20, 23, 56, *119*
Simons, K., 495, *570*
Simonsen, M., 219, 231, 249, 250, *262*
Singal, D. P., 382, 390, *442*
Singer, D. L., 383, *435*
Singer, S. J., 198, *268*, 389, 430, *445*
Singh, J., 201, *263*
Singh, M., 104, *111*
Siraganian, R. P., 293, *358*
Sirchia, G., 372, 374, 376, 382, 399, *438*, *441*, *445*
Siskind, G. W., 26, 89, *123*, 137, 163, 170, *184*, *186*
Sjaarda, J. R., 375, 380, *446*
Sjöberg, O., 93, *111*, *120*, 218, 232, 258, *261*, *266*, *268*
Sjöstedt, S. S., 103, *123*
Skehel, J. J., 490, *571*, *573*
Skidmore, B. J., 253, *262*
Skinsnes, O. K., 524, *573*
Sklarofsky, B., 276, *353*
Skurzak, H., 525, *572*
Slade, H. D., 43, 44, 49, *121*, *123*
Slettenmark-Wahren, B., 526, *571*
Slocum, D. R., 496, *569*
Slodki, M. E., 76, 80, 81, *115*, *123*
Sloneker, J. H., 4, 26, *121*, *122*, *123*
Slotnik, M., 542, *564*
Smale, C. J., 497, 498, 504, 514, *561*, *562*
Small, P. A., Jr., 96, *122*, 135, *184*, 204, *265*, 507, *573*
Smallmann, E., 107, *120*
Smit, M. R., 103, *125*

Author Index

Smith, C. B., 506, *571*
Smith, C. E., 548, *573*
Smith, C. W., 200, 201, *268*
Smith, E. E. B., 27, *120*
Smith, F., 4, 5, *110*, *114*, *115*, *123*, *124*
Smith, G. S., 362, 375, 383, 387, 432, *445*, *447*
Smith, H., 104, *123*
Smith, H. W., 104, *123*
Smith, J. W., 260, *268*
Smith, K. A., 527, 536, 539, *571*
Smith, K. O., 487, *571*
Smith, P. F., 455, 456, 460, 472, *478*
Smith, R. F., 166, *186*
Smith, R. T., 200, 219, 231, *263*, *266*
Smith, R. W., 525, 527, *571*
Smithies, O., 287, *358*, 420, 421, *445*
Smithwick, E. M., 550, *571*
Snell, G. D., 362, 363, 365, 368, 371, *445*
Snodgrass, M. J., 545, 552, 553, *564*, *571*
Snyderman, R., 516, *562*
Sober, H. A., 137, 139, 149, *183*, *282*, *356*
Sobotka, A. K., 288, 308, *354*, *358*
Sohier, R., 542, *563*
Sokol, F., 514, *573*
Solheim, B. G., *445*
Solnik, C., 554, *565*
Solowey, A. C., 400, *444*
Somers, P. J., 27, *111*, *134*, *183*
Somerson, N. L., 460, 461, 474, 475, *477*, *478*
Sondel, P. M., 533, *560*
Sonderkamp, H. J. A., 510, *572*
Soprey, P., 43, 44, *123*
Sorg, C., 73, 74, *123*
Souda, L. L., *122*
Soulsby, E. J. L., 279, *358*
South, M. A., 555, *568*
Spaich, D., 331, *358*
Spaun, J., 106, *123*
Spector, N. M., 508, *572*
Speechley, C. G., 104, *111*
Speel, L. F., 526, 536, *571*
Spencer, C. S., *573*
Spengler, H., *352*
Spicer, S. S., 388, 391, *447*
Spiegelberg, H. L., 178, 179, *185*, 225, *265*
Spieksma, F. T. M., 309, 310, *358*, *359*
Spiele, H., 549, *560*

Spies, J. R., 278, 290, 292, 293, 295, 332, *358*
Spitler, L., 167, *187*, 532, *571*
Spragg, J., 152, *187*, 202, *264*
Sprent, J., 171, *185*, 194, 205, 206, 213, 217, 242, 247, 248, *261*, *262*, *266*, *268*, 507, *568*
Springer, E. L., 25, *123*
Springer, G. F., 19, 52, 107, 108, *120*, *123*, 400, 433, *442*, 491, *571*
Springer, T., 420, 422, 423, 424, *439*
Squire, J. R., 287, *358*
Stacey, M., 27, 30, 32, 33, 53, 78, *111*, *114*, *116*, 134, *183*
Stanley, H. E., 197, *267*
Stanley, J. L., 496, *560*
Stanley, P. M., 489, 490, *571*
Stanworth, D. R., 286, 290, 292, 295, 311, 312, *358*
Stark, O., 366, *445*
Starr, S. E., 549, 550, 559, *561*, *571*
Starzl, T. E., 363, 401, *440*, *445*, 554, *569*
Stashak, P. W., 49, 87, 88, 90, 92, 93, 94, *110*, *111*, 557, *560*
Staub, A. M., 3, 6, 7, 9, 11, 12, 13, 17, 21, 38, 51, 52, 53, 55, 56, 57, 58, 59, 60, 61, 62, 63, 64, 66, 71, 72, 73, 74, 79, 104, *111*, *113*, *114*, *118*, *119*, *120*, *123*, *124*, 134, 136, *185*
Staub-Nielsen, L., 366, 370, 430, *445*
Steele, R. W., *572*
Steeves, R. A., 499, 549, 556, *561*, *567*, *572*
Steffen, G. I., 86, *121*
Stein, W. I., 293, *358*
Steinberg, S., 527, *564*
Steiner, A. L., 260, *268*
Steiner, L. A., 163, *187*
Steinman, H. G., 536, *564*
Steller, R., 100, *119*
Stellner, K., 72, 74, *124*
Stember, R. H., 336, *354*
Stephenson, J. R., 528, 545, 559, *572*
Stern, H., 523, *572*
Sternberg, M., 207, 248, *267*
Sternberger, L. A., 278, *358*
Stevan, M. A., 293, *358*
Stevens, A. H. J., 279, *357*
Stevens, D. A., 534, *563*
Stevens, H., 278, *358*

Stevens, J. G., 523, 542, 546, *568*, *572*
Stevens, R. H., 206, *268*
Steward, T. S., 47, *124*
Stewart, J. A., 396, *445*
Stewart, J. M., 152, *187*
Stierlin, H., 12, 16, 58, *118*, *125*
Stiffel, C., 217, 218, *261*, *266*, 434, *436*
Stimpfling, J. H., 363, 391, *437*, *445*
Stirm, S., 17, 21, 57, 58, 71, *119*, *121*, *124*
Stobo, J. D., 200, 201, 207, *268*
Stocker, B. A. D., 6, 7, 8, 13, 60, 63, 64, *119*, *120*, *124*
Stockert, E., 369, 387, 391, 392, *436*, *442*, 526, 531, *561*, *569*, *572*
Stollar, B. D., 137, *187*
Stoltenberg, I. M., 137, 139, *184*
Stone, S., 541, *566*
Storb, R., 366, *445*
Strand, M., 499, 544, 545, *565*, *572*, *574*
Strano, A. J., 542, *564*
Strauss, J. H., 495, 496, 497, *562*, *572*
Strejan, G. H., 307, 308, *350*, *358*
Strickland, A., 512, 518, *563*
Strober, S., 418, *441*
Stroehmann, I., 366, *436*, *445*
Strohl, W. A., 542, *572*
Strom, R., 213, *265*
Strom, T. B., 260, *268*
Strominger, J. L., 63, *120*, 250, 262, 397, 420, 422, 423, 424, 425, 431, *437*, *439*, *446*
Strong, D. M., 535, 537, *560*, *571*, *572*
Strosberg, A. D., 97, 102, *112*, *116*
Strouk, V., 525, *572*
Stuart, F., 538, *561*
Stuart-Harris, G. H., 507, *571*
Stull, A., 276, 318, *358*
Sturrock, R. D., 344, *351*
Stutman, O., 229, *268*
Sugg, J. Y., 77, *124*
Sulitzeanu, D., 219, 220, 226, 232, *266*, *268*, 527, *566*
Summers, D. F., 53, *124*, 387, *439*, 498, 530, 547, *564*, *568*
Sunayama, H., 47, 53, *124*
Suriano, J. R., 485, *567*
Surprenant, E. L., 323, *359*
Suszko, I. M., 319, *356*
Sutherland, C., 278, *358*
Sutherland, I. W., 33, 34, 41, *114*, *118*, *124*

Sutherland, J. C., 544, *567*
Suzuki, S., 47, 53, *124*
Svedberg, T., 4, *124*
Svehag, S. E., 204, *268*, 500, 501, 502, 512, 541, *572*
Svejgaard, A., 366, 370, 383, 398, 399, 430, *437*, *445*
Svensson, S., 5, 17, 29, 30, 60, 74, *111*, *115*, *116*, *118*
Sverak, L., 345, *357*
Svet-Moldavsky, G. T., 508, *572*
Swedlund, H. A., 273, *352*
Swift, D. L., 322, *357*
Swisher, S. N., 366, *445*
Swoveland, P., 542, *561*
Swyers, J., 535, *566*
Sysma, M. J., 43, 44, *125*
Szenberg, A., 170, *187*

T

Tachibana, D. K., 467, *478*
Tada, R., 542, *574*
Tada, T., 314, 320, 344, *378*
Tagaya, I., 527, *572*
Takagi, Y., 322, *357*
Takahashi, I., 102, *118*
Takahashi, T., 194, 207, 219, 249, *268*, 390, *445*
Takasugi, M., 373, 381, *442*, *445*
Takeichi, N., 526, 548, *566*, *571*
Takemoto, K., 527, *567*
Takeuchi, S., 526, *568*
Takeya, K., 508, *568*
Talmage, D. W., 192, *268*, 401, *440*
Tamura, A., 453, 455, *478*
Tanaka, A., 23, 24, *122*
Tanaka, N., 363, *441*
Tanayaki, N., 250, *268*
Tanford, C., 259, *263*
Tanigaki, N., 406, 420, 421, *442*, *445*
Taniguchi, M., 344, *358*
Taniguchi, S., 513, 515, 516, 542, *574*
Tannenbaum, S. W., 136, *183*
Tao, N., 301, 303, *354*
Taranta, A., 315, *356*
Tarcsay, L., 5, 37, *124*
Tarrow, A. B., 279, 311, *354*, *357*
Tasaki, T., 508, *568*
Taung, A. T., 387, *444*
Taussig, M. J., 247, 251, *268*
Taylor, D., 526, *569*

Taylor, J. M., 489, 572
Taylor, R. B., 176, 177, *185*, *187*, 200, 201, 207, 248, *263*, *267*, *268*, 389. 392, *445*, 508, 530, *560*, 572
Taylor-Robinson, D., 465, 466, *478*
Teichberg, I., 99, *124*
Teichmann, B., 68, 69, 70, 93, *116*
Teitelbaum, D., 164, *185*
Tennant, J. R., 433, *445*
Tennant, R. W., 545, *564*
Terasaki, P. I., 108, *116*, *120*, *123*, 341, 342, 343, 344, *356*, *357*, *358*, 362, 363, 364, 373, 374, 376, 380, 381, 382, 390, 391, 398, 399, 400, 401, 406, 416, 418, 427, 429, 432, 433, *435*, *436*, *438*, *440*, *441*, *442*, *443*, *445*, *446*
Terry, T. M., 468, *478*
Terry, W. D., 199, 203, *267*
Tevethia, S. S., 527, *572*
Thalenfeld, B., 372, *440*
Thé, T. H., 527, *572*
Theis, G. A., 249, *268*
Thieme, T. R., 48, *124*
Thies, D., 527, *568*
Thind, I. S., 508, *572*
Thirkill, C. E., 464, *478*
Thomas, D. B., 393, *443*
Thomas, E. D., 366, *445*
Thompson, J. L., 32, 34, *118*
Thompson, K., 146, 165, *184*, *187*, 243, *268*, 313, 348, *350*
Thomssen, R., 548, *560*
Thor, D. E., 168, *184*
Thorbecke, G. J., 214, 249, *268*
Thorne, H. V., 277, 282, 283, *351*, *353*
Thorsby, E., 364, 366, 368, 370, 398, 399, 430, *440*, *445*, *446*
Thrower, K. J., 468, *477*
Thurman, G. B., 535, 537, *560*, *571*, *572*
Thurow, H. D., 32, 34, *124*
Tigelaar, R. E., 173, *183*
Tillack, T. W., *268*
Tinelli, R., 17, 58, 60, 63, 64, 73, 74, *118*, *124*
Ting, A., 382, *446*
Ting, C. C., 386, *446*, 527, *572*
Ting, R. C., 508, 528, 567, *568*
Tips, R. L., 330, *358*
Todaro, G. J., 388, *440*, 499, 554, *560*, *569*, *572*
Todd, D. V., 96, *118*

Toffler, O., *352*
Tolh, E. K., 367, *435*
Tomasi, T. B., 101, *124*, 506, *572*
Tomasz, A., 31, *124*
Tomescu, N., 542, *563*
Tomioka, H., 273, *353*
Tomita, M., 258, *266*
Tompkins, W. A. F., 527, 534, *572*
Torii, M., 84, 93, *124*
Torres, E. J., 507, *573*
Torrigiani, G., 249, *263*
Tosi, R. M., 381, 384, 406, *438*, *446*
Tosolini, F. A., *572*
Tourtellotte, M. E., 198, *268*, 468, *477*
Toussaint, A. J., 515, *568*
Toy, S. T., 554, *573*
Tozawa, 494, *572*
Trabold, N., 366, *445*
Tralka, T. S., 542, *561*
Trapani, R. J., 374, *438*
Trasher, D. L., 382, *446*
Treffers, H. P., 104, *120*
Trefts, P., 178, *187*
Trinchieri, G., 200, *261*, 389, 390, 391, 392, 397, 431, *436*
Tripp, M., 363, 381, 431, *436*, *443*
Troup, G. M., 363, 373, 375, *446*
Truffa-Bachi, P., 233, *268*, *269*
Tsakraklides, E., 387, *446*
Tsuboi, S., 293, *354*
Turino, G. M., 279, 311, *354*
Turk, J. G., 533, *572*
Turner, H. C., 474, *476*
Turner, K. J., 107, *122*
Turner, M. J., 250, *262*, 397, 420, 422, 423, 424, 425, 431, *437*, *439*, *446*
Tyan, M. L., 333, *355*
Tyler, J. M., 27, 28, *124*, *125*
Tyndall, R. L., 552, *570*
Tyrrell, D. A. J., 491, 515, *563*, *566*

U

Uchida, T., 17, 60, 61, 63, 66, 74, *122*, *124*, 141, *187*, 529, *570*
Udomsakdi, S., 511, *563*
Ueda, Y., 527, *572*
Uemur, K., 106, *123*
Uetake, H., 60, 66, *124*
Uhlenbruck, G., 408, *446*
Uhr, J. W., 194, 201, 207, 211, 214, 215, 216, 246, 248, *261*, *269*, 500, *572*

Ukena, T. E., 528, *570*
Ukita, T., 258, *266*
Umberger, E. J., 278, *358*
Unanue, E. R., 176, *187*, 200, 201, 213, 215, 221, 237, 238, 239, 248, 250, *263*, *264*, *267*, *268*, *269*, 374, 377, 389, *440*, *446*
Underdown, B. J., 283, 295, 299, 303, *358*
Unger, L., 276, *358*
Unrau, A. M., 4, *124*

V

Vahlne, G., 103, *125*
Valdesuso, J. R., 460, *478*
Valentine, M. D., 308, *354*, *358*
Valentine, R. C., 202, 203, *269*
Vallotton, M., 202, *264*
Valtonen, M., 104, *119*, *125*
Valtonen, V. V., 104, *119*, *125*
Van Arsdel, P. P., 330, *358*
van den Tweel, J. G., 364, *446*
Vanderleeden, J. C., 236, *266*
van der Scheer, J., 132, 137, *185*
van der Steen, G. J., 364, *446*
van der Veen, J., 510, *572*
VanderVeer, A., 330, 331, *352*
van der Weerdt, C. H. M., 372, *446*
Vandvik, B., 494, *572*
Van Furth, R., 206, *269*
Van Holde, K. E., 287, *359*
van Hooff, J. P., 364, *446*
van Leeuwen, A., 363, 364, 374, 383, 387, 406, *435*, *437*, *446*
Vannier, W. E., 293, *359*
van Rood, J. J., 363, 364, 366, 374, 383, 387, 406, *435*, *436*, *437*, *446*
van Santen, M. C., 406, *446*
van Vreeswijk, W., 363, 367, *435*
Van Vunakis, H., 137, 139, *187*
Varekamp, H., 309, 310, *359*
Varga, J. M., 282, *352*
Vasconcelos-Costa, J., 527, *572*
Vassalli, P., 207, 215, 216, 217, 246, 248, *265*
Vaughan, W. T., 330, *359*
Vaz, N. M., 314, 329, 333, *354*, *359*
Verheij, H. M., 472, *478*
Vernon, C. A., 295, 299, 308, 328, *358*
Vernon, M. L., 551, *569*
Vesterberg, O., 286, 287, *359*

Vicari, G., 100, 102, *125*
Vincent, M. M., *572*
Vinuela, E., 287, *357*
Virelizier, J. L., 508, 509, 511, *572*
Vitetta, E. S., 194, 201, 207, 211, 214, 215, 216, 246, 248, *261*, *269*
Vladutin, A. O., 432, *446*
Vogt, A., 513, *572*
Vogt, M., 512, 518, *563*
Voigtmann, R., 406, 408, *436*, *446*
Vojtiskova, M., 385, 386, *446*
Volkert, M., 526, 540, 543, *567*, *573*
von Pirquet, C., 274, 311, *359*, 480, 483, 533, 549, *573*
Voorhorst, R., 293, 309, 310, *358*, *359*
Voracová, B., 368, *438*
Vosti, K. L., 106, 107, *125*
Vredevoe, D. L., 380, *446*
Vriesendorp, H. M., 366, *446*

W

Wadell, G., 487, 488, *568*, *573*
Wagner, H. C., 277, 306, *357*
Wagner, J. E., 42, 82, *117*
Wagner, R., 497, 514, *566*
Wahren, B., 538, 546, *573*
Wakim, K. C., 550, *573*
Waks, T., 194, 208, *263*
Waldman, R. H., 507, 536, *563*, *573*
Waldmann, T., *568*
Walford, R. L., 362, 363, 364, 373, 375, 380, 383, 387, 391, 432, *437*, *445*, *446*, *447*
Walker, D. L., 526, 536, 549, *569*, *571*
Wallach, D. F. H., 194, *263*
Wallenfels, B., 13, *122*
Wallis, V., 171, *184*
Walls, B. B., 460, *478*
Walters, C. S., 177, *186*
Walters, D., 344, *351*
Walz, M. A., 543, *573*
Walzer, M., 278, 279, *352*, *358*, *359*
Wang, A. C., 156, *187*
Wang, J. L., 421, 429, *437*
Wang, L., *571*
Wang, S. P., 451, 459, 464, 477, *478*
Ward, F. E., 376, 382, 387, *344*, *447*
Ward, J. R., 467, *476*
Warfield, D. T., 503, *562*
Warmsley, A. M. H., 393, *442*, *447*

Author Index

Warner, N. L., 170, *187*, 213, 214, 215, 221, 226, 230, 231, 232, 237, 238, 248, 249, *261, 263, 264, 266, 268, 269*
Warren, L., 412, *447*
Warren, S. A., 278, *358*
Warthin, A. S., 551, *573*
Warwick, A., 520, 521, *560, 566*
Wasserman, E., 49, *125*
Watanabe, M., 494, *572*
Waterfield, M. D., 96, 97, 98, *117*
Waterhouse, A. T., 278, *359*
Waters, H., 362, 375, 387, 432, *447*
Waterson, A. P., 516, *560*
Watkins, J. F., 529, 547, *573*
Watson, B., 103, *125*
Watson, D. H., 484, 485, 514, 535, *570, 573*
Watson, M. J., 28, *125*
Watson, R. O., 459, *476*
Watt, B. J., 292, 307, *353*
Wayne, F. M., 382, *439*
Webb, C., 164, *185*
Webb, D., 259, *269*
Webb, H. E., 548, *573*
Webb, S. R., 215, 217, 219, 249, *269*
Webb, T., 135, *185*
Webb, W. F., 373, *447*
Webley, D. M., 101, *111*
Webster, M. E., 42, *112, 125*
Webster, R. G., 493, 500, 515, *566, 567, 573*
Wecker, E., 172, *187*
Weckesser, J., 11, *120*
Wedderburn, N., 549, *571*
Weigert, M. G., 94, 100, *112, 119*, 160, *187*
Weigle, J., 363, *443*
Weigle, W. O., 87, 94, *112, 113*, 170, 178, 179, *185, 187*, 225, 231, 253, *262, 265*
Weiner, A., 330, *359*
Weinstein, R., 230, 231, *262*
Weinstein, W. J., 372, *440*
Weir, D. M., 49, *121*
Weisbart, R. H., 373, *447*
Weiss, E., 455, 456, *478*
Weller, T. H., 551, *562*
Wells, H. G., 128, *187*
Wells, J. V., 259, *263*
Welsh, K. I., 397, 407, 419, 429, *436, 444*
Werch, J., 555, *568*
Werner, T. C., 154, *183*, 203, *269*

Wessels, N. K., 396, *447*
Westaway, E. G., 511, *573*
Westbrook, D. L., 366, *446*
Westmoreland, D., 529, *573*
Westphal, O., 3, 4, 6, 7, 9, 11, 12, 13, 16, 17, 18, 19, 20, 21, 22, 23, 24, 25, 26, 37, 38, 49, 51, 52, 53, 55, 56, 57, 58, 59, 61, 62, 63, 64, 66, 68, 69, 70, 71, 72, 73, 74, 79, 80, 86, 93, 104, 105, 106, *111, 113, 114, 115, 116, 117, 118, 119, 120, 121, 122, 123, 124, 125*, 134, 136, *185*
Wetherbee, R. G., 536, *573*
Wetton, R., 549, *567*
Whang, H. Y., 7, *120, 125*
Wheat, R. W., 3, 6, 7, 12, 13, 16, 21, 25, 31, 32, 33, 36, 52, 53, 56, 104, *114, 119*
Wheeler, C. J., 523, *573*
Wheelock, E. F., 554, 555, *563, 573*
White, D. O., 489, 490, *571, 572*
White, D. S. G., 366, *447*
White, R. E., 106, *111*
White, R. G., 551, *573*
Whiteman, G. B., 307, 320, *357*
Whitford, H. W., 549, *567*
Wide, L., 273, 287, 288, 307, *353, 359*
Wiener, F., 212, *267*
Wigand, R., 488, *573*
Wigzell, H., 206, 212, 233, 249, *265, 269*
Wiktor, T. J., 497, 514, 526, *563, 565, 573*
Wilcox, W. C., 487, 514, *573*
Wildy, P., 484, *573*
Wilkins, M. H. F., 198, *269*
Wilkinson, J. F., 32, 33, 41, *113, 118, 124*
Wilkinson, J. M., 135, 140, 141, 160, *184, 186*
Wilkinson, R. G., 7, 8, 13, *120*
Willcox, N., 232, 236, 237, 238, 239, *264*
Willers, J. M. N., 43, 44, *125*
Williams, A. F., 208, 213, 215, 248, *264*
Williams, A. I. O., 200, *266*
Williams, B. M., 523, *572*
Williams, C. O., 454, 465, *476, 478*
Williams, E. B., 532, *571*
Williams, E. C., 129, 166, 167, 169, 173, 175, 182, *183, 187*
Williams, G. M., 401, *444*
Williams, R. C., 3, 95, 107, 108, *113, 118*
Williams, R. W., 375, *441*

Williams, T. D., 467, *478*
Williamson, A. R., 39, 40, *125*, 206, *268*
Williamson, P., 52, *123*
Willing, R. R., 327, *354*
Willingham, M. C., 388, 391, *447*
Wilson, A. B., 207, 262
Wilson, A. F., 323, *359*
Wilson, B. J., 316, *355*
Wilson, J. D., 201, 218, *269*
Wilson, S. K., 156, *187*
Wilt, F. H., 396, *447*
Winchurch, R., 259, *269*
Winkler, K. C., 43, 44, *125*
Winn, H. J., 391, 400, *444*, *447*
Winston, S. H., 526, 537, *570*
Winzler, R. J., 199, *264*, *269*
Wioland, M., 194, *269*
Wistar, R., 537, *560*
Witebsky, E., 462, *477*
Wittler, R. G., 454, 465, *476*, *478*
Wodehouse, R. P., 275, 277, 291, 300, 301, *359*
Woese, C., 468, *477*
Wofsy, L., 134, *184*, 233, *264*, *268*, *269*
Wohlenberg, C., 526, 527, 530, 535, *561*, *570*
Wolberg, C., 106, *125*
Wolf, H., 403, *447*
Wong, K. H., 106, *125*
Wood, H. A., 499, 526, 544, *560*
Wood, M. L., 554, *565*
Wood, P. A., 559, *571*
Wood, S. H., 507, *573*
Wood, W. B., Jr., 103, *125*
Woodbury, M. A., 337, *351*
Woodruff, J. F., 549, 554, *573*
Woodruff, J. J., 549, 554, *573*
Work, T. S., 398, *435*
Wraith, D. G., 309, 310, *355*
Wray, S. W., 505, *560*
Wrede, J., 68, 73, 93, *116*
Wright, A., 64, 66, 68, 74, *122*
Wright, G. L. T., 291, *359*
Wright, G. P., 278, *359*
Wright, P. W., 418, *441*, 526, 527, 540, *573*
Wrigley, N. G., 490, *573*
Wu, H., 301, 357, 528, *573*
Wu, T. T., 159, 160, *185*, *187*
Wunderlich, J. R., 249, *262*

Wyman, J., 150, *186*, 259, *266*
Wyman, M., 275, 329, *359*

Y

Yadomae, T., 27, *120*
Yagi, Y., 421, *442*
Yahara, I., 200, 201, *269*
Yamamoto, R., 467, *477*
Yamanouchi, K., 511, 526, 550, 552, *573*
Yang, H. Y., 524, *573*
Yang, Y., 34, *113*
Yaron, A., 137, 138, 149, 169, 175, *183*, *187*
Yasuda, J., 529, *573*
Yee, C. L., 542, *561*
Yin, H. H., 528, *570*
Yman, L., 293, *351*
Yonkovich, S. J., 160, *187*
Yoo, T. J., 158, *187*
Yoshikawa, Y., 511, 550, 552, *573*
Yoshiki, T., 499, 530, 544, 545, *565*, *574*
Yoshino, K., 513, 515, 516, 542, *574*
Young, B. G., 64, *125*
Young, E., 281, 295, 311, *351*, *356*
Young, J. D., 140, 141, 165, 168, *183*, *187*, 532, *571*
Young, L. E., 366, *445*
Young, N. M., 100, 101, 102, 103, *118*, *125*
Yowell, R. L., 233, *263*
Yphantis, D. A., 26, *125*
Yuhas, J. M., 545, *564*
Yunginger, J. W., 290, 301, *359*
Yunis, E. J., 337, *351*, 376, 382, 388, *439*, *440*, *447*
Yurconic, M., 545, *561*, *565*
Yurewicz, E. G., 26, *125*

Z

Zaalberg, O. B., 217, *269*
Zak, S., 169, 172, 174, *185*
Zamenhof, S., 38, 39, 40, 76, *122*, *125*
Zappacosta, S., 154, *186*
Zazepizki, E., 147, *187*
Zee, T. W., 373, *443*
Zeigel, R. F., 527, *563*
Zeiller, K., 194, *269*
Zeiss, C. R., 319, *356*
Zeller, E., 375, *446*

Author Index

Zeman, W., 542, 565
Zervas, J. D., 386, 432, *439, 447*
Zier, K. S., 533, *560*
Zieve, I., 330, *359*
Zinbar, S. N., 508, *572*
Zinder, N. D., 64, *125*
Zinkernagel, R. M., 244, *269*, 526, 531, 540, *574*
Zisman, B., 521, *574*
Zmijewski, C. M., 406, *436*
Zola, H., 3, 26, 83, 85, 86, 87, 91, 92, 93, 94, 103, *116*
Zolla, S. B., 134, *187*
Zucker-Franklin, D., *447*
Zupnik, J. S., 468, *478*
zur Hausen, H., 403, *447*

Subject Index

A

Acetolysis of sugar constituents, 4
Acholeplasma species, 450–451, 454, 457, 458, 461, 472, 473
Actinomycin D, and histocompatibility antigen, 395–396
Adenovirus, 485–489, 542
   A antigen, 487
   B antigen, 487
   C antigen, 487
   classification, 485
   fiber, 488
   penton, 488
   structure, 486
Agamma calf serum, 462
Alder pollen allergen, 306
Allergens, 271–359
   from *Alternaria* (mold), 278
   analysis
      biological, 286–287
      chemical, 286–287
      physical, 286–287
   areas of research, 273–274, 282–319
   from *Ascaris lumbricoides* (roundworm), 279, 307–308, 314
   atopic, 272
   from caddis fly, 315
   from castor bean, 278
   from codfish muscle, 294–295, 299, 306–307
   from cotton seed, 278
   dextran as, 278–279
   dosage, 272, 323
   egg white as, 294–295
   entry, route of, 272, 274–275
   food as, 279
   hapten, 315–317
   history, 274–280
   from horse antiserum, 278
   horse dander as, 294–295
   from housedust, 278, 309–310
   from *Hymenoptera* venom, 308
   for immunization, 319–322
   ingested, 279–280
   inhaled, 277–279
   injected, 278–279
   insects as, 278
   isolation methods, 282
   major, 281
   methodology, 282–290
      analysis, 286–290
      fractionations, 282–286
      methods, 287
   nomenclature, 280–282
   release from pollen, 324–327
      rate of, 324–327
   research areas, 273–274, 282–319
   route of entry, 272, 274–275
   sensitization by, 319–329
   size of, 322
   stimulation by, 319–329
   structure, 292
   types of, 275–282, 290–310
      Ascaris, 279–280, 299, 307–308, 314–315
      caddis fly, 315
      chlorogenic acid, 308–309
      codfish muscle, 306–307
      housedust, 309–310
      Hymenoptera venom, 308
      mite, 309–310
      pollens, 291–306
         from grass, 291–300
         from trees, 305–306
         from weeds, 300–305
   valence, 315–317
Allergenicity
   assay of, 286
   leukocyte histamine release technique, 288
   prick test, 288

Subject Index

scratch test, 288
theories, 311–315
  Berren's, 311
  bridging concept, 315
  lysine–sugar sites, 311
  reagin concept, 311
  Stanworth's, 312
  von Pirquet's (1906), 311
Allergoid, 317–319
  formaldehyde-treated, 319
  glutaraldehyde-treated, 319
  immunotherapy, 319
Allergy
  and allergens, 271–359
  family predisposition, 330
  family studies, 335–340
  genetics of, 329–345
    history, 329–332
  hayfever, 275–276
  history of, 274–280
  IgE mediated, 328–329, 332–333
  Ir gene, 332–333
  permeability theory, 331
  reactions, 322–324
  and ribonuclease (RNase), 332
  theories, 311–315
  three-gene hypothesis, 330
  Tips' theory, 330–331
  twin studies, 331
  von Pirquet (1906), 274
Alginate, 55
Alphavirus, 495
Ambrosia elatior, see Ragweed
Anaphylaxis, 315–316
Antibody
  and antigen, lock-and-key concept, 128, 153
  charge, 142–143
  combining site, 153–162
  complementarity, 136, 153–155
  –ferritin conjugation technique, 391
  –hapten interaction, 129–133
    structural specificity, 130–131
  heterogeneity, 133
    normal, 96
    restricted, 95–99
  hypervariable region, 158–162
  location of combining site, 158–162
  secretory, 506–507
  specificity, 142, 144

stereospecificity, 149
structure, 155–158
subsite, as concept, 148
Antigen
  A of adenovirus, 487
  A of *Escherichia coli*, 35, 38
  –antibody lock-and-key concept, 128
  artificial, 2, 68–74
  B of adenovirus, 487
  B of *Escherichia coli*, 35
  B of inbred rat, 365
  Boivin-type O, 85
  C of adenovirus, 487
  C (colorless) of virus, 484
  of *Candida*, 549–550
  capping, 530
  capsular polysaccharide, microbial, 25–45
  of *Chlamydia*, 467–475
  Creg HL-A8, 340–341, 345
  D (dense) of virus, 484
  D of timothy grass pollen, 316
  determinant, 127–187
  DL of dog, 366
  E of ragweed, 325–327, 336
  Forssman, 491
  galactan as, 468
  glucan as, 468
  GPL of guinea pig, 367
  H, 361–447
  H-1 of inbred rat, 365
  H-2, 265, 362, 368–369
  of *Haemophilus*, 38–40
  histocompatibility, 250–251, 361–447
  host, 528, 530
  II, 362
  immunobiology of, 83–108
  immunochemistry of, 49–83
  immunogenicity of, 83–95
  K, 31, 104, 106
  K of *Escherichia coli*, 35
  of *Klebsiella*, 31–35
  L of *Escherichia coli*, 35
  M (mucus), 40–42
  M of influenza virus, 492
  of *Mycoplasma*, 473–475
  O, 70
  O, Boivin-type, 85
  O of *Escherichia coli*, 19
  O of *Salmonella*, 17

O of *Shigella*, 19
pneumococcal, 26-31, 54-55, 86-88, 90-92, 95-98, 101-103
polysaccharide, microbial, as, 25-45
reaction with lymphocyte, 190
receptor complex, 251-257
  historical, 191-193
  IgM, 251-252
  lymphocytic, 189-269
recognition, as a concept, 174
RhL in rhesus monkey, 366
S of influenza virus, 492-493
specificity, 142, 144, 151
of *Staphylococcus*, 40
stimulating B lymphocytes, 252-254
of *Streptococcus*, 40, 42-45, 82
structure, 150
surface-coded, 525-527
synthetic, 147
TL (thymus-leukemia) in mouse, 531
transplantation, in inbred mouse, 362
tumor transplantation, 547
Vi of *Citrobacter ballerup*, 42
Vi of *Escherichia coli*, 42, 104, 106
virus-coded, 483-499, 507-510, 524-528
of *Xanthomonas campestris*, 26
Antigen-binding cells
  by B lymphocytes, 221-222, 239
  depletion, 233-235
  enrichment, 233-235
  hierarchy, 222
  in immune animals, 226-229
  immunocompetence, 232-242
  inactivation, specific, 235-240
  inhibition, 226, 228
  lymphocytes as, 217-232
  reduction in, 207
  specificity, 232-242
  suicide, 235-240
  by T lymphocytes, 221-222, 225-227, 239
  temperature effect, 222
  and tolerance, 231-232
Antigenicity, chemical basis of, 3
Apomyoglobin, 135
Arbovirus
  A, 495
  B, 495
Arenavirus, 540-541

Arginine deiminase, 475
Ascaris lumbricoides allergen, 279, 307-308, 314
Ascaris suum allergen, 299, 307-308, 314-315
  as a universal allergen, 280
Asterococcus, 451
Atopen, *see* Allergen atopic
Autoimmunity, 548-549
Autumnal catarrh, *see* Ragweed pollen hayfever

B

B cell, *see* Lymphocyte, B cell
$\beta_2\mu$, *see* β_2 Microglobulin
Bacillus anthracis poly-γ-D-glutamic acid capsule, 139
Bacillus palustris, 89
Bee sting, *see* Hymenoptera venom
Birch pollen as allergen, 324
  allergy in Scandinavia, 306
Blastogenesis of lymphocyte, 539-540
Boivin-type O antigen, 85
BPO-FLYS treatment, 317
Bradykinin, 152
Bridging theory of anaphylaxis, 315-316
Burkitt's lymphoma, 206
Burnet's clonal selection theory, 192
Burnet's self-nonself theory, 192
Bursectomy, 170

C

C (colorless) antigen, viral, 484
3-Caffeoylquinic acid, *see* Chlorogenic acid
Calf serum, agamma, 462
Candida antigen, 549-550
Capsule
  antigens of, 26-31
    Escherichia coli, 35-38
    Haemophilus, 38-40
    Klebsiella, 31-35
    Pneumococcus, 26-31, 54-55
    Staphylococcus, 40
  isolation, 25
  pathogenicity, 25
  polysaccharides, 25-42
  purification, 26
Castor bean as allergen, 294-295
Castor oil sensitivity in workers, 320

Subject Index

Cell death detection methods, 380–388
  by dye exclusion, 380
  by fluorochromasia test, 381
  by isotope marker, 381
Cell-mediated immunity (CMI), 549
  blastogenic response, 532
  migration inhibition factor (MIF) production, 532
  to viruses, 532–541
Chemotype
  as a concept, 12
  of Enterobacteriaceae, 14–16
  R, 23
Chikungunya virus, 496
Chlamydia, 449–478
  analysis of antigens, 464
  antigens, 467–475
    analysis, 464
    carbohydrate as, 468–469
    lipid as, 469–472
    protein as, 472–475
    structure, 467–475
  homogeneity, serological, 459
  host–parasite relationship, 453–454
  morphology, 453
Chlorogenic acid as allergen, from green coffee beans, 308–309
Cholesterol, 471
Chromium-release cell-mediated cytotoxicity assay, 534, 538
Citrobacter ballerup, Vi antigen, 42
Clonal selection theory tested, 219
Cobra venom, 253
Cod muscle as allergen, 294–295, 299, 306–307
Cohn–Bretscher hypothesis, 252–257
Colanic acid, *see* M antigen
Collagen, 151
Column chromatography, 233–234
Complement, 516–517
  and cytolysis, 207
  and lymphocytotoxicity test, 363, 372–383
  pathway of activation, 275–280
  -platelet fixation, 383
  -resistant bacteria, 104–105
  role of, 375–380
  sources of, 376
  and virolysis, 516
Concanavalin A, 491

Conversion, lysogenic, 63–64
  by phage, 64–66, 104
Core oligosaccharide
  defective, 22–23
  R-specific, 13–21
Corona virus, 516
Coxsackie virus, 503
Creg antigen, HL-A8, 340–341, 345
Cross-reactivity, 95, 97–99, 163–165, 170
  of HL-A, 398–401
Cycloheximide, and HL-A, 398
Cytolosis, complement-mediated, 207
Cytomegalovirus, 484, 535
  in mouse, 542
  posttransfusion syndrome, 555
Cytotoxic negative-absorption positive (CYNAP) reaction, 381, 387

D

D (dense) antigen, viral, 484
6-Deoxyhexosamine of *Escherichia coli*, 12
Dermatophagoides (mite)
  as allergen, 309–310
  in housedust, 309–310
Desensitization treatment, 316–317
  introduced by Noon (1911), 276
Detergent, 407
Determinant
  carbohydrate, 68–74
    disaccharide, 68
    monospecific, 68–73
    multispecific, 73–74
  carrier activity, 172–175
  conformational, 54–55
  and haptens, 162–164, 175–179
  noncarbohydrate, 74–76
    acetal substitution, 75–76
    acetyl substitution, 74
    ketal substitution, 74
    phosphate substitution, 76
    sulfate substitution, 76
Determinant, antigenic, 133–153
  Hc, 239
  Hv, 239
  identification, 133–136
  selection
    accessibility, 141–142
    charge, 142–143
    factors, 141–145

genetic, 143–145
sequential, 147
size, 136–141
Determinant, immunogenic, 129, 167–179
and haptens, 162–164, 175–179
Dextran, 3, 45–47, 84–85, 101, 137, 138, 148, 278–279
inhibition of precipitation of human anti-dextran, 50
3,6-Dideoxyhexose, 57–59, 71, 72
of *Salmonella*, 12
Diglyceride, 469–470, 472
Diplococcus pneumoniae capsular polysaccharide antigen, 26–31
composition, 27
cross-reacting, 77–80
oligosaccharide, 30
C polysaccharide, 31
structure, 28–29
DL antigen in dog, 366
α-DPN-lysine, 138
Dye exclusion, measuring cell death, 380

E

Ectromelia virus in mice, 504, 531
Egg white as allergen, 294–295
Ehrlich's side chain theory, 191
Electrophoresis, and altered motility, 207
Encephalomyocarditis virus, 521
Epitope, 251, 508
density, 255–256
Epstein–Barr virus, 484, 535, 542
in all lymphoid cell lines, 403
Escherichia coli
capsular polysaccharide antigens, 35–38, 53–54, 134
A, 35, 38
B, 35
composition, 36
K, 35
L, 35
O, 35
structure, 37–38
Vi, 42
core oligosaccharide, 20–21
6-deoxyhexosamine, 12
hexuronic acid, 12, 38
lipopolysaccharide, O-antigenic, 19

F

Fab subunit of immunoglobulin, 204–205, 514
Fc subunit of immunoglobulin, 205–206, 513
Ferritin antibody conjugation technique, 391
Fibroma virus in rabbit, 534
Flagellin, bacterial, 220, 222, 230, 232, 240–241, 252, 253, 255
Flavivirus, 495, 510–511, 521
Fluorochromasia test, 381
Food allergy in children, 322
Foot-and-mouth disease virus, 504, 514
Form variation, 63
Forssman antigen, 491
Fraction, persistent, 517

G

Gadus callarias, see Cod
Galactan as antigen, 468
Ganglioside, 529
Glucagon, 166–168
fragment, 166
structure, 166
Glucan as antigen, 468
Glycolipid, 469–472
Glycophospholipid, 471
Glycoprotein, viral, 514
GPL antigen in guinea pig, 367
Graft rejection, 363
Green coffee sensitivity in workers, 309
Gross leukemogenic virus, 528, 544–546, 548
Gumboro disease, 553

H

H-1 (antigen B) in inbred rat, 365
H-2 of inbred mouse, 265, 368–369
Haemophilus influenzae capsular polysaccharide antigen, 38–40
composition, 39
structure, 39
Haemophilus suis capsular polysaccharide antigen, structure, 40
Hapten, 191
–antibody interaction, 129–133
structural specificity, 130–131
–carrier conjugate, 164

Subject Index

and immunogen, 162–164
immunotherapy, 317
inhibition assay, 137
reactivity, 134
specificity, 130–133
synthetic, 136
Hayfever, see Allergy
Hemagglutination enhancement antibody consumption test, 487
Hemocyanin, 220, 223, 230, 232, 241
Hepatitis virus in mouse, 520–521, 553
Herpes simplex virus, 484–485, 521–523, 535
Histocompatibility antigen, 250–251, 361–447
  II, 362
  of dog, 366
  extraction of soluble, 407–414
    by potassium chloride, 408–414
  genetics, 368–371
  of guinea pig, 367–368
  H antigen, 361–447
    activity, biologic, 402–418
    on cell membrane, 388–392
    cell surface expression of, 385–398
    cross-reactivity, 398–401
    detection, serologic, 371–384
    expression during cell cycle, 392–395
    extraction, 402–418
    genetics, 368–369
    as genetic marker, 362
    on malignant cell, 386
    purification, 402–418
    sources, 402–407
    on spermatozoa, 385
    tissue distribution, 385–388
    on trophoblast cell, 386
    on virus-infected cell, 387–388
HL antigen (HL-A), 369–371
  alloantiserum, 374–375, 379–380
  cross-reactivity, 398–399
  from cultured cells, 403
  evaluation, serologic, 383–384
    by absorption test, 384
    by blocking test, 383–384
    by CYNAP reaction, 384
    by microadsorption, 384
  extraction, 407–414
  genetics, 369–371
  and glomerulonephritis, 364
  and Hodgkin's disease, 364
  and leukemia, 364
  named, 364
  and peripheral leukocytes, 404
  and platelets, 404–406
  polymorphism, 432
  and serum, 406–407
  solubilization, 364
  from spent medium, 403–404
  and susceptibility to disease, 433
  and virus infection, 432
HL-A8 Creg antigen, 340–341, 345
history, 362–365
and IgE regulating gene, see Ir gene
lymphocytotoxicity assay, 372–383
microcytotoxicity test, 373
and β_2 microglobulin, 420–430
of mouse, 365
of pig, 366
–platelet complement fixation, 383
properties
  chemical, 418–420
  molecular weight, 418
  physical, 418
purification, 414–416
  strategy, 414
of rat, 365–366
reactivity, biologic, 416–418
of rhesus monkey, 366
Histocompatibility Workshops, international, 364
Honey bee venom, see Hymenoptera venom
Horse dander as allergen, 294–295
Host-versus-graft reaction, 555–556
Housedust as allergen, 309–310
Hydrophobicity, 140
Hymenoptera venom
  as allergen, 294–295, 308
  bee sting, 321
  mellitin, 308
  phospholipase A, 299
Hypersensitivity
  delayed, 164, 238, 482
  immediate, 271–272

I

Immune response
  degenerate, 99

gene, 247–250, 332–333, 343–345, 505
  for E antigen, 337, 340–342
  on T cell, 249–250
  genetic control of, 94–95
  restricted, 97
  suppression by a virus, 483
  in virus infection, 479–574
Immunity
  cell cooperation in, 170–172
  cellular, 164–165, 172–175, *see also* Lymphocyte
  dichotomy of, 164–165
  humoral, 164–165
  persistence, 541–543
  specificity, 165–170
Immunochemistry of microbial polysaccharides, 49–83
  carbohydrate determinants, 50–55
  methods, serologic, 49
Immunodiffusion, double, 462–464
Immunodominance, 134, 145–153
  factors, 145–153
    accessibility, 147–149
    configuration, optical, 149–150
    conformation, 150–153
  of sugar, 51–52, 67
Immunofluorescence, 207
Immunogenicity, 162–163
  defined, 129
  of polysaccharide, 83–95
  versus tolerogenicity, 89–93
Immunoglobulin
  as antigen receptor, 243–247
    biologic function, 246–247
    specificity, 243–245
    synthesis, 245–246
  on B cell, 208–214
  function, 204–206
    Fab subunit, 204–205
    Fc subunit, 205–206
  on lymphocyte plasma membrane, 206–217
  properties, 201–206
    shape, 202–204
    size, 202–204
  quantitation, 212–213
  on T cell, 214–217
  use
    direct, 207
    indirect, 207
Immunoglobulin A, 506, 507

Immunoglobulin D, 211
Immunoglobulin E
  animal experiment, 333–334
  artificially induced, 328–329
  discovery, 273
  family studies, 335–339
  gene, regulating, 339–344
  genetic control of level in serum, 339–340
  —mediated sensitivity, 347
  population studies, 334–335
  radioimmunoassay (RIA), 273
  regulating gene, 339–344
Immunoglobulin G, 202–204, 206, 515
  blocking antibody, 318
  shape, 203
  size, 203
  structure, 155
    H chain, 156–158
    L chain, 156–158
  viral, 500–504
Immunoglobulin M, 203–206, 210–211, 506–507, 515
  on B cell, 208–209
  plasma membrane model, 205
  receptor, 258–259
  rheumatoid factor, 519
  7 S, 203, 206
  19 S, 204
  viral, 500–504
Immunopotency, 141, 145, 150
Immunoprophylaxis, 480
Immunotherapy in allergy, 276, 317
  with allergoid, 319
Influenza virus, 489–494, 504, 510, 536
  Forssman antigen, 491
  hemagglutinin, 489, 492, 509
  model, 491
  morphology, 490
  M protein, 492
  neuraminidase, 492, 493
  S antigen, 492–493
  spikes, 491
Interferon, 534
Isoallergen, 281
Isoantigen
  A, 547
  B, 547

J

Jerne's theory, 192
June cold, *see* Grass pollen hayfever

Subject Index

K

K antigen, 31, 104, 106
Kauffmann–White schema for *Salmonella*, 56
Klebsiella
    Capsular polysaccharide antigens, 31–35
        composition, 32–37
        structure, 36–37
    lipopolysaccharide, O-antigenic, 18
Kupffer cell, virus removal by, 519

L

Lactate dehydrogenase virus, 495, 549–552
Landsteiner's hapten, 191
Laurell's crossed immunoelectrophoresis technique, 346
Laurell's two-dimensional electrophoretic method, 464
LCM virus, *see* Lymphochoriomeningitis virus
LD_{50}, 103, 104
Lecithin, 471
Leukemia, 387
    virus, *see* Gross leukemogenic virus
Leukoagglutination, 363, 371
Leukoagglutinin, alloimmune, 363
Leukocyte
    agglutinin, 363
    alloantibody, 363
    peripheral, 404
Leukocyte histamine release technique, 274, 288–290
Levan, 47
Linkage disequilibrium, 343
Lipid A of *Salmonella*, 21–25
    constituents, 24
    structure, 24
Lipopolysaccharide
    bacterial, 5–25
    biochemistry, 7
    genetic determination, 7
    isolation, 8–11
    mutant, 7–8
    in R mutant of *Salmonella*, 22
    of *Salmonella typhimurium*, 25
    somatic, 2
    structure, 6–7
    regions I, II, III, 6–7
    sugar, 10–11, 14–16
Lolium perenne, *see* Perennial rye grass
Lymphocyte
    antigen binding on, 217–232
    receptor for, 242–251
    rosette formation, 217–219, 241
    B cell, 93–94, 171–173, 175, 178, 179, 182, 194, 481–482, 507–511, 543, 546, 556
    antigen binding, 239
    function, 196–197
    immunocompetence, depletion of, 235–238
    immunoglobulin, capped, 208
    immunoglobulin M (IgM) on, 208–212, 245
    inhibition by anti-Ig serum, 246
    inside of, 257–260
        allosteric change, 258
        cooperative effects, 258–259
        flip-flop mechanism, 257–258
    membrane marker, 194–196
    memory of, 512
    overloading, 245
    precursor cell, 214
    quantitation of, 212–213
    receptor
        number on, 223–224
        specificity of, 224–225
    rosette formation, 217–219
    sources, 195
    stimulation, 197
    tolerance, 231–232, 254–256
    classes, two, 193–197, *see also* Lymphocyte, B cell and T cell
    function, 196–197
    infection by latent virus, 554
    infection, persistent, 554
    plasma membrane, 197–201, 206–217
        immunoglobulin on, 206–217
        properties, 199–201
        structure, 197–199
    receptors for antigens, 189–269
    stimulation, 197
    T cell, 93–94, 171–182, 193, 243, 246, 481, 482, 507–511, 524, 531, 533, 543, 546, 556
    antigen binding by, 225–227, 239
    depletion, 509
    function, 196–197

Hc of flagellin, 244
helper cell, 247
immunocompentence, depletion of, 238–239
immunoglobulin detection on, 215–217
immunoglobulin formation, 214–215, 248
Ir gene, 249–250
membrane marker, 194–196
memory of, 512, 533
origin, 214–217
rosette formation, 219
sources, 195
stimulation, 197
transformation, 207
virus replication in, 554
Lymphocytic choriomeningitis virus (LCV), 540, 542, 543
Lymphocytotoxicity assay, 372–383, 533, 537
complement action on target lymphocyte, 372
indicator system, 380–381
limitations, 381–383
CYNAP, 381
microcytotoxicity test, 373
Lymphocyte reaction, mixed (MLC), 364
Lysozyme, 154, 165, 180

M

M antigen, 40–42
Macrophage
activation, 107
ontogeny, 522–524
supporting virus replication, 519–522
Maleate fumarate reciprocal system, 129
Mannan, 47–48, 52–53
bacterial, 47
structure, 48
of yeast, 47–48, 52–53
Mannose, 61
Marek's disease virus, 549
Measles virus, 494, 495, 530, 551, 552, 536–538, 556
antibody in multiple sclerosis, 505
on Faroe Islands (1847), 541
subacute sclerosing panencephalitis (SSPE), 536–538
and tuberculin reaction, 549
vaccination, 549
Medipest virus, 552–553
Medium, as a source of HL-A antigens, 403–404
Mellitin, 308
Membrane
capping, 200, 240–242
fluid mosaic model, 198–199, 389, 430
of lymphocyte, 197–201, 206–217
model of
fluid mosaic, 198–199, 389, 430
structure, 198–199
modulation, 199–201, 240–242
capping, 240–242
patching, 240–242
patches, 200, 240–242
release, 201
turnover, 201
Memory, immunologic (original antigenic sin), 501, 510–512
Microcytotoxicity assay, 538
β_2 Microglobulin, 420–430
Microlymphocytotoxicity, 367
Migration inhibition factor (MIF), 532–537
Mitogen, 251–257
MLC, see Lymphocyte reaction, mixed
Modulation of membrane components, 240–242
capping, 240–242
patching, 240–242
Mollicutes, 450
Mouse hepatitis virus, see Hepatitis virus
Mucus antigen, see M antigen
Multiple sclerosis, 505
and measles antibody, 505
Mumps virus, 503, 530, 536
Murine leukemogenic virus, 498–499, 538
antigen gs, 498
classification, 499
envelope antigen, 498
reverse transcriptase, 499
Mutants
R, 7–8, 13
rfa, 21
rfb, 13
SR, 13

Subject Index

Mycobacterium butyricum, 178
Mycoplasma species, 449–478
  analysis, antigenic, 459–464
  antigen preparation, 459–461
  antiserum preparation, 461–462
  assay, serologic, 462
    by double immunodiffusion, 462–464
  biochemistry, 455–456
  biology, 451–456
  classification, 450–451
  as contaminants in cell lines, 403
  disc inhibition on agar, 466
  glycolytic species, 458
  heterogeneity, serologic, 459
  host–parasite relationship, 453–454
  inhibition by serum, 464–467
    disc assay, 466
  metabolic inhibition testing, 465–466
  morphology, 451–453
  nomenclature, 450–451
  nonglycolytic arginine-utilizing species, 458
  phylogeny, 456–459
  serology, 456–459
  serum action on, 464–467
    growth inhibition on agar, 464–465
  structure, antigenic, 467–475
    carbohydrates, 468–469
    lipids, 469–472
    proteins, 472–475
  taxonomy, serologic, 458
  T strains, 459, 465
Mycoplasma bovigenitalium, 457, 458
Mycoplasma felis, 453, 457, 458
Mycoplasma gallisepticum, 453, 456, 458, 466, 468
Mycoplasma hominis, 454, 458, 468, 473
Mycoplasma mycoides, 450, 451, 455, 467
  galactan as antigen, 468
Mycoplasma pneumoniae, 452, 454, 456, 458, 460, 465, 466, 467
  diglyceride, 469–470
  lipid antigen, 469–471
  membrane antigen, 473–475
Myeloma protein, 99–103
  crystallization, 154
  IgA, 101, 102
  IgM, 103
  specificity, 100–103
Myxovirus, 536

N

Neuritis, optic, 505
Neutralization
  and antigen structure, 513
  complement dependent, 515–517
  a complex process, 512–515
  defined, 512
  mechanism, 512–515
  of virus, 481
Newcastle disease virus, 494, 548
Nuclease, staphylococcal, 151, 152

O

O factor, 57–68
Oligosaccharide
  inhibition with, 50–52
  specific antiserum, 52
Oncolysate, viral, 547, 548
Original antigenic sin, 481, 510–512
Orthomyxovirus, 489–494
  fowl plague virus, 489
  influenza virus, 489

P

Papain, 180
Paralysis, immunologic, 83, 87, 89–94
Paramyxovirus, 494–495, 536–538
  Newcastle disease virus, 494
  Sendai virus, 494
  simian 5 (SV5), 494
Pectin, 55
Penicillin sensitivity, 317
Perennial rye grass, 294–300
Pesistence
  of clones of immunocompetent cells, 483
  of virus, 483
Phagocytosis, 105
Phloroglucinol, triglycosylated, 52
Phosphatidyl glycerol, 471
Phospholipase A, 321
  from bee venom, 299
Phytagglutinin, 491
Plasma membrane, *see* Membrane
Platelet
  –complement fixation, 383
  as a source of HL-A, 404–406
Pneumococcus polysaccharide capsule,

26–31, 54–55, 86–88, 90–92, 95–98, 101–103, 106, 134
Poliomyelitis
  among eskimos, 541
  virus, 500–503, 507
Pollen as allergen, 275–277, 321
  of *Ambrosia elatior*, 283
  of grasses, 291–300, 321
  of orchard grass, 291, 293–295
  of perennial rye grass (*Lolium perenne*), 283–284, 294–300
  of short ragweed, 283, 321
  of timothy grass, 291, 294–296
Pollentoxin of rye grass, 275
Polylysine, 145
Polysaccharide, microbial
  antibodies with restricted heterogeneity, 95–99
  capsular, 25–42
    colanic acid, 40–42
    dextran, 45–47
    of *Diplococcus pneumoniae*, 2, 3, 26–31
    of *Escherichia coli*, 35–38
    of *Haemophilus*, 38–40
    of *Klebsiella*, 31–35
    levan, 47
    M antigen, 40–42
    mannan, 47–48
    of *Staphylococcus*, 40
    of *Streptococcus*, 42–45
    teichoic acid, 45
    Vi antigen, 42
  charge, 53–54
  chemistry of antigen, 3–48
    linkage, nature of, 5
    methods, 3–5
    sequence of sugar constituents, 4
    shape, 4
    size, 4
    sugar composition, 4
  core-defective mutant, 22, 23
  cross-reaction, 76–83
  determinant site, 52–53
  dose, 86–89
  Escherichia coli core structure, 20
  Escherichia coli B lipopolysaccharide structure, 23
  immunobiology of antigens, 83–108
  immunochemistry of antigens, 49–83

  antigen factor, 56–62
  artificial antigen, 68–74
  carbohydrate determinant, 50–55
  conversion, lysogenic, 62–68
  form variation, 62–68
  mutation, 62–68
  noncarbohydrate determinant, 74–76
  serology, 49
  immunogenicity, 83–95
  in infection, 103–108
  lipid A, 21–25
  lipopolysaccharide, bacterial, 5–25
    biochemistry, 7
    chemotype concept, 14–16
    core structure, 20, 22
    genetic determination, 7
    isolation, 8–11
    mutant, 7–8
    O-specific polysaccharide, 12–13, 18–19
    R-specific core oligosaccharide, 13–21
    from *Salmonella*, 17
    structure, 6–7
      of core, 20, 22
    sugar constituents, 10–11, 14–16
  molecular weight, 84–86
  myeloma protein, 99–103
  persistence, 86–89
  superstructure, 54–55
Potassium chloride and HL-A, soluble, 408–414, 417
Poxvirus, 533–534
PPLO, see *Mycoplasma*
Protease, 407, 409
Puromycin and HL-A, 396–398

R

Rabies virus, 496–498
  G protein, 497
  M protein, 497
Radiation leukemia virus, 556
Radioallergosorbent test (RAST), 228, 346
Ragweed pollen, 275, 294–295, 299–305, 324, 325
  allergen, 303–305
  antigen E, 325–327, 336
  antigen Ra5, 334–335
  isoelectrofocusing of allergen, 302

Subject Index

RAST, see Radioallergosorbent test
RAT, see L-Tyrosine-azobenzene-p-arsonate
Receptor
  Fc as, 529
  lecithin as, 528–529
Respiratory syncytial virus, 495
Rhabdovirus, 496–498
Rhinitis, allergic, 331
Rhizobium polysaccharide, 80, 82
RhL antigen in rhesus monkey, 336
Rift Valley fever virus, 541
Rinderpest virus, 494, 511, 552
Rosette formation, 207–219, 234, 241
Rous virus, 506
Rubella virus, 495, 539–540
Rye grass, perennial, 294–300

S

Salmonella, 57–67
  classification, serological, 2
  core defective mutant, 22
  core oligosaccharide, 20–21
  3,6-dideoxyhexose, 12, 57–59, 71, 72
  lipid A, 21–25
  lipopolysaccharide repeating units, 17, 19
  O factor, 17
  R mutant, 7–8, 22
Semliki forest virus, 496, 510
Sendai virus, 494, 548
Serum, human
  albumin, 135
  as source of HL-A, 406–407
Serum sickness, 278
Shigella lipopolysaccharide, O antigen, 19
Silk fibroin, 135
Simian virus, 5, 494
Sindbis virus, 496, 510, 539
Smith degradation of sugar, 4
Sound, low frequency, 407, 408
Specificity of polysaccharide
  O, 8, 9, 12–13
  R, 8
Split tolerance, 538
Sporoblomyces acetylphosphogalactan, 81
SSPE, see Measles virus
Streptococcus, capsular polysaccharide antigen, 40, 42–45, 82
Streptococcus MG, 420–471
Sugar
  composition of microbial polysaccharide, 4
  linkage, nature of, 5
  sequence methods, 4
Svedberg method, 4
Systemic lupus erythematosus, 549

T

T cell, see Lymphocyte, T cell
T coliphage, 515
Teichoic acid, 45, 46
Tetanus toxoid, 332
Tetrapeptide, 139–147
Thymectomy, 170–171
  neonatal, 508
Thymocyte, 214
Thymoma, 214
Thymus dependence, 508
  changes of, 551
Timothy grass pollen
  antigen D, 316
TL (thymus-leukemia) antigen in mouse, 531
Togavirus, 495–496, 511, 539–540
  alphavirus, 495
  arbovirus A, 495
  arbovirus B, 495
  flavivirus, 495
  lactate dehydrogenase virus, 495
  rubella virus, 495
  yellow fever virus, 494
Tolerance, see Paralysis, immunologic
  in B cells, 254–257
  high zone, 90, 92, 94
  immunologic, 483
  low zone, 89–90, 92, 94
  overloading, 254–255
  in T cells, 257
  to virus antigen, 543–546
  to virus infection, 557
Trachoma-inclusion conjunctivitis (TRIC), 451
Transplantation antigen in inbred mouse, 362
Transplantation immunity, induced, 547
Treadmill effect, 87, 90
Tree pollen as allergen, 306

Tuberculin sensitivity
  suppressed by virus, 549, 550
Tumor transplantation antigen, 547
L-Tyrosine-p-azobenzenearsonate
  (RAT), 243
L-Tyrosine-p-azobenzene derivatives, 169, 175, 182

V

Vaccinia virus, 533–534, 541
Varicella-zoster virus, 484, 542
Venezuelan equine encephalitis virus
  (VEE), 496, 539
Vesicular stomatitis virus, 496–498
Vi antigen, 42, 104, 106
Virolysis
  complement-dependent, 516
  complement-mediated, 516
Viropexis, 515
Virulence, bacterial, 103–104
Virus, see individual viruses
Virus infection
  antigens, 483–499, 507–510
    of adenovirus, 485–489
    of herpesvirus, 484–485
    of murine leukemogenic virus, 498–499
    of orthomyxovirus, 489–494
    of paramyxovirus, 494–495
    of rhabdovorus, 496–498
    thymus-dependent, 507–510
    of togavirus, 495–496
  and B lymphocyte memory, 510–512
  capping of viral antigen, 530
  cell-mediated immunity (CMI), 532–541
  determinant
    of host, 531–532
    of virus, 531–532
  and genetic control, 505–506
  and humoral response, 500–506
    by IgG, 500–504
    by IgM, 500–504
  immune response, 479–574
  immunity, cell-mediated, 532–541
  infectious complexes, 517–519
  and macrophage, 519–524
  modulation, antigenic, 531
  neutralization, 512–519
    of antiglobulin, 517–519
    complement-dependent, 515–517
    mechanism, 512–515
  and original antigenic sin, 510–512
  persistence of immunity, 541–543
  and receptor changes, 528–530
  secretory antibody response, 506–507
  surface changes on cell, 524–532
    by virus-coded antigen, 524–528
    nonvirion antigen, 528
    virion antigen, 524–528
  tolerance to virus antigen, 543–546

W

Waldenström protein, see Myeloma protein
Wart virus, 505
Wheat flour sensitivity
  in bakers, 320
  in millers, 320

X

Xanthomonas campestris capsular polysaccharide antigen, 26

Y

Yellow fever virus, 495, 520, 541